Chiropractic and Physical Therapies

Chiropractic and Physical Therapies

Edited by **Pete Edner**

SYRAWOOD
PUBLISHING HOUSE
New York

Published by Syrawood Publishing House,
750 Third Avenue, 9th Floor,
New York, NY 10017, USA
www.syrawoodpublishinghouse.com

Chiropractic and Physical Therapies
Edited by Pete Edner

International Standard Book Number: 978-1-68286-342-8 (Hardback)

Printed in China.

Contents

Preface

This book has been an outcome of determined endeavour from a group of educationists in the field. The primary objective was to involve a broad spectrum of professionals from diverse cultural background involved in the field for developing new researches. The book not only targets students but also scholars pursuing higher research for further enhancement of the theoretical and practical applications of the subject.

Chiropractic and manual therapies are some of the most successful forms of alternative medicine focused primarily on the musculoskeletal framework of the body. Most of the topics introduced in this book cover the latest studies in mobilisation, dry needling, lifestyle and dietary counselling, diagnostic practices in chiropractic, etc. The various studies that are constantly contributing towards the evolution of these fields are examined in detail. Researchers, students, chiropractors, manual therapists and related healthcare professionals will benefit alike from this book.

It was an honour to edit such a profound book and also a challenging task to compile and examine all the relevant data for accuracy and originality. I wish to acknowledge the efforts of the contributors for submitting such brilliant and diverse chapters in the field and for endlessly working for the completion of the book. Last, but not the least; I thank my family for being a constant source of support in all my research endeavours.

Editor

Delineating inflammatory and mechanical sub-types of low back pain: a pilot survey of fifty low back pain patients in a chiropractic setting

Janine S Riksman[1*], Owen D Williamson[2], Bruce F Walker[1]

Abstract

Background: An instrument known as the Mechanical and Inflammatory Low Back Pain (MAIL) Scale was drafted using the results of a previous expert opinion study. A pilot survey was conducted to test the feasibility of a larger study designed to determine the MAIL Scale's ability to distinguish two potential subgroups of low back pain: inflammatory and mechanical.

Methods: Patients with a primary complaint of low back pain (LBP) presenting to chiropractic clinics in Perth, Western Australia were asked to fill out the MAIL Scale questionnaire. The instrument's ability to separate patients into inflammatory and mechanical subgroups of LBP was examined using the mean score of each notional subgroup as an arbitrary cut-off point.

Results: Data were collected from 50 patients. The MAIL Scale did not appear to separate cases of LBP into the two notionally distinct groups of inflammatory (n = 6) or mechanical (n = 5). A larger "mixed symptom" group (n = 39) was revealed.

Conclusions: In this pilot study the MAIL Scale was unable to clearly discriminate between what is thought to be mechanical and inflammatory LBP in 50 cases seen in a chiropractic setting. However, the small sample size means any conclusions must be viewed with caution. Further research within a larger study population may be warranted and feasible.

Background

Low back pain (LBP) is a common condition, with about 79% of Australians experiencing LBP at some time in their lives [1]. In over 85% of cases presenting for primary care [2] a specific cause for pain cannot be identified [3]. In such cases, the LBP is often labelled as non-specific low back pain (NSLBP).

Over 90% of primary contact clinicians believe NSLBP is not a single condition, with three-quarters believing subgroups are already identifiable [4]. However there is little current evidence supporting the existence of these subgroups, or agreement between practitioners when defining their characteristics [5].

A recent study has shown that people diagnosed with NSLBP might be categorised as having mechanical (MLBP) or inflammatory (ILBP) low back pain [6]. In this study of expert opinion, a number of signs were identified as potentially indicating LBP of mechanical origin [6]. These were intermittent pain during the day, pain that develops later in the day, pain on standing for a while, pain with lifting, pain with bending forward a little, pain on trunk flexion or extension, pain on doing a sit up, pain when driving long distances, pain getting out of a chair and pain on repetitive bending, running, and coughing or sneezing.

Similarly, other studies suggest that ILBP might be defined by pain that wakes the person, pain on morning waking, pain associated with morning stiffness longer than 30 minutes and improvement of LBP with exercise but not rest [6-8].

Additionally, several studies into treatment-based classification have shown that people with certain clinical signs and symptoms may exhibit a preferential response to corresponding treatment modalities [9-12].

* Correspondence: janine_sr@hotmail.com
[1]School of Chiropractic and Sports Science, Murdoch University, South Street, Murdoch WA, 6151, Australia
Full list of author information is available at the end of the article

The aim of this study was to pilot a survey that tests the feasibility of discriminating cases of NSLBP into two subgroups, mechanical and inflammatory, based on clinical signs and symptoms.

Methods

Sample Population

This study included consecutive patients with a primary complaint of LBP who voluntarily presented for treatment to the Murdoch University Chiropractic Clinic and three private chiropractic practices in Perth, Western Australia, from March 2008 until July 2008. The study was approved by the Murdoch University Human Research Ethics Committee.

Any patient aged 18 years or older with a primary complaint of LBP, with or without referral to the lower extremity was eligible for inclusion. Exclusion criteria included those with the of presence any 'red flags' for serious spinal pathology (for example, tumour, fracture or infection), prior surgery to the lumbar spine, pregnancy, diagnosed bipolar disorder or schizophrenia, seeking legal advice regarding their condition or claiming treatment under a Worker's Compensation/Third Party insurance claim and finally chiropractic students. Chiropractic students were excluded as patient participants, as some had prior knowledge of the study methods.

LBP was defined as any pain in the region between the lower ribs and gluteal folds [13].

Patient Assessment

All patients received routine questions on LBP history and a physical examination of active lumbar range of motion, lower limb neurological examination (reflexes, sensation and motor strength), straight leg raise and various orthopaedic tests professed to identify dysfunction in the lumbopelvic region. Levels of pain, disability and fear avoidance beliefs were recorded using a numerical rating scale (NRS), Oswestry Disability Questionnaire (ODQ) and Fear Avoidance Beliefs Questionnaire (FABQ), respectively.

Measures of Health Status

Baseline demographics, self-reported pain and disability data were collected on all patients prior to treatment. The location of LBP was assessed using a body pain diagram. Current pain severity was assessed on an 11-point numerical rating scale (NRS), ranging from 0 (no pain) to 10 (worst pain imaginable) [14,15] and LBP-related disability was measured using an Oswestry Disability Questionnaire (ODQ) [16].

The Mechanical and Inflammatory Low Back Pain Scale (MAIL Scale)

Also at baseline, each study participant filled out the new instrument known as the Mechanical and Inflammatory Low Back Pain (MAIL) Scale, (Figures 1 and 2).

The MAIL Scale, comprised three parts and asked the patient to answer 'yes' or 'no' to a series of 19 questions relating to notional mechanical and inflammatory back pain.

Part A consists of 6 signs and symptoms thought to characterise inflammatory pain (Figure 1). Of these, questions 1 and 2 were derived from the clinical questionnaire administered by Rudwaleit et al [8], which showed morning stiffness and relief of pain with exercise (but not rest) to be independently associated with inflammatory back pain. Question 1b provides time frames to measure the duration of morning stiffness as Rudwaleit et al [8] found morning stiffness greater than 30 minutes distinguished inflammatory from mechanical pain. Questions 3 through 6 are those signs and symptoms thought to be associated with pain of a non-specific inflammatory nature by experts surveyed by Walker and Williamson [6]. Question 3b similarly provides time frames to measure the duration of morning pain. The potential answers were weighted in a subjective manner with weighting rising with increasing duration of morning pain or stiffness as this variable is thought to be strongly associated with ILBP [6,8].

Part B consists of 13 signs and symptoms thought to characterise MLBP (Figure 2) [6]. From the completed MAIL Scale, an arbitrary weighted score was generated for the number of mechanical and inflammatory characteristics exhibited by each patient. The spread of responses to the MAIL Scale was analysed in order to determine its preliminary ability to discriminate patients into categories.

Sample Size

For this pilot study, an arbitrary sample size of 50 was used. Sample size calculations for a fully powered study may be derived from the pilot study results.

Analysis

Data were entered, cleaned and analysed using Statistical Package for the Social Sciences (SPSS) version 16.0 [17]. Normality tests were performed on both MAIL Scale subgroups using a Shapiro-Wilk test in SPSS [17]. Descriptive statistics were used to analyse the scores and frequencies of responses to the MAIL Scale instrument questions. A Pearson's correlation test between the Inflammatory and Mechanical subscales was also performed.

Subject to normality being shown, the mean scores of each of the Inflammatory (Part A) and Mechanical (Part B) subscales of the MAIL Scale would be used as a notional and arbitrary cut-off point to indicate "Inflammatory LBP" and "Mechanical LBP". Those with scores greater than the mean in one subscale and less than the mean in the other subscale were categorised as either purely inflammatory or mechanical LBP. Any MAIL

The following questions relate to your current episode of ***low back pain***. Please tick the appropriate box for each statement.

PART A

	Yes	No
1. a) Do you experience <u>stiffness</u> in the mornings?		

b) If yes, how long does it last? *(tick box)*

☐ Less than 10 minutes
☐ 10-30 minutes
☐ 31-60 minutes
☐ 61-90 minutes
☐ longer than 90 minutes

2. Does your pain improve with exercise, ***but not*** with rest?		
3. a) Do you have <u>pain on waking</u> in the morning?		

b) If yes, how long does it last? *(tick box)*

☐ Less than 10 minutes
☐ 10-30 minutes
☐ 31-60 minutes
☐ 61-90 minutes
☐ longer than 90 minutes

4. Does your pain wake you up at night?		
5. Do you experience stiffness after resting (includes sitting)?		
6. Is your pain present at all times?		

Figure 1 Mechanical and Inflammatory Low Back (MAIL) Scale - Part A.

Scale scores that did not meet these criteria were categorised as "mixed" LBP.

Results

Patient Characteristics

Data were collected from all 50 patients in the pilot study; their main clinical features are presented in Table 1.

Of the 50 included patients, 38 were recruited through Murdoch University Chiropractic Clinic and 12 through private chiropractic practices in the Perth metropolitan area.

Mechanical and Inflammatory Low Back Pain Scale (MAIL Scale)

The MAIL Scale scores for all participants are shown in Table 1, with a mean inflammatory score of 6.9 (43.1%) out of a possible 16 and mean mechanical score of 7.7 (59.2%) out of a possible 13. Data were tested for normality using a Shapiro-Wilk calculation which showed the data for both subgroups were normally distributed (S-W 0.98, df 50, $p = 0.5$). An additional file containing MAIL Scale raw data for individual items is attached (See additional files 1 and 2: MAIL Scale Raw Scores and Mail Scale Variable Legend).

The number of positive and negative responses to each of the inflammatory and mechanical signs and symptoms are listed in Table 2.

'Morning stiffness' and 'Stiffness after resting' received the most positive responses in the inflammatory section, with 80% (n = 40) and 92% (n = 46) of patients answering "yes", respectively. In the mechanical section 'Pain on repetitive bending' (74%, n = 37), 'Pain on lifting'

The following questions relate to your current episode of ***low back pain***. Please tick the appropriate box for each statement.

PART B	Yes	No
1. Do you have pain intermittently during the day?		
2. Does your pain develop later in the day?		

Do you have pain associated with:	Yes	No
3. Standing for a while?		
4. Lifting?		
5. Bending forward a little?		
6. Bending forward as far as you can?		
7. Arching backwards?		
8. Doing or attempting to do a sit up?		
9. Driving long distances?		
10. Getting out of a chair?		
11. Repetitive bending?		
12. Running?		
13. Coughing or sneezing?		

Figure 2 Mechanical and Inflammatory Low Back (MAIL) Scale - Part B. Scoring key: SCORE: Part A ____/16 = ______% Part B ____/13 = ______% Scoring ■ Questions 1 and 3 in Part A attract 2 points each for a 'yes response'. ■ All other questions in Parts A and B attract one point for a 'yes' response, zero points for a 'no' response. ■ The five categories of questions 1b and 3b are scored from 0 to 4 points, with zero points for duration of <10 minutes, progressing to 4 points for >90 minute category. ■ The maximum score possible in Part A is 16 points and Part B is 13 points.

(70.8%, n = 34) and 'Pain on arching backwards' (70%, n = 35) were the most prevalent.

Seven patients (14%) responded "yes" and 1 (2%) responded "no" to all six inflammatory signs and symptoms. The number of patients responding "yes" to all 13 mechanical signs and symptoms was 2 (4%), with 1 (2%) patient responding "no" to all. There were no reports of participants having difficulty completing the MAIL Scale.

The Pearson correlation co-efficient assessing the general relationship between the MAIL Scale Part A Inflammatory and Part B Mechanical scores was calculated and showed a positive correlation of $r = 0.45$, $p = 0.01$. This is shown as a scatterplot in Figure 3.

The mean scores of the Inflammatory and Mechanical subscales of the MAIL Scale were used as an arbitrary cut-off point to classify "Inflammatory LBP" and "Mechanical LBP". Those with scores greater than the mean in one

Table 1 Baseline data and subject characteristics

	Mean (SD)
Age (years)	37.0 (15.5)
Gender	Male = 29 (58.0%)
NRS* *(0-10)*	5.3 (2.0)
ODQ†	22.5% (16.1%)
MAIL Scale‡ **- Inflammatory** *(0-16)*	6.9 (4.0)
MAIL Scale‡ **- Mechanical** *(0-13)*	7.7 (3.2)
FABQ§ **- Physical Activity** *(0-30)*	12.2 (5.2)

*Numerical Rating Scale.
†Oswestry Disability Questionnaire.
‡Mechanical and Inflammatory Low Back Pain Scale.
§Fear Avoidance Belief Questionnaire.

subscale and less than the mean in the other subscale were categorised as either purely inflammatory or mechanical LBP. By this method, 6 cases were classified as ILBP, 5 cases were classified as MLBP, with the remaining 39 cases classified as "mixed LBP". The frequency of each 'type' of LBP is shown in Figure 4.

Discussion

Introduction

This study found that the MAIL Scale was easy and relatively quick for participants to complete, but was unable to effectively categorise the majority of patients into either inflammatory or mechanical LBP. There are many reasons for this including that the sample size was too small to detect a difference (Type II error), the instrument is unable to distinguish between these two notional categories, the concept of mechanical and inflammatory causes in NSLBP is not valid, the population of patients did not have severe enough forms of NSLBP to be detected by the instrument or the majority of patients have mixed patterns of NSLBP. Of those 50 who entered the study, characteristics for age, sex and measures of health status (Table 1) are similar to those recorded in prior studies conducted in chiropractic teaching facilities [18].

Mechanical and Inflammatory Low Back Pain (MAIL) Scale

The items in this questionnaire were selected based on expert opinion and a search of current literature, and thereby have a level of both face and content validity [19].

While the MAIL Scale was unable to discriminate LBP into two groups, certain signs and symptoms appeared more prominently in each subscale and may be important for future research into this area.

Part A of the MAIL Scale dealt with those signs and symptoms thought to be associated with inflammatory LBP (Table 2). 'Stiffness after resting (includes sitting)' scored the highest "yes" response (92%) in this section. This sign is commonly regarded as an inflammatory symptom in a rheumatological context as the inflammatory mediators, cytokines, are strongly involved in the synovial immune and inflammatory response in conditions such as rheumatoid arthritis [20]. The presence of these cytokines may result in a "gelling" phenomenon, whereby a period of inactivity results in an accumulation of inflammatory mediators in the involved area. As the person then gets up to move, stiffness is experienced in the area until there has been sufficient movement to disperse the accumulated inflammation [20].

It is worthy of note that stiffness after seated rest may also have a mechanical cause as it has also been attributed to intervertebral disc herniation of the lumbar spine. The discs at the L4-5 and L5-S1 levels bear high loads [21,22] and in the seated position intradiscal pressure has shown increases to 100 kilograms of force (kgf), from 70 kgf in the standing position [23]. Therefore in a patient with a suspected lumbar spine disc lesion such as herniation, stiffness after resting (particularly in the seated position) may be a poor discriminating symptom of "mechanical" or "inflammatory" back pain in the absence of further clinical information.

'Morning stiffness' scored the second highest "yes" response (40 patients, 80%) and of those 40 patients, 28 (56.7%) experienced stiffness for 30 minutes or less, while for 11 (22.4%), the stiffness lasted over 30 minutes. Six of these 11 participants also experienced morning pain for longer than 30 minutes. In previous studies of morning stiffness, durations of greater than 30 minutes seemed to be the agreed threshold for determining the presence of inflammation [7,8,24]. As such, while a large number of LBP patients report experiencing morning stiffness in our study, less than a quarter were possibly attributable to an inflammatory aetiology based on the arbitrary scoring system used. It may be that systemic inflammation related to infection, or spondyloarthropathies are more likely to be associated with these symptoms and not those of similar symptoms in NSLBP. The inflammatory back pain criteria developed by Rudwaleit [12] were centred on back pain as a result systemic inflammation associated with ankylosing spondylitis. The use of these criteria in the development of the MAIL Scale makes the assumption that non-systemic inflammation would give similar but localised symptoms. However, this may not be the case. An alternate study design using blood inflammatory markers (i.e. ERS, CRP) as an external reference standard may assist in the detection of existing inflammation. However, while these markers will detect systemic inflammation, a study into chronic LBP has shown that significant systemic inflammatory reaction was absent in

Table 2 Frequency of MAIL Scale responses

Signs and symptoms	No	Yes	*n* responding
PART A - Inflammatory			
Morning stiffness	10 (20%)	40 (80%)	50
Duration of Morning stiffness			49
Did not have to answer	10 (20.0%)		
<10 mins	10 (20.0%)		
10-30 mins	18 (36.7%)		
31-60 mins	5 (10.2%)		
61-90 mins	0 (0.0%)		
>90 mins	6 (12.2%)		
Improvement of pain with exercise, but not rest	22 (44.9%)	27 (55.1%)	49
Morning pain on waking	19 (38.8%)	30 (61.2%)	49
Duration of morning pain			45
Did not have to answer	19 (42.2%)		
<10 mins	7 (15.6%)		
10-30 mins	10 (22.2%)		
31-60 mins	2 (4.4%)		
61-90 mins	0 (0.0%)		
>90 mins	7 (15.6%)		
Pain that wakes	31 (62%)	19 (38%)	50
Stiffness after resting (includes sitting)	4 (8%)	46 (92%)	50
Pain present at all times	30 (60%)	20 (40%)	50
PART B - Mechanical			
Intermittent pain during day	18 (36.7%)	31 (63.3%)	49
Pain developing later in the day	33 (68.8%)	15 (31.2%)	48
Pain with standing for a while	15 (30.6%)	34 (69.4%)	49
Pain with lifting	14 (29.2%)	34 (70.8%)	48
Pain with bending forward a little	16 (32.7%)	33 (67.3%)	49
Pain on bending forward as far as you can	19 (38%)	31 (62%)	50
Pain on arching backwards	15 (30%)	35 (70%)	50
Pain on doing or attempting a sit-up	16 (32%)	34 (68%)	50
Pain on driving long distances	18 (36%)	32 (64%)	50
Pain on getting out of a chair	23 (46%)	27 (54%)	50
Pain on repetitive bending	13 (26%)	37 (74%)	50
Pain on running	22 (44%)	28 (56%)	50
Pain on coughing or sneezing	34 (70.8%)	14 (29.2%)	48

the 273 participants sampled [25]. As such, while symptoms of apparent inflammation may be reported by these patients, objective signs may still yield sub-threshold measurements.

Part B of the MAIL Scale dealt with MLBP (Table 2). The relatively high proportion of patients responding "yes" to these "mechanical questions" is not unexpected when the biomechanics of these activities is considered. As mentioned previously, different activities result in varied loads and mechanical stresses to the spine. It is known that bending in various directions increases load on the elements of lumbar spine [23]. Repetition of this action may cause hysteresis [21] implying that the body is less protected against repetitive loads. This may also partly explain the high "yes" response rate to 'pain on driving long distances' due to the repetitive axial vibration in combination with the prolonged loading associated with sitting.

When lumbar flexion is coupled with lifting, the load increases significantly. Lifting a 20 kg weight with a flexed spine and straight knees results in 340 kgf load on the lumbar spine [23]. With proper lifting technique, limiting spinal flexion and 'lifting through' bent knees, the load on the spine is less (210 kgf), however this still represents a significant mechanical force on the spine. Similarly, activities such as performing a sit-up also

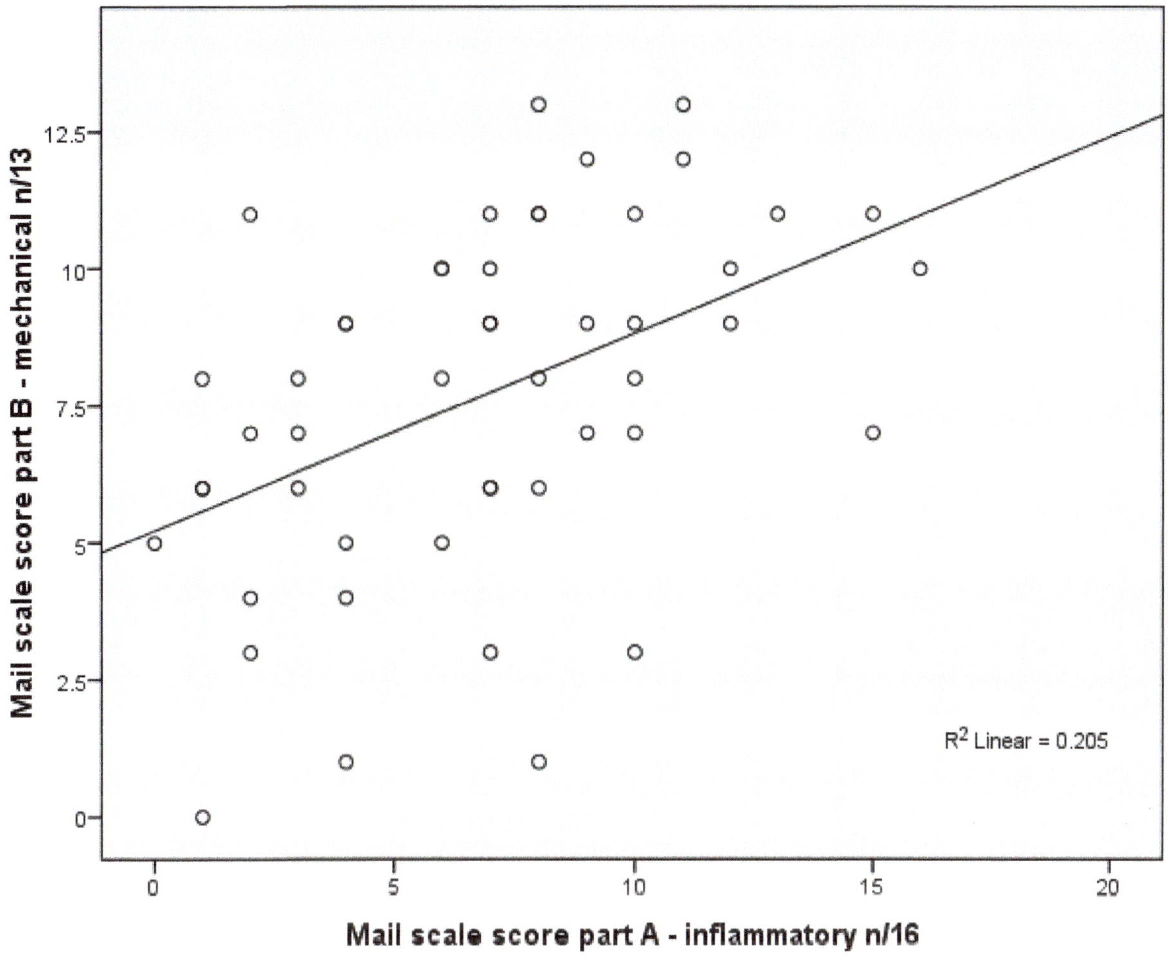

Figure 3 Scatterplot showing correlation between MAIL Scale Part A Inflammatory and Part B Mechanical scores.

increase the load on the spine, exerting 180 kgf to the lumbar discs.

'Pain developing later in the day' and 'Pain on coughing or sneezing' did not appear commonly, with only 15 (31.2%) and 14 (29.2%) of subjects responding "yes" respectively. The small number experiencing pain with coughing or sneezing may relate to the fact that only one respondent was diagnosed as having a disc herniation, and the presence of pain with these actions is commonly regarded as suggestive of a disc injury [26].

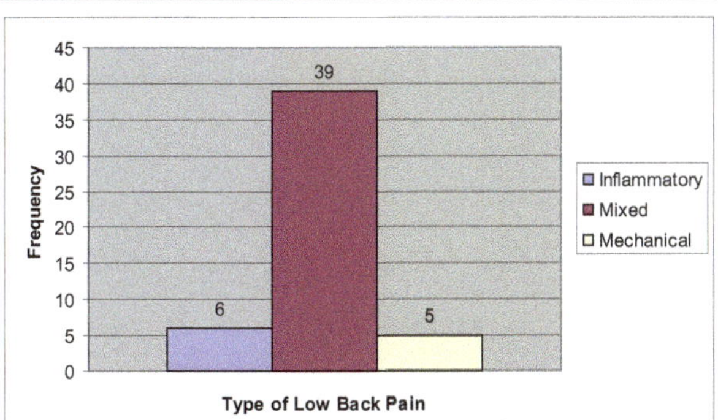

Figure 4 Frequency of "Inflammatory LBP" (MAILS A >7 and MAILS B < 8), "Mechanical LBP" (MAILS A < 7 and MAILS B > 8) and "Mixed" type of Low Back Pain.

The correlation between the mechanical and inflammatory subscales of the MAIL Scale showed a significant positive correlation of 0.45 (Figure 3). This suggests that a distinction between mechanical and inflammatory LBP may not exist, and that the MAIL Scale is unable to separate LBP into two groups. In addition a negative correlation would have been expected if the LBP was caused predominantly by an inflammatory or mechanical cause.

LBP was arbitrarily classified into "inflammatory", "mechanical" or "mixed" subgroups. Over three-quarters of the sample were classified into the "mixed" subgroup, with only 6 and 5 patients classified as "inflammatory" and "mechanical" cases, respectively (Figure 4). This difficulty in discriminating notional mechanical from inflammatory pain is consistent with the original research [6], where experts were unable to clearly delineate those characteristics that were exclusive to either type of pain. However, the small sample size in this study may limit the conclusions that can be drawn. With a larger more diverse study population, separation into subgroups may or may not become more evident.

Limitations and future research

The aim of this pilot study was to test the feasibility of a survey instrument that could potentially differentiate between the notional subgroups "inflammatory" and "mechanical" LBP. The results are not encouraging within the setting we chose.

We have shown that the frequency with which participants respond to each question in the MAIL Scale can be described, and their MAIL Scale scores derived. This can be used to assign them to an arbitrary subgroup classification, however it is less clear what contribution this makes.

The potential division of LBP into mechanical and inflammatory sub-groups based on an instrument of this type may rely on a much larger sample size. Analysis of a larger sample using an item-response theory approach such as Rasch analysis [27] would allow determination of which of these items are unidimensional, the hierarchy of those items and the most appropriate scoring system.

In any future research it may be best to recruit participants from other healthcare environments (such as clinics of physiotherapists, general practitioners and rheumatologists) as this may give a broader and more representative sample and decrease the potential for any selection bias. The broader spread of signs and symptoms may improve the ability of the instrument to discriminate between potential subgroups. In addition, consideration may be given to surveying active spondyloarthropathy patients from rheumatology clinics to ascertain whether they have a different frequency of the so-called mechanical signs and symptoms identified and present in the MAIL Scale instrument. It may be hypothesised that these patients have predominantly inflammatory pain and should exhibit less mechanical signs and symptoms that the NSLBP group.

Finally, it may be worth considering an alternative study design that uses an external reference standard, such as blood inflammatory markers which may assist the analysis by identifying systemic inflammatory cases. Depending on the study design selected, a sample size would need to be generated for a fully powered study. A power calculation has not been performed here, however the results shown in Table 1 may help with this calculation.

Conclusion

In this pilot study, the MAIL Scale was simple to administer but was unable to clearly discriminate between notional mechanical and inflammatory LBP in a chiropractic setting. Sample size restrictions and the research setting limit any conclusions from these findings. Further research with a larger and more diverse study population may be warranted. However, based on the findings in this pilot study, separation of NSLBP into mechanical and inflammatory subgroups may not be possible.

Additional material

Additional file 1: Mail Scale Raw Scores. An additional file containing the raw data of 50 subjects for individual items on the MAIL Scale.

Additional file 2: Mail Scale Variable Legend. An additional file containing the variable view of an SPSS data output and explanations of any abbreviations/numerical legends used within the MAIL Scale raw scores spreadsheet (additional file 1).

Author details

[1]School of Chiropractic and Sports Science, Murdoch University, South Street, Murdoch WA, 6151, Australia. [2]Department of Epidemiology and Preventive Medicine Monash University, The Alfred Centre, 99 Commercial Road, Melbourne VIC, 3004, Australia.

Authors' contributions

JR contributed to the design, carried out the data collection, performed the literature search, and drafted and wrote the manuscript which is based on her Honours thesis. BW and OW contributed to the supervision, concept and design, and editing and revision for the intellectual content of the article. BW provided statistical advice, and critical review of the manuscript. All authors read and approved the final manuscript.

Competing interests

BW is the Editor in Chief of the journal Chiropractic & Osteopathy. JR and OW declare that they have no competing interests.

References

1. Walker B, Muller R, Grant W: **Low Back Pain in Australian Adults. Prevalence and Associated Disability.** *Journal of Manipulative and Physiological Therapeutics* 2004, **27**:236-244.
2. Deyo R, Rainville J, Kent D: **What can the history and physical examination tell us about low back pain.** *Journal of the American Medical Association* 1992, **268**:760-765.
3. Australian Acute Musculoskeletal Pain Guidelines Group (AAMPGG): **Evidence-Based Management of Acute Musculoskeletal Pain.** Australian Academic Press: Brisbane; 2003 [http://www.nhmrc.gov.au], Retreived 03 August 2007.
4. Kent P, Keating J: **Do Primary-Care Clinicians Think That Nonspecific Low Back Pain Is One Condition?** *Spine* 2004, **29**:1022-1031.
5. Kent P, Keating J: **Classification in nonspecific low back pain: What methods do primary care clinicians currently use?** *Spine* 2005, **30**:1433-1440.
6. Walker B, Williamson O: **Mechanical or inflammatory low back pain. What are the potential signs and symptoms?** *Manual Therapy* 2008.
7. Calin A, Porta J, Fries J, Schurman D: **Clinical history as a screening test for ankylosing spondylitis.** *Journal of the American Medical Association* 1977, **237**:2613-2614.

8. Rudwaleit M, Metter A, Listing J: **Inflammatory Back Pain in Ankylosing Spondylitis. A Reassessment of the Clincial and Diagnostic Criteria.** *Arthritis and Rheumatism* 2006, **54**:569-578.
9. Fritz J, Brennan G, Clifford S, Hunter S, Thackeray A: **An Examination of the Reliability of a Classification Algorithm for Subgrouping Patients with Low Back Pain.** *Spine* 2006, **31**:77-82.
10. Fritz J, Lindsay W, Matheson J, Brennan G: **Is there a subgroup of patients with low back pain likely to benefit from mechanical traction? Results of a randomized clinical trial and subgrouping analysis.** *Spine* 2007, **32**: E793-800.
11. Fritz J, Delitto A, Erhard R: **Comparison of Classification-Based Physical therapy With Therapy Based on Clinical Practice Guidelines for Patients with Acute Low Back Pain. A Randomized Clinical Trial.** *Spine* 2003, **28**:1363-1372.
12. Childs J, Fritz J, Flynn T: **A Clinical Prediction Rule to Identify Patients with Low back Pain Most Likely to Benefit from Spinal Manipulation: A Validation Study.** *Annals of Internal Medicine* 2004, **141**:920-928.
13. Van Tulder M, Becker A, Bekkering T, Breen A: **Chapter 3. European Guidelines for the Management of Acute Non-Specific Low Back Pain in Primary Care.** *European Spine Journal* 2006, **15**:S169-191.
14. Jensen M, Turner J, Romano J: **What is the maximum number of levels needed in pain intensity measurement?** *Pain* 1994, **58**:387-392.
15. Katz J, Melzack R: **Measurement of pain.** *Surg Clin North Am* 1999, **79**:231-252.
16. Fritz J, Irrgang J: **A comparison of a modified Oswestry Low Back Pain Disability Questionnaire and the Quebec Back Pain Disability Scale.** *Physical Therapy* 2001, **81**:776-788.
17. **SPSS 16.0 for Windows.** Chicago: SPSS Inc; 2008, Release 16.0.2.
18. Hoiriis K, Pfleger B, McDuffie F, Cotsonis G, Elsangak O, Hinson R, Verzosa G: **A randomized clinical trial comparing chiropractic adjustments to muscle relaxants for subacute low back pain.** *Journal of Manipulative and Physiological Therapeutics* 2004, **27**:388-398.
19. Streiner D, Norman G: *Health Measurement Scales. A practical guide to their development and use* New York: Oxford University Press; 1993.
20. Sulli A, Maestroni G, Villaggio B, Hertens E: **Melatonin Serum Levels in Rheumatoid Arthritis.** *Annals of the New York Academy of Science* 2002, **966**:276-283.
21. White A, Punjabi M: *Clinical Biomechanics of the Spine* Philadelphia: J.B. Lippincott Company; 1978.
22. Souza I: *Differential Diagnosis and Management for the Chiropractor. Protocols and Algorithms 3rd Edition.* 3 edition. Boston: Jones and Bartlett Publishers Inc; 2005.
23. Nachemson A: **The lumbar spine, an orthopaedic challenge.** *Spine* 1976, **1**.
24. Gran J: **An epidemiological survey of the signs and symptoms of ankylosing spondylitis.** *Clinical Rheumatology* 1985, **4**:161-169.
25. Park H, Lee S: **Investigation of High-Sensitivity C-reactive Protein and Erythrocyte Sedimentation Rate in Low Back Pain Patients.** *The Korean Journal of Pain* 2010, **23**:147-150.
26. Cipriano J: *Photographic manual of regional orthopaedic and neurological tests. Fourth Edition.* Fourth edition. Sydney: Lippincott Williams and Wilkins; 2003.
27. Rasch G: *Probabilistic models for some intelligence and attainment tests* Chicago: University of Chicago Press; 1960, (reprinted 1980).

Chiropractic at the crossroads or are we just going around in circles?

John W Reggars[1,2]

Abstract

Background: Chiropractic in Australia has seen many changes over the past 30 years. Some of these changes have advanced the professional status of chiropractic, improved undergraduate training and paved the way for a research culture. Unfortunately, other changes or lack of changes, have hindered the growth, public utilisation and professional standing of chiropractic in Australia. This article explores what influences have impacted on the credibility, advancement and public utilisation of chiropractic in Australia.

Discussion: The 1970's and 1980's saw a dramatic change within the chiropractic profession in Australia. With the advent of government regulation, came government funded teaching institutions, quality research and increased public acceptance and utilisation of chiropractic services. However, since that time the profession appears to have taken a backward step, which in the author's opinion, is directly linked to a shift by sections of the profession to the fundamentalist approach to chiropractic and the vertebral subluxation complex. The abandonment, by some groups, of a scientific and evidenced based approach to practice for one founded on ideological dogma is beginning to take its toll.

Summary: The future of chiropractic in Australia is at a crossroads. For the profession to move forward it must base its future on science and not ideological dogma. The push by some for it to become a unique and all encompassing alternative system of healthcare is both misguided and irrational.

Background

This article is based on the inaugural FG Roberts Memorial Lecture, delivered by the author at the Annual Conference of the Chiropractic & Osteopathic College of Australasia, Melbourne, Australia 2010.

Frederick George Roberts was a natural health practitioner embracing chiropractic, osteopathy and naturopathy, who operated many clinics throughout Australia during the 1950's and 1960's. He visited all these clinics regularly and gave public lectures on natural healing. From 1959, his interest turned more to chiropractic and osteopathy and he founded the Chiropractic and Osteopathic College of Australasia in 1959.

This paper is the author's perception of the many changes which have impacted, both positively and negatively, on chiropractic and the chiropractic profession over the past 30 years. Some of those changes have advanced the professional status of chiropractic, improved undergraduate training and paved the way for a research culture. Unfortunately, other changes, or lack of changes, have adversely affected the profession's growth, credibility and the public utilisation of chiropractic services in Australia. It would also appear, that the crossroads confronting the profession in Australia are not unique, as there are many parallels with what has occurred or is occurring internationally.

Discussion

Introduction

In order to appreciate and fully comprehend what I perceive to be the crossroads currently confronting the chiropractic profession in Australia, it is necessary to reflect on where the profession has come from, and the roads it has taken to reach these crossroads.

Furthermore, this is not first time the literature has referred to chiropractic being at some sort of crossroads. Others have also opined on similar circumstances facing the profession [1-3]. These three references will be

Correspondence: reggars@chirofirst.com.au
[1]Suite1/593 Whitehorse Road, Mitcham, Victoria, 3132 Australia
Full list of author information is available at the end of the article

discussed in this article, in the context of the current status of chiropractic in Australia.

Pre-registration

The author graduated from the Chiropractic College of Australasia (Melbourne) in 1972, and at that time, in all but one Australian State or Territory, chiropractic was not afforded any formal recognition by governments and there was no regulation or registration of chiropractors or osteopaths. Also, at that time, at least within the field of chiropractic, little to no research was being undertaken, and that which was being conducted, was of dubious quality.

As a young student I, like most of my peers, believed without question what I was told by my lecturers, what was written in scholarly journals, and even more so, what was written in books about chiropractic. However, there were some theories that tested the bounds of credibility and were difficult to accept as fact. For example, Fred Stoner in his book "The eclectic approach to chiropractic" [4], discusses the theory of "Vivaxis", which refers to a relationship between the geographical location where one is born and the earth's energy fields. Stoner cites the work of Goodheart, founder of Applied Kinesiology, and writes: *"Dr. Goodheart noted that the direction in which the patient faces may affect the strength of his muscles. After examining over 500 patients, he found that if a patient faces toward the town in which he was born, a definite increase in muscle strength can be noted (as demonstrated through muscle testing). Furthermore, the body often seems to lunge forward when faced toward this direction."*

While to any reasonable person the theory of "Vivaxis" is absurd, it is no more fanciful than some of the contemporary and accepted diagnostic and therapeutic protocols used by many chiropractors today, in the detection and correction of the vertebral subluxation complex (VSC).

Professional recognition

As an unregulated profession, chiropractic in Australia was, in many respects, the master of its own destiny. However, in 1977 a dramatic change occurred that in many ways changed the future direction of chiropractic in Australia. In that year Edwin Webb and his colleagues compiled and published the "Report of the Committee of Inquiry into Chiropractic, Osteopathy, Homoeopathy and Naturopathy", commonly called "The Webb Report" [5].

This government report paved the way for registration of chiropractors, Australia wide, the establishment of government funded teaching institutions, the beginnings of a research culture and acceptance by mainstream health professions. Webb and his committee recommended that chiropractors and osteopaths be registered but with a proviso: *"The Committee recommends that chiropractic and osteopathy should not be given legal recognition in any form which would imply that they are alternative health systems."* This suggested caveat on the registration of chiropractors and osteopaths in 1977 has equal relevance today, particularly when one considers the road by which the fundamentalists of this profession would have it travel into the future.

The Report also noted: *"Plenty of anecdotal evidence has been published both as to the "cures" produced by chiropractic, osteopathy ..... Virtually none of this arises from properly controlled experiments or from the statistical analysis of large samples. Evidence it may be, but not scientific evidence..."*

It is now over 30 years since that report was written, yet the "subluxationists" [6] in the profession still rely on such anecdotal research to support the "Palmer" theory of "dis-ease" [7].

The cross roads

Chiropractic practice in Australia in the 1970's was much like it is today. Most chiropractors focused on and promoted treatment for musculoskeletal conditions. However, there is today, as there was then, another group of chiropractors, which were indoctrinated with the "true belief" that subluxations were the root of all man's ills.

They were the pseudo religious zealots whose ideology alienated chiropractic from science-based healthcare and prevented it from gaining the level of credibility and cultural authority required to establish itself on equal ground with other mainstream health professions [8]. The "subluxationists" of today appear to be no different and as Keating et al [9] write: *"The dogma of subluxation is perhaps the greatest single barrier to professional development for chiropractors. It skews the practice of the art in directions that bring ridicule from the scientific community and uncertainty among the public. Failure to challenge subluxation dogma perpetuates a marketing tradition that inevitably prompts charges of quackery. Subluxation dogma leads to legal and political strategies that may amount to a house of cards and warp the profession's sense of self and of mission."*

But around 1991 a change was occurring, which commenced with the publication of the RAND report, "The Appropriateness of Spinal Manipulation for Low Back Pain" [10]. This report gave support for the use of manipulation in the treatment of acute low back pain: *"...support is consistent for the use of spinal manipulation as a treatment for patients with acute low back pain and an absence of other signs or symptoms of lower limb nerve root involvement."*

This sound scientific study conducted by an internationally recognised research organisation, and headed by a renowned epidemiologist, showed that spinal manipulation seemed to be effective for acute low back pain. This independent study provided the public, governments, third party payers and mainstream healthcare professions, the proof that spinal manipulation really worked.

Unfortunately, this study was hijacked by an overzealous section of the chiropractic profession, who wrongly broadcast that it was chiropractic, rather than manipulation, that was shown to be beneficial and the authors were forced to publicly admonish this section of the profession by stating: *"Misrepresentation of the RAND study undermines chiropractic's credibility"* and *"Our results have been seriously misrepresented by chiropractors"* [11].

Also around this time a keynote address was given in Melbourne, Australia, at the Chiropractors & Osteopaths Musculoskeletal Interest Group (COMSIG) Conference [1]. This was the first reference to the profession being at a "crossroads" and it was provided by Professor Evan Willis, a sociologist from Latrobe University, Melbourne, whose special interest was in health policies and the social structure of healthcare. Willis concluded: *"So finally which way at the crossroads? If research is the name of the game then chiropractic needs to be in it and urgently so. Patient testimonials have long ceased to be effective in persuading."*

Even then, Willis recognised that the profession could not continue down the same road as it had in the past and expect to prosper, as it was no longer the master of its own destiny. Chiropractic was now becoming more accountable to both government and the public and to survive, inter-professional co-operation was required: *"... chiropractic cannot continue down the same path as previously and expect it to serve them as well has been the case in the past. An increasingly informed consumer orientated public and governments wishing to scrutinize every cent of public expenditure is the name of the game.[sic] Seeking to build bridges with other practitioners interested in musculoskeletal medicine is an important objective."* [1]

The road to ideology or science

The early 1990's also saw a resurgence of "chiropractic philosophy" in Australia and, with it, the VSC. The source of this philosophical push was the Chiropractors Association of Australia (CAA). Through the CAA's "Core Values" and "Vision Statement" [12], the profession was once again torn between the pursuit of science or the adherence to ideological dogma. Chiropractic fundamentalist "Core Values" (Appendix 1), such as, *"that subluxations compromise the expression of innate intelligence, and that prevention and removal of subluxations will facilitate the expression of optimal health"*, regrettably underpin and dictate the policies and actions of this organisation.

Juxtaposed to this return to ideology, the 1990's saw a push for an evidence-based approach to practice from Australia's mainstream healthcare industry.

It also appeared that the CAA came to a realisation that what was needed was more than just anecdotal evidence to legitimize and support its "Vision" and "Core Values" and therefore amended its research grant guidelines in order to match its "Core Values" and "Vision". Also at this time, the Australian Spinal Research Foundation (ASRF) narrowed and promoted its research grant focus to studies concerned only with the VSC. The Vision Statement of the ASRF [13] states, *"We are the Research Foundation which demonstrates that subluxation-based chiropractic care enhances quality of life and improves human performance."* The ASRF's Research Culture Statement [13] states: *"Our focus is on funding research that investigates the nature of vertebral subluxation and its impact on physiology, health and quality of life."*

However, quality scientific research on spinal manipulation and chiropractic care continued throughout Australia, and internationally, by highly skilled and dedicated chiropractic and other health care researchers [14]. Through this research chiropractic gained an increasing but reserved acceptance and recognition by Australian governments, third party payers, other health disciplines and the public.

Chiropractic achieved this improved standing, not by proclaiming the evils of the ubiquitous VSC and the benefits from removing such an evil entity, nor by relying on the scant and feeble research base supporting this theoretical construct but by good scientific investigation and the publication of high quality research.

The second reference to chiropractic and crossroads came in 2002 when Meeker and Haldeman [2] highlighted the positive changes that had occurred in the profession in the preceding 20 years. They highlighted changes over the past two decades, such as changes in perception from alternative and unorthodoxy to mainstream, both within and outside the profession. Chiropractic was used more than any other complementary and alternative medicine (CAM) group; chiropractic usage in the USA tripled from 3.6% to 11%; patient satisfaction was high; there would be an estimated 100,000 chiropractors in the US by 2010, and, chiropractic care was now included in US Medicare and the majority of private health insurers.

Meeker and Haldeman also discussed how the profession could abandon its alternative tag and become fully integrated into mainstream health care: *"The next decade should determine whether chiropractic maintains the trappings of an alternative healthcare profession or becomes fully integrated into all healthcare systems."* Also, *"In today's dynamic health care milieu, chiropractic stands at the crossroads of mainstream and alternative medicine. Its future role will probably be determined by its commitment to interdisciplinary cooperation and science-based practice."* These are the same crossroads referred to, and the same recommendations, made by Evan Willis, some 10 years earlier [1].

The third reference to chiropractic and crossroads was in 2009 when Ebrall [3] saw the situation quite differently. He saw the crossroads as really a fork in the road, and suggested that our profession drove over the crossroads sometime ago and that they are now, *"but a diminishing dot in our collective rear-view mirror"* and that chiropractic is, *"a dynamic and decidedly unique paradigm of enhanced health and well-being centred on the identification and adjustment of spinal subluxations."*

While it may well be that one group of Australian chiropractors travelled down a fork in the road on their quest to validate the theoretical construct of the VSC, that road has inevitably taken them back to the crossroads and the stark choice of science or ideology.

Chiropractic today

So what is the state of chiropractic in Australia today? There are over 4300 registered chiropractors in Australia; there are three government funded chiropractic educational programs; chiropractic care is recognised and paid for by government funded workers compensation and transport accident insurers; the cost of chiropractic care is reimbursed by all major private health insurers, and chiropractors are publishing high level research in prestigious national and international journals.

That's the positive, encouraging and illuminating side. But there is a negative, disheartening and dark side.

While Australian data are lacking, the US adult use of chiropractic services declined from 9.9% in 1997 to 7.4% in 2002. This was the largest relative decrease among CAM professions and, as of 2007, only 7% of the US population was being reached by chiropractic [15].

Chiropractic does not have the same level of mainstream credibility as other healthcare professions. Public perception of chiropractic compares unfavourably with mainstream medicine, with regard to ethics and honesty. In a 2006 Gallup Poll of US adults, chiropractors rated last among seven healthcare professions for being very high or high in honesty and ethical standards [16,17].

In 2006, Australian Readers Digest conducted a poll on the most trusted professions [18]. Chiropractors were placed 13th on a list of 30 professions. Placed at 13th, I suppose the profession can console itself in the knowledge that they rated higher in trust than psychics, ministers of religion, car salesmen and politicians but poorer for the knowledge that the public trusts hairdressers more than chiropractors. And while such polls may not be good scientific evidence, they agree with similar polls on the public's perception of chiropractors [19].

The last Newsletter of the Chiropractors Registration Board of Victoria (CRBV), Australia, noted a total of 42 formal complaints against registered chiropractors in Victoria [20]. From personal experience, as a former member of the CRBV, many complaints emanated from the widespread use of false and misleading advertising or advertising designed to engender fear and distress. The use of terms such as, "silent deadly killers" and "spinal decay", when referring to subluxations, do little to promote the profession in a positive light.

Vertebral Subluxation Complex: use and misuse

What has fuelled this diminishing market share, public distrust and numerous complaints of misconduct? The answer is the road to the VSC. However, it is not this theoretical construct itself that has created this situation and led us back to the crossroads, but rather the way it is taught, sold and promoted, to not only chiropractors but the general public.

In Australia, the "Peak Body" of the chiropractic profession, the CAA, actively promotes subluxation based chiropractic via its previously mentioned "Core Values" (Appendix 1) [12]. Based on the VSC, the CAA's "Vision Statement" [12] envisages chiropractic as a separate and distinct alternative health system: *"To achieve a fundamental paradigm shift in healthcare direction where chiropractic is recognised as the most cost efficient and effective health regime of first choice that is readily accessible to all people."* In light of this "Vision Statement", it is worthwhile remembering the recommendation of the Webb Report, thirty three years ago [5], *"The Committee recommends that chiropractic and osteopathy should not be given legal recognition in any form which would imply that they are alternative health systems."*

Chiropractic trade publications and so-called educational seminar promotion material often abound with advertisements of how practitioners can effectively sell the VSC to an ignorant public. Phrases such as "double your income", "attract new patients" and "keep your patients longer in care", are common enticements for chiropractors to attend technique and practice management seminars. Selling such concepts as lifetime chiropractic care, the use contracts of care, the misuse of diagnostic equipment such as thermography and surface electromyography and the x-raying of every new patient, all contribute to our poor reputation, public distrust and official complaints.

To illustrate how the VSC dogma and ideology can be misused by some chiropractors, it is worth reviewing the case of Dr. Mark Pearson-Gills, who was disciplined by the CRBV for advocating a 60 visit, 12 month treatment plan for a 41/2 week old infant. The defendant later appealed the decision in the Victorian Civil and Administrative Tribunal (VCAT) and the transcript of the proceedings is on the public record [21]. The facts of the case were that "Baby CC was approximately 41/2 weeks old, when her mother brought her to see Dr. Pearson-Gills, after reading an advertisement promoting the applicant's practice and offering a first session at a reduced rate of $20. Dr. Pearson-Gills explained in a clinic handout that, *"The SOLE purpose of your chiropractic examination and care is to locate and correct subluxations."* After examining the baby, using thermography and other means, Dr. Pearson-Gills recommended a 60-visit 12-month plan of care.

It is likely that any reasonable person presented with this scenario would find such a plan indefensible and a prima facie case of professional misconduct.

However, Dr. Pearson-Gills produced expert witnesses and several of his peers to defend his actions. The defence rested not on scientific evidence but the philosophical underpinning of finding and correcting subluxations.

In summing up, the Presiding Member of the tribunal discredited the testimony of one expert witness, Dr. Matthew McCoy, from the USA: *"Dr McCoy gave evidence at the request of Dr. Pearson-Gills and his solicitor and his attendance in Australia was funded by Dr Pearson-Gills. Despite his protestations that he appeared against chiropractors, the inescapable conclusion is that Dr McCoy is a partisan witness committed to defending the practices of subluxation based chiropractors against malpractice claims and registration board investigation." and ".... I will discount any evidence that Dr McCoy gave, which supported the applicant's case. I gained the impression watching him that he had flown to Australia to give evidence to VCAT as part of his job in supporting WCA (World Chiropractic Alliance) practitioners."*

In my view, Smith's words of 1999 [19] resonate today, with the same clarity: *"Why do we tolerate the charlatans, hucksters, profiteers, and wild-eyed 'philosophers' who taint our profession's image, who obstruct political unity and espouse untrue science that cannot withstand the test of research; who recruit patients with gimmicks, and who mislead naive students and young practitioners with dogma and promises of great wealth? Is it because profession ethics is mostly lacking in chiropractic? Is it due to a laissez faire attitude within chiropractic where anyone can say anything under the guise of "philosophy"? Or is mainstream chiropractic simply scared to confront these fringe elements, fearful of litigation or argument? Have we become a profession ruled by a vocal minority (the Ouiji board practitioners), hellbent on keeping our profession in the past with dogma dominating over science, with leaders who espouse anti-scientific rhetoric, with practitioners who give free spinal exams and $10 office visits, all the while masquerading as "principled" chiropractors who preach unproved health gospel? Is this characterization wrong, or painfully accurate? You tell me."*

For the true believer, the naive practitioner or undergraduate chiropractic student, who accepts in good faith the propaganda and pseudo-science peddled by the VSC teachers, mentors and professional organisations, the result is the same, a sense of belonging and an unshakable and unwavering faith in their ideology.

Others use the propaganda and pseudo-science as a convenient way to justify the exploitation of their patients, and diminish their social and ethical responsibilities as a registered health practitioners, and because their peers are doing the same thing, they reason that they are less accountable; "et to quoque".

Subluxation: fact and fiction

The CAA and ASRF continue their search for the "holy grail" of evidence to support their subluxation based ideology, but they, and their international counterparts, have failed to produce any worthwhile evidence that subluxations actually exist, let alone adversely impact on a person's health or well-being. Nor have they shown that removal of such an entity has any positive impact on health [9,22,23]. The reality is that the VSC remains a theoretical construct.

Today's culture of evidence based practice has reluctantly led those who promote the VSC, to do so via "research evidence". However, this so-called evidence, is invariably a congealed mix of reality, half truths and "cherry picked quotes" that are misused, misrepresented or overstated. As Phillips [24] writes: *"Chiropractic fundamentalists have sought to make their philosophy more acceptable in today's world by guising scientific rationality under the cloak of emotionality. They selectively incorporate scientific findings that support their "major premise" while shunning or ignoring scientific findings incongruent with their way of thinking".*

A recent article published in the ASRF Newsletter, known as Illuminate, highlights this point [25]: *"Flu prevention should include chiropractic. Tell your patients why"* and *"Through research we know that chiropractic has beneficial effects on........ pulmonary function and other immune system processes, stated Matthew McCoy, DC, MPH, Editor of the Journal of Pediatric, Maternal & Family Health - Chiropractic."* Dr. McCoy then goes on to quote one study, by *"Patricia Brennan PhD and her team"* [26]. This is the same Matthew McCoy, who is also the Editor of the Journal of Vertebral Subluxation Research and whose testimony was rejected in the aforementioned Pearson-Gills case.

The study by Brenann et al [26], quoted above and a couple of other similar studies, are often cited by the VSC proponents, as proof that correction of VSC's improves immune function. However, this particular study provided no such proof or even a connection between subluxations and immune function. All that the Brennan study showed was that if you push on someone's back hard enough you will get a temporary change in the blood levels of certain biochemical markers.

The changes had nothing to do with subluxations, rather the study identified what happens when you apply different force levels during a manipulative thrust. In other words, you may have well got the same result if you had hit someone in the middle of the back with a piece of 4 × 2 timber. Brennan et al state in the conclusion of their paper, that their results cannot be extrapolated to show improved immune function after spinal manipulation: *"Although it is tempting to speculate on the possible biological significance of our results in terms of the potential for improved host defense against invading microorganisms and in terms of the implications in mild inflammatory processes such as hypomobile joints we believe such speculation to be unjustified by the data presented."* But these facts have not stopped the zealots and others from misrepresenting the results of this study.

Currently the CAA and the ASRF in Australia are promoting "wellness care", which involves the detection and adjustment of VSC's. Last year in ASRF's Newsletter, Illuminate [27], Dr. James Chestnut proclaimed: *".... it is not possible to be well if vertebral subluxation complex is present as a vertebral subluxation complex represents a non-homeostatic state ..... which makes a state of wellness impossible."* So, under the paradigm, published by the CAA, it is easy to make the next step and conclude that everyone needs life time chiropractic care to rid their bodies of subluxations in order to stay healthy. Once again, no evidence just belief and rhetoric.

Chiropractic education

There are currently three undergraduate chiropractic teaching institutions in Australia. All are government funded and part of Australia's mainstream tertiary education system.

The undergraduate chiropractic program at RMIT University [23] promotes the subluxation myth by defining its model of chiropractic to include: *"Functional derangement of the spine and other articulations may occur; where spinal we call this a vertebral subluxation complex (VSC)."* and *"Such derangements may affect the functioning of the neurological system in a variety of ways through a variety of mechanisms; we see such altered function as ranging from the Newtonian and quantifiable findings of pain and altered sensation to the Quantum and qualitative findings of altered cognitive and affective dimensions;"* The author suggests that such existential rhetoric is more suited to a degree in philosophy than a degree in science.

In contrast, in the United Kingdom (UK), the General Chiropractic Council (GCC), a regulatory authority similar to the Chiropractic Board of Australia (CBA), recently sought position statements on the VSC, from the three chiropractic teaching institutions in the UK. Unlike Australia, not one of these institutions taught the VSC theory in the context of modern health care delivery [23].

Associate Professor Phillip Ebrall, Head of the Chiropractic Unit, at RMIT University, has also written extensively about the VSC and, in particular, how it should be taught to chiropractic students [28]. He writes: *"Inspired by a visit to Disneyland this paper explores the challenges associated with the need to teach something that may not exist. It reports lessons learned by viewing a successful commercial illusion that has capacity to inform a pedagogical approach to abstract objects."*

What is the point of teaching something that does not exist? Could it be that the VSC itself is just "successful commercial illusion"?

To illustrate the belief in the VSC and chiropractic fundamentalism, at its extreme, the founder and former President of the largest college of chiropractic in the world was once quoted as saying, *"Rigor mortis is the only thing we can't help!"* [29]. It comes as no surprise that this university is now the subject of a class action law suit, by former students, which alleges breach of contract, for the failure of the university to teach differential diagnosis [30].

Murphy in his paper comparing and contrasting the evolution of chiropractic to the acceptance and integration of podiatry into mainstream healthcare wrote about the teaching of subluxation [31]: *"These concepts are lacking in a scientific foundation and should not be permitted to be taught at our chiropractic institutions as part of the standard curriculum."* and *"Faculty members who hold to and teach these belief systems should be replaced by instructors who are knowledgeable in the evidence-based approach to spine care..."*

The irony of this fervent belief in the VSC and chiropractic philosophy is that its development was not founded on vitalistic theory but rather as a legal strategy, conjured up by an attorney, in the defence of a chiropractor charged with practicing medicine [7,32,33]: *"Many in chiropractic never learned the origin of the pseudo-region or chiropractic philosophy. It was nothing more than a legal tactic used in the Morriubo's case."* [34], and *"B.J. Palmer probably developed his dis-ease theory as a result of the winning strategy used by his attorney Thomas Morris to defend Japanese chiropractor Shegatoro Morijubo in Wisconsin in 1907"* [35].

Back to the crossroads

So where to from here, which road will the chiropractic profession take, subluxation or science?

If we take the path of the VSC, then I have no doubt that whatever acceptance, credibility and privileges the profession has gained in the last 35 years will be rapidly lost.

Chiropractors will be further alienated from mainstream healthcare. The profession will survive but it will again be dumped into the unscientific quack bin with homeopathy and iridology. Others within mainstream healthcare, who are trained in spinal manipulation, will continue to progress and fill the void.

As Nelson et al [36] rightly put it, we have an obligation as licensed health care providers not to promote unscientifically unreasonable beliefs as clinical truths: *"Neither a chiropractor nor any other healthcare provider practicing under the protection of a licensed profession has the ethical right to promote unscientifically unreasonable beliefs. The principle of fidelity and the state of scientific knowledge regarding certain historical chiropractic beliefs should not allow the expression of these beliefs to the patient as clinical truths."*

Further, on subluxation they write, *"A number of models are impractical, implausible or even indefensible from a purely scientific point of view (e.g., subluxation- based healthcare), from a professional practice perspective (e.g., the primary care model), or simply from common sense (e.g. Innate Intelligence as an operational system for influencing health)."*

If we take the road of science, we may still have a chance to establish ourselves as spine care specialists. Murphy [31] writes: *"We see a tremendous opportunity for chiropractic medicine to become what it can and should be: a profession of non-surgical spine specialists who not only offer one useful modality of treatment for spinal pain (manipulation), but offer something much greater and more important - expertise in the diagnosis and management of spinal pain patients."*

A recent decision in the UK by the GCC, may provide us with a road map [23]. A position statement published in early 2010 states:

- *"The chiropractic vertebral subluxation complex is an historical concept but it remains a theoretical model.*
- *It is not supported by any clinical research evidence that would allow claims to be made that it is the cause of disease or health concerns.*
- *Chiropractors are reminded that they must make sure their own beliefs and values do not prejudice the patients' care.*
- *They must provide evidence based care, which is clinical practice that incorporates the best available evidence from research, the preferences of the patient and the expertise of practitioners, including the individual chiropractor her/himself."*

This position statement was also endorsed by the British Chiropractic Association (BCA) [37], the equivalent body in the UK, to the CAA in Australia:

- *"The BCA welcomes today's statement from the General Chiropractic Council (GCC) on Vertebral Subluxation Complex.*
- *For many years, the BCA has not supported the concept of the Vertebral Subluxation Complex.*
- *To facilitate the integration of chiropractic, unsubstantiated historical concepts and ambiguous terminology must be discarded in favour of an emphasis on delivering an evidence-based care model that is easily understood by other members of the healthcare team"*

The decision by the GCC and the BCA followed the failed court case of Simon Singh, a science writer, who was sued for libel by the BCA for claiming that chiropractors used bogus treatments [38].

As a consequence of this libel suit Singh's supporters made complaints to the GCC and the UK's Advertising Standards Authority [29], over the use of the term subluxation and the unsubstantiated claims, made by some chiropractors, of the successful treatment of various diseases such as colic, asthma, irritable bowel syndrome etc., that were purportedly caused by subluxations. These complaints and the subsequent investigations, have led some chiropractic organisations to advise their members to remove references to subluxation and the treatment of a number of diseases in their advertising [39].

There are also some parallels between the GCC position statement and the recent release of the Code of Conduct for Chiropractors, by the newly formed CBA [40]. The CBA's Code of Conduct defines good care as, involving evidence informed care, and that chiropractors should avoid expressing their personal beliefs to patients in ways that exploit their vulnerability or that are likely to cause them distress.

In response to the GCC's and CBA's positions, it would appear that the true believers and others are attempting to marshal their forces. At the forefront is Dr. McCoy whose article, *"The death of subluxation."*, published in the ASRF Newsletter, Illuminate, [41]: encourages like minded chiropractors to, *"Pick up your pitch forks and torches and get ready to storm the castle"* and *"Subluxation, family wellness focused chiropractors need to take over the regulatory boards, agencies and organisations in this profession."*

Summary

So it would appear, that for the past thirty odd years all we have done is gone around in circles and we are once again back at the crossroads," Science or Subluxation."

The "subluxationists" see chiropractic as a unique system of healthcare supported not by science, but an ideology and pseudo-science, yet they still want to be accepted into mainstream healthcare and enjoy all the benefits that come with the acceptance and credibility of a science based discipline. If this profession is to move forward it has to base its future on science and not ideological dogma.

In a recent commentary, Scott Haldeman [42] highlighted the need to base therapy on evidence: *"It does not serve patients to provide treatment that has been shown to be ineffective or where there is insufficient evidence to reach a conclusion when there are other options available that have been demonstrated to be beneficial."* and *"It is not acceptable today to claim that a treatment is effective in helping patients when there is no evidence to support these claims."*

Finally, Haldeman concludes: *"It does not help the reputation of a profession that is striving to be considered the authority in a field, if practitioners are unwilling to understand and practice according to the latest clinical evidence".*

Hopefully, Dr McCoy is right and the "subluxation" will die or at least assume a more credible identity. But similar to what happened in the UK, it may require clear and decisive action on the part of the CBA and/or the Australian Competition and Consumer Commission (ACCC) to finally put it to rest.

However, I also think it is time for the moderates and conservatives within our profession to become more involved with shaping its future. For too long now the "the near empty tin has made far too much noise". It is about time government, other health care providers and the public were made aware that not all chiropractors are pseudo religious zealots who have abandoned science for ideology: *"Chiropractic does have a large silent majority which seems content to tolerate the fringe elements and to let other people fight their political battles, allthewhile wondering why our situation doesn't seem to be improving."* [19].

Maybe it's time for the silent majority to pick up their pitch forks and torches, and get ready to storm the castle, and to take over the regulatory boards, agencies and organisations of this profession?

Appendix 1

Chiropractors Association of Australia

Core Values

We recognise...

• *and respect a universal intelligence (or order) in all matter and an innate intelligence within a living organism that strives to preserve life and, if uninhibited, will express optimal well being.*

• *that the practice of chiropractic focuses on the relationship between structure (primarily the spine) and function (as coordinated by the nervous system) and how that relationship affects the preservation and restoration of health.*

• *that subluxations compromise the expression of innate intelligence, and that prevention and removal of subluxations will facilitate the expression of optimal health.*

We respect, care about and are committed to the individual's holistic well being and emphasise the inherent recuperative power of the body to heal itself without the use of drugs or surgery and value the importance of intellectual honesty, scientific and academic excellence and the maintenance of integrity in serving the individual, the community and the profession.

Vision Statement

To achieve a fundamental paradigm shift in healthcare direction where chiropractic is recognised as the most cost efficient and effective health regime of first choice that is readily accessible to all people.

Author details

[1]Suite1/593 Whitehorse Road, Mitcham, Victoria, 3132 Australia. [2]School of Chiropractic and Sports Science, Faculty of Health Sciences, Murdoch University. Murdoch, Western Australia, 6150.

Competing interests

The author declares that they have no competing interests.

References

1. Willis E: **Chiropractic & osteopathy at the crossroads: opening address to COMSIG Chiropractic Conference–7th November, 1992.** *COMSIG Rev* 1993, **2**:1-4.
2. Meeker WC, Haldeman S: **Chiropractic: a profession at the crossroads of mainstream and alternative medicine.** *Ann Intern Med* 2002, **136**:216-227.
3. Ebrall P: **The crossroad was really a fork.** *Chiropractic Journal of Australia* 2009, **39**:15.
4. Stoner F: *The eclectic approach to chiropractic.* 2 edition. Las Vegas, Nevada USA: FLS Publishing; 1976.
5. Webb E: **Report of Committee of Inquiry into Chiropractic, Osteopathy, Homeopathy and Naturopathy.** Government of Australia; 1977.
6. Homola S: **Chiropractic vertebral subluxations: Science vs. pseudoscience.** [http://www.sciencebasedmedicine.org/?p=6839].
7. Keating J: *Early Palmer Theories of Dis-ease* Whittier CA: Los Angeles College of Chiropractic; 1996.
8. Johnson C, Baird R, Dougherty PE, Globe G, Green BN, Haneline M, Hawk C, Injeyan HS, Killinger L, Kopansky-Giles D, *et al*: **Chiropractic and public health: current state and future vision.** *J Manipulative Physiol Ther* 2008, **31**:397-410.
9. Keating JC Jr, Charlton KH, Grod JP, Perle SM, Sikorski D, Winterstein JF: **Subluxation: dogma or science?** *Chiropr Osteopat* 2005, **13**:17.
10. Shekelle P, Adams AH, Chassin MR, Hurwitz E, Park RE, Phillips RB, Brook RH: **The Appropriateness of Spinal Manipulation for Low-Back Pain, Indications and Ratings by a Multidisciplinary Expert Panel.** Santa Monica, CA: Rand Corporation; 1991.
11. Shekelle P: **Misinterpretation of RAND study undermines chiropractic credibility.** *ACA Journal of Chiropractic* 1993, 59-63.
12. **Chiropractors Association of Australia - Core Values and Vision Statement.** [http://chiropractors.asn.au], Members only access.
13. **Australian Spinal Research Foundation - Mission Statement.** [http://www.spinalresearch.com.au/Research/tabid/148/language/enAU/Default.aspx].
14. Phillips RB, Adams AH, Sandefur R: **Chiropractic Research.** In *Chiropractic in the United States: Training, Practice, and Research.* Edited by: Cherkin DC, Mootz RD. Washington: Agency for Healthcare Policy and Research; 1998:92-100.
15. Tindle HA, Davis RB, Phillips RS, Eisenberg DM: **Trends in the use of complementary and alternative medicine by US adults: 1997-2002.** *Alternative Therapies in Health and Medicine* 2005, **11**:42-49.
16. Gallup: **Honesty/Ethics in Professions.** [http://www.gallup.com/poll/1654/Honesty-Ethics-Professionas.aspx].

17. Editorial Staff: **Gallup Poll: Americans Have Low Opinion of Chiropractors' Honesty and Ethics Medical Doctors, Five Other Health Occupations Rate Higher.** *Dynamic Chiropractic* 2007, **28.**
18. Readers Digest: **Australia's Most Trusted 2006.** [http://www.readersdigest.com.au/australias-most-trusted-2006].
19. Smith JC: **Chiropractic ethics: an oxymoron? Contemporary ethical issues in chiropractic.** *Journal of chiropractic humanities* 2000, **9**:1-17 [http://archive.journalchirohumanities.com/Vol%209/SmithComtemp.pdf].
20. Courtin J: **Chiropractors Registration Board of Victoria, News.** 2010, **22**:1.
21. Victorian Civil and Administrative Tribunal: **Pearson-Gills versus Chiropractors Registration Board of Victoria.** Tribunal VCAT 436 (22 March 2006): Government of Victoria; 2006 [http://www.austlii.edu.au/au/cases/vic/VCAT/2006/436.html].
22. Mirtz TA, Morgan L, Wyatt LH, Greene L: **An epidemiological examination of the subluxation construct using Hill's criteria of causation.** *Chiropr Osteopat* 2009, **17**:13.
23. General Chiropractic Council, UK: **Guidance on claims made for the chiropractic vertebral subluxation complex.** General Chiropractic Council, United Kingdom; 2010 [http://www.gcc-uk.org/page.cfm?page_id=437&fc=1&hi=subluxation#hi].
24. Phillips RB, Adams RH, Sandefur R: **The battle for innate: A perspective on fundamentalism in chiropractic.** *Journal of Chiropractic Humanities* 2004, **11**:1-10 [http://archive.journalchirohumanities.com/Vol%2011/JChiroprHumanit2004-11-2-10.pdf].
25. Chestnut J: **Flu plan should include chiropractic: Let your patients know why.** In *Illuminate, Chiropractic News. Volume 3.* Australian Spinal Research Foundation; 2009.
26. Brennan PC, Triano JJ, McGregor M, Kokjohn K, Hondras MA, Brennan DC: **Enhanced neutrophil respiratory burst as a biological marker for manipulation forces: duration of the effect and association with substance P and tumor necrosis factor.** *J Manipulative Physiol Ther* 1992, **15**:83-89.
27. Chestnut J: **Wellness and chiropractic: Oxymoronic, redundant, synonymous or simply a perfect marriage.** In *Illuminate Chiropractic News. Volume 2.* Australian Spinal Research Foundation; 2010.
28. Ebrall P: **Towards better teaching about the vertebral subluxation complex.** *Chiropractic Journal of Australia* 2009, **39**:165-170.
29. Williams SE: **Interview with Syd E Williams DC.** *Health Magazine* Health Media Ventures Inc; 1993, 44-53.
30. **Life University class action law suit now official.** [http://www.ebm-first.com/chiropractic/latest-news.html].
31. Murphy DR, Schneider MJ, Seaman DR, Perle SM, Nelson CF: **How can chiropractic become a respected mainstream profession? The example of podiatry.** *Chiropr Osteopat* 2008, **16**:10.
32. Leach RA: *The Chiropractic Theories: A textbook of scientific research.* 4 edition. Baltimore, Maryland: Lippincott, Williams & Wilkins; 2004.
33. Keating J: **Ain't got enough philosophy. Dynamic chiropractic 16 June 2003.** In *Dynamic Chiropractic. Volume 21.* MPA Media; 2003.
34. Perle S: **Foundation for Anachronistic Chiropractic Pseudo-Religion.** [http://smperle.blogspot.com/2009/07/foundation-for-anachronistic.html].
35. Leach RA: **Subluxation Theory Quiz.** Lippincott, Williams & Wilkins; 2009 [http://www.chiroaccess.com/surveys/TakeSurveyPage.aspx?s=c27e654274ea4ea2856591f64c1aa92b&tsid=c7f3087ee6ea4b0cb021ee4efd3de28a&c=en-US].
36. Nelson CF, Lawrence DJ, Triano JJ, Bronfort G, Perle SM, Metz RD, Hegetschweiler K, LaBrot T: **Chiropractic as spine care: a model for the profession.** *Chiropr Osteopat* 2005, **13**:9.
37. British Chiropractic Association: **BCA statement on vertebral subluxation complex.** [http://www.chiropractic-uk.co.uk/default.aspx?m=8&mi=14&title=For+Chiropractors].
38. Coghlan A: **Simon Singh wins libel battle against chiropractors.** In *Science in Society. Volume 15.* New Scientist; 2010, [http://www.newscientist.com/article/dn18780-simon-singh-wins-libel-battle-against-chiropractors.html].
39. **McTimony chiropractors told to take down their websites.** [http://www.quackometer.net/blog/2009/06/chiropractors-told-to-take-down-their.html].
40. **Chiropractic Board of Australia - Code of Conduct for Chiropractors.** [http://www.chiropracticboard.gov.au/Codes-and-Guidelines.aspx].
41. McCoy M: **The death of subluxation.** In *Illuminate Chiropractic News. Volume 2.* Australian Spinal Research Foundation; 2010.
42. Haldeman S, Underwood M: **Commentary on the United Kingdom evidence report about the effectiveness of manual therapies.** *Chiropr Osteopat* 2010, **18**:4.

3

International web survey of chiropractic students about evidence-based practice: a pilot study

Ryunosuke Banzai[1], Dustin C Derby[2], Cynthia R Long[1], Maria A Hondras[1*]

Abstract

Background: Positive attitude toward evidence-based practice (EBP) principles in healthcare education may be one of the first steps for motivating a healthcare professional student to later apply EBP principles in clinical decision-making. The objectives for this project were to pilot an international web-based survey of chiropractic students and to describe student attitudes, behaviors, and knowledge about EBP principles.

Methods: We used SurveyMonkey™ to develop our survey based on an existing questionnaire used to measure basic knowledge, skills and beliefs about EBP among allied healthcare professionals and CAM practitioners. We invited 26 chiropractic educational institutions teaching in English and accredited by official organizations to participate. Academic officials and registrars at participating institutions forwarded an invitation email and two reminders to students between July and September 2010. The invitation contained a link to the 38-item web-based questionnaire. Descriptive statistics were performed for analysis.

Results: Fourteen institutions from Australia, Canada, US, Denmark and New Zealand participated. Among an estimated 7,142 student recipients of invitation letters, 674 participated in the survey for an estimated response rate of 9.4%. Most respondents reported having access to medical/healthcare literature through the internet, but only 11% read literature every week and 21% did not read literature at all. Respondents generally agreed that the use of research evidence in chiropractic was important. Although 76% of respondents found it easy to understand research evidence and 81% had some level of confidence assessing the general worth of research articles, 71% felt they needed more training in EBP to be able to apply evidence in chiropractic care. Respondents without previous training in research methods had lower confidence in assessing published papers. While more than 60% marked the correct answer for two knowledge items, the mean number of correct answers to the five knowledge questions was 1.3 (SD 0.9).

Conclusions: Although it is feasible to conduct an international web survey of chiropractic students, significant stakeholder participation is important to improve response rates. Students had relatively positive attitudes toward EBP. However, participants felt they needed more training in EBP and based on the knowledge questions they may need further training about basic research concepts.

Background

Since the early 1990's when the Evidence-Based Medicine Working Group at McMaster University [1] established explicit methodologies to determine "best evidence" for clinical medicine, many professional groups and organizations have emphasized the importance of evidence-based practice (EBP) for their practitioners [2-6]. The EBP movement emerged to facilitate clinical decision-making by healthcare professionals and their patients; however, both groups are challenged to know how, where, and when to seek out the best evidence to bridge gaps between research evidence and practical health outcomes [7].

Djulbegovic et al. [8] recently stated that "we should regard evidence-based medicine as a constantly evolving heuristic foundation for optimizing clinical practice, rather than a new scientific or philosophical theory that changes the nature of medicine." By virtue of the exponential growth of healthcare information of both high and low quality, acquisition of EBP principles requires

* Correspondence: maria.hondras@palmer.edu
[1]Palmer Center for Chiropractic Research, Palmer College of Chiropractic, 741 Brady Street, Davenport, IA 52803-5209, USA
Full list of author information is available at the end of the article

certain knowledge and skills to synthesize the best available research evidence with other factors in clinical decision-making [9,10].

There are a number of ways available to deal with the difficulties and barriers of teaching EBP principles [11-18] and exposure to EBP principles in healthcare education has received considerable attention during the past decade [5,19-23]. The Accreditation Council for Graduate Medical Education [5] requires medical residents to demonstrate the ability to appraise and to integrate scientific evidence. Similarly, an understanding of the principles of EBP and the application of evidence into practice is part of the core training both of medical doctors and complementary and alternative medicine (CAM) healthcare practitioners in the United Kingdom [6]. Smith et al. [23] stated that the development of "evidence-based skills" should include early exposure and experience with fundamental literature searching and critical appraisal skills. Novice clinicians may then develop critical thinking skills and learn to apply those skills to clinical decision-making. Because scientific evidence application plays such a critical role in the clinical decision-making process, healthcare students should learn and implement best practices using EBP during their professional course of study. Chiropractic, one of the most widely used CAM disciplines, [24] is no exception.

Research on the inclusion of EBP principles in chiropractic curricula is lacking. Chiropractic students receive little formal instruction to generate searchable questions, conduct literature searches, critically appraise the literature or apply evidence to patient management [25,26]. Wyatt et al. [27] posited that instruction for EBP principles in chiropractic curricula in the US appeared to be deficient and an emphasis on "chiropractic philosophy" may promote unsupported beliefs and theories without research evidence. Other studies have found that chiropractic students have little interest in reading clinical research literature [23,28]. Understanding chiropractic student attitudes toward, knowledge of, and potential barriers and facilitators of using EBP principles may better inform curricular management and implementation of EBP at chiropractic educational institutions. Although several surveys of EBP have targeted health professionals, these data are lacking for health professional students, in general, and chiropractic students in particular.

The objectives of this study were to pilot a web-based survey of chiropractic students worldwide and to describe their attitudes, behaviors, and knowledge about EBP. Positive attitude toward EBP principles in healthcare education may be one of the first steps for motivating a healthcare professional student to later apply EBP principles in individual practice.

Methods

We conducted an anonymous, cross-sectional, web-based international survey of chiropractic students. The Palmer College of Chiropractic Institutional Review Board approved this project.

Eligibility Criteria

We set institutional and individual criteria for this project. Eligible institutions taught their curriculum in English and met criteria for accreditation from official organizations such as the Council on Chiropractic Education (CCE), the European CCE and CCE Australia. The CCE ensures the quality of chiropractic education by means of accreditation, educational improvement and public information, and requires institutions to teach research methods and procedures [29]. Of the 41 chiropractic educational institutions listed on the World Federation of Chiropractic quarterly report published on 30 September 2009, [30] 26 institutions met the eligibility criteria and were invited to participate in the study. Next, we invited students at least 18 years old who were enrolled in the chiropractic degree program at participating institutions. Students were not eligible if they were enrolled in bachelor programs other than chiropractic or in prerequisite studies to matriculate in a chiropractic program.

Recruitment

We used both institutional and student recruitment strategies to reach our target population. First, we sent an invitation email to the Academic Deans or equivalent at the 26 eligible institutions asking for support of the project and permission to contact their registrar or their designee who maintains the chiropractic program student email distribution list. The institutional invitation described the purpose of the project, the secure and anonymous nature of data collection from students, and provided investigator contact information. We sent a second institutional invitation to non-responder institutions approximately three weeks later. Next, we prepared a similar communication to each institutional registrar of the institutions who granted permission and asked them to forward the student recruitment email invitation to all chiropractic students via their electronic distribution lists. Approximately three and five weeks later, we sent second and third invitation emails to the registrars to distribute to students.

Survey Questionnaire

We used SurveyMonkey™to develop our survey based on the existing questionnaire that Hadley et al. [6] used to measure basic knowledge, skills and beliefs about EBP among allied healthcare professionals and CAM practitioners. First, we revised the instructions and items from the original questionnaire to target chiropractic students as opposed to practitioners. Second, we added five multiple choice knowledge questions that assessed fundamental critical appraisal concepts and four facilitator questions of interest with this student population. Third, our new questionnaire was a web-based version of the original paper questionnaire with the new items. Finally, we pre-tested and refined the questionnaire by inviting graduate clinical research fellows, research clinicians and clinical research project managers at our institutional research center to complete the survey; we incorporated feedback to improve clarity and readability of the instrument.

The final questionnaire had 38 items arranged in seven categories: attitudes, behaviors, facilitators, confidence, barriers, knowledge, and background information [see Additional file 1]. While the student respondents were anonymous, the invitation emails directed recipients to institution-specific Uniform Resource Locators (URLs) on SurveyMonkey™to track and estimate response rates by institution. The Consent to Participate page, the first screen of the questionnaire, included the title and purpose of the project, procedures for the anonymous and voluntary nature of the survey, and the potential risks and benefits to participants. Three questions followed the informed consent page to assess eligibility based on participant age, program of study, and whether or not they had already received a doctor of chiropractic or equivalent degree. Eligible participants were asked if they would like to participate in the survey with two choices; (1) No thank you, I decline to participate in this survey, and (2) Yes, I agree to participate in this survey. Choosing the second choice constituted participant consent to begin the survey. No questions other than those regarding eligibility required response. Despite a potential for duplication, we allowed multiple responses from the same computer to increase convenience for participants. There was neither password-protected access to the survey nor restriction for the range of the Internet Protocol (IP) address. The last page of the questionnaire thanked respondents for their participation and closed the window at the completion of the survey.

Data Analysis

RB monitored the SurveyMonkey™web pages on a daily basis. RB downloaded data collected from survey participants from SurveyMonkey™, stored these data on the college's secure network, and transferred these data into SPSS statistical package version 17.0 (Chicago, IL) through Microsoft Office Excel® for descriptive analysis. In addition to descriptive statistics for the recruitment process, we summarized the data as percentages and calculated means and standard deviations (SD) where appropriate.

Results

Figure 1 displays the institutional and student recruitment efforts between July 8 and September 2, 2010. We sent invitation letters to the 26 eligible institutions on July 8 and 27, 2010. Fifteen institutions granted permission to contact their registrars and students. Of these, two institutions requested to review the ethics approval for the project before granting permission while 13 institutions granted permission based on our own institutional ethics approval. Among the 11 non-participating institutions, 10 did not respond to the institutional invitation while one refused due to perceived confidentiality concerns. We asked 15 registrars or their designee to forward the invitation letters to chiropractic students via their local distribution lists. One registrar did not respond. Of the 14 institutions who forwarded student invitations, nine institutions (87.5%) were from the US while the other five were from Australia, Canada, Denmark and New Zealand. Twelve institutions provided the exact number of students while the other two provided approximate numbers, for a total estimate of

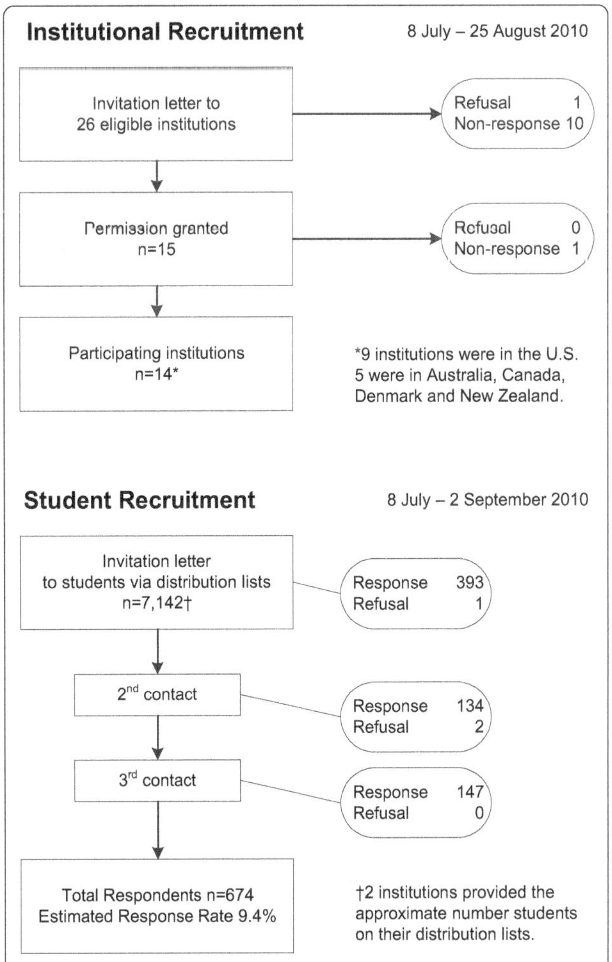

Figure 1 **Institutional and student recruitment efforts.**

7,142 students attending chiropractic programs at 14 institutions.

Of 740 persons who opened the link to the web survey, 674 were eligible and agreed to participate in the survey for an estimated 9.4% response rate. Three respondents declined to participate in the survey. Sixty three respondents were ineligible, some for multiple reasons: nine were younger than 18 years old, 32 were not students in a chiropractic program, and 38 had already received a doctor of chiropractic or equivalent degree. For the three waves of student recruitment, 393, 134 and 147 opened the survey link at the first, second and third contact, respectively. Students at Canadian Memorial College of Chiropractic received only one invitation because of summer recess during the recruitment process. Of 674 respondents, 171 (25.4%), 146 (21.7%) and 146 (21.7%) were from Life University, Palmer College of Chiropractic Davenport campus and New Zealand College of Chiropractic, respectively. Beyond the eligibility criteria, there were no additional required fields for the survey, so some items were incomplete.

The mean age of student respondents was 27.2 years (range 18-60). Table 1 displays additional respondent background information. While nearly three-fourths (72.5%) of respondents had no experience in the medical/healthcare field, two-thirds (66.6%) of respondents had taken at least one course about EBP or research methodology in their chiropractic education. There were 226 respondents (33.5%) who reported no formal education or training in research methods, epidemiology or statistics outside of the chiropractic curriculum, while 143 reported outside training in research methods, 52 in epidemiology, and 208 in statistics. Seventy-five students reported no EBP training either inside or outside of the chiropractic curriculum.

Table 1 Background information of respondents

Variable	Category	Percent
Gender (*n* = 476)	Female	48.9
	Male	51.1
Primary Language (*n* = 475)	English	88.4
	Others	11.6
What academic year are you in your chiropractic program? (*n* = 475)	Year1	25.7
	Year2	27.4
	Year3	26.7
	Year4	13.5
	Year5	6.7
Do you have any experience in the medical/ healthcare field? (*n* = 477)	No	72.5
	Yes	27.5
Have you already taken a course related to evidence-based practice or research methodology in your chiropractic education? (*n* = 476)	None	33.4
	Once	46.4
	Twice	15.8
	> Twice	4.4
Have you been personally involved in conducting any kind of research? (*n* = 478)	None	58.8
	Once	27.4
	Twice	6.5
	> Twice	7.3

Among 571 respondents, 545 (95.6%) reported having access to medical/healthcare literature through the internet. There were 348/612 (56.9%) and 370/609 (60.8%) who searched for and read research evidence more than once a month, respectively. Only 69 of 611 respondents (11.3%) answered that they read every week regularly to keep up to date with medical/healthcare literature, while 229 (37.5%) read occasionally, 184 (30.1%) read only for specific information, and the remaining 129 (21.1%) answered that they do not keep up to date with medical/ healthcare literature. Almost half of respondents (284/ 591, 48.1%) agreed that their institutions balanced philosophy, art and research evidence well.

Table 2 shows the mean (SD) and percentages of responses to each question about attitudes toward, facilitators, barriers and confidence of using EBP principles. Respondents had a mean of 4.8 (1 = Strongly Disagree, 6 = Strongly Agree) regarding the importance of the use of research evidence in chiropractic care and a mean of 4.2 regarding their ease in understanding research evidence. Almost all of the respondents (96%) reported being comfortable reading research evidence in English, and half of the respondents agreed that they had enough time to search and read research literature. Further, the mean confidence (1 = Not confident at all, 6 = Very confident) ranged from 3.6 in evaluating statistical tests in the open literature to 4.3 in assessing the general worth of research articles. However, the 75 respondents who had no previous training in research methods, epidemiology, statistics or EBP had lower confidence ranging from a mean of 3.2 in assessing study design to 3.8 in assessing the general worth of research articles.

Table 3 displays the results of the five items aimed to assess students' knowledge of fundamental research concepts. While more than 60% marked the correct answer for two knowledge items, less than half answered correctly for the other three items. In addition, approximately 30% of all participants elected not to answer any of the knowledge questions. The mean number of correct answers to the 5 knowledge questions was 1.3 (SD 0.9) for the 461 respondents who answered all 5 questions; only one individual answered all 5 questions correctly. Evaluating this by whether or not the respondent reported previous training in research methods, epidemiology, statistics or EBP showed that the mean number of correct responses was lowest for those who had no previous training (n = 69;

Table 2 Attitudes, facilitators, barriers and confidence of using EBP

	Strongly Disagree	Disagree	Slightly Disagree	Slightly Agree	Agree	Strongly Agree	Mean*	SD
Attitudes								
1.I think that chiropractic is composed of a balanced combination between philosophy, art and science. (*n* = 636)	2.2	7.2	5.0	13.1	36.2	36.3	4.8	1.3
2. I think that the use of research evidence is an important factor in chiropractic care. (*n* = 636)	0.6	1.4	1.3	8.2	33.3	55.2	5.4	0.9
3. I think that research evidence has little impact on chiropractic care. (*n* = 631)	37.6	36.1	12.7	6.2	4.6	2.9	2.1	1.3
4. I think that evidence- based practice is a temporary fad. (*n* = 631)	38.4	35.8	13.2	6.8	3.6	1.9	2.1	1.2
5. I feel that I need more training in evidence- based practice to be able to apply research evidence into chiropractic care. (*n* = 635)	5.7	11.5	12.1	25.0	30.9	14.8	4.1	1.4
6. I find it easy to understand research evidence. (*n* = 635)	2.4	6.3	15.0	32.0	34.6	9.8	4.2	1.1
Facilitators								
1. I feel that my institution incorporates research evidence into chiropractic education well. (*n* = 592)	4.2	7.4	11.5	27.4	38.0	11.5	4.2	1.3
2. I have a good teacher(s) at my institution who is(are) familiar with evidence-based practice principles.(*n* = 591)	2.5	3.0	6.4	18.8	41.8	27.4	4.8	1.2
3. I have at least one good role model of chiropractor who is familiar with evidence-based practice principles.(*n* = 592)	1.7	6.6	7.1	16.0	37.3	31.3	4.7	1.2
Barriers								
1. I am comfortable reading research evidence in English. (*n* = 572)	2.8	0.2	1.0	7.0	32.5	56.5	5.4	1.0
2. I have enough time to search medical/healthcare literature. (*n* = 570)	9.8	21.4	19.5	28.8	17.2	3.3	3.3	1.3
3. I have enough time to read medical/healthcare literature. (*n* = 570)	8.4	20.5	23.0	30.2	15.6	2.3	3.3	1.3
	Not confident at all	Not very confident	Slightly not Confident	Slightly Confident	Confident	Very Confident	Mean†	SD
Confidence								
1. Assessing study design (*n* = 572)	7.2	12.5	11.6	36.6	26.5	5.6	3.8	1.3
2. Evaluating bias (*n* = 572)	4.7	7.4	10.4	31.8	37.1	8.6	4.2	1.2
3. Evaluating the adequacy of sample size (*n* = 570)	5.5	6.7	10.8	28.0	39.2	9.9	4.2	1.3
4. Assessing generalisability (*n* = 572)	5.4	8.6	14.8	30.4	34.3	6.5	4.0	1.3
5. Evaluating statistical tests/principles (*n* = 570)	7.4	14.1	18.2	33.2	22.2	4.9	3.6	1.3
6. Assessing the general worth of research articles (*n* = 570)	4.1	5.6	9.7	30.9	41.8	7.9	4.3	1.2

Numbers listed are percentages unless otherwise noted.
*Mean scores for Attitudes, Facilitators and Barriers: Likert scale where 1 = Strongly Disagree and 6 = Strongly Agree.
†Mean scores for Confidence: Likert scale where 1 = Not confident at all and 6 = Very confident.

mean 1.1; SD 0.8) and highest for those who reported two or more courses in their chiropractic program in addition to at least one course outside of their chiropractic program (n = 51; mean 1.5; SD 0.9).

At the end of the questionnaire, participants had the opportunity to provide comments about the survey. Of 74 who entered comments, 12 liked the survey while six commented that the instructions and items in the questionnaire were unclear and confusing. Fifteen respondents suggested areas for survey improvement, such as adding a question to assess one's understanding of the definition of EBP and including more items related to background information. Another respondent stated that the use of the term 'doctor of chiropractic' may not be relevant in some regions.

Discussion

The results of this pilot study indicate that while it is feasible to conduct a web-based international survey of students attending chiropractic educational institutions in a relatively short period of time, institutional and student recruitment will require significant effort to improve response rates. Despite the low estimated response rate (9.4%), the number of respondents was 674 which allowed us to describe student attitudes, behaviors and basic knowledge of EBP principles.

Table 3 Knowledge questions with correct answers in bold

Questions	Answers	Respons
Which section of an article is the best section to evaluate when critical analysis of information is needed? (*n* = 479)	1. Abstract	17.1
	2. Introduction section	3.1
	3. Methods section	**48.0**
	4. Conclusions section	28.8
	5. References	2.9
Because three cases of a very rare brain cancer have been detected in children living in a small community located near a hazardous waste disposal site, local clinicians want to determine if they can identify risk factors associated with cancer development. They should conduct a _______ to address this question. (*n* = 474)	1. Case series	25.7
	2. Randomized clinical trial	7.4
	3. Prospective cohort study	22.6
	4. Cross-sectional study	16.9
	5. Case-control study	**27.4**
A randomized clinical trial is designed to compare two different treatment approaches for a disease/condition of interest. The purpose of randomization is to: (*n* = 470)	1. Obtain treatment groups of similar size	2.3
	2. Select a representative sample of patients for study	53.8
	3. Increase patient compliance with treatment	4.0
	4. Obtain treatment groups with coparable baseline prognoses	**37.4**
	5. Increase the prevalence of disease in both groups	2.3
A controversy occurred between the proponents of drug therapy and spinal manipulation for patients with asthma. To support their position, one party wrote, "Of 119 patients with asthma, 97 showed improvement following spinal manipulation." The inference that in patients with asthma, spinal manipulation is the therapy of choice is: (*n* = 470)	1. Correct	13.6
	2. Incorrect because the comparison is not based on rates	3.4
	3. Incorrect because no control or comparison group is being used	**60.9**
	4. Incorrect because no test of statistical significance is being made	16.6
	5. Incorrect because a cohort effect may be operating	5.5
The following spinal manipulation research was performed: 1,000 randomly selected children two years of age were given full spine manipulation once per month for 12 consecutive months, and then followed for 10 years. Of these, 80% were never afflicted with spine pain or spine related disease. Which is the most correct conclusion regarding the efficacy of spinal manipulation? (*n* = 466)	1. Spinal manipulation is an excellent preventive therapy because of the high rate of healthy children.	16.5
	2. No conclusion is possible because no follow-up was made of children who did not receive spinal manipulation.	**66.7**
	3. Spinal manipulation is not very effective because it should have produced a higher rate of healthy children.	1.7
	4. No conclusion is possible because no test of statistical significance was performed.	11.8
	5. The significant figure is 100% - 80% = 20%, the rate of acquiring spine pain or illness.	3.2

Numbers listed are percentages.

Hadley's survey [6] of allied healthcare professionals and CAM practitioners found that the majority felt that EBP was essential to their practice. Similarly, the majority of our chiropractic student respondents felt that use of research evidence is an important factor in chiropractic care (96.7%), that evidence-based practice is not a temporary fad (87.4%), that they need more training in EBP to apply the evidence in practice (70.7%), and had little to no exposure to research methods, epidemiology and statistics outside of the chiropractic curriculum (33.5%). Unlike Hadley's survey, our chiropractic student respondents had greater confidence in their ability to assess research study design, generalisability, evaluate bias, sample size and statistical tests. However, student responses to very basic critical appraisal concepts revealed low levels of knowledge that did not match confidence levels. In addition, nearly one-third of the survey respondents did not attempt to answer any of the knowledge questions.

Similar to other health professional training programs, EBP training must be included in chiropractic curricula to prepare future chiropractors to effectively practice evidence-based clinical decision-making. The minimum requirement listed in CCE standards (p. 18) states that doctor of chiropractic degree programs must include research methods and procedures, and "document how each subject appears in the curriculum and is integrated into a coherent degree program." [29] Historically, chiropractic college curricula met this criterion by including one 2-or 3-credit course in research methods or critical appraisal. Little has been published regarding the most effective strategies for EBP training in chiropractic educational institutions. Research of other health professional training programs shows that EBP concepts provided in a stand-alone course improve student knowledge but may not change student behavior and attitudes toward using evidence if it is not tied to clinical application [31]. Recent studies suggest that evidence-based clinical skills can be taught, but they are not necessarily continued into future practice [32,33]. Most educators advocate for a "whole-program approach" and clinically integrated teaching of EBP seeded throughout a curriculum is likely required for truly meaningful learning and application [34-37].

In the US, the National Center for Complementary and Alternative Medicine at the National Institutes of Health created a research education grant program to increase the quality and quantity of research content in institutions that train CAM physicians and practitioners. Four chiropractic educational institutions were awarded grants through this program in the past 5 years (PAR-040-97 and PAR-080996) and have worked toward integrating EBP concepts and practice into their curricula [38]. Evidence that EBP is now being weaved through coursework and extra-curricular activities at the awarded campuses is suggested in their 13 presentations and 1 workshop on these topics scheduled for the 2011 Association of Chiropractic Colleges-Research Agenda Conference [39].

Students' perceived competencies in EBP principles may overestimate the actual skill sets essential for clinical decision-making [19]. In our survey, students had a positive attitude about EBP, had some training in EBP or research methods in their chiropractic program, but did not demonstrate good knowledge in research evidence principles. Regardless of whether or not respondents reported previous training in research methods, epidemiology, statistics or EBP, the mean knowledge scores were very low. Given the positive attitude toward the value of EBP principles, the perceived need for additional EBP training, and the low level of knowledge demonstrated by respondents, it was surprising that half of respondents agreed they had enough time to search and read research literature. Future surveys with higher response rates may inform academic administrators at chiropractic educational institutions about the current perspectives of their students related to EBP principles and may inform decisions about implementing EBP principles in their curricula. Furthermore, they may capture shifts in the knowledge of students due to initiatives such as those in the US described above.

Several surveying recommendations flow from the current research. First, surveyors conducting research with students attending chiropractic institutions should gather baseline information about registrar recordkeeping. For instance, two institutions in the current study could not report accurate enrollment numbers for their institution. Second, researchers should negotiate access to student email lists. By doing so, they can more actively target survey solicitations and follow-up messages as well as assert better control for potential survey duplication. The use of student email lists also allows the researcher to accurately calculate response rates to the survey, as well as to better gauge respondent representativeness to the population post-data collection. If these recommendations are followed, it is likely that future efforts will require ethics approval at all institutions surveyed.

Future surveys of this population should consider questionnaire translation into other languages and use multiple recruitment methods. We only used one method of student recruitment, namely three waves of invitations from the institutional contacts who maintain student email distribution lists. Institution-specific and more creative student recruitment methods may increase the response rate because some students may not check college email regularly, but might respond to other recruitment methods.

Limitations

Similar to other surveys, limitations of this study include survey error regarding coverage and non-response [40]. Being denied access to survey students within some of the chiropractic institutions, as well as simply not hearing back from others, means that the current study possessed a certain level of coverage error. The high levels of non-response for certain items, coupled with the overall low response rate for the survey, indicates a certain degree of response bias, i.e., those students who chose to respond to those items may significantly differ from those who omitted a response. Furthermore, the demographic items, including whether or not students had previous training or education in EBP or research methodology either within or outside the chiropractic curriculum, were positioned at the end of the survey following the knowledge items. If respondents closed their browser before answering the knowledge items, then these records included missing data for the demographic and training information, which prevented further assessments of response bias and generalisability. A final limitation of this study concerns the self-report nature of the data. Significant issues are associated with many types of self-report data, especially when the responses solicited by this instrument could be perceived as personal in nature, and in some cases could invite social criticism or social reprimand.

Conclusion

The results of this survey indicate that although it appears feasible to conduct a web-based survey with chiropractic students, significant stakeholder participation is crucial to improve response rates. Students had relatively positive attitudes toward EBP. However, they felt they needed more training in EBP and based on the knowledge questions they may need further training about basic research concepts.

Additional material

Additional file 1: A copy of the questionnaire developed to measure chiropractic students' attitudes, behaviors and knowledge of EBP principles.

Acknowledgements

This investigation was conducted in a facility constructed with support from Research Facilities Improvement Program Grant Number 06 RR15433-01 from the National Center for Research Resources, National Institutes of Health (NIH). CRL's work was supported in part from Grant Number 1R25AT003580 from the NIH National Center for Complementary and Alternative Medicine. Special thanks to all institutions and students who participated in this survey. We also thank Stacie S. Lyons and Dana J. Lawrence for editorial assistance and comments to earlier manuscript drafts. The Clinical Research graduate program at Palmer College of Chiropractic funded $200 to purchase the SurveyMonkey™ license.

Author details

[1]Palmer Center for Chiropractic Research, Palmer College of Chiropractic, 741 Brady Street, Davenport, IA 52803-5209, USA. [2]Institutional Planning & Research, Palmer College of Chiropractic, 723 Brady Street, Davenport, IA 52803-5209, USA.

Authors' contributions

RB conceived the idea for the survey. RB, MAH and DCD contributed to project design. RB and MAH prepared the invitation letters to institutions and students and replied to queries about the project. RB managed the data and prepared the first manuscript draft. RB and CRL analyzed the data. MAH, DCD, and CRL provided critical and constructive support for data analysis, interpretation and manuscript preparation. All authors edited and approved the final version of the manuscript.

Competing interests

The authors declare that they have no competing interests. None of the authors teach, employ, nor supervise students eligible for this project.

References

1. Evidence-Based Medicine Working Group: **Evidence-based medicine. A new approach to teaching the practice of medicine.** *JAMA* 1992, **269**:2420-2425.
2. **ICN position statement on Nursing Research.** [http://www.icn.ch/networks/nursing-research-a-tool-for-action/].
3. **University of Iowa.** [http://www.uihealthcare.com/depts/nursing/rqom/evidencebasedpractice/indes.html].
4. **Agency for Healthcare Research and Quality.** [http://www.ahrq.gov].
5. Outcome Project: **General Competencies. Accreditation Council for Graduate Medical Education.**[http://www.acgme.org/acWebsite/home/home.asp].
6. Hadley J, Hassan I, Khan KS: **Knowledge and beliefs concerning evidence-based practice amongst complementary and alternative medicine health care practitioners and allied health care professionals: a questionnaire survey.** *BMC Complement Altern Med* 2008, **8**:45.
7. Malone DE, Staunton M: **Evidence-based practice in radiology: step 5 (evaluate)–caveats and common questions.** *Radiology* 2007, **243**:319-328.
8. Djulbegovic B, Guyatt GH, Ashcroft RE: **Epistemologic inquiries in evidence-based medicine.** *Cancer Control* 2009, **16**:158-168.
9. Humphreys BL: **The 1994 Unified Medical Language System knowledge sources.** *Health Libr Rev* 1994, **11**:200-203.
10. Hook O: **Scientific communications. History, electronic journals and impact factors.** *Scand J Rehabil Med* 1999, **31**:3-7.
11. Taheri H, Mirmohamadsadeghi M, Adibi I, Ashorion V, Sadeghizade A, Adibi P: **Evidence-based medicine (EBM) for undergraduate medical students.** *Ann Acad Med Singapore* 2008, **37**:764-768.
12. Scherrer CS, Dorsch JL, Weller AC: **An evaluation of a collaborative model for preparing evidence-based medicine teachers.** *J Med Libr Assoc* 2006, **94**:159-165.
13. Schardt C, Adams MB, Owens T, Keitz S, Fontelo P: **Utilization of the PICO framework to improve searching PubMed for clinical questions.** *BMC Med Inform Decis Mak* 2007, **7**:16.
14. Nicholson LJ, Warde CM, Boker JR: **Faculty training in evidence-based medicine: improving evidence acquisition and critical appraisal.** *J Contin Educ Health Prof* 2007, **27**:28-33.
15. Hatala R, Keitz SA, Wilson MC, Guyatt G: **Beyond journal clubs. Moving toward an integrated evidence-based medicine curriculum.** *J Gen Intern Med* 2006, **21**:538-541.
16. Hadley JA, Wall D, Khan KS: **Learning needs analysis to guide teaching evidence-based medicine: knowledge and beliefs amongst trainees from various specialities.** *BMC Med Educ* 2007, **7**:11.
17. Green ML: **A train-the-trainer model for integrating evidence-based medicine training into podiatric medical education.** *J Am Podiatr Med Assoc* 2005, **95**:497-504.
18. Davis D, Evans M, Jadad A, Perrier L, Rath D, Ryan D, *et al*: **The case for knowledge translation: shortening the journey from evidence to effect.** *BMJ* 2003, **327**:33-35.
19. Caspi O, McKnight P, Kruse L, Cunningham V, Figueredo AJ, Sechrest L: **Evidence-based medicine: discrepancy between perceived competence and actual performance among graduating medical students.** *Med Teach* 2006, **28**:318-325.
20. Fernandez CE, Delaney PM: **Applying evidence-based health care to musculoskeletal patients as an educational strategy for chiropractic interns (a one-group pretest-posttest study).** *J Manipulative Physiol Ther* 2004, **27**:253-261.
21. Green ML: **Evidence-based medicine training in internal medicine residency programs a national survey.** *J Gen Intern Med* 2000, **15**:129-133.
22. Morris J, Maynard V: **The value of an evidence based practice module to skill development.** *Nurse Educ Today* 2007, **27**:534-541.
23. Smith M, Long C, Henderson C, Marchiori D, Hawk C, Meeker W, *et al*: **Report on the development, implementation, and evaluation of evidence-based skills course.** *J Chiropr Educ* 2004, 116-126.

24. Barnes PM, Bloom B, Nahin RL: **Complementary and alternative medicine use among adults and children: United States, 2007.** *Natl Health Stat Report* 2008, 1-23.
25. Rose KA, Adams A: **A survey of the use of evidence-based health care in chiropractic college clinics.** *J Chiropr Educ* 2000, **14**:71-77.
26. Fernandez CE, Delaney PM: **Evidence-based health care in medical and chiropractic education: A literature review.** *J Chiropr Educ* 2004, **18**:103-115.
27. Wyatt LH, Perle SM, Murphy DR, Hyde TE: **The necessary future of chiropractic education: a North American perspective.** *Chiropr Osteopat* 2005, **13**:10.
28. Newell D, Cunliffe C: **Attitudes toward research in undergraduate chiropractic students.** *Clinical Chiropractic* 2009, **6**:109-119.
29. **The council on chiropractic education.** [http://www.cce-usa.org].
30. **WFC Quarterly World Report.** [http://www.wfc.org/website/images/wfcqwr/qwr_200909.pdf].
31. Coomarasamy A, Khan KS: **What is the evidence that postgraduate teaching in evidence based medicine changes anything? A systematic review.** *BMJ* 2004, **329**:1017.
32. McGinn T, Seltz M, Korenstein D: **A method for real-time, evidence-based general medical attending rounds.** *Acad Med* 2002, **77**:1150-1152.
33. Bradley P, Oterholt C, Herrin J, Nordheim L, Bjorndal A: **Comparison of directed and self-directed learning in evidence-based medicine: a randomised controlled trial.** *Med Educ* 2005, **39**:1027-1035.
34. Aiyer MK, Dorsch JL: **The transformation of an EBM curriculum: a 10-year experience.** *Med Teach* 2008, **30**:377-383.
35. Coomarasamy A, Taylor R, Khan KS: **A systematic review of postgraduate teaching in evidence-based medicine and critical appraisal.** *Med Teach* 2003, **25**:77-81.
36. Khan KS, Coomarasamy A: **A hierarchy of effective teaching and learning to acquire competence in evidenced-based medicine.** *BMC Med Educ* 2006, **6**:59.
37. Agrawal S, Szatmari P, Hanson M: **Teaching evidence-based psychiatry: integrating and aligning the formal and hidden curricula.** *Acad Psychiatry* 2008, **32**:470-474.
38. **National Center for Complementary and Alternative Medicine.** [http://nccam.nih.gov/cgi-bin/grants/funding.pl].
39. **Association of Chiropractic Colleges-Research Agenda Conference.** [http://www.chirocolleges.org/accrac/].
40. Dillman DA: **1941-, Mail and Internet surveys.** *Internet, mail, and mixed-mode surveys: the tailored design method* Hoboken, N.J.: Wiley & Sons; 2009

A survey of accessibility and utilisation of chiropractic services for wheelchair-users in the United Kingdom: What are the issues?

Naomi D McKay* and Jennifer Langworthy

Abstract

Background: People with physical disabilities experience barriers to healthcare across all services despite a legal and moral obligation to the contrary. Complementary medicine is considered as supplementary to conventional care and integration of these approaches is essential to achieve optimal care. This paper explores the utilisation of chiropractic services and practitioner experiences of treating wheelchair-users which appears under-reported.

Methods: A 20 item questionnaire was posted to 250 randomly selected chiropractors registered with the General Chiropractic Council. Follow-up questionnaires were sent 7 days after the initial return date. Quantitative data were subjected to frequency analysis.

Results: The response rate was 64% (n = 161). The majority (66%) of chiropractors had been in practice less than 10 years and were practice owners (50%). Fifty-two percent of chiropractors sampled had treated a patient in a wheelchair in the previous 5 years. The majority (87%) had treated between 1 and 5 such patients. Patients with multiple sclerosis, stroke and cerebral palsy most commonly presented for treatment. The majority of patients' presenting complaint was musculoskeletal in origin, primarily for pain control. Only 13% of respondents worked in a fully accessible clinic. Impracticality of alterations was the most common reason for inaccessibility.

Conclusions: Wheelchair-users seem to be an underserved patient group in relation to chiropractic services. Chiropractic management is primarily utilised for pain control in patients with physical disabilities in which mobility may be improved or maintained. Co-management of wheelchair-users with GPs appears to be desirable in order to achieve optimal patient care however more research is required regarding the efficacy of chiropractic treatment for a range of disabling conditions. Physical access was identified as a key barrier to accessing care.

Keywords: chiropractic, wheelchair-user, disabilities, complementary and alternative medicine, access

Background

The aim of all healthcare practitioners is to provide patients with the best possible service. However, in 2008, 32% of the 10.2 million people covered by the Disability Discrimination Act (DDA) experienced problems in the previous 12 months accessing pubic services, including healthcare [1,2]. There is a shortage of literature documenting the experiences of patients with physical disabilities when accessing healthcare however disabled patients have reported problems getting appointments at short notice and also at a time they have access to transport. In some cases patients have to battle the inaccurate assumption that their symptoms are somehow related to their disability [3]. Other barriers to healthcare include poor practitioner attitudes towards disability and limited physical access. These barriers have been linked to the development of preventable health complications [4].

Disability is defined by law [5] as "someone who has a physical or mental impairment that has a substantial and long-term adverse effect on his or her ability to carry out normal everyday activities." Although limited, evidence suggests that patients with physical disabilities consult complementary and alternative medicine (CAM) therapists including chiropractors, more often than the

* Correspondence: naomi.chiro@gmail.com
Anglo-European College of Chiropractic, 13-15 Parkwood Road, Bournemouth, UK

general population. Furthermore, they visited these practitioners more frequently, primarily for complaints of chronic pain and depression [6]. The majority of patients with physical disabilities appear to utilise CAM therapies that are manual rather than herbal in nature. This may be related to the symptoms commonly experienced by this patient group. Common therapies used by these patients include physiotherapy, aquatherapy, relaxation techniques, massage and chiropractic [6-8].

Evidence suggests that patients with disabilities consider complementary therapies as supplementary to, not a replacement for conventional care [7]. One study found that wheelchair-users with multiple sclerosis (MS) considered conventional care to be more beneficial than some CAM therapies for the treatment of their condition [9]. The integration of CAM with conventional medicine is however important as patients are entitled to full disclosure on all possible treatment options as a matter of autonomy [10].

While research exists which documents the experiences of wheelchair-users accessing CAM providers, the experiences of practitioners treating these patients appear under-reported. This study explored the utilisation of chiropractic services and potential barriers to care for wheelchair-users in the United Kingdom (UK) from the practitioner's perspective. Hitherto the term 'disability' is limited to someone who is reliant on a wheelchair for mobility.

Methods

This study was internally reviewed by a review panel for ethics and feasibility. Following a ruling by the ethics committee that the study was sufficiently low risk, a 20 item questionnaire was constructed and subsequently piloted by 10 registered chiropractors. These data were excluded from final analysis. Using the random number generator 250 chiropractors were selected within SPSS version 17.0 for Windows XP. This was to represent 10% of the 2500 chiropractors registered with the General Chiropractic Council (GCC) in October 2009. Questionnaires were coded prior to distribution to enable follow-up of non-responders.

The questionnaire was posted to subjects with a cover letter and stamped addressed return envelope. Chiropractors who had treated a patient in a wheelchair since 2004 were eligible to answer the entire questionnaire. Those who had not could answer 9 out of the 20 questions. Participants were requested to return the questionnaire within 17 days of receipt. A second questionnaire was sent to non-respondents one week after the initial deadline, allowing a further 14 days for return. Participants were assured of confidentiality. Chiropractors were able to decline participation in the study by non-return of the questionnaire.

Data were collated using SPSS version 17.0 for Windows XP and were subjected to frequency analysis. Data were not used if a question had not been answered, if respondents had selected multiple responses inappropriately or where only one practitioner had reported a feature which did not appear in the choices provided. As such, none of the qualitative data gained was included in this study.

Results

Demographic

One-hundred and sixty-one of 250 chiropractors returned the questionnaire, providing a response rate of 64%. This represented only 6% of chiropractors registered with the GCC at the time of the study therefore the results cannot be assumed to be representative of chiropractors throughout the UK. Despite this, the issues identified in this paper may well exist beyond the sample studied. In this study 96 (60%) chiropractors sampled worked more than 37.5 hours per week. Eighty (50%) were practice owners, 56 (35%) associates, 6 (4%) partners in the practice and 18 (11%) rented a treatment room in another establishment. Fifty-eight (36%) of the chiropractors had been in practice for 5 years or less, 48 (30%) 6-10 years and 54 (34%) for 11 years or more. All results below are reported from the practitioner's perspective.

Treatment numbers, presenting complaints and challenges

Approximately half (n = 83, 52%) of chiropractors sampled had treated a patient in a wheelchair in the previous 5 years. The majority (n = 72, 87%) had treated between 1 and 5 such patients, 9 (11%) between 6 and 10, while 2 (2%) had treated more than 10. Forty-three (52%) chiropractors reported the patient's general practitioner (GP) had been informed the patient was receiving chiropractic care. Table 1 identifies the specific disabling conditions and Table 2 details the primary presenting complaints of the wheelchair-users seen by the responding chiropractors.

Table 2 Most common presenting complaints in wheelchair-users encountered by chiropractors sampled

Table 1 Most common disabling conditions in wheelchair-users encountered by chiropractors sampled (not exclusive)

Condition	n (%)
Multiple sclerosis	44 (53%)
Stroke	26 (31%)
Paralysis	24 (29%)
Cerebral palsy	23 (28%)
Trauma	20 (24%)
Congenital deformity	8 (10%)
Spina bifida	6 (7%)

Table 2 Most common presenting complaints in wheelchair-users encountered by chiropractors sampled (not exclusive)

Presenting complaint	n (%)
Neck pain	45 (54%)
Low back pain	41 (49%)
Other muscular pain	25 (30%)
Headache	10 (12%)
Depression	6 (7%)
Insomnia	5 (6%)

Fifty-one (61%) chiropractors experienced challenges related to the management and treatment of this patient group and these are shown in Table 3. It is not known however whether these issues prevented or restricted the treatment of the patient.

Motivation for treatment and key expectations

From the practitioner's perspective, the main motivation for wheelchair-users seeking chiropractic treatment is the patient's desire to utilise multiple therapies to manage their condition. The majority of patients sought care for pain control however the source of pain was not identified in this study. The main motivations for wheelchair-users seeking care and their key expectations of treatment are outlined in Tables 4 and 5 respectively.

Access to Chiropractic Care

Since being in practise, 8 (5%) respondents had refused to treat a wheelchair-user due to lack of access. A wheelchair user had never presented to 48 (30%) chiropractors surveyed at any point in their career. The availability of facilities for wheelchair-users in the sampled chiropractic clinics is outlined in Figure 1.

Factors that chiropractors identified which may prevent the adaptation of their clinic to increase disabled access are given in Table 6.

Discussion

Treatment of wheelchair-users

This study found that wheelchair-users are not commonly treated by the chiropractors sampled. In addition, the likelihood of treating such a patient does not appear to increase with time in practice.

The most common conditions encountered by chiropractors sampled were those in which mobility can be maintained or improved such as in MS and cerebral palsy. The presenting complaints encountered by chiropractors were primarily musculoskeletal in nature, which concurs with the findings of Rose [11] who found 38% of chiropractors sampled believed wheelchair-users require more treatment for musculoskeletal disorders. While more research is required regarding the efficacy of chiropractic treatment in wheelchair-users common sense dictates that a wheelchair user with normal anatomy receiving treatment has the potential to experience the same benefits as the general population. In addition, wheelchair-users may utilise chiropractic services more than the general population as although the health needs in disabled and able-bodied people are mostly the same, disabled patients are more prone to secondary conditions giving them a greater need of additional services [3].

In the current study, pain control was the most common reason patients in wheelchairs sought chiropractic treatment. Chiropractic care has already been found to be an effective treatment for chronic pain syndrome in MS [12]. This suggests chiropractic management may be effective in managing pain in other disabling conditions. Carson et al [8] found that 42% (n = 97) of 231 people with MS sampled used chiropractic care regularly. Of these, 81% (n = 79) use chiropractic to manage the symptoms of the disease. This is almost double the number of chiropractors who had treated a wheelchair-user for symptoms associated with their condition in the current study. However, the apparent high use of chiropractic services among MS patients compared to those

Table 4 Practitioner-perceived motivations of wheelchair-users to seek chiropractic treatment (not exclusive)

Motivation	n (%)
Desire/need for multiple therapies for effective treatment	48 (58%)
Dissatisfaction with conventional care	30 (36%)
Trying something new/experimental	30 (36%)
Expectation of a chiropractic 'cure' or improvement	13 (16%)

Table 3 Specific challenges faced by chiropractors in the treatment of wheelchair-users (not exclusive)

Motivation	n (%)
Modifying treatment due to restriction of patient mobility	24 (29%)
Manoeuvring patients on and off treatment bench	20 (24%)
Accessing clinic and treatment room	8 (10%)
Managing increased physical load and manual handling	6 (7%)
Fitting treatment into standard appointment time	4 (5%)

Table 5 Key expectations for treatment of wheelchair-users seeking chiropractic care (not exclusive)

Key expectation	n (%)
Pain control	60 (72%)
Maintenance/improvement of mobility	36 (43%)
Relief of symptoms associated with their condition	35 (42%)
Relief of symptoms associated with wheelchair use	24 (29%)
Resolution of muscular problems	17 (20%)

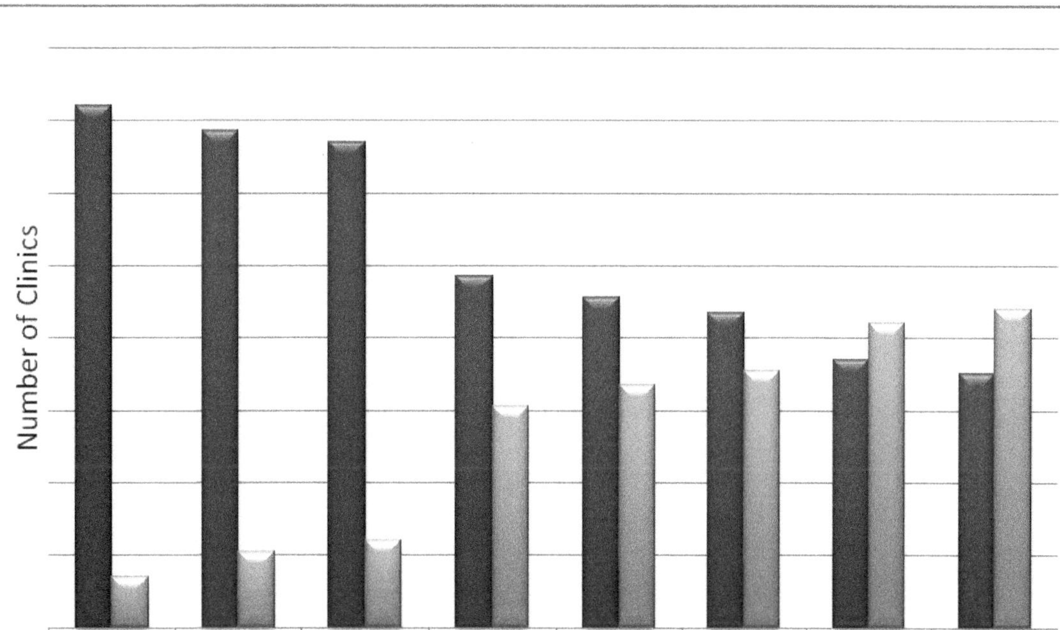

	Height adjustable treatment bench	All facilities present	Sizeable treatment room	Disabled parking	Widened doorways	Ramp at entrance	Lift to upper floors	Disabled toilets
Not Present	144	137	134	97	91	87	74	70
Present	14	21	24	61	67	71	84	88

* missing data n=3

Figure 1 Availability of Wheelchair Friendly Facilities in Chiropractic Clinic.

with other disabling conditions may be misleading as the majority of research concerns these patients.

In the current study, 24 (29%) chiropractors had treated a wheelchair-user to relieve symptoms associated with their wheelchair use. Sitting for long periods in a confined space puts these patients at risk of developing muscle imbalances, fatigue and contraction, trigger points and pain [13]. Chiropractic has been shown to be effective in the treatment of myofascial complaints [14]. This may therefore be an area in which chiropractors can apply evidence-based treatment methods to wheelchair-users. The perceived key expectations of treatment of wheelchair-users in the current study included a combination of the factors listed as respondents were invited to select more than one option. This is important in the interpretation of results in which expectations may appear misleadingly distinct. In addition, it would have been useful for chiropractors to rate the importance of each expected treatment outcome in relation to each individual patient they had treated in order to increase accuracy of results. This however was beyond the scope of this study.

Table 6 Factors preventing the adaptation of chiropractic clinics to increase disabled access (not exclusive)

Factor	n (%)
Impracticality of alterations	86 (56%)
Limited funds	55 (36%)
Would not increase patient numbers	39 (25%)
Unaware of need to change	13 (8%)
Lack of time to make changes	11 (7%)

Treatment Challenges

Fifty-one (61%) chiropractors surveyed experienced challenges specific to the treatment of wheelchair-users. According to the GCC, chiropractors should consider how services can be provided to anyone who may want to use them, including giving extra help for disabled users [15]. In order to achieve optimal care, practitioners are generally required to allow additional time and to have basic understanding of the nature of their patient's disability. Shinto et al [9] reported CAM therapists spend significantly more time with patients during treatment visits compared to their National Health Service (NHS) counterparts. While allowing extra time presented a challenge to a small minority of chiropractors in the current study, no chiropractor identified it as a reason to refuse treatment.

Manoeuvring a patient on and off the treatment bench presented a challenge for a substantial proportion of the chiropractors in the current study. Manual handling tasks are physically demanding, often unpredictable in nature and in the chiropractic setting, take place in an unfavourable environment [16]. However, while practitioner and patient safety is paramount, chiropractors must look to overcome these barriers. Of the chiropractors sampled, over one-quarter claimed to have modified their treatment in order to accommodate a wheelchair-user. Limited mobility does not therefore appear to be a factor which would prevent the treatment of wheelchair-users in chiropractic clinics. Indeed according to the GCC to do so would be unethical.

The Role of Chiropractic Services

It is important to define the role of chiropractic services in the treatment of wheelchair-users. Iezzoni et al [17] concluded that people with disabilities were generally satisfied with conventional care and any dissatisfaction was largely related to quality of care in terms of physical access and practitioner knowledge regarding their condition. This would appear to be borne out by the view of a significant proportion of the practitioners in the current study. Nonetheless, this statement is somewhat ambiguous as it is not clear whether these patients sought chiropractic care in addition to, or instead of, conventional care. In addition, more than half of the respondents recognised the need for patients in wheelchairs to use multiple therapies to effectively manage their condition, suggesting that the chiropractor's perceived role is to co-manage these patients with their GP or other healthcare professional. Of note, such an integrated approach has been cited as the preferred model from the disabled patient's perspective [9].

GP Awareness

GPs are the gatekeepers of healthcare for patients with disabilities [18]. However there is conflicting evidence regarding the availability of CAM via GP referral [8,19]. Schmit et al [19] found that GPs in the UK were reluctant to refer patients to CAM practitioners due to a perceived lack of scientific evidence regarding their usefulness and safety. The GPs also believed establishing a scientific base would help them determine which therapy would be most appropriate for a particular patient. These concerns are therefore likely to negatively impact on the number of wheelchair-users referred to chiropractors particularly as GPs are the most frequently accessed healthcare professional by these patients [18]. In the current study approximately half of chiropractors sampled believed the GP of the wheelchair-user was aware their patient was receiving chiropractic care. This figure may be inaccurate as it is not known whether the practitioner informed the GP themselves. Greater inter-professional communication between chiropractors and GPs are vital however, to facilitate optimal care for wheelchair-users.

Access Issues

The first step in achieving equal access to healthcare is to recognise how disabled patients experience barriers [11]. It is therefore difficult to assess the true accessibility of the clinics in the current study as only practitioner opinion was sought. Moreover, a wheelchair-user had never presented to approximately one third of the respondents. Thus chiropractors may be unaware of potential difficulties for wheelchair-users trying to utilise their services. Accessibility is an important consideration for healthcare providers as delay in receiving care may lead to increased chronicity of new conditions, seriousness of symptoms and an overall reduction in health status. Furthermore, facilities which provide good access are likely to have high levels of patient satisfaction in terms of the provision of care [20].

The criteria for accessibility in the current survey were based on the recommendations of the Office for Disability Issues (ODI) [21]. These requirements were used as the DDA requirements were considered too broad and would therefore not give specific insight into the facilities currently available in the clinics sampled. In the current study there appeared to be a disparity between practitioner perceptions of accessibility and true accessibility. For example, clinics which had disabled parking and ramp access did not always have doorways or treatment rooms large enough to accommodate a wheelchair. Therefore the usefulness of the former is negated. Only 21 (13%) clinics had all features recommended by the ODI in the current study. However, more than half of chiropractors surveyed denied any potential barriers to the treatment of a wheelchair-user despite working in clinics with limited facilities which may prevent access.

Access and the Law

Approximately half (51%) of the chiropractors in the current study were clinic owners and therefore responsible for the compliance of their clinic with disability law. Under part III of the DDA 1995, healthcare providers are required to take all reasonable steps to avoid physical features that would make it difficult or impossible for a person with a physical disability to access their service [5]. It is outside the scope of the current study to determine whether clinics sampled were compliant with the DDA. Approximately half of the chiropractors in this study cited impracticality of alterations as a reason not to increase the accessibility of their clinic. High costs and structural limitations have been identified as potential barriers to achieving accessibility [20]. In light of this, it would have been interesting to know what equates to impracticality in the current sample. Furthermore, approximately one third of chiropractors cited lack of funds as a primary limiting factor to improved access. Despite these limitations, chiropractors should seek to maximise ease of access in whichever ways they can to ensure they do not fall short of their legal and moral obligations to these patients.

The concept of universal accessibility is a philosophy that describes full access for all people and is realised through the elimination of barriers to access for all potential users. Furthermore, it is most useful when considering moving to, or building a new clinic [20]. As a result, it is essential that new graduates or practitioners looking to open new clinics should do so with the ODI recommendations in mind. In the current study 39 (25%) chiropractors sampled would not improve access to their clinic as it would not increase patient numbers. This does not appear to be consistent with the moral code to which the profession subscribes particularly as wheelchair-users cannot become patients of a clinic they cannot access.

Limitations of Study

There are several limitations to this study which must be considered in the interpretation of results. Firstly, the number of responses received prevents the results being generalised to other chiropractors in the UK. However, the issues raised may well exist beyond the sample studied. The reliability and validity of the questionnaire is unknown. This requires cautious analysis of the insights gained. Chiropractors were not specifically asked to consult patient files in their reporting of results therefore responses which relied on memories spanning five years increases the likihood of inaccurate recollection of information. In addition, respondents were only asked to approximate some data in order to maximise response rate which may reduce accuracy of results. Approximately one third of respondents had been in practice for less than five years. This may affect the data as they have had less patient exposure and therefore opportunity to encounter a wheelchair-user. Subjective findings must also be interpreted with caution as these were given from a practitioner point of view while in certain instances, they related more to the personal experience of the patient.

Conclusions

Wheelchair-users appear to be an underserved patient group in relation to chiropractic services. Improvements are needed particularly in terms of physical accessibility to care, an area in which chiropractors may be viewed as failing to fulfil their ethical obligations to such patients. Among wheelchair-users who have received treatment, chiropractic management appears to be primarily utilised for pain control in patients with physical disabilities in which mobility may be improved or maintained. More research is required however regarding the effectiveness of chiropractic treatment across a range of disabilities. It would appear that in treating these patients, an integrated approach between chiropractors and GPs may well provide optimal care to wheelchair-users.

Acknowledgements
The authors would like to thank all the practitioners who took part in this survey.

Authors' contributions
NM conceived the study and collected and analyzed the data. Both authors designed the study and contributed to and approved the final manuscript.

Competing interests
The authors declare that they have no competing interests.

References

1. **Family Resources Survey (FRS) Disability Prevalence Estimates 2007-2008.** [http://www.officefordisability.gov.uk/research/facts-and-figures.php#gd].
2. **Difficulties in Accessing Goods and Services.** [http://www.officefordisability.gov.uk/research/research-reports.php#rea].
3. Scheer J, Kroll T, Neri MT, Beatty P: **Access barriers for persons with disabilities: the consumer's perspective.** *Journal of Disability Policy Studies* 2003, **13**:221-230.
4. Beatty PW, Hagglund KJ, Neri MT, Dhont KR, Clark MJ, Hilton SA: **Access to health care services among people with chronic or disabling conditions: patterns and predictors.** *Arch Phys Med Rehabil* 2003, **84**:1417-1425.
5. **GREAT BRITAIN. Department for Education and Employment, 1999.** *Disability Discrimination Act 1995. Code of practice. Rights of access. Good, facilities, services and premises* London: The Stationary Office Limited.
6. Krauss HH, Godfrey C, Kirk J, Eisenberg DM: **Alternative health care: its use by individuals with physical disabilities.** *Arch Phys Med Rehabil* 1998, **79**:1440-1447.
7. Hurvitz EA, Leonard C, Ayyangar R, Nelson VS: **Complementary and alternative medicine use in families of children with cerebral palsy.** *Dev Med Child Neurol* 2003, **11**:107-109.
8. Carson EA, Swait G, Johnson IP, Cunliffe C: **Chiropractic care amongst people with multiple sclerosis: A survey of MS therapy centres in the UK.** *Clinical Chiropractic* 2009, **12**:23-27.
9. Shinto L, Yadav V, Morris C, Lapidus JA, Senders A, Bourdette D: **The perceived benefit and satisfaction from conventional and complementary and alternative medicine (CAM) in people with multiple sclerosis.** *Complement Ther Med* 2005, **13**:264-272.
10. Liptak GS: **Complementary and alternative therapies for cerebral palsy.** *Ment Retard Dev Disabil Res Rev* 2005, **11**:156-163.
11. Rose K: **A survey of the accessibility of chiropractic clinics to the disabled.** *J Manipulative Physiol Ther* 1999, **22**:523-527.
12. Dougherty P, Lawerence D: **Chiropractic management of musculoskeletal pain in the multiple sclerosis patient.** *Clinical Chiropractic* 2005, **8**:57-65.
13. Todd AI, Bennett AI, Christie CJ: **Physical implications of prolonged sitting in a confined posture - A literature review.** *Ergonomics* 2007, **19**:7-21.
14. Vernon H, Schneider M: **Chiropractic management of myofascial trigger points and myofascial pain syndrome: a systematic review of the literature.** *J Manipulative Physiol Ther* 2009, **32**:14-24.

15. **The GCC code of practice and standard of proficiency required for the competent and safe practice of chiropractic: effective from 30th June 2010.** [http://www.gcc-uk.org/chiro_search.cfm].
16. Nelson A, Baptiste AS: **Update on evidence-based practices for safe patient handling and movement.** *Orthop Nurs* 2006, **25**:367-368.
17. Iezzoni LI, Davis RB, Soukup J, O'Day B: **Satisfaction with quality and access to health care among people with disabling conditions.** *Int J Qual Health Care* 2002, **14**:369-381.
18. Hogg J: **Essential healthcare for people with learning disabilities: barriers and opportunities.** *J R Soc Med* 2001, **94**:333-336.
19. Schmidt K, Jacobs PA, Barton A: **Cross-cultural differences in GP's attitudes towards complementary and alternative medicine: a survey comparing regions of the UK and Germany.** *Complement Ther Med* 2002, **10**:141-147.
20. Jones KE, Tamari IE: **Making our offices universally accessible: guidelines for physicians.** *Can Med Assoc J* 1997, **156**:647-656.
21. **Experiences and Expectations of Disabled People.** [http://www.officefordisability.gov.uk/research/facts-and-figures.php#gd].

5

Prevalence of pain-free weeks in chiropractic subjects with low back pain - a longitudinal study using data gathered with text messages

Nadège Lemeunier[1*], Alice Kongsted[2] and Iben Axén[3]

Abstract

Introduction: The use of automated text messages has made it possible to identify different courses of low back pain (LBP), and it has been observed that pain often fluctuates and that absolute recovery is rather rare. The purpose of this study was to describe the prevalence of pain-free weeks and pain-free periods in subjects with non-specific LBP treated by chiropractors, and to compare subjects from two different countries in these aspects.

Methods: Data were obtained from two practice-based multicentre prospective outcome studies, one Danish and one Swedish, involving subjects being treated by chiropractors for non-specific LBP. Over 18 weeks, subjects answered a weekly automated text message question on the number of days in the past week that they had experienced bothersome LBP, i.e. a number between 0 and 7. The number of weeks in a row without any LBP at all ("zero weeks") as well as the maximum number of zero weeks in a row was determined for each individual. Comparisons were made between the two study samples. Estimates are presented as percentages with 95% confidence intervals.

Results: In the Danish and the Swedish populations respectively, 93/110 (85%) and 233/262 (89%) of the subjects were eligible for analysis. In both groups, zero weeks were rather rare and were most commonly (in 40% of the zero weeks) reported as a single isolated week. The prevalence of pain free periods, i.e. reporting a maximum of 0, 1 or 2, or 3-6 zero weeks in a row, were similar in the two populations (20-31%). Smaller percentages were reported for ≥ 7 zero weeks in a row. There were no significant differences between the two study groups.

Conclusion: It was uncommon that chiropractic subjects treated for non-specific LBP experienced an entire week without any LBP at all over 18 weeks. When this occurred, it was most commonly reported for brief periods only. Hence, recovery in the sense that patients become absolutely pain free is rare, even in a primary care population.

Introduction

Low back pain (LBP) is a very common condition with an annual prevalence of at least 50% [1]. However, approximately 80% of patients suffering from LBP are diagnosed with non-specific LBP [2] because the specific causes are rather rare. One consequence is that it is difficult to find an effective treatment for this large, heterogeneous group of patients, which probably explains the limited treatment effect generally obtained in scientific trials[3,4].

Traditionally, randomized clinical trials and outcome studies have the disadvantage of measuring outcome at only a few points in time, leaving an absence of data for the periods in between. However, for patients the time "in between" is as important as some arbitrarily selected points in time, such as at 6 or 12 months after treatment. Further, LBP often runs an episodic or fluctuating course [5-8] which is ignored by follow ups measured only at one or a few points in time. Commonly, the proportion of subjects who are improved at these time points is estimated. This approach fails to take the trajectory of pain into account, thereby not fully describing recovery or improvement. With the use of diaries or automated text messages it is possible to follow the course of a disease more closely, whether treated or not.

* Correspondence: nadege.franco@sfr.fr
[1]Institut Franco-Européen de Chiropratique, Toulouse, France
Full list of author information is available at the end of the article

In this study, text messaging was used to record weekly follow-ups over a period of 18 weeks in two populations of chiropractic subjects with LBP, one in Denmark and another in Sweden. By means of these data, it was possible to identify individual clinical courses of LBP. It was confirmed that pain often fluctuated [9,10] and that, although the majority of subjects improved to some degree, absolute recovery was rather rare [6,11]. Presumably, this is contrary to what clinicians in primary care expect, namely a gradual more or less stable path of improvement. The expectations of clinicians have been found to be considerably higher than the patient-reported outcomes in a quality assurance study of a secondary care spine centre [12]. Obviously, if the care-giver and the patient have higher expectations of the outcome than what they will experience, both will be dissatisfied. For patients, this may result in a lengthy period of doctor shopping. For the clinician, it may result in a prolonged treatment course, because unrealistic effects are aimed for. More evidence concerning course and recovery patterns of non-specific LBP is therefore needed [13]. The frequently collected data from the two mentioned LBP studies [6,11] made it possible to study the frequency with which chiropractic subjects experienced pain free periods over a stretch of time as well as the length of such periods. The purpose of this study was to perform secondary analyses of these data in order to describe the prevalence of pain-free weeks and periods in subjects with non-specific LBP treated by chiropractors, and to compare two populations of different nationalities in these aspects. In the primary analyses, the aim was to describe the clinical course without focus on pain-free weeks.

Knowledge of this type will make it possible for practitioners to inform patients about the most likely evolution of his/her LBP problem. By analysing prospective data from different populations and countries, wider generalisations regarding clinical outcome would be possible.

Methods

Data were obtained from two practice-based multicentre prospective outcome studies involving subjects being treated by chiropractors for non-specific LBP; one was conducted in Denmark and one in Sweden. Both studies have been reported elsewhere [6,9-11].

Prior to inclusion, subjects received written and verbal information about the study. The projects were presented to the relevant local ethics committees. In Denmark, the committee stated that the study did not need approval. In Sweden, approval was granted by the local ethics committee at the Karolinska Institutet (2007/1458-31/4).

Study populations

Seven chiropractors were invited to participate in the Danish study on the condition that they followed an instruction program on how to examine and diagnose their patients according to an evidence-based classification system [9,14]. Subjects aged 18-65 years with non-specific LBP, who had not had chiropractic treatment for the present episode of LBP prior to the consultation in the present clinic, were consecutively included (n = 110).

In the Swedish study, 35 chiropractors who had been compliant in a previous practice-based study were recruited. These chiropractors were found to be similar to the members of the Swedish Chiropractors' Association (In Swedish: Legitimerade Kiropraktorers Riksorganisation) regarding age, gender and years in practice [11]. Altogether, 262 subjects with non-specific LBP were enrolled. The age range of these subjects was 16-69 years and they had not been under chiropractic care for the past 3 months.

In both populations, subjects were considered to have non-specific LBP as cases of significant pathologies would have been referred out. Other exclusion or non-inclusion criteria were: previous back surgery (Danish study), pregnancy, and inability to read Danish/Swedish. Not having a mobile phone, not knowing how to use the text message function or not wanting to participate in the study obviously also precluded participation in the studies.

The gender distribution was fairly similar in the two studies with 45% and 48% females, respectively [9,11]. Most subjects had LBP only, but 46% in the Danish and 50% in the Swedish study had also leg pain. Twenty five per cent of the Danish study participants had experienced LBP for more than 3 months and 57% of the Swedish participants reported to have had LBP for more than 30 days in the past year. Further detailed information concerning LBP duration was not collected at baseline.

Six of the seven Danish chiropractors had graduated from the University of Southern Denmark whereas the majority (56%) of the Swedish chiropractors had graduated from a chiropractic college in England (Anglo-European College of Chiropractic in Bournemouth) and a further 13% from the University of Southern Denmark. The remaining Swedish chiropractors had an American or Australian chiropractic degree.

Previous studies of chiropractors in the Scandinavian countries have shown that their treatment will consist of spinal manipulative therapy (SMT), mobilization, soft tissue treatment, massage, advice, exercise therapy and information [15-17]. The SMT can be either purely manual or assisted by mechanical devices (drop-piece tables and activators). The appropriate treatment was decided by the chiropractors in the two studies and not taken into account in our analyses.

Previous comparisons between drop-outs and participants in the two original studies revealed that the drop-outs in the Danish study were more likely to be men, to have leg pain and to report short duration LBP [9]. In the Swedish study, however, gender and leg pain were not significantly different between drop-outs and those who stayed in the study, but the Swedish drop-outs had a shorter duration of LBP in the past year and reported lower pain intensity [10].

Clinical procedures, data collection and validity of data

In the Danish study, the chiropractors collected baseline data using a standardized physical examination protocol [14], as described in detail elsewhere [6], treated "as usual" and followed every week over 18 weeks with the help of automated text messages, using the SMS-Track-Q program [18]. Eighteen weeks follow- up was chosen for practical reasons. The data collection took place from February till October 2008.

In the Swedish study, after recording base-line data, the clinical examination and treatment were decided by the chiropractors according to usual practice. Subjects were followed by weekly text messages using the same data collection method as in Denmark but over 6 months[11]. In the present study, to allow comparisons with the Danish study, only data from the first 18 weeks have been included. The data collection took place from May 2008 to June 2009.

Thus in both studies subjects received a weekly automated text message question concerning the number of days in the past week that they had 1) been bothered by LBP (Danish study) or 2) experienced bothersome LBP (Swedish study). The subjects replied via a text message with a number between 0 and 7. If no reply message had been received within 4 days, a reminder was automatically sent. If no reply had been received when the next week's text message question was sent, the data was recorded as "missing".

The text message questions were:

In Denmark: "Using a number from 0 to 7, please answer how many days you have been bothered by your low back pain this week." In Sweden: "How many days during this previous week has your low back pain been bothersome (i.e. affected your daily activities or routines?). Please answer by a number from 0 to 7."

A thorough scrutiny of the SMS-Track method using data from the Swedish study indicated that the SMS-Track system yields high response rates not affected by season, is user friendly and has good compliance [10]. An inter-reliability study showed the SMS-Track method to be superior to retrospective data collection in subjects with non-specific LBP [19]. A comparison between pain intensity (none/moderate/severe) and number of days with pain per week revealed almost identical profiles of these two variables over 18 weeks in the Danish study [9]. The outcome measure used herein, "zero weeks", i.e. the weeks a subject reports zero days of bothersome LBP, is therefore assumed to describe the absence of pain.

Data analysis

The weekly text message replies were automatically transferred into a data file to be used for analysis. The resulting spread sheets were analysed by hand in the following manner:

- First, each row (representing one subject) was checked for number of weeks without a response, "missing" data. Subjects who had missing data for altogether 11 weeks or more were arbitrarily defined as below a minimally satisfactory compliance level. They were excluded from the analyses because it was considered impossible to obtain a truthful impression of their clinical course. The remaining missing values were considered to represent at least one day with LBP in order to evaluate a "worst case" scenario.
- Second, the number of weeks in a row without pain ("zero weeks") was counted during the 18 weeks in each of the two populations. Thus, every zero week was classified in relation to the number of zero weeks in a row, regardless if several such periods were found in the same individual. For ease of presentation, these results were then reduced into six categories: 1, 2, 3, 4, 5-9, and 10-18 weeks in a row with no LBP.
- Third, the maximum number of zero weeks in a row per subject was counted and grouped into one of five categories: 0, 1 or 2, 3-6, 7-10, or 11-18 weeks in a row with no LBP. This means that only one value, the maximum number of zero weeks, was calculated for each individual, with possible values from 0 to 18.
- Finally, two additional analyses were performed. First, a more generous definition of no pain was used, allowing for 1 or 2 days of pain in a week also to be counted as a zero week ("best case") in subjects originally included in the analysis. Second, no subjects were withdrawn from the analysis and all missing data were simply interpreted as not being zero-weeks ("worst case"). A best and a worst case scenario have been chosen to illuminate the effect of: on the one hand, keeping to a strict definition of no pain, and on the other hand, keeping to a strict definition of compliance.

Results are displayed as bar graphs including 95% confidence intervals (CIs). The two study samples were compared and differences between estimates considered statistically significant when the CIs did not overlap.

Results

Participants

Seventeen individuals from the Danish study were excluded because they had more than 11 missing answers. The corresponding number in the Swedish study was 29 (Figure 1). The number of subjects with valid data was therefore 93 (85%) and 233 (89%) respectively, in the final Danish and Swedish data files.

Missing data in the two study populations

In the two populations, 49 Danish patients (53%) and 145 Swedish patients (32%) had some missing data. The frequency distribution of the missing data is reported in Figure 2. In both populations, the number of missing data rarely exceeded 9 for any individual.

Number of "zero weeks" in a row in the two populations

Throughout the study period, the reported weekly number of days with LBP was rarely zero. When a zero week was present, it appeared as a single week in about 40% of cases (Figure 3). The proportion of subjects with more than one zero week in a row diminished as the number of weeks in a row increased (Figure 3). Almost identical results were found in the two populations and the 95% CIs always overlapped (Figure 3).

Maximum number of "zero weeks" in a row per subject in the two populations

As can be seen in Figure 4, the proportions of subjects reporting a maximum of 0, 1 or 2, or 3-6 zero weeks in a row were similar in the two populations (20-31%) regardless category. Smaller percentages were reported for 7-10 weeks (8% and 15% in the two cohorts, respectively), and for 11-18 zero weeks in a row (11% and 13%, respectively) (Figure 4). There were no statistically significant differences between the two study groups, as the 95% CIs overlapped.

Additional analyses

The two additional analyses did not alter the picture revealed in the original results. This was true both when

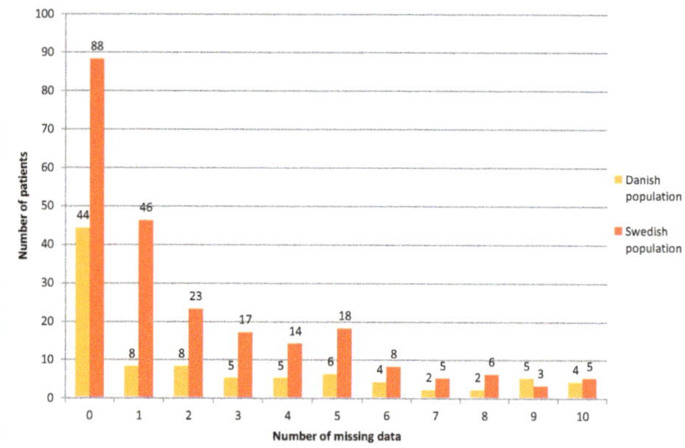

Figure 2 Frequency distribution of missing data. The numbers of patients are shown for the Danish and the Swedish populations separately.

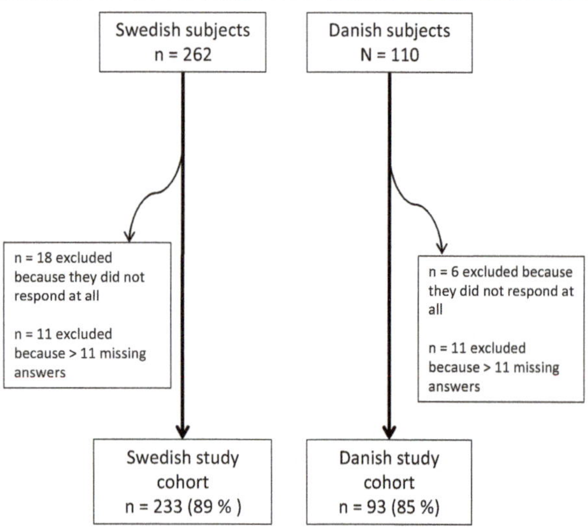

Figure 1 Flowchart showing the number of participants in two clinical outcome studies.

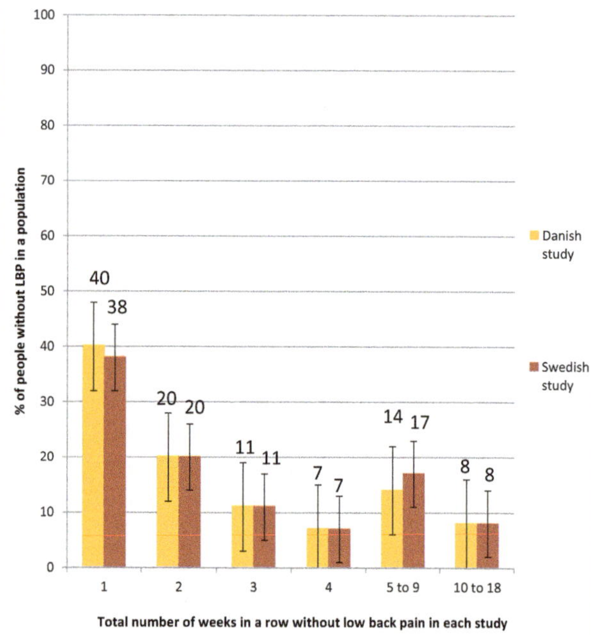

Figure 3 Number of weeks in a row with 0 days of low back pain for 326 subjects in two clinical outcome studies. The percentages are shown for the Danish and Swedish populations separately. Bars indicate the 95% confidence intervals.

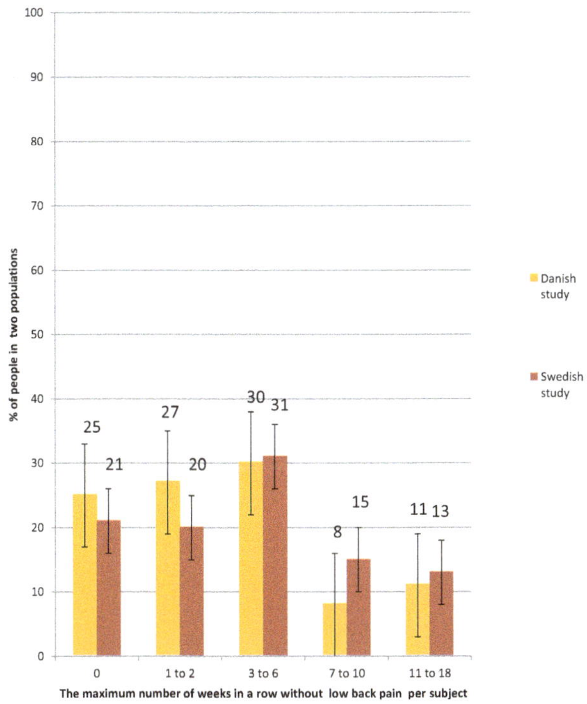

Figure 4 Maximum number of weeks in a row without low back pain per subject in two clinical outcome studies. The percentages are shown for the Danish and Swedish populations separately. Bars indicate the 95% confidence intervals.

allowing for a more generous definition of the absence of pain, namely also 1 or 2 days of LBP in the week and when assuming that all missing data represented weeks with LBP (data available on request).

Discussion

Summary of findings

This study showed that weeks with no LBP days at all were rare during an 18 week period following a first visit to a chiropractor. Most often, the subjects reported to have had at least one day with LBP in any given week. Furthermore, having a pain free week most commonly occurred on its own as an isolated event. In fact, one third and one fourth of subjects, respectively, in the Danish and Swedish studies, never experienced a single zero week during 18 weeks. Despite the fact that most patients were expected to improve fairly quickly [6,11] very few reported being absolutely pain free for any longer periods. This finding raises the question whether the pain free episodes can be predicted from baseline variables. However, this was not one of our aims but should be investigated in future studies.

Methodological considerations

As this was not a randomized study with an untreated control group, it is not possible to determine whether there were any associations between the therapeutic approach and the observed course of LBP. The results observed here may therefore have occurred as a result of treatment but may also merely reflect the natural course. However, it is reasonable to assume that each chiropractor did his/her best at tailoring the treatment to the needs of each subject in order to obtain an optimal result and that the outcome truthfully reflects what generally happens in daily clinical practice. No similar studies were found in the literature for comparison.

In all, 15% and 11% of the original Danish and Swedish participants were not included in our analysis due to missing data. Further, as is often the case, previous analyses had demonstrated some differences between participants and drop-outs [6,10], and revealed that the drop-outs tended to report short duration of LBP [9]. This would possibly lead to an underestimation of pain-free weeks. However, the number of drop-outs in each population was very low (11 and 15%), thus rendering this risk minimal. We consider the final study samples fairly representative of the typical chiropractic patient with non-specific LBP, due to the nature of the studies and the high participation rates.

These analyses were performed according to the worst case principle, in the sense that missing data were never interpreted as a zero week, not even if an isolated week with missing data was surrounded by one or several zero weeks. This approach ensures that subjects did at least as well as our result suggests. Obviously, missing data could be both LBP and no LBP, but we chose this approach instead of imputing data for missing values, since a majority (53% and 62% respectively) of the included subjects had some missing values. However, the missing data did not alter the results as the majority of the respondents only had 1 to 5 weeks of missing data, and few patients had more than 5 weeks of missing data (17/93 and 27/233 respectively in the Danish and the Swedish populations).

In the additional analysis, the findings were similar regardless definition of zero week. A more lenient definition of "LBP free", including both 1 and 2 days of pain in one week did not change the results. This indicates that LBP, when present, usually consist of more than the occasional pain. A more "severe" interpretation of data did not influence our findings either, indicating that our results provide a good picture of reality.

Limitations of gathering data with SMS

Frequent monitoring of patients with LBP using a few simple questions can obviously provide information on clinical course. The text message method is, however, not a suitable technique to obtain more detailed data on the state of the LBP problem. Indeed, only limited amounts of data can be sent in a text message.

Therefore, by choosing the term "bothersomeness", which has been found to be associated with pain intensity, disability and psychological health [20], it is believed that the relevant clinical features of the LBP condition is covered in one single question.

Comparison of the two study populations

The fact that the results were similar between the two cohorts, even though the questions to the subjects were somewhat differently worded in the two studies, strengthens the validity of these findings.

The similar results in the two studies might seem surprising as the involved chiropractors worked differently. The Danish chiropractors had been selected on quite special criteria and had to put considerable effort into the clinical examination of their patients with the purpose of obtaining an evidence-based diagnosis. This may have resulted in a selection of a more academically minded, well-informed and skilled type of clinician. It is also possible that their evidence-based diagnoses would have resulted in a more effective treatment and therefore more zero weeks. Also the Swedish chiropractors had been selected on some criteria of "excellence", as they had been compliant in a previous practice-based study, and therefore perhaps were typical of more competent clinicians. Their examination and diagnostic procedures had not, however, been "streamlined" in any fashion. Therefore we suspected that they might produce less favourable results than their Danish colleagues, but this could not be demonstrated from the simple outcome "zero weeks". Possibly, other outcomes could have revealed some differences between the cohorts.

Conclusion

It was uncommon that chiropractic subjects with non-specific LBP experienced an entire week without bothersome LBP during a course of 18 weeks. When this occurred, it was most commonly reported for brief periods only. Hence, recovery in the short term, in the sense that patients become absolutely pain free for longer periods, is rare, even in a primary care population.

Recommendations

- To learn more about the patterns of the clinical and the natural courses of non-specific LBP, it would be relevant to study this phenomenon for a range of patient populations, in the general population and for different types of treatment.
- Moreover, these results emphasize the importance of measuring recovery over a time-span rather that at one given point. This applies both to researchers and to clinicians who want to undertake quality assurance projects in their own clinic.
- It is essential that these findings are taken into account by teaching institutions in order to prepare students for the clinical reality already at the undergraduate level.

Acknowledgements

The authors gratefully acknowledge Professor Charlotte Lebœuf-Yde, DC, MPH, PhD, for editorial assistance.

The Danish study was funded by 'The Foundation for Chiropractic Research and Education' in Denmark and the Swedish study was funded in part by the Swedish Chiropractors' Association and in part by the European Chiropractors' Union.

Author details

[1]Institut Franco-Européen de Chiropratique, Toulouse, France. [2]Nordic Institute of Chiropractic and Clinical Biomechanics, Odense, Denmark. [3]Unit of Intervention and Implementation Research, Institute of Environmental Medicine, The Karolinska Institutet, Stockholm, Sweden.

Authors' contributions

NL was responsible for the analysis of data and participated in the manuscript preparation. AK was responsible for the design of the Danish study and the supervision of data collection. IA was responsible for the design of the Swedish study and the supervision of data collection. AK and IA were supervising the study process and were involved in the manuscript preparation. All the authors revised and approved the final manuscript.

Author's information

1: Institut Franco-Européen de Chiropratique, Toulouse, France

2: Nordic Institute of Chiropractic and Clinical Biomechanics, Odense, Denmark

3: Unit of Intervention and Implementation Research, Institute of Environmental Medicine, The Karolinska Institutet, Stockholm, Sweden

Competing interests

The authors declare that they have no competing interests.

References

1. Leboeuf-Yde C, Fejer R, Nielsen J, Kyvik KO, Hartvigsen J: **Consequences of spinal pain: do age and gender matter? A Danish cross-sectional population-based study of 34,902 individuals 20-71 years of age.** *BMC Musculoskelet Disord* 2011, **12**:39.
2. Deyo RA, Rainville J, Kent DL: **What can the history and physical examination tell us about low back pain?** *JAMA* 1992, **268(6)**:760-765.
3. Brealey SCS, Farrin A, Morton V, Torgerson D, Burton AK, Garratt A, Harvey E, Letley L, Martin J, Vickers M, Whyte K, Manca A, Klaber Moffett J, Russell I, Underwood M, Williams M: **United Kingdom Back Pain and Exercise and manipulation (UK BEAM) randomised trial: effectiveness of physical treatments for back pain in primary care.** *BMJ* 2004, **329(7479)**:1377.
4. COST, B, 13: **Working Group on Guidelines for Chronic Low Back Pain. European guidelines for the management of chronic nonspecific LBP.** *Eur Spine J* 2006, **15(Suppl 2)**:S192-S300.
5. Dunn KM, Jordan K, Croft PR: **Characterizing the course of low back pain: a latent class analysis.** *American journal of epidemiology* 2006, **163(8)**:754-761.
6. Kongsted A, Leboeuf-Yde C: **The Nordic back pain subpopulation program - individual patterns of low back pain established by means of text messaging: a longitudinal pilot study.** *Chiropractic & osteopathy* 2009, **17**:11.
7. Leboeuf-Yde C, Gronstvedt A, Borge JA, Lothe J, Magnesen E, Nilsson O, Rosok G, Stig LC, Larsen K: **The Nordic back pain subpopulation program: a 1-year prospective multicenter study of outcomes of persistent low-back pain in chiropractic patients.** *Journal of manipulative and physiological therapeutics* 2005, **28(2)**:90-96.

8. Hestbaek L, Leboeuf-Yde C, Engberg M, Lauritzen T, Bruun NH, Manniche C: **The course of low back pain in a general population. Results from a 5-year prospective study.** *Journal of manipulative and physiological therapeutics* 2003, **26(4)**:213-219.
9. Kongsted A, Leboeuf-Yde C: **The Nordic back pain subpopulation program: course patterns established through weekly follow-ups in patients treated for low back pain.** *Chiropractic & osteopathy* 2010, **18**:2.
10. Axén I, Bodin L, Bergström G, Halasz L, Lange F, Lövgren PW, Rosenbaum A, Leboeuf-Yde C, Jensen I: **The use of weekly text messaging over six months was a feasible method for monitoring the clinical course of low back pain in patients seeking chiropractic care.** *Journal of Clinical Epidemiology* 2011.
11. Axen I, Bodin L, Bergstrom G, Halasz L, Lange F, Lovgren PW, Rosenbaum A, Leboeuf-Yde C, Jensen I: **Clustering patients on the basis of their individual course of low back pain over a six month period.** *BMC Musculoskelet Disord* 2011, **12(1)**:99.
12. Johansen B, Mainz J, Sabroe S, Manniche C, Leboeuf-Yde C: **Quality improvement in an outpatient department for subacute low back pain patients: prospective surveillance by outcome and performance measures in a health technology assessment perspective.** *Spine (Phila Pa 1976)* 2004, **29(8)**:925-931.
13. Wasiak R, Young AE, Dunn KM, Cote P, Gross DP, Heymans MW, von Korff M: **Back pain recurrence: an evaluation of existing indicators and direction for future research.** *Spine (Phila Pa 1976)* 2009, **34(9)**:970-977.
14. Petersen T, Laslett M, Thorsen H, Manniche C, Ekdahl C, Jacobsen S: **Diagnostic classification of non specific low back pain. A new system integrating patho-anatomical and chemical categories.** *Physiotherapy Theory and Practice* 2007, **19**:213-237.
15. Senstad O, Leboeuf-Yde C, Borchgrevink C: **Frequency and characteristics of side effects of spinal manipulative therapy.** *Spine (Phila Pa 1976)* 1997, **22(4)**:435-440, discussion 440-431.
16. Leboeuf-Yde C, Hennius B, Rudberg E, Leufvenmark P, Thunman M: **Side effects of chiropractic treatment: a prospective study.** *Journal of manipulative and physiological therapeutics* 1997, **20(8)**:511-515.
17. Malmqvist S, Leboeuf-Yde C: **Chiropractors in Finland–a demographic survey.** *Chiropractic & osteopathy* 2008, **16**:9.
18. **SMS -Track Questionnaire 1.1.3.** *New Agenda Solutions* 2007.
19. Johansen B, Wedderkopp N: **Comparison between data obtained through real-time data capture by SMS and a retrospective telephone interview.** *Chiropractic & osteopathy* 2010, **18(1)**:10.
20. Dunn KM, Croft PR. **Classification of low back pain in primary care: using "bothersomeness" to identify the most severe cases.** *Spine* 2005, **30(16)**:1887-1892.

Burnout among chiropractic practitioners: real or imagined an exploratory study protocol

Shawn Williams[1*] and Stanley Innes[2]

Abstract

Burnout is a psychological syndrome of emotional exhaustion, depersonalization and reduced personal accomplishment that has been found to exist in a significant number of healthcare and helping professionals. It imposes a significant societal burden by shortened practitioner lifespan, decreased efficiency, negative health outcomes and poorer levels of patient care. Theoretical models suggest that it appears to be the result of a complex interaction between job resources and job demands. It may be reasonable to conclude that Chiropractic professionals experience similar vocational demands and thus experience significant levels of occupational stress and subsequent burnout. However the data on burnout within the chiropractic profession is limited. It is possible that this results in significant negative outcomes on chiropractors and their patients. Therefore, the objective of this paper is to demonstrate the need to explore burnout in chiropractic practice and offer a research protocol for a potential study.

Keywords: Burnout, Chiropractic, Exploratory

Background

Past research has sought to explore and quantify the elevated levels of stress and susceptibility to burnout found in the helping professions. This has been demonstrated in professionals that share many similar characteristics to chiropractic such as medical practitioners [1,2], dentists [3-5], nurses [6-9], physical therapists [10-15], and occupational therapists [16-18]. However, this subject has never been studied in the chiropractic profession.

Factors that have been identified which increase levels of stress and susceptibility to burnout include constantly focusing on the needs of others, which may lead to fatigue, feelings of frustration and anger, a sense of ineffectiveness and failure, and the onset of depression and associated co-morbidities [2,19-22]. Other factors include physical workload, quality of recipient contact, physical environment, type of patient feedback, financial pressures and supervisor support [22]. These factors have been shown to vary across geographic locations [10-13,23].

* Correspondence: swilliams2@york.cuny.edu
[1]Department of Health Professions, CUNY York College, 94 - 20 Guy R. Brewer Blvd, Jamaica, NY 11451, USA
Full list of author information is available at the end of the article

With this body of evidence available for comparison it would seem logical to explore those significant factors already identified. Therefore, the objective of this paper is to demonstrate the need to explore burnout in chiropractic practice and to propose a research protocol for a potential study. Thus we would seek to question a representative selection of chiropractors from varying locations on their perceptions of the impact of these factors using an established and validated questionnaire.

Literature review

In 2008 there were 49,100 registered chiropractors in the U.S.; of these approximately 44% were self-employed [24]. While there is a trend of increasing numbers of chiropractors there is counter pattern of declining use of chiropractic. In the U.S., 9.9% of U.S. adults reported having seen a chiropractor in 1997 vs. 7.4% in 2002. This was the largest relative decrease among CAM professions, which overall had a stable use rate [25].

Against this backdrop is the unfavourable public perception of chiropractic when compared with mainstream medicine with regard to ethics and honesty: in a 2006 Gallup Poll of U.S. adults, chiropractors were rated last among seven health care professions for being very high or high in honesty and ethical standards [26].

CareerCast.com rates chiropractic as the 10th least stressful occupation in the USA in 2011 [27]. They based this on their perception that chiropractic involves low levels of physical demands, healthy offices, low levels of required stamina, low levels of competitiveness, no travel, few deadlines, no personal hazards, solid levels of income, and a positive outlook for employment and income growth. No significant sampling of chiropractors was undertaken in obtaining these results.

This perception would stand in contrast to a retrospective analysis [28] of licensed chiropractors in California. Here, alarmingly, the authors identified that the attrition in the first 10 years of practice rose from 10% to 25% in the past decade. The authors hypothesized that the rising attrition rate of chiropractors may be linked to a number of forces such as changes in population, an oversupply of chiropractors, changes in reimbursement, the cost of education, and chiropractors' general dissatisfaction with their own profession [28]. In addition, data from a recent pilot study [29] exploring the attitudes of non-practicing chiropractors suggest that business ethics, overhead expenses and salaries were contributing factors of attrition in the chiropractic profession.

A cursory glance on affiliated contemporary chiropractic material suggests that stress and burnout are salient and important issues. The first discussion on burnout was noted in 1987 in an ICA Review of Chiropractic [30]. Shelley Simon also wrote of this syndrome and its likely increasing prevalence in the Chiropractic newspaper Dynamic Chiropractic [31]. More recently it was raised in the American Chiropractors Association News [32] as an occupation whose practitioners are more prone to job burnout. A web search reveals a multitude of chiropractic associated organizations/assistants offering to help reduce stress levels by altering practice methods.

The authors contend that this milieu, and other factors, create high levels of vocational stress and may generate high levels of burnout. However there are mixed messages from the available information sources and to date there has been no research into this sizable and significant occupational group.

Although burnout and stress are separate concepts, it has been a commonly held belief that the cumulative effect of chronic stress often results in a condition known as burnout [33]. This has been particularly prevalent in the health care service industry [34]. If stress and burnout in the delivering of chiropractic care are at similar levels to that of other helping professions then accurate data, as opposed to anecdotal information, are required for a number of reasons.

First, burnout can negatively affect the chiropractic professional and in turn the quality of care delivered to the patient. Burnout has been implicated in poor patient outcomes in other caring professions [11,12]. It is, therefore, possible that higher burnout levels result in poorer clinical decisions and treatment applications with an increased incidence of adverse outcomes.

Second, Mertz et al. (2010) suggest that most non-practicing chiropractors believed that the practice of chiropractic medicine was not a good career choice and would not recommend someone choosing chiropractic as a vocation [29]. Research has suggested that chiropractic colleges rely on practicing chiropractors as major recruiters of students [35]. Increasing levels of burnout in the chiropractic profession may impact on this avenue of student recruitment for chiropractic colleges.

Third, this is a preventable syndrome [36,37]. Early recognition and intervention have been shown to reduce the negative impact on individuals, families, communities and health resources [36,37]. Similar actions may be needed in the chiropractic profession. Finally, the impact of stress and burnout on health care professionals may have significant consequences also on the provider [38]. On a personal level this has included a depletion of emotional and physical resources, an increased likelihood of feelings of incompetence, a lack of achievement (negative self-image) and neglect of self, coupled with family and broader societal obligations [39]. It has also been implicated in higher levels of mental illness, substance abuse, absenteeism, reduced productivity and compromised patient care [6,10,19,39-43].

The authors contend that with such potentially serious and long-term consequences, this issue can no longer be left unexplored in the chiropractic profession.

Purpose and objectives of the study

The purpose of the intended study is to learn more about the levels of stress and burnout in the chiropractic profession. The specific objectives are to measure their prevalence and to compare those to levels previously identified and quantified in helping professions similar to the chiropractic profession.

Methods/Design

Study population and sampling

The authors intend to approach the appropriate chiropractic registration bodies with a request for assistance in distributing a mail out questionnaire to their membership. A pre-paid envelope with return address will be included. An alternative on-line survey option will also be made available.

For example, access to email listings of chiropractors is available for academic/educational purposes via a request through the State Board of Chiropractic Examiners, NJ. The investigators could request the email contact information of a randomized sample of licensed chiropractors from the State of New Jersey, State Board of Chiropractic Examiners, thus ensuring a systematic random sampling of the population of interest.

Subjects will include any Doctor of Chiropractic currently licensed to practice chiropractic and whom is at least 21 years old; with no limit on maximum age criteria.

Assuming a 60% return rate, the investigators will request the email contact information of a randomized sample of at least 500 licensed chiropractors in order to obtain sufficient numbers for the appropriate statistical analysis to be performed.

Variables of interest and their rationale

While the term "burnout" has become quite common in both research and practice, it has been ill defined historically. Initially, the term burnout was introduced by Freudenberger in the 1970's, and was used as an informal expression by lawyers, social workers, psychiatrists, teachers and hospice counsellors, to denote their gradual energy depletion and loss of motivation and commitment that was often associated with a wide array of other physical and mental symptoms [41,44].

Maslach's (1982) definition of burnout is now the most influential and widely referenced [33]. It is described in their self-titled inventory (Maslach Burnout Inventory- MBI) as a psychological syndrome of emotional exhaustion (EE), depersonalization (DP), and reduced personal accomplishment (PA) that can occur among people who work with other people in some helping capacity. Here emotional exhaustion is seen to reduce a workers ability to provide support at a psychological level [45]. Depersonalization results in a negative and/or cynical attitude towards his or her client and/or work related responsibilities. The third aspect of burnout, reduced personal accomplishment, refers to the tendency to evaluate oneself negatively, such that one is no longer effective in working with clients and in fulfilling one's job responsibilities [2,45]. Their inventory has been shown to be both a reliable and valid tool in evaluating job burnout [2]. To date, the primary form of this instrument used to measure burnout among helping professionals is the MBI-HSS [2,11,38,44,46]. Three dimensions EE, DP and PA are rated on a 7-point likert scale (ranging from 0, "never" to 6, "every day"). Scores on each subscale are computed by summing the numeric responses. Permission to use the MBI-HSS will be obtained from Consulting Psychologists Press http://www.mindgarden.com/products/mbi.htm.

Respondents will also be asked to complete a second questionnaire that contains demographic questions (including gender, age, income levels and absenteeism) and open-ended questions related to chiropractic-specific stressors, as previously found in the literature. Examples of these include issues such as poor public perception, professional-identity inconsistencies, philosophical dissonance, negative media coverage, workplace injury levels from unique physical demands, market competition from other manual therapists, student loan default rates in North America and threats to autonomy [26,47,48].

Data collection and management

An email letter of solicitation will be send to the random sample of emails via a group email distribution. This letter of solicitation will be in the body of the email and contain a link to an online version of the Maslach Burnout Inventory-Human Services Survey (MBI-HSS) and a brief demographic questionnaire developed by the primary investigator. SURVEY MONKEY (Gold member) software will be the electronic medium used. The Consent to Participate page shall include the title and purpose of the project, procedures for the anonymous and voluntary nature of the survey and potential risks and benefits to participants. The participants will complete the surveys in a place of their choice (e.g., their office, home or place of work), which has access to a computer. The Principal Investigator (PI) will conduct his portion of the research at York College, 94-20 Guy R. Brewer Blvd, Jamaica, NY 11451.

All survey related data will be stored on a thumb drive, which will be stored in locked cabinet at the place of research. After a minimum of 3 years, the PI will destroy the information on the thumb drive.

Analysis of data

This study is conducted with an observational research design that will involve the use cross-sectional data collection as a means of establishing the prevalence of burnout among chiropractors and to examine its association with some potential risk factors.

The primary analysis will involve descriptive summary statistics (means, standard deviations) and inferential statistics (confidence intervals) for estimating the prevalence of burnout. The use of univariate analysis using t-tests and chi-square statistic will be utilized to compare the rate of burnout with the factors under investigation. Chiropractic-specific stressors will be correlated using Pearson correlation. Moreover, the relationship between the dimensions of burnout and ratio-level demographic variables will be tested using bivariate Pearson correlational analyses. Spearman's rho analyses will we used for ordinal-level data. To control for possible confounding factors, a multiple logistic regression will be utilized with burnout as the dependent variable.

Ethical considerations

Research ethics and ethics approval will be sought from the principal investigators academic institution at the School of Health & Behavioral Sciences, CUNY - York College, New York, United States of America. All responses will be kept completely confidential and investigator(s) will be blinded to response and subject identity connectors.

Discussion

Summary of proposed study, need for the study and benefits of the study

Chiropractors are significant members of the health care community. Past studies have shown that the health care profession population experiences high levels of stress and burnout. Previous studies have identified ameliorable factors, which can result in the implementation of effective interventions with outcomes that include improved levels of patient care and practitioner health measures. No such exploration has been offered in the chiropractic profession; consequently an evidence-based intervention is not possible. The authors contend that now is the time.

Abbreviations

U.S.: United States: EE: Emotional exhaustion; DP: Depersonalization; PA: Personal accomplishment; PI: Principle investigator.

Author details

[1]Department of Health Professions, CUNY York College, 94 - 20 Guy R Brewer Blvd, Jamaica, NY 11451, USA. [2]35 Maroondah Highway, Lilydale 3140, Australia.

Authors' contributions

SW is the PI of the proposed study, and the original proposal author. SI added content expertise and editorial modifications. Both authors read and approve the final version of the manuscript.

Competing interests

The authors declare that they have no competing interests.

References

1. Grembowski D, Paschane D, Diehr P, Katon W, Martin D, Patrick DL: **Managed care, physician job satisfaction, and the quality of primary care.** *J Gen Intern Med* 2005, **20(3)**:271-277.
2. Maslach C, Jackson S, Leiter M: *Maslach Burnout Inventory Manual.* 3 edition. California: Consulting Psychologist Press; 1996.
3. Gunn SM, Woolfolk M, Maxson B: **Dentists: satisfaction and attitudes on the future.** *J Am Coll Dent* 1990, **57(1)**:12-15.
4. Humphris G: **A review of burnout in dentists.** *Dent Update* 1998, **25(9)**:392-396.
5. Te Brake H, Bouman AM, Gorter R, Hoogstraten J, Eijkman M: **Professional burnout and work engagement among dentists.** *Eur J Oral Sci* 2007, **115(3)**:180-185.
6. Piko BF: **Burnout, role conflict, job satisfaction and psychosocial health among Hungarian health care staff: a questionnaire survey.** *Int J Nurs Stud* 2006, **43(3)**:311-318.
7. Kumar S, Fischer J, Robinson E, Hatcher S, Bhagat RN: **Burnout and job satisfaction in New Zealand psychiatrists: A national study.** *Int J Soc Psychiatry* 2007, **53(4)**:306-316.
8. Maslach C, Schaufeli WB, Leiter MP: **Job burnout.** *Annu Rev Psychol* 2001, **52**:397-422.
9. Ilhan MN, Durukan E, Taner E, Maral I, Bumin MA: **Burnout and its correlates among nursing staff: questionnaire survey.** *J Adv Nurs* 2008, **61(1)**:100-106.
10. Wandling BJ, Smith BS: **Burnout in orthopaedic physical therapists.** *J Orthop Sports Phys Ther* 1997, **26(3)**:124-130.
11. Balogun JA, Titiloye V, Balogun A, Oyeyemi A, Katz J: **Prevalence and determinants of burnout among physical and occupational therapists.** *J Allied Health* 2002, **31(3)**:131-139.
12. Donohoe E, Nawawi A, Wilker L, Schindler T, Jette DU: **Factors associated with burnout of physical therapists in Massachusetts rehabilitation hospitals.** *Phys Ther* 1993, **73(11)**:756-61, 750. 6; discussion.
13. Li Calzi S, Farinelli M, Ercolani M, Alianti M, Manigrasso V, Taroni AM: **Physical rehabilitation and burnout: different aspects of the syndrome and comparison between healthcare professionals involved.** *Eura Medicophys* 2006, **42(1)**:27-36.
14. Ogiwara S, Hayashi H: **Burnout amongst physiotherapists in Ishikawa Prefecture.** *J Phys Ther Sci* 2002, **14(1)**:7-13.
15. Schuster ND, Nelson DL, Quisling C: **Burnout among physical therapists.** *Phys Ther* 1984, **64(3)**:299-303.
16. Painter J, Akroyd D, Elliot S, Adam RD: **Burnout among occupational therapists.** *Occup Ther Health Care* 2003, **17(1)**:63-78.
17. Meade I, Brown T, Trevan-Hawke J: **Female and male occupational therapists: a comparison of their job satisfaction level.** *Aust Occup Ther J* 2005, **52**:136-148.
18. Rogers JC, Dodson SC: **Burnout in occupational therapists.** *Am J Occup Ther* 1988, **42(12)**:787-792.
19. Wolfe GA: **Burnout of therapists: inevitable or preventable?** *Phys Ther* 1981, **61(7)**:1046-1050.
20. Leiter MP, Maslach C: **Burnout and health.** In *Handbook of health psychology.* Edited by: Baum A, Revenson TA, Singer JE. Mahwah, NJ: Erlbaum; 2001:415-426.
21. Ahola K, Hakanen J: **Job strain, burnout, and depressive symptoms: a prospective study among dentists.** *J Affect Disord* 2007, **104(1-3)**:103-110.
22. Demerouti E, Bakker AB, Nachreiner F, Schaufeli WB: **The job demands-resources model of burnout.** *J Appl Psychol* 2001, **86(3)**:499-512.
23. Pavlakis A, Raftopoulos V, Theodorou M: **Burnout syndrome in Cypriot physiotherapists: a national survey.** *BMC Health Serv Res* 2010, **10**:63.
24. **Occupational outlook handbook, 2010-11 edition, chiropractors.** 2009, [Internet]; Available from: http://www.bls.gov/oco/ocos071.htm..
25. Tindle HA, Davis RB, Phillips RS, Eisenberg DM: **Trends in use of complementary and alternative medicine by US adults: 1997-2002.** *Altern Ther Health Med* 2005, **11(1)**:42-49.
26. Editoral Staff: **Gullop poll: Americans have low opinion of chiropractors' honesty and ethics.** *Dyn Chiropr* 2007, **25(03)**[http://dynamicchiropractic.com/mpacms/dc/article.php?id=52038].
27. **Careercast.com releases 2011 stressful job report.** 2011, [Internet]; April 19, Available from: http://green.tmcnet.com/news/2011/04/19/5454753.htm..
28. Foreman SM, Stahl MJ: **The attrition rate of licensed chiropractors in California: an exploratory ecological investigation of time-trend data.** *Chiropr Osteopat* 2010, **18**:24.
29. Mirtz TA, Hebert JJ, Wyatt LH: **Attitudes of non-practicing chiropractors: a pilot survey concerning factors related to attrition.** *Chiropr Osteopat* 2010, **18**:29.
30. Garte SH: **The cost of caring - staying on the fire: The chiropractor's guide to burnout.** *ICA Rev* 1987, **43(4)**:9-13.
31. Simon S: **Primary prevention for career burnout: building resilience.** *Dynamic Chiropractic* 2008, **26(13)**:1-10.
32. **Extinguishing job burnout.** 2010, [Internet]; Available from: http://www.acatoday.org/content_css.cfm?CID=2283..
33. Schaufeli W, Enzmann D: *The burnout companion to study and practice: A critical analysis* London: Taylor & Francis; 1998.
34. Felton JS: **Burnout as a clinical entity-its importance in health care workers.** *Occup Med (Lond)* 1998, **48(4)**:237-250.
35. Coulter I, Adams A, Coggan P, Wilkes M, Gonyea M: **A comparative study of chiropractic and medical education.** *Altern Ther Health Med* 1998, **4(5)**:64-75.

36. Balch CM, Shanafelt T: **Combating stress and burnout in surgical practice: a review.** *Thorac Surg Clin* 2011, **21(3)**:417-430.
37. Ybema JF, Evers MS, van Scheppingen AR: **A longitudinal study on the effects of health policy in organizations on job satisfaction, burnout, and sickness absence.** *J Occup Environ Med* 2011, **53(11)**:1251-1257.
38. Maslach C, Florian V: **Burnout, job setting, and self-evaluation among rehabilitation counsellors.** *Rehabil Psychology* 1988, **33**:85-93.
39. Blust L: **Health professional burnout: Part I #167.** *J Palliative Med* 2009, **12(7)**:639-640.
40. Dyrbye LN, Thomas MR, Massie FS, Power DV, Eacker A, Harper W, *et al*: **Burnout and suicidal ideation among U.S. medical students.** *Ann Intern Med* 2008, **149(5)**:334-341.
41. Freudenberger HJ: **Staff burn-out.** *J Soc Issues* 1974, **30**:159-165.
42. Kompier MAJ, Marcelissen FHG: *Handbook work stress* Amsterdam: NIA; 1990.
43. Maslach C: **Burned-out.** *Human Behavior* 1976, **5(9)**:16-22.
44. Schaufeli WB: **Past performance and future perspectives of burnout research.** *SA J Ind Psychol* 2003, **29(4)**:1-15.
45. In *Evaluating Stress: A book of resources.* Edited by: Zalaquett CP, Wood RJ. Lanham, Md., 1997:.
46. Maslach C, Jackson SE: **The measurement of experienced burnout.** *J Occup Behav* 1981, **2(2)**:99-113.
47. Copper R, McKee HJ: **Chiropractic in the United States: trends and issues.** *Milbank Q* 2003, **81(1)**:107-138.
48. Foreman SM, Stahl MJ: **Chiropractors disciplined by a state chiropractic board and a comparison with disciplined medical physicians.** *J Manipulative Physiol Ther* 2004, **27(7)**:472-477.

7

A descriptive study of chiropractors' opinions and practices regarding office-based health product sales

Stacey A Page[1*], Jaroslaw P Grod[2] and D Gordon McMorland[3]

Abstract

Background: Although the sale of non-prescription health products is ubiquitous, the views of health professionals, such as chiropractors, regarding the sale of such products are not well known. Practitioner opinion is important to understand and inform professional practice. The purpose of this study was to describe chiropractors' perspectives and practices on the sale of health care products from practitioners' offices.

Methods: Chiropractors were invited to provide written comments about health product sales at the end of a fixed choice, mailed survey. Respondents' comments were analyzed using qualitative description. Ethics approval was received from the Conjoint Health Research Ethics Board at the University of Calgary.

Results: One hundred seven of the 265 respondents (response rate of 51%) provided written comments. Approximately 30 pages of double-spaced, typed text were gathered. Respondents did not consistently endorse or condemn health product sales, and engaged in the practice to greater and lesser extents. While some were opposed to health products sales, some accepted the practice with a degree of ambivalence whereas others clearly embraced it. Some respondents acknowledged a professional conflict of interest in such sales and marketing, and described strategies used to mitigate it. Others provided a range of justifications for the practice. Personal integrity and professional standards were discussed and a need for monitoring identified.

Conclusions: A wide range of opinions and practices were described and this is consistent with resulting variation in practice. In light of this, standards that facilitate consistency in practice may benefit professionals and the public alike.

Keywords: Chiropractic, Professional ethics, Codes of ethics, Marketing

Background

The sale of non-prescription health products is ubiquitous, meeting a significant consumer demand [1,2]. Natural health products, such as vitamins, minerals, herbal remedies, homeopathic and traditional medicines, nutritional supplements, and products such as cosmeceuticals, rehabilitation and fitness aids can be found online, in major retail chains, mall kiosks and in the offices of health professionals. A recent report estimated the total retail sales of natural health products in Canada to be worth $2.5 billion dollars in 2005, growing to an estimated $2.75 billion by 2010 [1]. Distributors identified healthcare practitioners as among their top three current and future most important distribution channels [1]. The regulation of and evidence base for many of these products are uneven or non-existent, leaving consumers to fend for themselves in a "buyer beware" market [3-5].

The roles and responsibilities of health professionals regarding the sale of non-prescription health products are unclear [5-7]. Should health professionals be marketing health goods to their patients? If so, to what standards should they adhere? Should there be any limits placed upon this practice? How are such sales monitored by professional bodies?

* Correspondence: sapage@ucalgary.ca
[1]Office of Medical Bioethics, RM 93, HMRB, Faculty of Medicine, University of Calgary, 3330 Hospital Drive NW, Calgary AB. T2N-4N1, Canada
Full list of author information is available at the end of the article

Research considering the sale of health products by health professional is limited. There have been a few studies that have explored the practice among dermatologists [7,8], dentists [9] and most recently chiropractors [6,10]. Together, these studies suggest product retailing by health professionals is prevalent. Proponents believe that it affords control over product quality, that it is a service patients appreciate, and that treatment compliance is enhanced [11]. Opponents argue that product sales are undertaken for profit, thus presenting a conflict of interest compromising the therapeutic relationship and professional integrity [12-14].

Considering chiropractic specifically, studies have suggested that the majority of practitioners (54-89%) sell a range of products [6,10,15]. Chiropractic trade reports and publications suggest product sales are a major revenue source, improving practice profitability for chiropractors [16-18].

Relative to other disciplines, the public trust in the healing professions is high [19]. Such trust is dependent upon practioners upholding their duties to act in their patients' best interests and is central to the effectiveness of the patient-practitioner relationship. Professional practice is guided in part by codes of ethics and conduct. As the health product market place continues to grow, so too will the potential for ethical conflicts faced by practitioners choosing to retail health products. Little is known about chiropractors' individual considerations of this practice

This study reports on the qualitative findings of a previous [10] survey where chiropractors had the opportunity to comment on the sale of health products. Guidance offered by the Alberta Chiropractic Association and College and the Canadian Chiropractic College are considered.

Methods

A random sample of 518 chiropractors (of 929 total population) in the province of Alberta, Canada received an initial survey package with a follow-up package sent out three weeks later., The four-page survey contained 34 fixed-choice questions about chiropractors opinions and practices surrounding health product sales. Subjects were invited to provide written comments about the sale of health products by chiropractors. Subjects were assured their data would be de-identified. The confidentiality of study responses was preserved by replacing respondents' names with codes and be reporting all findings in aggregate. This study received ethics approval from the Conjoint Health Research Ethics Board at the University of Calgary.

Results

Two hundred sixty five chiropractors (51.2%) completed and returned the survey. Respondents were mostly men (N = 207; 78.1%) and had been in practice for a median of 12 years (IQR 8-20 years). Most were in multidisciplinary group practices (N = 204; 77.3%) and most (N = 208; 78.5%) were satisfied with their number of weekly patient contact hours. The majority (N = 247; 95.0%) believed that chiropractors should sell health products and 89.4% (N = 236) currently sold health products from their practices. The quantitative survey results are presented elsewhere [10]. This paper reports on the analysis of the volunteered, qualitative comments.

The written comments of 107 respondents were transcribed, yielding approximately 30 pages of double-spaced typed text. The text was entered into the Ethnograph (qualitative analytic) software [20]. The first author (SP) reviewed, coded and summarized the textual data using qualitative description. Qualitative description is a low-inference interpretation that focuses on describing "the facts [21]". codes and summary was reviewed against the raw data by the two other authors (JG, GM). No discrepancies in interpretation occurred.

The following themes emerged.

Conflict of interest

Several commentators readily acknowledged the potential for a conflict of interest to exist when treating chiropractors were also involved in health product sales. Respondents spoke generally about the potential for conflict of interest to occur when any health care practitioner "over treats" a patient.

Some respondents were very clear in their opinion that product sales crossed an ethical line *(2-165 They are unethical and inappropriate when they are central to revenue generating strategies).* Several were aware of instances in which chiropractors appeared to push products sales (e.g., *2-149 "I have some concern with practices which profess to be strongly "anti-allopathic" against the "pill and a bill" practices of medicine yet you always leave the clinic with a bag of supplements to assist this and prevent that;" 2-187 "The concern I have is when it is dispensed/promoted as a profit centre. This has created lots of bad will when patients are encouraged to buy bags of products...")*

Others held a more ambivalent position, where the motivations toward practitioner profit or patient well being were sometimes described as "hard to distinguish. Some likened keeping these interests in balance as a fine line or something that one had to be constantly mindful of (2-220), while others admitted feeling uncomfortable about engaging in the practice (e.g., *2-149 "I try to satisfy my guilt for carrying this type of stuff by having a low margin").*

Finally, some respondents experienced no conflict of interest at all and felt that health product sales fit well within their practices. (e.g., *"...The feedback I got from patients describing the knowledge base I had was greater than anyone they had met got me to realize the time and money spent on my education was not only valuable but that it was worth charging a full fee. I am exceptionally comfortable with this position.")*

Mitigating actions

A second category of responses centred on practices or behaviours that respondents believed mitigated potential conflict of interest.

To this end, chiropractors described provisions to minimize perceived conflicts of interest. Most often, chiropractors talked about the mark-up they placed on products sold, attempting to minimize conflict of interest by selling products at cost or for a very small mark up. Others acknowledged a profit margin. The descriptions ranged from statements like the practitioner was "not out to make money (2-35)" to a "very modest mark-up" to a "small profit" to "fair market value." The labor costs associated with maintaining a product inventory, and for spending the time discussing such products with patients were also presented as justifications for how costs were structured (*2-21 "Keeping stock and dealing with GST is laborious...." 2-581 "It is time consuming to advise patients on why these products are helpful and to advise them on proper consumption levels* etc. *to advance their recovery. The mark-up on products 20-30% is poor compensation for the time"*).

Despite supporting sales generally, several respondents expressed their opposition to multi-level marketing.

A second initiative undertaken to alleviate the perception of competing interests was the efforts to ensure products were purchased voluntarily. Chiropractors used terms like '"don't hard sell" and "unpushy" to emphasize that purchases were at the patient's discretion. Some noted they directed patients to other places where such purchases could be made (*2-08 "When I make recommendations to patients re: products I always advise them that they don't need to purchase them from our clinic and I provide other potential sources"*). A few acknowledged they had observed aggressive marketing among their colleagues (e.g., *2-74 Some DCs are very pushy about selling products and thus make good money from it)*.

Justifications

Another theme that emerged in the comments was how product sales were justified by the respondents. Several arguments were identified including professional role, scope of practice and quality assurance considerations.

Most commonly, respondents believed that product sales were consistent with their duty or obligation to act in patient's best interest. Products that promoted health or healing were viewed as enhancements to patient care and in line with the chiropractor's role (e.g., *2-219 "I feel I use health care products the same way I use my adjustments - that is for the good of the patient)*. Within this argument, a range of perspectives was again evident. While some viewed any contribution to health as a justification for product sales (e.g.,*2-339 In regards to supports* (e.g., *in-soles, pillows) they are a mandatory prerequisite to patient health and if I do not carry them, I would be doing my patients a disservice)* others suggested that product sales should be based on clinical need and response to a presenting condition only.

Some chiropractors further argued that sales were well within their scope of practice and fields of expertise (e. g., *2-137 Chiropractors...receive extensive training in the appropriate use of those health products and as such have the right and responsibility to prescribe these products to patients if they would be of benefit)*. A few suggested that the training and resulting expertise that chiropractors had with respect to the use of health products generally, and nutritional products specifically, is far superior to other disciplines, in particular medicine.

Contrasting with these perspectives, some cautioned that chiropractors might not have the necessary expertise to support certain product sales (e.g., *2-103 I think some chiropractors overstep their boundaries and make nutritional supplements a huge part of their practice without proper educational back-up)*. Others believed that there were limits to what chiropractors should be offering to enhance patient well-being (*2-551 "As chiropractors do not take kindly to other practitioners doing spinal manipulation, I think it reflects poorly on our profession when we get excessively involved by areas better served by naturopaths* (e.g., *supplements) and podiatrists (foot assessment and orthotics))*

Some practitioners asserted that they could attest to the quality of the products they sold, in contrast to the potentially unknown quality available on the general market. References were made to products being of "very good quality," or "best quality available."

Practitioners also spoke of having researched the products that they sold, with a few citing specific sources such as peer reviewed literature or manufacturers' standards.

Some believed that product sales were a convenience offered to patients and were justified on the basis of patient demand. Further to this, some chiropractors noted they only sold products available to health practitioners or that were otherwise hard to find or unavailable. A few suggested that having products readily available enhanced treatment compliance.

Ethics and regulation

A group of respondents averred that professionalism and ethics in practice were a matter of individual integrity. If a chiropractor was ethical as an individual, there was no reason to doubt his or her integrity in professional practice. Similarly, respondents acknowledged that there are typically a few people in any professional group whose actions are not consistent with the values of the whole. Specifically considering product sales, respondents focused on the practitioner's intent, that is, where engaging in sales clearly for the patient's well being was acceptable whereas engaging in it for profit was not.

Finally, although individual integrity was noted to be critical in the maintenance of professionalism in practice, some spoke of the need for the profession to monitor individual practices and sanction those who clearly violated standards of practice. A need for guidelines, education and awareness for chiropractors relating to product sales was identified.

Discussion

Chiropractors who responded to this survey did not uniformly support or condemn the practice of health product sale and, consistent with this engaged in product sales to varying extents. While a few chiropractors were implacably opposed to health product sales, most accepted the practice under various conditions and with varying degrees of comfort. Some clearly embraced the practice. Consistent with arguments in the literature, those engaged in the health product sales believed it was a convenience for patients and part of their role and responsibility as health care providers. Those who offered comments recognizing potential harms spoke of the practice as compromising professional integrity and described strategies to minimize negative effects.

Conflict of interest relates to a set of conditions or a situation such that professional judgment about a primary interest may be unduly influenced by a secondary interest [22]. Conflict of interest in selling health products from within a professional practice occurs if the potential sale of a product causes practitioners to deviate from their professional obligations to their patients in anticipation of economic gain. Assuming products are safe and efficacious, selling them is ethically neutral. Selling products primarily for profit rather than for patient necessity violates the practitioner's fiduciary duty to act in patient's best interests as their own interests prevail [12]

Recommended strategies to address conflict of interest involve taking steps to avoid or prevent the set of conditions provoking it [22]. Indeed, a few respondents stated that they did not engage in product sales or minimized the conflict by maintaining no/low profit margins.

Others emphasized that purchases were made voluntarily by patients, arguing that they had no influence over the patient's actions, a disingenuous claim at best in view of the nature of the therapeutic relationship and its inherent power imbalance. Patients may feel that purchases are necessary in order to maintain a positive relationship with the practitioner or to receive future care. Little research has investigated this area however one small study of patient opinion indicated that patients reason for purchasing products from practitioners was their trust in the practitioner [8]. Anecdotal reports suggest that such purchases may leave patients feeling exploited by practitioners [23]. While subtle influence may be pervasive, more worrisome is the allegation of aggressive sales strategies used by some of the respondents' colleagues.

Conflict of interest rules are a means of acknowledging that such problems may arise and offering guidance for individuals in managing these circumstances. Conflict of interest involving health product sales is recognized within the Canadian Chiropractic Association's (CCA) national code of ethics and conduct of chiropractors and also within Alberta College and Association of Chiropractors (ACAC), both of which permit health products sales provided certain conditions are met. The relevant section from the CCA's Code of Ethics and Conduct (Article 21) states:

It is not unethical to dispense items providing; it does not create a conflict of interest, they serve the best interests of the patient, clinical value has been demonstrated, and the item is available at a fair market price [24].

The Alberta College and Association of Chiropractors Code of Ethics provides the following guidelines:

A chiropractor who sells or markets professional products to their patients must:

- Ensure that they do not exploit the trust inherent in the chiropractor-patient relationship
- Not misrepresent or exaggerate the value of the products
- Prior to the sales of the product, have thoroughly evaluated the information related to the product and must be satisfied that the therapeutic value represented is rational
- Make available to patients all information necessary for the patients to make an informed choice as to whether to purchase the products, including whether the product is available elsewhere [25]

The guidance offered by these codes is limited. Neither provides a clear definition of, or restriction on, the types of products chiropractors may choose to sell, leaving the interpretation and resulting choice up to individual practitioners. At a minimum, products should be related to the practitioner's area of expertise. However, there is debate within the profession as to where the boundaries of this expertise lie, as illustrated by the comments provided for this study.

Both the provincial and national codes stop short of requiring that a scientific evidence base exist for products sold from offices, recommending instead that subjective review is sufficient. Although some respondents cited reviews of scientific evidence, others referenced manufacturer's data or simply stated they promoted things they used/liked or knew worked. The widely recognized lack of scientific evidence and uneven regulatory oversight for many health products [26-28], mean that reliance on an individual practitioner's opinion or preference may leave consumers further at risk. Others have proposed that members of their profession establish a board of peers charged with the review of evidence and approval of products for in-office dispensing based on established criteria [14].

The Canadian Code makes reference to product cost, arguably the issue at the centre of the potential conflict of interest. The standard recommended is "fair market price" which may be interpreted as what the market or, more accurately, consumers will bear, and is inconsistent with no profit-taking or cost-recovery transactions, leaving room for financial exploitation. While many respondents spoke of products retailing at cost, variation in product pricing was clear leaving consumers with inconsistency in practice standards. The provincial code is silent with respect to product pricing.

Limitations

Despite the number of comments and the range of opinions expressed, the findings arising from the comments volunteered are not necessarily reflected of the chiro practic profession as a whole and may not generalize to practitioners in other areas, or to those who chose not to respond.

Conclusion

Product sales in chiropractic appear well-established both provincially and nationally in Canada. As noted by some respondents, ethics and integrity are individual attributes. While this may be true, the actions of individual practitioners may affect public perception of the profession as a whole. To facilitate the integrity of professional judgment and to protect patient best interests, clearly articulated standards and consistency in practice are paramount.

The comments provided by the respondents suggest that existing guidelines may not be sufficiently detailed or stringent to adequately guide practice, or possibly that practitioners are simply not aware of these standards. It does not appear as though the profession has monitoring mechanism in place to assess compliance and enforce standards although several respondents suggested this would be a worthwhile undertaking on the part of the governing body. It would be worthwhile to systematically investigate how often complaints are received in this area by the provincial colleges or national association, and to determine whether disciplinary action has been taken.

Future research gathering data from a national sample of practitioners and examining patient perspectives will further inform the profession.

Acknowledgements

This study was funded by a Research Grant from the University of Calgary, University Research Grants Committee. The survey respondent's participation is gratefully acknowledged. Dr. Michael C. King's review of manuscript drafts is sincerely appreciated.

Author details

[1]Office of Medical Bioethics, RM 93, HMRB, Faculty of Medicine, University of Calgary, 3330 Hospital Drive NW, Calgary AB. T2N-4N1, Canada. [2]Private practice, Toronto, ON. [3]National Spine Care, #300 - 301 14th Street NW, Calgary, Alberta T2N 2A1, Canada.

Authors' contributions

SP designed and administered the study, conducted the preliminary data analysis and drafted the manuscript. JG contributed to the study design, data analysis and manuscript review. DGM contributed to the study design, data analysis and manuscript review. All authors read and approved the final manuscript.

Competing interests

The authors declare that they have no competing interests.

References

1. Canadian Health Food Association: **Natural Health Products State of the Industry Report.** 2005.
2. Gold MD: **Clinical case: dispensing cosmeceuticals from the office (commentary).** *Virtual Mentor* 2006, **8**:503-508.
3. Angell M, Kassirer JP: **Alternative Medicine - The Risks of Untested and Unregulated Remedies.** *NEJM* 1998, **339**:839-841.
4. Raynor D, Dickinson R, Knapp P, Long A, Nicolson D: **Buyer beware? Does the information provided with herbal products available over the counter enable safe use?** *BMC Medicine* 2011, **9**:94.
5. Boon H, Hirschkorn K, Griener G, Cali M: **The ethics of dietary supplements and natural health products in pharmacy practice: a systematic documentary analysis.** *Int J Pharm Pract* 2010, **17**:31-38.
6. Page SA, Grod JP: **An audit of health products advertised for sale on chiropractic websites in Canada and consideration of these practices in the context of Canadian Chiropractic codes of ethics and conduct.** *JMPT* 2009, **32**:485-492.
7. Castanedo-Tardan MP, Baumann L: **Ethics of selling skin care.** *Clin Dermatol* 2009, **27**:355-358.
8. Ogbogu P, Fleischer AB Jr, Brodell RT, Bhalla G, Draelos ZD, Feldman SR: **Physicians' and Patients' Perspectives on Office-Based Dispensing: The Central Role of the Physician-Patient Relationship.** *Arch Dermatol* 2001, **137**:151-154.
9. Ratcliff R: **Retailing home care products within the dental office: a future dental service?** *J Dent Pract Admin* 1990, **7**:56-64.
10. Page SA, Grod JP, McMorland DG: **The perspectives and practices of Alberta chiropractors regarding the sale of health care products in chiropractic offices.** *J Manipulative Physiol Ther* 2011, **34**:476-482.
11. Gormley DE: **There Is Nothing Wrong With Dermatologists Selling Products to Patients!** *Arch Dermatol* 1999, **135**:765-766.
12. American Medical Association: **Council on Ethical and Judicial Affairs. Sale of health-related products from physicians' offices. CEJA-1-A-99.** American Medical Association; 1999.
13. BenefitsWorld: **Drastic health cuts increase pressure on benefits rates. BenefitsWorld eNews Dec 1, 2001.A Periodic Newsletter about the World of Canadian Benefit Plans, Sponsors and Providers.** 2005, Howard Kettner.

14. Draelos ZD: **The dermatology dispensing debate.** *Skin Therapy Lett* 2007, **12**:1-3.
15. Page SA: **An audit of health products and services marketed on chiropractic websites in Alberta and consideration of these practices in the context of chiropractic codes of conduct and ethics.** *J Can Chiropr Assoc* 2007, **51**:91-98.
16. Newswire Today: **Retail product sales at point of service improve chiropractic clinic revenues and patient loyalty.** 2007 [http:// Newswiretoday.com].
17. Pelletier N: **Increase revenue by $200 K with nutritional and postural analysis.** *Chiropr Economics* 1999, **41**:64-67.
18. Friedman D: **Liquid Vitamins: The Wave of the Future.** 1998, Chiropractic Economics Magazine March/April, 36,38,40-41.
19. GALLUP: **Honesty/Ethics in Professions.** 2011 [http://www.gallup.com/ home.aspx].
20. Seidel J: **The Ethnograph. [5].** Thousand Oaks CA, Scolari, Sage Publications Software, Inc; 1998.
21. Sandelowski M: **Whatever happened to qualitative description?** *Res Nurs Health* 2000, **23**:334-340.
22. Thompson DF: **Understanding Financial Conflicts of Interest.** *N Engl J Med* 1993, **329**:573-576.
23. Ulene V: **Medical Merchants.** Los Angeles Times; 2007.
24. Canadian Chiropractic Association: **Code of Conduct, Code of Ethics. Canadian Chiropractic Association website. 1996.** 2008.
25. Alberta College and Association of Chiropractors: **Code of Ethics. Alberta College and Association of Chiropractors Website, Legislation.**, 11-13-2007. 6-10-2008.
26. Breen KJ: **Ethical issues in the use of complementary medicines.** *Climacteric* 2003, **6**:268-272.
27. Kondro W: **Debate over credibility of natural health product claims.** *Can Med Assoc J* 2005, **172**:983.
28. Moquin B, Blackman MR, Mitty E, Flores S: **Complementary and Alternative Medicine (CAM).** *Geriatric Nursing* 2005, **30**:196-203.

Predictors of outcome in neck pain patients undergoing chiropractic care: comparison of acute and chronic patients

Cynthia Peterson[1*], Jennifer Bolton[2] and B Kim Humphreys[1]

Abstract

Background: Neck pain is a common complaint in patients presenting for chiropractic treatment. The few studies on predictors for improvement in patients while undergoing treatment identify duration of symptoms, neck stiffness and number of previous episodes as the strong predictor variables. The purpose of this study is to continue the research for predictors of a positive outcome in neck pain patients undergoing chiropractic treatment.

Methods: Acute (< 4 weeks) (n = 274) and chronic (> 3 months) (n = 255) neck pain patients with no chiropractic or manual therapy in the prior 3 months were included. Patients completed the numerical pain rating scale (NRS) and Bournemouth questionnaire (BQ) at baseline prior to treatment. At 1 week, 1 month and 3 months after start of treatment the NRS and BQ were completed along with the Patient Global Impression of Change (PGIC) scale. Demographic information was provided by the clinician. Improvement at each of the follow up points was categorized using the PGIC. Multivariate regression analyses were done to determine significant independent predictors of improvement.

Results: Baseline mean neck pain and total disability scores were significantly ($p < 0.001$and $p < 0.008$ respectively) higher in acute patients. Both groups reported significant improvement at all data collection time points, but was significantly larger for acute patients. The PGIC score at 1 week (OR = 3.35, 95% CI = 1.13-9.92) and the baseline to 1 month BQ total change score (OR = 1.07, 95% CI = 1.03-1.11) were identified as independent predictors of improvement at 3 months for acute patients. Chronic patients who reported improvement on the PGIC at 1 month were more likely to be improved at 3 months (OR = 6.04, 95% CI = 2.76-13.69). The presence of cervical radiculopathy or dizziness was not predictive of a negative outcome in these patients.

Conclusions: The most consistent predictor of clinically relevant improvement at both 1 and 3 months after the start of chiropractic treatment for both acute and chronic patients is if they report improvement early in the course of treatment. The co-existence of either radiculopathy or dizziness however do not imply poorer prognosis in these patients.

Keywords: Neck pain, Chiropractic, Outcomes, Prognostic factors

Background

Patients suffering from neck pain are second only to low back pain patients in terms of the frequency of presentation for chiropractic treatment [1-4]. For many of these patients the precise diagnosis is difficult to ascertain and thus becomes labeled 'non-specific' neck pain or neck pain from mechanical dysfunction [1,3-5]. Research evidence has yet to determine with clarity whether spinal manipulative therapy (SMT) or mobilization of the neck is the superior treatment for these patients [1-9] although it appears that both of these treatments have better outcomes when combined with exercise [5,10].

Manipulative therapy to the cervical spine has traditionally been considered somewhat controversial by certain health care practitioners. Recent high quality research evidence supports the relative safety of chiropractic SMT to

* Correspondence: cynthia.peterson@balgrist.ch
[1]University of Zürich and Orthopaedic University Hospital Balgrist, Forchstrasse 340, 8008 Zürich, Switzerland
Full list of author information is available at the end of the article

the cervical spine with no increased risk of vertebral artery injury compared to patients seeking care from other primary medical physicians who do not manipulate the neck [11-13]. A few studies have begun to investigate specific predictors for a positive response to chiropractic SMT in neck pain patients and have identified the duration of symptoms, stiffness of the neck and the number of previous episodes of neck pain as some of the strongest predictors of an immediate positive response [7,8,14]. Therefore, the purpose of this study is to continue the research for predictors of positive outcomes in neck pain patients undergoing chiropractic treatment and to determine if these differ between acute and chronic patients.

Methods

This is a prospective cohort study with three month follow-up. Ethics approval was obtained from the Canton of Zürich Switzerland ethics committee (EK-19/2009) and written informed consent was obtained from all patients.

Patients

Consecutive new patients over the age of 18 with neck pain of any duration who had not undergone chiropractic or manual therapy in the prior 3 months were recruited from multiple chiropractic practices in Switzerland. Patients with specific pathologies of the cervical spine that are contraindications to chiropractic manipulative therapy, such as tumours, infections, inflammatory arthropathies, acute fractures, Paget's disease, anti-coagulation therapy, cervical spondylotic myelopathy, known unstable congenital anomalies and severe osteoporosis, were excluded. Although the data was collected for subacute patients (symptoms between 4 and 12 weeks), for this study these patients were not used due to the small sample size (19% of total patients).

All active members of the Association of Swiss Chiropractors (ASC) (260 in total) were asked to contribute patients to this study. Notification and instructions about this study as well as the study protocol were sent to all chiropractors by email as well as discussed verbally during the annual mandatory post-graduate continuing education (CE) convention held immediately prior to the start of data collection. Workshops were also conducted during the CE convention by one of the authors on the use of outcome measures in clinical practice. It was emphasized via email and verbally that there should be no changes in the treatment methods used by the contributing chiropractors as the purpose of this study was to evaluate outcomes as would be found in routine chiropractic practice. Therefore, standardization of treatment method or treatment number was not desired. It is known however, from the data collected for the 'Swiss Job Analysis' study done in 2009 that the 'diversified' technique is applied to between 76 and 100% of chiropractic patients in Switzerland. The other commonly used treatments used include advice on the activities of daily living, trigger point therapy, therapeutic exercises and mobilization techniques [15].

Outcome measures

The numerical rating scale (NRS) for neck pain and a separate NRS for arm pain as well as the Bournemouth Questionnaire for neck (BQN) disability, which has been translated and validated in German [16], were administered to the patient immediately prior to the first treatment by the office staff of each practice. The BQN is a multidimensional instrument covering 7 domains with each domain evaluated using an 11-point numerical rating scale (0 through 10). The seven domains include: (i) pain; (ii) disability (activities of daily living (ADL)); (iii) disability (social activities); (iv) anxiety; (v) depression; (vi) work, both inside and outside the home, fear avoidance; and (vii) locus of control. In addition to each domain, the total score (maximum 70 points) is also calculated. The BQN was shown to be much more sensitive to change compared to the German versions of the Neck Pain and Disability (NPAD) questionnaire and the Neck Disability Index (NDI) for all subscales[16].

One week after the first treatment, data from the NRS (neck), NRS (arm), Patient Global Impression of Change (PGIC) scale [17], and the BQN were collected from the patient via a short telephone interview. Similarly, these same data were collected at 1 month and 3 months after the start of treatment via telephone interviews. These telephone interviews were conducted by research assistants at the university hospital who were unknown to the patients.

Demographic and clinical baseline data

Additional information provided by the treating chiropractor at the initial consultation included: patient age, gender, marital status, paid employment, whether or not the onset of pain was due to trauma, whether or not the patient smokes, whether or not the patient was currently taking pain medication, duration of current complaint, number of previous episodes, whether or not the patient also had signs and symptoms of cervical radiculopathy, whether or not the patient also complained of dizziness and the patient's general health status. This information was completed on a baseline information form.

Prognostic (predictor) variables

All variables were identified in advance and were taken from information completed by the chiropractor on the baseline information form at the first consultation and from changes in variables between baseline and the data collection time points (1 week, 1 month and 3 months).

Continuous variables consisted of patient age, NRS (neck), NRS (arm), BQN scores and change scores. All other variables, with the exception of 'number of previous episodes' and 'general health', were dichotomized for ease of interpretation (yes/no or present/absent as appropriate). The 'number of previous episodes' was divided into 3 categories: none, 1 to 3 episodes, and 4 or more episodes. 'General health' was categorized as 'good', 'average', or 'poor' as determined by the treating chiropractor.

Patients whose symptoms were less than 4 weeks in duration were classified as 'acute' and those whose symptoms were longer than 12 weeks were classified as 'chronic'. Sub-acute patients were not included in this study to make a clear distinction between acute and chronic patients. Acute vs. chronic patients were analyzed separately as previous research has shown that length of complaint is a strong predictor of outcome [7]. Moreover, there is a clear rationale to expect that predictors may well be different between acute and chronic patients given the differences in the course of their condition. This is borne out by recent research investigating prediction of outcomes in acute and chronic pain patients as separate groups [18].

Outcomes

Outcomes were evaluated using the NRS (neck), NRS (arm) and the BQN total and sub-scale raw change (i.e. baseline minus 1 week, 1 month or 3 month) scores. For the prediction analysis the outcome 'improvement' was defined as scores of 1 (much better) or 2 (better) on the PGIC scale. Scores of 3 (slightly better), 4 (no change), 5 (slightly worse), 6 (worse) and 7 (much worse) were categorized as 'not improved'.

Statistical analysis

Baseline factors were compared between acute (symptoms < 4 weeks) and chronic (symptoms > 12 weeks) patients using the chi^2 test for categorical variables and the unpaired t-test for continuous variables. Within patient differences for continuous variables were analysed using the paired t-test.

Multivariate regression analyses were carried out to determine statistically significant independent predictors of improvement. 'Improvement' as the dependent variable in the regression analysis was categorized as scores of 1 (much better) or 2 (better) on the PGIC. First, all potential predictors were separately entered into a univariate model and those significantly associated with improvement ($p < 0.1$) were entered in a forward stepwise multivariate model, which entered only those variables independently associated with 'improvement' ($p < 0.05$). Variables in the model were checked for redundancy by noting the correlation coefficients (>0.8) between variables in the presence of the other variables in the model. The properties of the final predictive model were ascertained by calculating the sensitivity, specificity, % correctly classified, and the area under the Receiver Operator Characteristic (ROC) curve. A value of at least 70% for the area under the ROC was considered acceptable for discriminative accuracy [19]. The adjusted $\%R^2$ was used as the index of the percentage of the variance in the outcome explained by the model. SPSS version 17 was used for all data analyses.

Results

Baseline characteristics

Of the 260 active members of the Association of Swiss Chiropractors, 81 (31%) recruited patients for this study. Six hundred fifty seven neck pain patients provided baseline data with 274 being acute (< 4 weeks), 124 being subacute (4 – 12 weeks) and 255 being chronic (> 12 weeks). The 124 subacute patients in the database were not included in this study and 4 other patients were deleted from the database because they could not be reached for the three consecutive follow-up telephone calls. This resulted in baseline data for 529 total acute and chronic patients (Table 1). The mean age was 40.0 (SD ± 12.58) and 41.8 (±13.87) years for acute and chronic patients respectively. The majority of acute and especially chronic patients were female. Acute patients were significantly more likely to be in paid employment, to be taking pain medication and to be in 'good health' compared to chronic patients. There was a significant difference in the number of previous episodes of neck pain between the acute and chronic patients with chronic patients more likely to report four or more

Table 1 Baseline characteristics for acute and chronic patients

	ACUTE (< 4 WEEKS) (N = 274)	CHRONIC (> 12 WEEKS) (N = 255)	P-VALUE
Gender (Male)	112 (40.9)	89 (34.9)	0.157
Age (years)	40.0 (±12.58)	41.8 (±13.87)	0.114
In paid employment	235 (86.7)	200 (79.1)	0.020*
Taking pain meds	101 (37.0)	66 (25.9)	0.006*
Radiculopathy present	34 (12.5)	29 (11.4)	0.691
Previous episodes:			
None	109 (40.5)	116 (47.5)	0.0001*
1–3	82 (30.5)	25 (10.2)	
4 or more	78 (29.0)	103 (42.2)	
Trauma onset	32 (11.7)	40 (15.7)	0.179
Smoker	61 (22.8)	56 (22.6)	0.96
In good health	197 (73.0)	138 (54.4)	0.001*
Dizziness present	51 (44.7)	64 (45.1)	0.957

Values are numbers (%). N = number of observations. * = p < 0.05.

previous episodes (p = 0.001). There was no difference between acute and chronic patients for the proportion presenting with radiculopathy, pain onset due to trauma, smoking, or symptomatic for dizziness.

Table 2 compares the baseline NRS (neck and arm) scores as well as the BQN subscale and total scores for acute and chronic patients. Acute patients reported significantly higher baseline values for neck pain, disability in activities of daily living, disability in social activities and the total BQN score.

General outcomes

At 1 week after the start of treatment 77.8% of acute patients and 37.6% of chronic patients reported that they were significantly 'improved'. By 1 month 86.6% of acute patients and 62.4% of chronic patients reported being 'improved and at 3 months 84.3% of acute patients and 70.1% of chronic patients stated that they were 'improved'. Actual 'worsening' of their condition was reported by less than 4% of acute patients and less than 9% of chronic patients at any time point. Figure 1 shows the number of patients with available data at each data collection time point as well as the sources of missing data. The reasons for the smaller sample sizes at the 1 week, 1 month and 3 month data collection time points are two fold. First, there is a narrow window within which these telephone calls are allowed in this study (e.g. between days 6 and 8 for 1 week data). If patients are not able to be contacted after several attempts during the data collection window, missing data are recorded for that time point but these patients remain in the study. However, if a patient cannot be contacted for 3 consecutive time points, they are removed from the study, including their baseline data. Second, this is still an ongoing study with new patients recruited weekly in order to establish a large database for future research. Thus for several of the patients with baseline and 1 week follow-up data, the dates for the 1 and 3 month follow-up telephone calls were not yet reached in the data captured in this particular study.

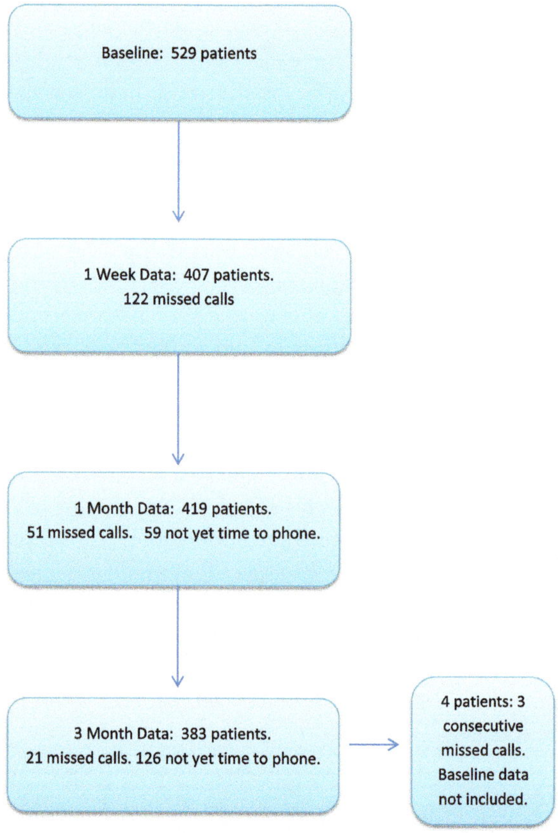

Figure 1 Flow chart of available patient data and source of missing data at each collection time point.

Table 2 Numerical rating scale (NRS) for pain and Bournemouth Questionnaire (BQ) baseline scores for acute and chronic patients

	Acute Baseline (N =272)	Chronic Baseline (N = 255)	p- Value
NRS neck	6.12 (±2.01)	5.5 (±2.29)	0.001*
NRS arm	2.28 (±2.20)	2.23 (±2.70)	0.838
BQ pain	5.91 (±2.34)	5.53 (±2.23)	0.06
BQ Disability in activities of daily living	4.81 (±2.86)	3.75 (±2.58)	0.0001*
BQ Disability in social activities	4.32 (±3.17)	3.03 (±2.95)	0.0001*
BQ Anxiety	5.41 (±2.88)	5.63 (±2.69)	0.366
BQ Depression	3.44 (±3.16)	3.41 (±3.04)	0.918
BQ Fear-avoidance beliefs	4.80 (±2.94)	4.43 (±2.93)	0.148
BQ Locus of control	4.80 (±2.94)	4.43 (±2.93)	0.091
BQ Total score	33.96 (±15.26)	30.50 (±14.18)	0.008*

Values are means (±SD). N = numbers of observations. * = p < 0.05.

Prognostic variables

Outcome at 1 Week

Univariate logistic regression analysis of potential predictors at baseline for improvement at 1 week for acute and chronic patients is shown in Table 3. No factors were associated with improvement for the acute patients and only 3 factors, namely the BQN pain and depression subscales as well as the total BQN score, were associated for improvement in the chronic patients. In view of a lack of strong association between baseline variables and early improvement at 1 week no further analysis was conducted.

Outcome at 1 Month

Univariate logistic regression analysis was also carried out to determine the unadjusted associations between

Table 3 Univariate logistic regression analysis of potential predictors at baseline for improvement at 1 week in acute and chronic patients

Predictor variable	Acute (N = 217)		Chronic (N = 190)	
	Unadjusted OR (95% CI)	p-value	Unadjusted OR (95% CI)	p-value
Gender (male)	0.84 (0.44 to 1.61)	0.61	0.85 (0.46 to 1.59)	0.62
*Age (higher)	0.99 (0.97 to 1.02)	0.60	1.00 (0.98 to 1.02)	0.87
Dizziness present	1.63 (0.24 to 1.69)	0.36	1.08 (0.48 to 2.41)	0.86
Radiculopathy present	1.69 (0.55 to 5.18)	0.36	0.53 (0.18 to 1.52)	0.24
Trauma	0.91 (0.32 to 2.59)	0.86	0.90 (0.40 to 2.06)	0.81
Previous episodes category (higher)	1.10 (0.50 to 2.42)	0.82	1.23 (0.65 to 2.35)	0.52
Taking medication	0.86 (0.44 to 1.66)	0.64	1.38 (0.71 to 2.68)	0.35
Paid employment	1.01 (0.41 to 2.51)	0.98	1.00 (0.76 to 1.33)	0.981
Smoke	1.11 (0.50 to 2.43)	0.80	1.78 (0.87 to 3.61)	0.12
In good health	1.22 (0.61 to 2.46)	0.57	1.08 (0.60 to 1.96)	0.79
*BQ Pain	0.98 (0.85 to 1.12)	0.73	**1.13 (0.99 to 1.29)**	**0.08**
*BQ Disability	1.06 (0.94 to 1.18)	0.35	1.09 (0.97 to 1.23)	0.15
*BQ Social disability	1.08 (0.98 to 1.19)	0.14	1.07 (0.96 to 1.19)	0.21
*BQ Anxiety	1.02 (0.91 to 1.14)	0.74	1.10 (0.98 to 1.24)	0.11
*BQ Depression	0.99 (0.89 to 1.10)	0.83	**1.12 (1.01 to 1.24)**	**0.03**
*BQ Fear avoidance beliefs	0.96 (0.85 to 1.07)	0.44	1.09 (0.98 to 1.21)	0.69
*BQ Locus of control	1.05 (0.94 to 1.18)	0.37	0.98 (0.88 to 1.09)	0.69
*BQ Total	1.01 (0.98 to 1.03)	0.64	**1.02 (1.00 to 1.04)**	**0.07**
*NRS Neck	1.02 (0.98 to 1.03)	0.79	1.03 (0.91 to 1.17)	0.65
*NRS Arm	0.96 (0.86 to 1.08)	0.48	0.99 (0.88 to 1.12)	0.92

*Continuous variables. BQ = Bournemouth Questionnaire. NRS = Numerical rating scale. OR = odds ratio (95% Confidence intervals). N = Number of observations.

baseline variables and 1 week outcomes with improvement at 1 month for the acute and chronic patients (Table 4). For the acute patients, six variables were associated with improvement at 1 month. These were the 'social disability' subscale, 'depression' subscale, PGIC at 1 week, the baseline to 1 week 'pain' subscale change score, the baseline to 1 week 'locus of control' subscale change score, and the baseline to 1 week NRS neck pain change score.

Only two variables in the univariate logistic regression analysis were associated with 1 month improvement for the chronic patients. These were being in paid employment and the PGIC score at 1 week.

The subsequent multivariate analysis for predictors of improvement at 1 month resulted in four variables independently associated with the outcome for the acute patients (Table 5). These were the PGIC at 1 week, baseline to 1 week NRS neck pain change score, baseline to 1 week BQ 'pain' subscale change score and the baseline 'depression' subscale score. Acute patients who reported significant improvement at 1 week on the PGIC were almost 3 times more likely to report improvement at 1 month. For every 1 point change (decrease) on the baseline to 1 week BQ 'pain' subscale score, acute patients were approximately 20% more likely to be improved at 1 month. For every 1 point change (decrease) in the baseline to 1 week NRS neck pain score, these patients were 36% more likely to be improved at 1 month. For every 1 point increase in the baseline 'depression' subscale score, acute patients were 16% less likely to report improvement at 1 month. This final model explained 21.7% of the variance in improvement at 1 month.

Only 1 factor, the PGIC at 1 week, remained independently predictive of improvement in chronic patients at 1 month. Patients improved at 1 week were approximately 4 times more likely to be improved at 1 month. However, the final model explained very little (12.7%) of the variance in improvement at 1 month.

Outcome at 3 months

Table 6 shows the univariate logistic regression analyses to determine the associations between baseline variables, 1 week outcomes and 1 month outcomes and improvement at 3 months for both acute and chronic patients. Sixteen variables were predictors of improvement for acute patients and eight variables for chronic patients.

In the subsequent multivariate model for improvement at 3 months, only two variables remained as independent predictors in the acute patients and one variable in

Table 4 Univariate logistic regression analysis of potential predictors at baseline and 1 week for improvement at 1 month in acute and chronic patients

Predictor variable	Acute (N = 215)		Chronic (N = 204)	
	Unadjusted OR (95% CI)	**p-value**	**Unadjusted OR (95% CI)**	**p-value**
Gender (male)	0.69 (0.32-1.51)	0.36	0.75 (0.42 to 1.35)	0.34
*Age (higher)	0.98 (0.95 to 1.01)	0.13	1.00 (0.98 to 1.02)	0.85
Dizziness present	1.54 (0.47 to 5.02)	0.47	1.02 (0.45 to 2.31)	0.96
Radiculopathy present	2.19 (0.49 to 9.78)	0.30	0.60 (0.25 to 1.44)	0.25
Trauma	0.74 (0.24 to 2.36)	0.62	1.29 (0.59 to 2.83)	0.52
Previous episodes category (higher)	1.18 (0.47 to 2.93)	0.73	1.31 (0.71 to 2.43)	0.39
Taking medication	1.76 (0.74 to 4.18)	0.20	1.04 (0.54 to 2.00)	0.40
Paid employment	0.90 (0.29 to 2.78)	0.85	**0.55 (0.27 to 1.13)**	**0.10**
Smoke	1.43 (0.51 to 3.98)	0.49	1.01 (0.50 to 2.03)	0.98
In good health	1.72 (0.76 to 3.90)	0.19	1.58 (0.89 to 2.81)	0.12
*BQ Pain	1.09 (0.83 to 1.28)	0.31	1.00 (0.89 to 1.13)	0.98
*BQ Disability	1.08 (0.94 to 1.24)	0.29	1.01 (0.90 to 1.13)	0.87
*BQ Social disability	**1.12 (0.98 to 1.27)**	**0.09**	1.07 (0.97 to 1.19)	0.18
*BQ Anxiety	0.97 (0.85 to 1.12)	0.69	1.06 (0.75 to 1.17)	0.31
*BQ Depression	**0.90 (0.80 to 1.01)**	**0.08**	0.96 (0.88 to 1.06)	0.42
*BQ Fear avoidance beliefs	1.05 (0.92 to 1.20)	0.51	1.03 (0.94 to 1.14)	0.52
*BQ Locus of control	1.08 (0.95 to 1.24)	0.25	0.96 (0.87 to 1.07)	0.46
*BQ Total	1.01 (0.98 to 1.04)	0.49	1.00 (0.98 to 1.02)	0.83
*NRS Neck	1.08 (0.90 to 1.30)	0.39	1.00 (0.88 to 1.13)	0.93
*NRS Arm	1.05 (0.90 to 1.22)	0.53	0.98 (0.89 to 1.09)	0.76
PGIC @ 1 week	**4.04 (1.63 to 10.07)**	**.003**	**4.60 (2.04 to 10.38)**	**.0001**
*Baseline: 1 Week BQ Pain Change Score	**1.14 (0.99 to 1.32)**	**0.08**	1.01 (0.88 to 1.15)	0.88
*Baseline:1 Week BQ Disability Change Score	1.09 (0.95 to 1.26)	0.23	0.99 (0.88 to 1.12)	0.90
*Baseline: 1 Week BQ Social disability Change Score	1.10 (0.95 to 1.28)	0.20	1.10 (0.98 to 1.25)	0.12
*Baseline: 1 Week BQ Anxiety Change Score	1.13 (0.96 to 1.32)	0.14	1.08 (0.93 to 1.25)	0.31
*Baseline: 1 Week BQ Depression Change Score	0.99 (0.85 to 1.16)	0.93	1.01 (0.90 to 1.14)	0.84
*Baseline: 1 Week BQ Fear avoidance beliefs Change Score	0.99 (0.86 to 1.16)	0.88	1.08 (0.96 to 1.22)	0.21
*Baseline: 1 Week BQ Locus of control Change Score	**1.12 (1.00 to 1.26)**	**0.05**	1.03 (0.94 to 1.13)	0.58
*Baseline: 1 Week BQ Total Change Score	1.02 (0.99 to 1.05)	0.13	1.01 (0.92 to 1.21)	0.43
*Baseline: 1 Week NRS Neck Change Score	**1.42 (1.14 to 1.77)**	**0.002**	1.06 (0.92 to 1.21)	0.43
*Baseline: 1 Week NRS Arm Change Score	1.12 (0.92 to 1.36)	0.27	0.95 (0.82 to 1.10)	0.49

*Continuous variables. BQ = Bournemouth Questionnaire. NRS = Numerical rating scale. OR = odds ratio (95% Confidence intervals). N = Number of observations. PGIC = Patient global impression of change scale.

the chronic patients (Table 7). The PGIC score at 1 week and the baseline to 1 month BQN total change score were independent predictors in acute patients and the PGIC at 1 month was the only predictor of improvement at 3 months in the chronic patients. Acute patients who reported being improved on the PGIC at 1 week were approximately 3 times more likely to be improved at 3 months. For every 1 point change (decrease) in the BQN baseline to 1 month total score, acute patients were 7% more likely to be improved at 3 months. Chronic patients who reported being improved on the PGIC at 1 month were 6 times more likely to be improved at 3 months. The models explained 28.8% and 19.9%% of the variance in outcome at 3 months for acute and chronic patients respectively.

Discussion

The predictors of improvement in acute and chronic neck pain patients undergoing chiropractic treatment appear to be very similar to those found for patients suffering from low back pain [18-25]. The most consistent predictor of improvement for both acute and chronic neck pain patients was reported prior improvement. Acute patients who reported being improved 1 week after the start of treatment were approximately 3 times more likely to be improved at 3 months while chronic

Table 5 Multivariate logistic regression analysis of prognostic predictors at baseline and at 1 week for improvement at 1 month in acute and chronic patients

	Coefficient	OR	95% CI	p-value	Sensitivity; Specificity; Percentage correctly predicted; Area under ROC (95% CI); Adjusted R^2
Acute N = 180					
BQ 5: Baseline Depression	−0.18	0.84	0.71 to 0.98	0.024	99.4%; 4.3%; 87.2%; 0.79 (0.70 to 0.88); 21.7%
Baseline to 1 Week BQ Pain change score	0.19	1.21	1.02 to 1.44	0.032	
Baseline to1 Week NRS Neck Change Score	0.31	1.36	1.10 to 1.75	0.017	
PGIC @ 1 Week	1.05	2.87	1.08 to 7.64	0.035	
Chronic N = 156					
PGIC @ 1 Week	1.48	4.41	1.95 to 9.96	0.001	100.0%; 0%; 67.3%; 0.66 (0.57 to 0.75); 12.7%

BQ = Bournemouth Questionnaire. NRS = Numerical pain rating scale. OR = odds ratio (95% Confidence intervals). N = Number of observations. PGIC = Patient global impression of change scale.

neck pain patients who reported being improved at 1 month were over 6 times more likely to also report improvement at 3 months.

Although the various demographic details collected at baseline in this study were largely not predictive of improvement at 1 week, 1 month or 3 months, it is important to emphasize two clinical conditions that were not predictive of a worse outcome. Thus neck pain patients who also had cervical radiculopathy (34 acute and 29 chronic patients) or who reported associated dizziness (51 acute and 64 chronic patients) improved as much as neck pain patients without these additional signs or symptoms. Previous studies on low back pain patients undergoing chiropractic treatment reported that the presence of additional leg pain was a negative predictor of improvement [25-27]. The Swiss chiropractors contributing patients to this current study were specifically informed prior to the start of data collection that the presence of arm pain alone was not sufficient to diagnose radiculopathy and that clinical signs of nerve root compression were also required. However, it was left up to the individual chiropractor to make this diagnosis based on clinical experience. There was no attempt to determine whether or not their diagnosis was correct. Swiss chiropractors have a significant amount of exposure to patients with radiculopathy in their mandatory two year post-graduate program and were therefore assumed competent in their diagnosis.

Acute neck pain sufferers (symptoms < 4 weeks) presented with higher levels of pain and disability compared to chronic patients (symptoms > 12 weeks), but improved more quickly and in a higher proportion than chronic patients. Although the acute patients did better than the chronic patients (in part due to the natural history of neck pain), it is important to point out that many of the chronic patients also improved. Additionally, the percentage of chronic patients reporting improvement continued to rise at each data collection time point whereas this appeared to level off at 1 month for acute patients. This study intentionally analyzed acute and chronic patients separately rather than including duration of neck pain into the prediction model. Previous research has already shown that duration of neck pain is a strong predictor of outcome [7] and it was particularly desired to assess the outcomes of chronic patients as they are the ones who are often more challenging and expensive to treat.

Although there was no significant age difference between the acute and chronic neck pain patients in this study, the chronic patients were significantly less likely to be in paid employment, reported significantly more prior episodes of neck pain and were less likely to be in good general health. The duration of symptoms and the number of previous episodes of neck pain have been found to be predictors of outcome in previous studies [7,8,14]. Surprisingly, this study did not find that the number of previous episodes of neck pain was linked with improvement as reported by Rubinstein et al. [7]. However, there was a difference between the Rubinstein et al. study and this current study in the way previous neck pain episodes were classified. This variable was dichotomized (yes/no) in the Rubenstien et al. study compared to categorizing previous episodes into one of three groups (none, 1–3, 4 or more) in this current study. It was hoped that providing more specific detail about the number of previous episodes would prove to be predictive of improvement. However, this was not the case. Also as reported in other studies, the majority of patients in this study were women, particularly in the chronic category [1,3]. This may be one reason why chronic patients were less likely to be in paid employment. Women, particularly with children, are less likely to work outside of the home in Switzerland compared to some other western countries [28].

Limitations

There are several limitations to this study. Although a high proportion of both acute and chronic neck pain patients improved at all time points, without a control group this improvement cannot be attributed to treatment. It is also

Table 6 Univariate logistic regression analysis of potential predictors at baseline, at 1 week and at 1 month for improvement at 3 months in acute and chronic patients

Predictor variable	Acute (N = 197)		Chronic (N = 185)	
	Unadjusted OR (95% CI)	**p-value**	**Unadjusted OR (95% CI)**	**p-value**
Gender (male)	1.31 (0.60-2.85)	0.50	0.63 (0.33 to 1.23)	0.18
*Age (higher)	0.98 (0.96 to 1.01)	0.29	1.00 (0.98 to 1.02)	0.99
Dizziness present	1.40 (0.42 to 4.65)	0.58	1.06 (0.42 to 2.67)	0.90
Radiculopathy present	0.89 (0.31 to 2.54)	0.82	1.34 (0.46 to 3.89)	0.59
Trauma	0.87 (0.36 to 2.12)	0.76	0.78 (0.34 to 1.82)	0.56
Previous episodes category (higher)	0.65 (0.30 to 1.39)	0.27	1.41 (0.71 to 2.78)	0.33
Taking medication	0.65 (0.30 to 1.39)	0.27	0.89 (0.4 to 1.82)	0.75
Paid employment	1.30 (0.45 to 3.75)	0.63	0.61 (0.28 to 1.34)	0.22
Smoke	1.88 (0.62 to 5.72)	0.27	0.96 (0.45 to 2.08)	0.93
In good health	1.42 (0.63 to 3.18)	0.40	0.74 (0.39 to 1.42)	0.37
*BQ Pain	0.98 (0.82 to 1.15)	0.77	1.00 (0.87 to 1.15)	0.98
*BQ Disability	1.10 (0.96 to 1.26)	0.18	1.05 (0.92 to 1.219)	0.49
*BQ Social disability	**1.13 (0.99 to 1.28)**	**0.06**	1.09 (0.97 to 1.22)	0.16
*BQ Anxiety	1.02 (0.89 to 1.17)	0.76	**1.12 (0.99 to 1.26)**	**0.08**
*BQ Depression	0.91 (0.81 to 1.02)	0.11	0.97 (0.88 to 1.08)	0.63
*BQ Fear avoidance beliefs	**1.14 (0.99 to 1.30)**	**0.07**	1.02 (0.91 to 1.14)	0.70
*BQ Locus of control	1.02 (0.89 to 1.17)	0.77	1.03 (0.91 to 1.15)	0.66
*BQ Total	1.01 (0.98 to 1.04)	0.47	1.01 (0.99 to 1.04)	0.37
*NRS Neck	1.09 (0.91 to 1.30)	0.36	1.02 (0.89 to 1.18)	0.73
*NRS Arm	**0.90 (0.79 to 1.02)**	**0.09**	1.901 (0.89 to 1.14)	0.93
PGIC @ 1 week	**3.61 (1.47 to 8.89)**	**0.005**	**3.37 (1.42 to 8.00)**	**0.006**
*Baseline: 1 Week BQ Pain Change Score	1.13 (0.96 to 1.32)	0.15	1.06 (0.91 to 1.24)	0.43
*Baseline: 1 Week BQ Disability Change Score	1.05 (0.91 to 1.21)	0.49	0.98 (0.85 to 1.13)	0.79
*Baseline:1 Week BQ Social Disability Change Score	1.06 (0.92 to 1.22)	0.42	0.99 (0.87 to 1.12)	0.83
*Baseline: 1 Week BQ Anxiety Change Score	1.06 (0.92 to 1.23)	0.42	1.12 (0.98 to 1.27)	0.11
*Baseline: 1 Week BQ Depression Change Score	0.89 (0.77 to 1.04)	0.14	1.09 (0.95 to 1.24)	0.21
*Baseline: 1 Week BQ Fear avoidance beliefs Change Score	**1.20 (1.02 to 1.40)**	**0.026**	0.98 (0.87 to 1.12)	0.81
*Baseline: 1 Week BQ Locus of control Change Score	1.06 (0.95 to 1.19)	0.29	1.00 (0.90 to 1.12)	0.96
*Baseline: 1 Week BQ Total Change Score	1.02 (0.99 to 1.05)	0.24	1.01 (0.98 to 1.05)	0.38
*Baseline: 1 Week NRS Neck Change Score	**1.25 (1.04 to 1.51)**	**0.02**	1.10 (0.87 to 1.17)	0.94
*Baseline: 1 Week NRS Arm Change Score	0.94 (0.79 to 1.12)	0.48	1.03 (0.87 to 1.22)	0.72
PGIC @ 1 Month	**3.94 (1.47 to 10.60)**	**0.007**	**5.82 (2.83 to 11.97)**	**0.001**
*Baseline: 1 Month BQ Pain Change Score	**1.30 (1.11 to 1.52)**	**0.001**	**1.22 (1.06 to 1.41)**	**0.006**
*Baseline: 1 Month BQ Disability Change Score	**1.41 (1.18 to 1.68)**	**0.001**	**1.15 (1.02 to 1.30)**	**0.02**
*Baseline:1 Month BQ Social Disability Change Score	**1.44 (1.22 to 1.71)**	**0.001**	1.06 (0.95 to 1.18)	0.33
*Baseline: 1 Month BQ Anxiety Change Score	**1.26 (1.09 to 1.46)**	**0.001**	**1.16 (1.04 to 1.30)**	**0.008**
*Baseline: 1 Month BQ Depression Change Score	**1.15 (0.99 to 1.33)**	**0.08**	1.05 (0.94 to 1.19)	0.40
*Baseline: 1 Month BQ Fear avoidance beliefs Change Score	**1.33 (1.14 to 1.55)**	**0.001**	1.04 (0.94 to 1.14)	0.49
*Baseline: 1 Month BQ Locus of control Change Score	**1.36 (1.16 to 1.60)**	**0.001**	**1.18 (1.07 to 1.30)**	**0.001**
*Baseline: 1 Month BQ Total Change Score	**1.08 (1.04 to 1.11)**	**0.001**	**1.03 (1.01 to 1.06)**	**0.004**
*Baseline: 1 Month NRS Neck Change Score	**1.30 (1.10 to 1.54)**	**0.002**	**1.18 (1.03 to 1.36)**	**0.02**
*Baseline: 1 Month NRS Arm Change Score	1.10 (0.93 to 1.31)	0.26	1.12 (0.94 to 1.33)	0.22

*Continuous variables. BQ = Bournemouth Questionnaire. NRS = Numerical rating scale. OR = odds ratio (95% Confidence intervals). N = Number of observations. PGIC = Patient global impression of change.

Table 7 Multivariate logistic regression analysis of prognostic predictors at baseline, at 1 week and at 1 month for improvement at 3 months

	Coefficient	OR	95% CI	p-value	Sensitivity; Specificity; Percentage correctly predicted; Area under ROC (95% CI); Adjusted R^2
Acute N = 146					
Baseline to 1 Month BQN total Change Score	0.66	1.07	1.03 to 1.11	0.001	97.6%; 35.0%; 89%; 0.82 (0.72 to 0.92); 28.8%
PGIC @ 1 Week	1.21	3.35	1.13 to 9.92	0.029	
ChronicN = 133					
PGIC @ 1 Month	1.80	6.04	2.76 to 13.69	0.001	77.9%; 63.2%; 73.7%; 0.71 (0.62 to 0.79); 19.9%

BQ = Bournemouth Questionnaire. PGIC = Patient global impression of change. N = number of observations.

acknowledged that the improvement for many of the acute patients was most likely due to natural history. In this study we collected baseline variables using paper questionnaires but subsequent outcomes were collected through telephone interviews. It has been shown that telephone interview data may have a slightly positive effect on outcomes encouraging patients to report more favorably [29-31]. An attempt was made to minimize this effect by employing anonymous research assistants, unknown to the patients, who collected the telephone data from the university rather than from the practice setting where the patient was being treated.

Data was also purposely not collected on specific treatments applied or frequency of chiropractic treatment. It would be interesting and important for the education of chiropractors to compare treatment and technique methods with patient outcomes in the future. Data was collected in this study on the date of the last treatment however, and this will be evaluated and reported when the 1 year outcomes data is assessed in the near future.

Another limitation to the study may be the validity of the Bournemouth Questionnaire to adequately measure the psychosocial domains such as depression, anxiety, etc. as these variables were not predictive of improvement at 3 months. However, when compared to the NPAD and NDI the BQ was much more sensitive to change on all domains [16], including the domains of anxiety, depression, fear avoidance and pain locus of control. Certainly 'depression' was identified as a negative predictor of improvement at 1 month in the multivariate analysis for acute patients which suggests that for depression, at least, the BQN is sensitive as a predictor of outcome.

A further limitation may be the fact that most of the variables that were not continuous variables were dichotomized into yes/no or present/absent with the exception of 'number of previous episodes' and 'general health'. This was done to facilitate the clinical utility of this study and assist in interpretation of the results. In most cases there was a straightforward yes/no (i.e. smoking, paid employment, etc.) answer. In those few variables where this was not the case, we used clinical experience to make the decision and it is fair to say that we may have made the wrong judgment on those two variables which were categorized with three options. This is the same model used in a similar research study done on low back pain patients however [18].

Although this study found that neither the presence of radiculopathy nor dizziness were negative predictors of outcome, no power analysis was done to determine whether the 115 patients with dizziness or the 63 patients with radiculopathy were adequate sample sizes to definitively draw these conclusions. However, at least for the dizziness patients, 115 is approximately one fifth of the total sample of 529 patients.

Previous research has identified 'stiffness' as a predictor of outcome (8) in neck pain patients treated with SMT. This was not included in the baseline evaluations done by the treating chiropractors and is therefore another limitation in this study.

The final possible limitation to this study may be the fact that compared to baseline there were fewer patients at the 1 and 3 month analyses. This was primarily due to the fact that it was not yet time for the 1 month and 3 month telephone calls for several patients. However, both the acute and chronic groups at 3 months had nearly 200 patients each. The first author of this study is directly in charge of large medical databases in two departments at this hospital. Experience of periodically calculating and monitoring pain scores, PGIC scores, proportions of patients improving or worsening with various treatments in these databases has consistently demonstrated that once a threshold of approximately 100 patients in a cohort is reached, additional patients make minimal difference in the statistical results calculated. Therefore this missing data is unlikely to have changed the outcomes with sample sizes this large. If outcome data was available for any of the follow-up time periods, the patient and their baseline data remained in this study.

Conclusions

For the most part, baseline variables were not predictive of outcome in neck pain patients and as a consequence prediction of outcome at 1 week was not possible using the potential predictors measured in this study. Instead, the most consistent predictor of improvement at both 1 and 3 months for both acute and chronic neck pain patients undergoing chiropractic treatment is significant self-reported improvement early on. Importantly, the co-existence of cervical radiculopathy or dizziness in addition to neck pain was not associated with a negative outcome for either acute or chronic patients.

Competing interests

The authors declare that they have no competing interests.

Authors' contributions

CP: Concept and design of the study, collection and entry of data, analysis and interpretation of data, drafting and revising the manuscript, final approval of the manuscript. JB: Concept and design of the study, data analysis and interpretation, revising the manuscript, final approval of the manuscript. BKH: Concept and design of the study, data analysis, revising the manuscript, final approval of the manuscript. All authors read and approved the final manuscript.

Acknowledgements

The authors thank the numerous Swiss chiropractors contributing patients for this study.

Author details

[1]University of Zürich and Orthopaedic University Hospital Balgrist, Forchstrasse 340, 8008 Zürich, Switzerland. [2]Anglo-European College of Chiropractic, 13-15 Parkwood Road, Bournemouth, England BH5 2DF, UK.

References

1. Fejer R, Kyvik KO, Hartvigsen J: **The prevalence of neck pain in the world population: a systematic critical review of the literature.** *Eur Spine J* 2006, **15**:834–848.
2. Vernon H, Humphreys K, Hagino C: **Chronic mechanical neck pain in adults treated by manual therapy: a systematic review of change scores in randomized clinical trials.** *J Manipulative Physiol Ther* 2007, **30**:215–227.
3. Hurwitz EL, Morgenstern H, Harber P, Kominski GF, Yu F, Adams AH: **A randomized trial of chiropractic manipulation and mobilization for patients with neck pain: clinical outcomes from the UCLA neck-pain study.** *Am J Public Health* 2002, **92**:1634–1641.
4. Vernon HT, Humphreys BK, Hagino CA: **A systematic review of conservative treatments for acute neck pain not due to whiplash.** *J Manipulative Physiol Ther* 2005, **28**:443–448.
5. Gross A, Miller J, D'Sylva J, Burnie SJ, Goldsmith CH, Graham N, Haines T, Brønfort G, Hoving JL: **Manipulation and mobilization for mechanical neck disorders.** *Man Ther* 2010, **15**:315–333.
6. Hemmilä HM: **Bone setting for prolonged neck pain: a randomized clinical trail.** *J Manipulative Physiol Ther* 2005, **28**:508–515.
7. Rubinstein SM, Knol DL, Lebouef-Yde C, de Koekkoek TE, Pfeifle CE, van Tulder MW: **Predictors of a favorable outcome in patients treated by chiropractors for neck pain.** *Spine* 2008, **33**:1451–1458.
8. Thiel HW, Bolton JE: **Predictors for immediate and global responses to chiropractic manipulation of the cervical spine.** *J Manipulative Physiol Ther* 2008, **31**:172–183.
9. Martínez-Segura R, Fernández-de-las Peñas C, Ruiz-Sáez M, López-Jiménez C, Rodríguez-Blanco C: **Immediate effects on neck pain and active range of motion after a single cervical high-velocity low-amplitude manipulation in subjects presenting with mechanical neck pain: a randomized controlled trial.** *J Manipulative Physiol Ther* 2006, **29**:511–517.
10. Evans R, Bronfort G, Nelson B, Goldsmith CH: **Two-year follow-up of a randomized clinical trial of spinal manipulation and two types of exercise for patients with chronic neck pain.** *Spine* 2002, **27**:2383–2389.
11. Thiel HW, Bolton JE, Docherty S, Portlock HC: **Safety of chiropractic manipulation of the cervical spine.** *Spine* 2007, **32**:2375–2378.
12. Rubinstein SM, Leboeuf-Yde C, Knol DL, de Koekkoek TE, Pfiefle CE, van Tulder MW: **The benefits outweigh the risks for patients undergoing chiropractic care for neck pain: a prospective, multicenter, cohort study.** *J Manipulative Physiol Ther* 2007, **30**:408–418.
13. Cassidy JD, Boyle E, Côté P, He Y, Hogg-Johnson S, Silver FL, Bondy SJ: **Risk of vertebrobasilar stroke and chiropractic care: results of a population-based case–control and case-crossover study.** *Spine* 2008, **33**:S176–183.
14. Tseng YL, Wang WTJ, Chen WY, Hou TJ, Chen TC, Lieu FK: **Predictors for the immediate responders to cervical manipulation in patients with neck pain.** *Manual Therapy* 2006, **11**:306–315.
15. Humphreys BK, Peterson CK, Muehlemann D, Haueter P: **Are Swiss Chiropractors so Different? Results from the Swiss Job Analysis Survey 2009.** *J Manipulative Physiol Ther* 2010, **33**:519–535.
16. Soklic M, Peterson CK, Humphreys BK: **Translation and validation of the German version of the Bournemouth questionnaire for neck pain.** *Chiropractic & Manual Therapies* 2012, **20**:2.
17. Fischer D, Stewart AL, Bloch DA, Lorig K, Laurent D, Holman H: **Capturing the patient's view of change as a clinical outcome measure.** *JAMA* 1999, **282**:1157–1162.
18. Peterson CK, Bolton J, Humphreys BK: **Predictors of improvement in acute and chronic low back pain patients undergoing chiropractic treatment.** *Accepted for publication J Manipulative Physiol Ther* 2012, April.
19. Malmqvist S, LeBoeuf-Yde C, Ahola T, Andersson O, Ekström K, Pekkarinen H, Turpeinen M, Wedderkopp N: **The Nordic back pain subpopulation program: predicting outcome among chiropractic patients in Finland.** *Chiropr Osteopat* 2008, **16**:13.
20. LeBoeuf-Yde C, Grønstvedt A, Borge JA, Lothe J, Magnesen E, Nilsson Ø, Røsok G, Stig LC, Larsen K: **The Nordic back pain subpopulation program: a 1-year prospective multicenter study of outcomes of persistent low-back pain in chiropractic patients.** *J Manipulative Physiol Ther* 2005, **28**:90–96.
21. LeBoeuf-Yde C, Grønstvedt A, Borge JA, Lothe J, Magnesen E, Nilsson Ø, Røsok G, Stig LC, Larsen K: **The Nordic back pain subpopulation program: demographic and clinical predictors for outcome in patients receiving chiropractic treatment for persistent low-back pain.** *J Manipulative Physiol Ther* 2004, **27**:493–502.
22. Lawrence DJ, Meeker W, Branson R, Bronfort G, Cates JR, Haas M, Haneline M, Micozzi M, Updyke W, Mootz R, Triano JJ, Hawk C: **Chiropractic management of low back pain and low back-related leg complaints: A literature synthesis.** *J Manipulative Physiol Ther* 2008, **31**:659–674.
23. Kongsted A, Leboeuf-Yde C: **The Nordic back pain subpopulation program – individual patterns of low back pain established by means of text messaging: A longitudinal pilot study.** *Chiropr Osteopat* 2009, **17**:11.
24. Kongsted A, Leboeuf-Yde C: **The Nordic back pain subpopulation program: Course patterns established through weekly follow-ups in patients treated for low back pain.** *Chiropr Osteopat* 2010, **18**:2.
25. Axén I, Rosenbaum A, Röbech R, Wren T, Leboeuf-Yde C: **Can patient reactions to the first chiropractic treatment predict early favorable treatment outcome in persistent low back pain?** *J Manipulative Physiol Ther* 2002, **25**:450–454.
26. Childs JD, Fritz JM, Flynn TW, Irrgang JJ, Johnson KK, Majkowske M, Delitto A: **A clinical prediction rule to identify patients with low back pain most likely to benefit from spinal manipulation: A validation study.** *Ann Intern Med* 2004, **141**:920–928.
27. Axén I, Jones JJ, Rosenbaum A, Lövgren PW, Halasz L, Larsen K, Leboeuf-Yde C: **The Nordic back pain subpopulation program: Validation and improvement of a predictive model for treatment outcome in patients with low back pain receiving chiropractic treatment.** *J Manipulative Physiol Ther* 2005, **28**:381–385.
28. Mandel H, Semyonov M: **A welfare state paradox: State interventions and women's employment opportunities in 22 countries.** *Am J of Sociology* 2006, **111**:1910–1949.
29. Hays RD, Kim S, Spritzer KL, Kaplan RM, *et al*: **Effects of mode and order of administration on generic health-related quality of life scores.** *Value Health* 2009, **12**:1035–1039.

30. Hanmer J, Hays RD, Fryback DG: **Mode of administration is important in US national estimates of health-related quality of life.** *Medical Care* 2007, **45**:1171–1179.
31. Power JR, Mishra G, Young AF: **Differences in mail and telephone responses to self-rated health: use of multiple imputation in correcting for response bias.** *Aust N Z J Public Health* 2005, **29**:149–154.

How do chiropractors manage clinical risk? A questionnaire study

Martin Wangler[1], Cynthia Peterson[2,3], Beatrice Zaugg[4], Haymo Thiel[5] and Rob Finch[6*]

Abstract

Background: The literature on chiropractic safety tends to focus on adverse events and little is known about how chiropractors ensure safety and manage risk in the course of their daily practice. The purpose of this study was to investigate how chiropractors manage potentially risky clinical scenarios. We also sought to establish how chiropractors perceive the safety climate in their workplace and thus whether there is an observable culture of safety within the profession.

Methods: An online questionnaire was designed to determine which of nine management options would be chosen by the respondent in response to four defined clinical case scenarios. Safety climate within the respondent's practice setting was measured by seeking the level of agreement with 23 statements relating to six different safety dimensions. 260 licensed chiropractors in Switzerland and 1258 UK members of The Royal College of Chiropractors were invited to complete the questionnaire. Questionnaire responses were analysed quantitatively in respect of the four clinical scenarios and the nine management options to determine the likelihood of each option being undertaken, with results recorded in terms of % likelihood. Gender differences in response to the management options for each scenario were evaluated using the Mann–Whitney U (MWU) test. Positive agreement with elements comprising each of the six safety dimensions contributed to a composite '% positive agreement' score calculated for each dimension.

Results: Questionnaire responses were received from 76% (200/260) of Swiss participants and 31% (393/1258) of UK members of The Royal College of Chiropractors. There was a general trend for Swiss and UK chiropractors to manage clinical scenarios where treatment appears not to be successful, not indicated, possibly harmful or where a patient is apparently getting worse, by re-evaluating their care. Stopping treatment and/or incident reporting to a safety incident reporting and learning system were generally found to be unlikely courses of action. Gender differences were observed with female chiropractors appearing to be more risk averse.

Conclusions: Swiss and UK chiropractors tend to manage potentially risky clinical scenarios by re-evaluating the case. The unlikeliness of safety incident reporting is probably due to a range of recognised barriers, although Swiss and UK chiropractors are positive about local communication and openness which are important tenets for safety incident reporting. The observed positivity towards key aspects of clinic safety indicates a developing safety culture within the Swiss and UK chiropractic professions.

Keywords: Chiropractic, Safety, Risk, Incident-reporting

* Correspondence: rob.finch@rcc-uk.org
[6]The Royal College of Chiropractors, Chiltern Chambers, St Peters Avenue, Reading RG4 7DH, UK
Full list of author information is available at the end of the article

Background

It stands to reason that chiropractors aim to ensure their patients experience a comfortable and hazard-free environment, and provide treatment modalities that are safe. But do chiropractors routinely implement safety measures when managing patients? Clinical situations where safety would be expected to be an issue include:

- Treating a patient when it is not indicated.
- Treating a patient when it is *contra*-indicated.
- Failing to refer to another healthcare provider when required.
- Undertaking inappropriate/failing to undertake appropriate diagnostic tests.
- Continuing treatment when the patient is not getting better.

Any of the above could lead to injury or an undesired reaction, so it is important to be mindful of the risk of these situations arising.

The literature on safety in relation to chiropractic tends to focus on adverse events [1], and while safety incident reporting programmes are now available to the chiropractic profession in some countries as an educational risk-management measure [2], little is known about how chiropractors routinely ensure safety and manage risk in the course of their daily practice.

Our aim in the study reported here was to investigate how chiropractors manage potentially risky clinical scenarios. We did this by determining how chiropractors in Switzerland and the UK, where we had ready access to a population of chiropractors of reasonable size, would handle a range of defined clinical scenarios. These scenarios were devised to prompt reflection on patient management in the context of the safety considerations listed above, including whether to stop treatment (for reasons of safety) and/or report to a safety incident reporting and learning system. We also sought to establish how chiropractors perceive the safety climate in their workplace.

Methods

Questionnaire design and data collection

An anonymous, two-part, online questionnaire was developed using SurveyMonkey®. The first part of the questionnaire was designed to determine how respondents would handle four defined clinical scenarios, designed by us to prompt reflection on typical safety considerations. The scenarios were designed to be plausible and realistic and we tested this by seeking the views of a group of 16 experienced chiropractors. After adjustment, the final questionnaire included the four scenarios with the respondent able to choose from nine management options, with multiple answers possible, and provision for adding free-text comments. The nine management options were themed around either continuing, pausing or stopping treatment. We were interested to determine what the respondents felt was appropriate, and to look for consensus, without making any judgements ourselves.

The second part of the questionnaire, which was based closely on the validated Medical Office Survey on Patient Safety [3], aimed to determine how positive respondents were towards six safety climate dimensions within their clinic.

To ensure compliance with the Helsinki Declaration, the questionnaire was submitted to the Cantonal Research Ethics Committee (KEK), Bern, where it was confirmed to be ethically unproblematic due to its anonymous nature. A permit was not required. Questionnaire responses were retained in a SurveyMonkey® account which was password-protected in order to ensure data security. Potential respondents were assured of the complete anonymity of their responses and the investigators' intention to publish the findings of their study. Submission of the completed questionnaire implied consent from the respondent.

The final version of the questionnaire listed the following four clinical scenarios:

1. A patient with non-specific low-back pain has not improved at all after 4–6 treatments.
2. A patient, who has a simple neck problem with no previous long-term problems, has now improved at least 80% and stayed at this level for a couple of weeks.
3. A patient returns from the last treatment with a new distal pain (e.g. sciatica when treated only for localized LBP, or brachialgia when treated only for local neck pain).
4. An elderly woman complains about immediate chest pain on inspiration after manual treatment directed to her thoracic spine.

The nine management options provided were as follows:

- I would re-evaluate the patient with a view to establishing a better diagnosis.
- I would send the patient for diagnostic imaging.
- I would change my treatment approach and use another technique.
- I would send the patient for a second opinion to another healthcare professional but keep on monitoring their condition.
- I would try a few times more.
- I would encourage the patient to continue the treatment until their spine is subluxation-free.

- I would stop treatment and monitor the patient regularly.
- I would stop the treatment, apologise and report the event to the chiropractic reporting and learning system.
- I would stop the treatment, but tell the patient that s/he is welcome to return if they feel the need.

Each of these management options had four different possible responses: 'never', 'unlikely', 'likely' and 'most likely'. Respondents were also invited to provide comments on their choice from which we were particularly interested to identify views and attitudes in relation to safety incident reporting.

The second part of the questionnaire measured the safety climate within the practice setting by seeking the level of agreement on a five-point scale, with the responses 'strongly disagree', 'disagree', 'neither agree nor disagree', 'agree' and 'strongly agree', with 23 statements relating to six different safety dimensions, as follows:

- Teamwork – helping out, relationships, respect, teamwork-emphasis.
- Work pressure – rushing, overwork, staff contingent, patient numbers.
- Staff training – in response to new processes, on-the-job, appropriateness of tasks.
- Process and standardisation – organisation, procedures, workflow, processes.
- Communication openness – ideas for improvement, alternative views, asking questions, voicing disagreement.
- Patient tracking/follow-up – reminders, documentation, reports, monitoring.

The questionnaire also included a section to enable collection of the following demographic data: gender, age, college of graduation, number of years in practice and practice setting (alone or with others) to provide an opportunity to explore differences among groups within the responding cohort.

The link to the finalised online questionnaire was emailed to all 260 licensed chiropractors in Switzerland and 1258 UK members of The Royal College of Chiropractors. These Swiss and UK groups are each known to have access to a national online safety incident reporting and learning system ('CIRLS' [4] and 'CPiRLS' [5] respectively).

Data analysis

The questionnaire responses were analysed quantitatively in respect of the four clinical scenarios and the nine management options described above. Management options identified as either 'most likely' or 'likely' by 75% or more of the respondents were arbitrarily designated, overall, as *likely* to be undertaken, and those options identified as either 'most likely' or 'likely' by 25% or fewer respondents were arbitrarily designated, overall, as *unlikely* to be undertaken. Thus, results were recorded in terms of '% likelihood'.

Positive agreement (strongly agree/agree with a positive statement or strongly disagree/disagree with a negative statement) with elements comprising each of the six safety dimensions contributed to a composite '% positive agreement' score calculated for each dimension. A score greater than 60%, but less than 75%, was arbitrarily considered to indicate that respondents were *moderately positive* about the given safety dimension. A score of 75% or more was arbitrarily considered to indicate that respondents were *highly positive* about the given safety dimension.

Demographic differences in the responses to the management options for each of the four clinical scenarios were explored using the Mann–Whitney U (MWU) test [6]; $P < 0.05$ was considered statistically significant. The mean scores and standard deviations (SD) were also calculated for each management decision in these groups. SPSS version 17.0 was used for this data analysis.

We made general observations in respect of apparent differences in the responses from Swiss and UK-based chiropractors but did not statistically analyse these differences. Demographic differences were explored using a combined dataset.

Results

Response rate and demographic characteristics of respondents

The questionnaire response rate was 76% (200/260) for Swiss participants and 31% (393/1258) for UK participants.

The demographic data collected is shown in Table 1. In summary, among the Swiss responders there were more male responders than females (70:30) whereas, among the UK responders, the cohort was almost equally divided by gender. The most common age group for responders from both countries was 41–50 years. More than 90% of UK chiropractors had graduated from a UK institution, while all but 0.5% of respondents practising in Switzerland had qualified in the USA or Canada. In comparison to their UK colleagues, a greater proportion of those practising in Switzerland work on their own.

Case scenarios

The likelihood of the nine clinical management options being undertaken in response to the four case scenarios is presented in Figures 1, 2, 3, and 4.

Scenario 1 (*a patient with non-specific low-back pain has not improved at all after 4–6 treatments),* suggests a case where treatment has not been successful. Figure 1 illustrates that under these circumstances:

Table 1 Demographic details of the Swiss and UK respondents

Respondent characteristics		Swiss respondents (n = 200)	UK respondents (n = 393)
Gender	Male	70.0%	47.6%
	Female	30.0%	52.4%
Age group	21-30 years	2.5%	20.9%
	31-40 years	30.5%	27.5%
	41-50 years	37.0%	31.0%
	51-60 years	22.0%	15.5%
	61 years or above	8.0%	5.1%
College of graduation	Anglo-European College of Chiropractic	0.5%	51.6%
	McTimoney College of Chiropractic	0.0%	18.8%
	Welsh Institute of Chiropractic	0.0%	21.1%
	Other (Europe)	0.0%	0.0%
	Other (USA/Canada)	99.5%	8.5%
Number of years in practice	1-2 years	2.0%	13.5%
	3-5 years	9.5%	15.9%
	5-10 years	22.5%	21.9%
	10+ years	66.0%	48.7%
Practice setting	On your own	48.5%	32.8%
	With other chiropractor(s)	49.5%	66.2%
	With other health care practitioners	15.0%	37.9%

- Swiss and UK chiropractors were likely to re-evaluate, send for imaging, and change the treatment approach.
- UK chiropractors were likely to refer to another healthcare professional.
- Both groups were unlikely to continue the treatment until the patient is subluxation-free.
- Both groups were unlikely to stop and then monitor regularly.
- Both groups were unlikely to stop to apologise and report to the incident reporting system.
- Swiss chiropractors were unlikely to stop and invite the patient to return as needed.

Additional comments highlighted that incident reporting may not be considered relevant in cases where there is a lack of progress (Table 2).

Scenario 2 *(a patient, who has a simple neck problem with no previous long-term problems, has now improved at least 80% and stayed at this level for a couple of weeks)* is a case where no further improvement is apparent. Figure 2 illustrates that under these circumstances:

- None of the management options suggested are categorised by our criteria as *likely* for either Swiss or UK chiropractors.
- Both groups were unlikely to stop to apologise and report to the incident reporting system.
- UK chiropractors were unlikely to try a few more times, or stop treatment and invite the patient to return as needed.

Again, additional comments highlighted that incident reporting may not be considered relevant in cases where there is a lack of progress (Table 2).

Scenario 3 *(a patient returns from the last treatment with a new distal pain (e.g. sciatica when treated only for localized LBP, or brachialgia when treated only for local neck pain)),* suggests the patient is getting worse following treatment. Figure 3 illustrates that under these circumstances:

- Swiss and UK chiropractors were likely to re-evaluate, send for imaging, and change the treatment approach.
- Both groups were unlikely to continue the treatment until the patient is subluxation-free.
- Both groups were unlikely to stop and invite the patient to return as needed.
- Both groups were unlikely to stop and then monitor regularly.
- Both groups were unlikely to stop to apologise and report to the incident reporting system.

Additional comments revealed differing views about the need to report such an incident, a perception that incident reporting is relevant only when the chiropractor is at fault, and also that incident reporting may not necessarily lead to cessation of treatment (Table 2).

Scenario 4 *(an elderly woman complains about immediate chest pain on inspiration after manual treatment directed to her thoracic spine),* suggests that treatment has caused injury. Figure 4 illustrates that under these circumstances:

- Swiss and UK chiropractors were likely to re-evaluate, and send for imaging.
- UK chiropractors were likely to refer to another healthcare professional.
- Swiss chiropractors were unlikely to continue the treatment until the patient is subluxation-free.
- Swiss chiropractors were unlikely to stop and invite the patient to return as needed.
- Both groups were unlikely to stop to monitor regularly.
- Both groups were unlikely to stop to apologise and report to the incident reporting system.

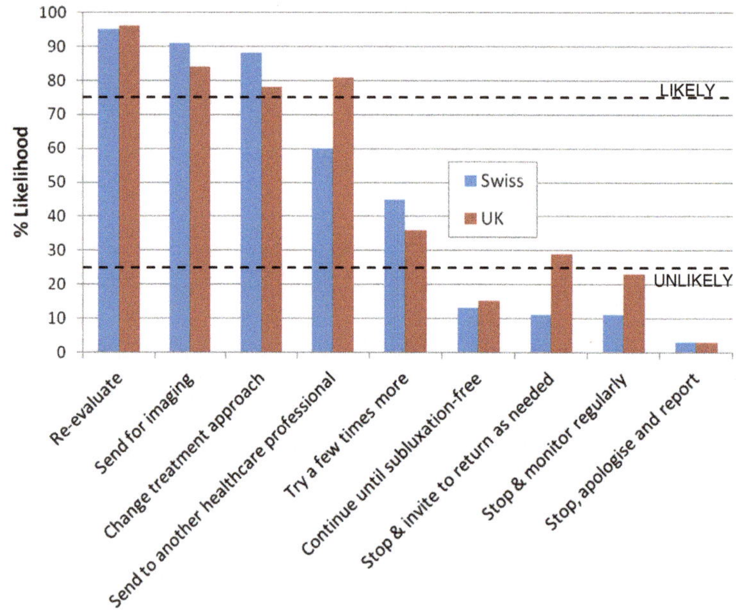

Figure 1 Clinical management options in response to case scenario 1. Likelihood of nine given clinical management options being followed in response to *Case Scenario 1: A patient with non-specific low-back pain has not improved at all after 4–6 treatments.* The dotted lines demarcate a region of the chart outside of which management options were arbitrarily designated as 'likely' (upper line) or 'unlikely' (lower line) to be undertaken. Thus, in this instance, Swiss and UK chiropractors are likely to re-evaluate, send for imaging, and change the treatment approach; UK chiropractors were likely to refer to another healthcare professional; both groups were unlikely to continue the treatment until the patient is subluxation-free, stop and then monitor regularly or stop to apologise and report to the incident reporting system; Swiss chiropractors were unlikely to stop and invite the patient to return as needed.

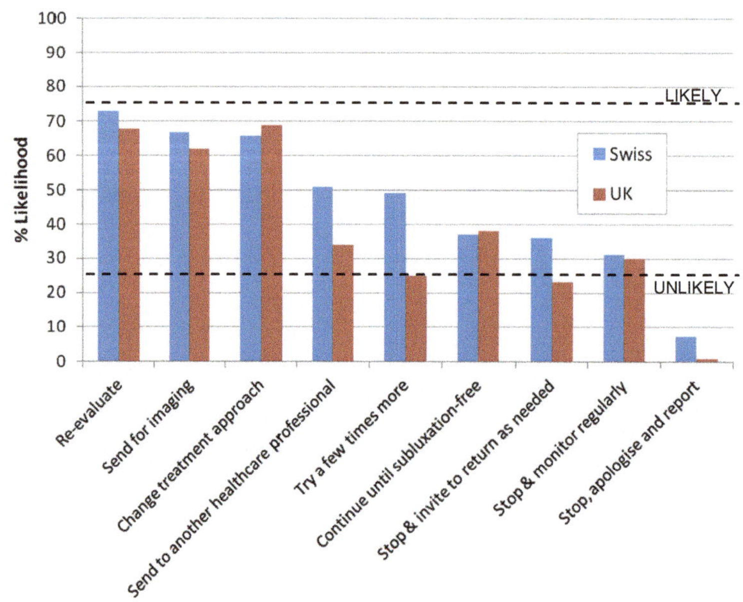

Figure 2 Clinical management options in response to case scenario 2. Likelihood of nine given clinical management options being followed in response to *Case Scenario 2: A patient, who has a simple neck problem with no previous long-term problems, has now improved at least 80% and stayed at this level for a couple of weeks.* The dotted lines demarcate a region of the chart outside of which management options were arbitrarily designated as 'likely' (upper line) or 'unlikely' (lower line) to be undertaken. In this instance, none of the management options were categorised by our criteria as *likely* by either Swiss or UK chiropractors; both groups were unlikely to stop to apologise and report to the incident reporting system; UK chiropractors were unlikely to try a few more times, or stop treatment and invite the patient to return as needed.

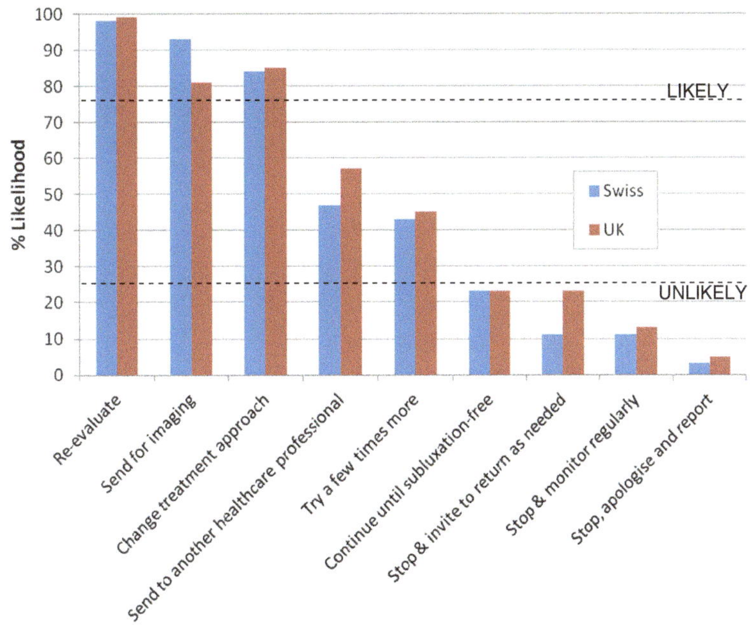

Figure 3 Clinical management options in response to case scenario 3. Likelihood of nine given clinical management options being followed in response to *Case Scenario 3*: *A patient returns from the last treatment with a new distal pain (e.g. sciatica when he was treated only for localized LBP, or brachialgia when he was treated only for local neck pain)*. The dotted lines demarcate a region of the chart outside of which management options were arbitrarily designated as 'likely' (upper line) or 'unlikely' (lower line) to be undertaken. In this instance, Swiss and UK chiropractors were likely to re-evaluate, send for imaging, and change the treatment approach; both groups were unlikely to continue the treatment until the patient is subluxation-free, stop and invite the patient to return as needed, stop and then monitor regularly or stop to apologise and report to the incident reporting system.

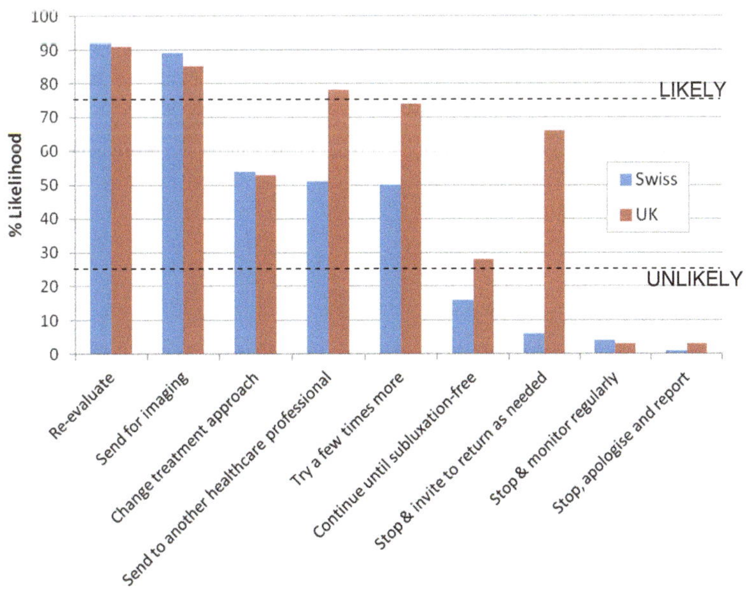

Figure 4 Clinical management options in response to case scenario 4. Likelihood of nine given clinical management options being followed in response to *Case Scenario 4*: *An elderly woman complains about immediate chest pain on inspiration after manual treatment directed to her thoracic spine*. The dotted lines demarcate a region of the chart outside of which management options were arbitrarily designated as 'likely' (upper line) or 'unlikely' (lower line) to be undertaken. Swiss and UK chiropractors were likely to re-evaluate, and send for imaging; UK chiropractors were likely to refer to another healthcare professional, Swiss chiropractors were unlikely to continue the treatment until the patient is subluxation-free; Swiss chiropractors were unlikely to stop and invite the patient to return as needed; both groups were unlikely to stop to monitor regularly or stop to apologise and report to the incident reporting system.

Table 2 Respondents' comments on incident reporting considerations in the context of the case scenarios indicated

Scenario 1. A patient with non-specific low-back pain has not improved at all after 4–6 treatments.	Scenario 2. A patient, who has a simple neck problem with no previous long-term problems, has now improved at least 80% and stayed at this level for a couple of weeks.
'It wouldn't have occured to me to report it to CPiRLS, in a case of - "not responded to treatment" unless they had had a reaction to treatment"	*'It makes no sense to me to stop treatment, apologise and report it to CPiRLS, which I consider more in the context of serious incidences and not lack of progress.'*
'There has been no incident why would one report to CPiRLS?'	
'Report to CPiRLS but continue'	
Scenario 3. A patient returns from the last treatment with a new distal pain (e.g. sciatica when treated only for localized LBP, or brachialgia when treated only for local neck pain).	**Scenario 4. An elderly woman complains about immediate chest pain on inspiration after manual treatment directed to her thoracic spine.**
'The case might possibly be considered to be material for CIRLS.'	*'I would still report it to the CPiRLS - but would continue with treatment, I don't feel they are mutually inclusive.'*
'I would report to CPiRLS if the exacerbation was significant and sustained, but would rarely apologise unless I was clearly at fault.'	*'I would report the event to CPiRLS but I would not apologise as this suggests I have done something wrong.'*
'I would only report to the CIRLS when I made a bad judgement or didn't access the findings properly.'	*'If it's only a broken rib, with no pulmonary complication, I would not think of reporting to CIRLS so far, but maybe in the future I will.'*
'I don't see reporting an incident on CPiRLS as necessarily being linked with stopping treatment.'	*'If (the patient's pain) is extreme, and would not get better within a few days, I would report it to the CIRLS. Otherwise I would not.'*
'I would be most likely to re-examine the patient and if I felt I was the most likely cause of the increase in symptoms I would report to CPiRLS'	

Additional comments revealed the view that incident reporting is only relevant in relatively extreme cases of injury or fault, and also that reporting does not necessarily lead to treatment being stopped (Table 2).

Demographic differences in respect of case scenario responses

When we explored combined data from the Swiss and UK groups across all four clinical case scenarios, we identified a significant difference in the management option "to re-evaluate the patient with a view to establishing a better diagnosis" between practitioners with one to two years in practice and those with over 10 years in practice [the less experienced practitioners had a mean score of 3.18 (SD = .79) and the more experienced clinicians had a mean score of 3.49 (SD = .71) (p = 0.014)]. No other statistically-significant differences were observed in respect of age, college of graduation, years in practice or practice-setting. However, we identified numerous statistically-significant differences, for combined Swiss and UK data, between males and females for some of the management decisions for Scenarios 1–4:

With Scenario 1 *(a patient with non-specific low-back pain has not improved at all after 4–6 treatments),* female practitioners were significantly more likely to:

- send the patient for diagnostic imaging.
- send the patient for a second opinion to another healthcare professional but keep on monitoring their condition (see Table 3).

With Scenario 2 *(a patient, who has a simple neck problem with no previous long-term problems, has now improved at least 80% and stayed at this level for a couple of weeks)*, female practitioners were significantly more likely to:

- re-evaluate the patient with a view to establishing a better diagnosis.
- send the patient for diagnostic imaging.
- change their treatment approach and use another technique.
- send the patient for a second opinion to another healthcare professional but keep on monitoring their condition.
- encourage the patient to continue the treatment until their spine is subluxation-free.
- stop the treatment, apologise and report the event to the chiropractic reporting and learning system (See Table 4).

Table 3 Significant gender differences in management decisions for scenario 1 *(a patient with non-specific low-back pain has not improved at all after 4–6 treatments)*

Management choice	Males mean (SD)	Females mean (SD)	P value
"I would send the patient for a second opinion to another healthcare professional but keep on monitoring their condition"	3.01 (.73)	3.24 (.74)	0.003
"I would send the patient for diagnostic imaging"	3.02 (.70)	3.24 (.66)	0.003

Table 4 Significant gender differences in management decisions for scenario 2 *(a patient, who has a simple neck problem with no previous long-term problems, has now improved at least 80% and stayed at this level for a couple of weeks)*

Management choice	Males mean (SD)	Females mean (SD)	P value
"I would encourage the patient to continue the treatment until their spine is subluxation free"	1.92 (.97)	2.23 (.95)	0.002
"I would change my treatment approach and use another technique"	2.76 (.80)	3.03 (.78)	0.002
"I would re-evaluate the patient with a view to establishing a better diagnosis."	2.74 (.81)	2.98 (.79)	0.01
"I would send the patient for a second opinion to another health care professional but keep on monitoring their condition."	2.13 (.68)	2.30 (.73)	0.04
"I would send the patient for diagnostic imaging."	2.01 (.69)	2.21 (.72)	0.03
"I would stop the treatment, apologize and report the event to the chiropractic reporting and learning system"	1.38 (.49)	1.52 (.54)	0.03

With Scenario 3 (*a patient returns from the last treatment with a new distal pain (e.g. sciatica when treated only for localized LBP, or brachialgia when treated only for local neck pain)*), female practitioners were significantly more likely to:

- change their treatment approach and use another technique.
- send the patient for a second opinion to another healthcare professional but keep on monitoring their condition.
- encourage the patient to continue the treatment until their spine is subluxation-free (See Table 5).

With Scenario 4 (*an elderly woman complains about immediate chest pain on inspiration after manual treatment directed to her thoracic spine*), female practitioners were significantly more likely to stop the treatment, but tell the patient that they are welcome to return if they feel the need (Table 6).

No specific management options were identified where male practitioners were significantly more likely to agree than females.

Safety dimensions

The level of agreement of respondents with respect to the six safety dimensions measured is shown in Figure 5. This illustrates that:

- Swiss and UK chiropractors were highly positive about teamwork and work pressure as they relate to safety culture.
- Swiss chiropractors were highly positive about staff training, process and standardisation, and communication openness as they relate to safety culture.
- Swiss chiropractors were moderately positive about patient tracking/following-up as it relates to safety culture.
- UK chiropractors were moderately positive about staff training, process and standardisation, communication openness and patient tracking/following-up as it relates to safety culture.

Discussion

Case scenarios

For the case scenarios presented, there was a general trend that chiropractors were *unlikely* to stop treatment but were *likely* to re-evaluate, reflect on the diagnosis and alter the treatment approach.

For Scenario 1, where improvement has not been achieved after 4–6 treatments, some practitioners opted to cease treatment. However, there is a strong case to continue here despite the apparent lack of progress since NICE evidence-based guidance recommends up to 9 treatments over 12 weeks for persistent, non-specific low-back pain [7]. Reporting this scenario as a safety

Table 5 Significant gender differences in management decisions for scenario 3 *(a patient returns from the last treatment with a new distal pain (e.g. sciatica when treated only for localized LBP, or brachialgia when treated only for local neck pain)*

Management choice	Males mean (SD)	Females mean (SD)	P value
"I would encourage the patient to continue the treatment until their spine is subluxation free"	1.72 (.90)	1.93 (.90)	0.03
"I would change my approach and use another technique"	3.03 (.67)	3.21 (.71)	0.01
"I would send the patient for a second opinion to another healthcare professional but keep on monitoring their condition"	2.52 (.69)	2.78 (.72)	0.001

Table 6 Significant gender differences in management decisions for scenario 4 *(an elderly woman complains about immediate chest pain on inspiration after manual treatment directed to her thoracic spine)*

Management	Males mean (SD)	Females mean (SD)	P value
"I would send the patient for a second opinion to another healthcare professional but keep on monitoring their condition"	2.91 (.88)	3.21 (.82)	0.003
"I would send the patient for diagnostic imaging"	3.21 (.81)	3.43 (.71)	0.011
"I would stop the treatment, but tell the patient that she is welcome to return if she feels the need"	1.95 (.87)	2.20 (.82)	0.02

incident was found to be an unlikely course of action and two comments highlighted that such a case is not viewed as one that would prompt an incident report. However, one respondent commented that they would report the incident and also continue treatment. This revealed an attitude which recognises that harm and blame are not necessary triggers for an incident report, and perhaps that sharing an apparent lack of treatment success with colleagues may have learning value. We recognise the need for practitioners to be clear about what is meant by 'safety incident' and what should be reported; an issue that has been clearly identified by others as a barrier to incident reporting [8]. However, as far as CPiRLS and CRLS are concerned, there is guidance but no rules about what does and does not constitute a reportable incident. Use of these systems as general learning and care improvement tools is to be encouraged, particularly during a period when chiropractic incident reporting is a relatively new process and still becoming integrated into usual practice.

Scenario 4 suggested rib injury, such as a fracture or costo-chondral sprain, with osteoporosis as a possible risk factor. There is a strong argument for such an incident to be reported because patient injury occurred and because reflection on the detailed circumstances of the case, shared with colleagues, might serve to minimise the risk of such an occurrence happening elsewhere. However, incident reporting was found to be an unlikely option and comments revealed that this may be due to a perceived connection of reporting with guilt and error, as has been identified with other healthcare reporting initiatives [8], or only warranted in extreme cases. UK chiropractors appeared more likely to refer the patient in this case. This was presumably in the context of the injury rather than the original complaint since they also appeared much more likely to stop treatment and invite

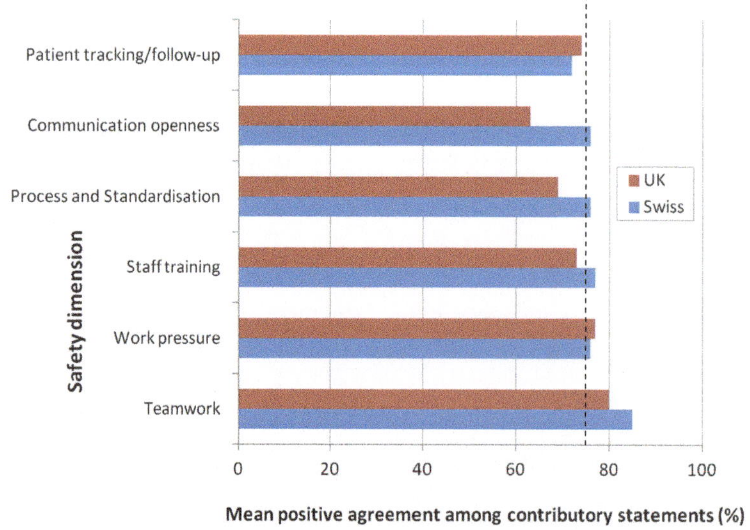

Figure 5 Agreement with safety dimensions. Degree of positive agreement among respondents with respect to six safety dimensions. A score greater than 60% but less than 75% was arbitrarily considered to indicate that respondents were moderately positive about the given safety dimension. A score of 75% (indicated by the dotted line), or greater, was arbitrarily considered to indicate that respondents were highly positive about the given safety dimension. Thus, it was established in this study that Swiss chiropractors were moderately positive about patient tracking/follow-up, and highly positive about all other safety dimensions. UK chiropractors were highly positive about work pressure and teamwork and moderately positive about all other safety dimensions.

the patient to return as needed. This was supported by the comment:

> 'In this scenario I would re-exam and most likely refer her back to her GP for further examination/diagnostic imagery. Treatment would stop until the results were in. Treatment would then commence depending on these results, perhaps this area would either be left or Activator technique utilised. Other areas of complaint would continue to be treated.'

Gender differences in respect of case scenario responses

The fact that men and women have differing perceptions of risk is well documented with women having a lower propensity towards risky choices in most domains of life [9]. It is perhaps not surprising, therefore, that we identified gender differences in chiropractors' management of potentially risky clinical scenarios. In our study, female chiropractors were more likely to refer patients for another opinion, and hence mitigate for risk, in three of the four scenarios. They were also more likely to stop treatment in two of the scenarios. However, interestingly, only in the case of Scenario 2 were they were more likely to report the incident to CPiRLS/CRLS. This may suggest that incident reporting is not viewed as an effective risk reduction measure; a finding observed in other studies [8].

Safety dimensions

Our questionnaire also prompted chiropractors to reflect on safety culture and it was encouraging to note the positivity towards all workplace safety culture dimensions. Communication openness and professional collaboration are known to help prevent critical incidents [10] so the fact that Swiss respondents were highly positive and UK respondents moderately positive about communication openness, and both groups were highly positive about teamwork, bodes well. Respondents' comments highlighted a number of contributory factors important for patient safety in the clinic environment, for example:

> 'Regular meeting with the whole team helps to keep up with the quality and safety'.

However, some respondents also highlighted the fact that a high proportion of chiropractors (33% of UK respondents and 48% of Swiss respondents in our study) work alone, limiting opportunities for fostering a safety culture through activities such as teamwork.

Limitations and further study

Caution should be exercised when drawing general conclusions about the UK chiropractic profession from the findings presented in this article since the response rate of 31% means the respondent group may not comprise a representative sample. We did not investigate, further, the reasons for this low response rate.

While we determined the demographic characteristics of the respondents, we do not know how well these characteristics represent those of the entire chiropractic populations in Switzerland and the UK.

While there were some apparent differences between respondents from Switzerland and those from the UK, we did not statistically analyse these possible differences.

Further studies specifically designed to investigate the attitudes towards and the barriers to using online chiropractic safety incident reporting and learning systems are now required in order to develop measures to increase participation.

Conclusions

- This study prompted chiropractors to reflect on aspects of clinical risk.
- Swiss and UK chiropractors tend to manage potentially risky clinical scenarios by re-evaluating their care and changing their approach.
- Safety incident reporting to an online system is currently an unlikely course of action, probably due to previously recognised barriers, although Swiss and UK chiropractors are positive about local communication and openness which are important tenets for safety incident reporting.
- Barriers to the use of safety incident reporting systems need to be addressed in order to encourage wider use of the existing systems.
- A significant proportion of Swiss and UK chiropractors practice in a single-handed environment. We suggest that single-handed practitioners have most to gain from participation in a national safety incident reporting and learning system.
- Female chiropractors appear to be more risk-averse than male chiropractors.
- Positivity towards key aspects of clinic safety indicate a developing safety culture within the Swiss and UK chiropractic professions.

Competing interests

The authors declare that they have no competing interests.

Authors' contributions

MW instigated this study and designed the first draft of the questionnaire. All authors provided general expertise on the topic and critical comments on the draft questionnaire. MW collected the questionnaire data and collated the findings, CP advised on and undertook the statistical analysis and RF drafted the manuscript. All authors reviewed the manuscript, provided critical comments and approved the final version. All authors read and approved the final manuscript.

Author details
[1]European Academy of Chiropractic, Bahnhofstrasse 15, CH-3400 Burgdorf, Switzerland. [2]University of Zürich and Orthopaedic University Hospital Balgrist, Forchstrasse 340, 8008 Zürich, Switzerland. [3]Swiss Academy for Chiropractic, Sulgenauweg 38, 3007 Bern, Switzerland. [4]ChiroSuisse, Eidgenössische Prüfung Chiropraktik, Johann-Verresisus Strasse 18, CH-2502 Biel, Switzerland. [5]Anglo-European College of Chiropractic, 13-15 Parkwood Road, Bournemouth BH5 2DF, UK. [6]The Royal College of Chiropractors, Chiltern Chambers, St Peters Avenue, Reading RG4 7DH, UK.

References

1. Gouveia LO, Castanho P, Ferreira JJ: **Safety of chiropractic interventions: a systematic review.** *Spine* 2009, **34**(11):E405–E413.
2. Thiel H: **Incident reporting and learning systems for chiropractors – developments in Europe.** *J Can Chiropr Assoc* 2011, **55**:155–158.
3. Sorra J, Franklin M, Streagle S: **Survey user's guide: medical office survey on patient safety culture.** *AHRQ Publication* 2008, **08**(09):0059.
4. Wangler M, Zaugg B: *Promotion of Patient Safety Competence among Licensed Chiropractors: Four Instructional Approaches*, MME Thesis. Switzerland: University of Berne; 2008. http://www.mme-alumni.uzh.ch/masterthesen/thesen_anzeige.php?ID=70&sprache=de.
5. Finch RP, Bolton J, Cunliffe C, Jay TC, Thiel HW, Webster M, Connor C: **Development of CPiRLS: the future of patient safety incident reporting and learning in the UK [abstract].** In *Proceedings of the World Federation of Chiropractic Congress.* Montreal; 2009.
6. Mann HB, Whitney DR: **On a test of whether one of two random variables is stochastically larger than the other.** *Ann Math Stat* 1947, **18**:50–60.
7. National Institute for Health and Clinical Excellence (NICE, UK): *Early management of persistent non-specific low back pain - CG88.* London: National Institute for Health and Clinical Excellence; 2009.
8. Pfeiffer Y, Manser T, Wehner T: **Conceptualising barriers to incident reporting: a psychological framework.** *Qual Saf Health Care* 2010, **19**:e60.
9. Harris CR, Jenkins M, Glaser D: **Gender differences in risk asssessment: why do women take fewer risks than men?** *Judgment and Decision Making* 2006, **1**:48–63.
10. Taylor-Adam S, Vincent C: *Systems analysis of clinical incidents: the London protocol, 2004.* London: Clinical Safety Research Unit, Imperial College London, Department of Surgical Oncology and Technology. Clinical Safety Research Unit; 2004.

10

The Five Eras of Chiropractic & the future of chiropractic as seen through the eyes of a participant observer

J Keith Simpson

Abstract

Chiropractic has endured a turbulent history, marked by tremendous advances in areas such as education and licensing while marred by interprofessional conflict and a poor public image. The prolonged interprofessional conflict was instrumental in shaping the culture of chiropractic. These obstacles have long-since been removed although there are lingering effects from them.

This article examines the chiropractic profession's history by dividing it into five Eras and suggests that there are three options available for the future of the profession. One: maintaining the status quo. Two: uniting under an evidence based scientific approach as partners in the health care delivery system that has buried the "one-cause, one-cure" sacred cow. The steps required to achieve this outcome are outlined. Three: openly dividing the profession into evidence based practitioners and subluxation based practitioners. Adopting this option would allow each branch of the profession to move forward in the health care delivery system unhindered by the other.

It is unclear which option the profession will choose and whether the profession is mature enough to follow option two remains to be seen. What is evident is that the time to act is now.

Background

This article is based on the second FG Roberts Memorial Lecture, delivered by the author at the Annual Conference of the Chiropractic & Osteopathic College of Australasia, Melbourne, Australia 2011.

In the initial FG Roberts Memorial Lecture and the subsequent paper, Dr Reggars recounted some of the many accomplishments that the chiropractic profession has achieved over the past 30 years and how the changes have impacted on chiropractic and the chiropractic profession [1].

This paper reviews the origins of chiropractic from the unregulated 19th century health care system in the United States of America and its frequently turbulent journey into the 21st century. It is the author's contention that the culture of chiropractic as it stands is for a large part the result of external forces and that unless and until the profession recognizes how these forces have influenced its development, progression of chiropractic into the 21st century health care system will not occur. Whilst some within the profession may consider this to be a good thing, it will be argued that the survival of the profession hinges upon its acceptance of science and seizing upon the tremendous opportunity ahead.

The author came into chiropractic with an exercise physiology background and graduated from Canadian Memorial Chiropractic College in 1982 with no understanding of 'The Big Idea' [2]. Following 24 years in private practice, a PhD in sociology and 7 more years in chiropractic academia, the author still wonders what all the fuss is about, but certainly recognizes the difficulties that The Big Idea has presented [3].

Discussion

For the purpose of debate, the history of the profession will be divided into five distinct and at times overlapping eras:

1. The Era of Free trade in Medicine: 1860 ~ 1900
2. The Era of Prosecution: 1900 ~ 1950
3. The Era of Persecution: 1920 ~ 2000
4. The Era of Legitimation: 1960 - present
5. The Era of Opportunity: 2000 - present

Correspondence: k.simpson@murdoch.edu.au
School of Chiropractic & Sports Science Murdoch University, Perth, Australia

The Era of Free Trade in Medicine (1860 - 1900)

Chiropractic emerged out of what is recognized as The Era of Free Trade in Medicine (1860-1900). This was a time when all and sundry could ply their trade because there was no legislation governing health care in the United States of America [4,5].

Three predominant groups of "healers" were represented in the first half of the 19th century:

1. Orthodox medicine (physicians), whose principal treatment methods included bloodletting, blistering, purgatives (massive doses of compounds of mercury, antimony and other mineral poisons) and tonics (arsenical compounds);
2. Thomsonian/eclectics, whose principal treatment methods were botanical remedies, steam baths and rest; and
3. Homeopaths, whose principal treatment methods were homeopathic remedies, fresh air, sunshine, bed rest, proper diet, and personal hygiene [6].

Health care provision was not limited to members of these three groups however. This was also the time of the 'isms':

- Spiritualism
- Vitalism
- Mesmerism
- Mysticism

Add to the mix Christian Scientists, magnetic healers and manual therapists (osteopaths, chiropractors, bone setters) and we begin to appreciate the health care landscape of the time. It is noteworthy that, during this deregulated period, the United States became one of the healthiest nations in the world, boasting the world's lowest infant mortality rate [7]. This came about largely as a result of the work of a non-medical practitioner, Lemuel Shattuck. Shattuck's 1850 Report to the Sanitary Commission of Massachusetts has been hailed as one of the most significant documents in the history of public health and ultimately led to widespread adoption of public health and sanitation measures that were responsible for saving thousands of lives [8,9]. From within this prescientific era [10], chiropractic emerged in 1895 as an empirical "health science" interested in the spine and its possible relationship to disease states [11,12]. It is important to remember that chiropractic was not the only group interested in the notion of spinal irritation (aka: rachialgia) and that this was a very controversial subject [13,14].

The Era of Free Trade in Medicine gave way to the Golden Age of Medicine and The Golden Age of Scientific Advancement (1890 - 1950). Because chiropractic was heavily influenced by both of these Golden Ages, they will be considered briefly.

The Golden Age of Scientific Advancement largely drove the Golden Age of Medicine.

These ages brought with them what were considered miraculous medical breakthroughs, including vaccination and antibiotics. There were dramatic declines in the mortality rate for infectious diseases as well as increases in expected lifespan. No disease seemed incapable of being defeated by science. The medical profession enjoyed the benefits of these advancements with rapid progression to the top of the professional hierarchy and a concomitant increase in cultural authority [15,16].

This was also the era of medical education reform, which saw a science-based curriculum introduced concomitant with university affiliation as directed by the Flexner Report [17]. The American Medical Association's Medical Education Committee promoted the Flexner Report to the 168 institutions providing 'medical' education. Schools that agreed to adopt the Flexner recommendations received generous funding via the Rockefeller Foundation while schools that did not assent, simply ceased operation due to lack of funding. The result was that, by 1930, only 76 of the 168 medical schools remained [15]. In this manner, virtually all healing arts other than allopathic medicine were effectively eliminated, and the number of new medical graduates entering the profession was dramatically reduced from over 5440 per year to 3536 [15].

In part because of the rejection of science by a significant element within the chiropractic profession [18], and in part because the Flexner Report dismissed the chiropractors as "unconscionable quacks who should be dealt with by the public prosecutor and the grand jury" [17], the chiropractic profession bypassed the era of educational reform.

With Flexner's simple phrase, the chiropractic profession found itself mired in The Era of Prosecution, which was closely overlapped by The Era of Persecution.

The Era of Prosecution: 1900 ~ 1950

Practically from its very origins in 1895, the chiropractic profession was in conflict with allopathic medicine [19]. The relationship between political medicine and chiropractic was described by Scotton as a "holy war between the forces of good and evil"[20] and Carter [21] referred to "the libel and slander campaign of dirty tricks" when describing political medicine's dealings with the chiropractic profession.

The Era of Prosecution began in 1902, less than a decade after Daniel David Palmer (DD) 'discovered' chiropractic. DD was charged with practising medicine without a licence in 1902 and 1903, however the charges were either dismissed, or the prosecution simply did not proceed [22]. In 1906, DD was the first chiropractor jailed following his conviction for practising medicine without a licence. He was fined $350.00 plus court costs, and incarcerated until the fine was paid. After serving 23 days, DD paid the fine and was released [23].

In the first thirty years of the chiropractic profession's existence, there were more than 15,000 prosecutions, about 20 percent of which resulted in incarceration [24]. In fact, "Go to jail for chiropractic" was the advice given to members of the Federated Chiropractors of California, and the Alameda County (California) Chiropractors' Association deemed it mandatory for its members to go to jail rather than pay a fine if convicted for practising medicine without a license [12]. On one occasion there was a mass arrest of 100 chiropractors in New York City [25]. In 1921 alone, 450 of the 600 California chiropractors chose jail over a fine following convictions for practising medicine without a licence [26] and such prosecutions continued well past mid-century [27].

With DD's conviction, his son, BJ Palmer, determined that a means of defending the profession was required and the Universal Chiropractor's Association (UCA) was founded, primarily as a protective association for all chiropractors. Shortly after its formation, the UCA officially condemned the "mixer" policies of the American Chiropractic Association, a rival association that had been formed by Langworthy in 1922 [28]. The condemnation was significant because, in a strictly pragmatic legal move, the UCA's legal counsel used Langworthy's textbook, *Modernized Chiropractic*, and the paradigm espoused therein, as the basis for successfully defending chiropractors charged with practising medicine without a licence [28].

The UCA's first case was the defence of Shegataro Morikubo, a graduate of the Palmer School and Infirmary of Chiropractic, who was charged in 1907 with the unlicensed practice of medicine, surgery and osteopathy. Upon learning of Morikubo's indictment, BJ Palmer travelled to Lacross, Wisconsin where the case was to be heard, and hired State Senator Tom Morris, LL.B., senior partner in the law firm of Morris and Hartwell, for the defence of Morikubo. The first step in the defence was to suggest to the prosecution that, because Morikubo had neither used any surgical procedure nor prescribed or used any drugs, the trial should be limited to the unlicensed practice of osteopathy. The prosecutor agreed and the trial proceeded on the sole charge of unlicensed practice of osteopathy. In presenting the defence arguments, Morris used *Modernized Chiropractic*, which stated that chiropractic had a separate and distinct philosophy and practice that was unlike any other method of treatment. He reinforced this argument by calling several witnesses, including practitioners trained in both osteopathy and chiropractic. Following a 30-minute deliberation, Morikubo was unanimously acquitted [29].

Using similar tactics, Morris oversaw the defence of more than 3300 chiropractors, with a win rate approaching 90 percent [28]. The Morris defense strategy was as simple as it was effective. It involved four clear concepts:

1. Chiropractic is <u>not</u> medicine; chiropractic has a "separate and distinct philosophy and practice".
2. Chiropractors do not diagnose, but analyze the spine for the cause of dis-ease.
3. Chiropractors do not "treat," but adjust the spine for the cause of dis-ease.
4. The Chiropractic profession has been built upon success in cases where medical doctors failed [28].

Morris has been acknowledged as the architect of "chiropractic philosophy" because of his demonstration of how to use chiropractic theories or philosophy in the courtroom to defend against charges of the unlicensed practice of medicine. In recognition of this, he was awarded the first "Philosopher of Chiropractic" (PhC) degree from BJ Palmer's chiropractic school in 1907 [30]. Following Morris' success in the Morikubo case, BJ Palmer embraced "chiropractic philosophy" with evangelical zeal, and thus the courtroom experience of Morikubo became a powerful determinant of the chiropractic profession's development [29].

It is noteworthy that the above interpretation has been questioned. Peters and Chance contend that Morikubo himself established the defense used by Morris [31]. It is clear that Morikubo and Morris consulted prior to the trial, and considering the recognition afforded Morris, it seems likely that Morris was the originator of the defense strategy used, and most certainly the record shows that he used it repeatedly and with great success.

Wardwell considered the Morikubo case the "third major event in chiropractic history", again because this was the point at which BJ Palmer began his "straight philosophical journey"[32]. During this journey, the chiropractic community developed and embraced a distinct lexicon and rationale toward health and its maintenance in order to emphasise the difference between medicine and chiropractic [33]. Thus the "philosophy of chiropractic" became "an unyielding dogma" [30].

The Era of Persecution: 1920 - 2000

This Era began shortly after the Era of Prosecution and can be divided into an informal and a formal era.

Dr Morris Fishbein was labelled the "Medical Mussolini" and described as the most important non-chiropractor to influence the chiropractic profession because he was responsible for beginning the informal medical campaign against chiropractors and orchestrated the American Medical Association's (AMA) anti-chiropractic crusade for over fifty years [34]. From his position of power as editor of the Journal of the American Medical Association (JAMA) and secretary of the AMA (1924 to 1949) he determined the tone of articles appearing in JAMA and ensured that anti-chiropractic pieces regularly appeared [34].

In spite of, or perhaps because of having achieved market dominance, the AMA launched an "all-out war on chiropractic, the most successful of contemporary alternatives" [35]. This war constitutes the formal Era of Persecution. It began in 1962 with the adoption of The Iowa Plan and the formation of the Committee on Quackery to implement same [36]. Simply put, the Iowa Plan's overall goal was to "contain and eventually eliminate the cult of chiropractic as a health hazard in the United States" [36].

Chiropractors and chiropractic training institutions were in abundance during this time. To put things into perspective, by 1910 there were some 392 schools in the USA offering chiropractic training [37] with up to 16,000 practising chiropractors in the country [19]. This is in contrast to the 76 medical schools at the time.

The Committee on Quackery was well funded, and operated a highly successful campaign that was centred on three main strategies:

1. An ethics based boycott, which deemed it unethical for AMA members to have professional dealings with chiropractors;
2. Convincing other organizations to adopt or adapt the AMA's anti-chiropractic policy; and
3. Instituting a comprehensive political campaign to thwart chiropractic progress on several fronts, including but not limited to education, research and insurance funding [36].

The chiropractic profession's response to the formal campaign was launched in 1976 when five chiropractors, Drs Chester A Wilk, James W Bryden, Patricia B Arthur, Michael D Pedigo, and Steven Lumsden filed an antitrust lawsuit against the American Medical Association (AMA) and fourteen other defendants [38].

The Era of Persecution officially ended in the United States in 1987 when the presiding Judge, Susan Getzendanner, issued a permanent injunction order against the AMA because she correctly recognized that there would be lingering effects of the decades long AMA boycott: the culture of political medicine had become anti-chiropractic and the AMA would possibly re-offend [39,40].

The Iowa Plan was not confined to the United States. In Australia, the Australian Medical Association had adopted the Iowa Plan's ethics based boycott as well as a very negative 'exclusive dogma' policy on chiropractic. The Association was very active and successful in blocking the advancement of chiropractic within Australia [3]. While there was no trial or injunction order issued within Australia, the Australian Medical Association formally ended its ethics based boycott and rescinded its exclusive dogma policy on chiropractic following the intervention of the Australian Consumer and Competition Commission [41,42].

Clearly, opposition to the growing profession of chiropractic was formidable, prolonged and widespread. The profession's survival resembles the history of early social protest and reform movements in western history. Like the abolitionists, early chiropractors were victims of systematic persecution and often banished from one town to another. Similar to the feminists and suffragettes, pioneer chiropractors were often ostracised in the community [43]. While the persecution and prosecution might have been seen as impediments to the profession, the contrary was the case. Gibbons reminds us that "phase of real persecution and enforced poverty" afforded chiropractors "much of their identity and motivation" [44].

Importantly, from a sociological perspective, the sustained campaign by the AMA crystalized chiropractic culture into one with a unique lexicon and a siege mentality.

With the end of the Eras of Prosecution and Persecution came the Era of Legitimation during which the chiropractic profession enjoyed advancements on many fronts [32].

The Era of Legitimation: 1960 - present

The Era of Legitimation saw inquiries into chiropractic - lots of inquiries - 18 in all. The New Zealand Royal Commission, the Webb Royal Commission in Australia, the LaCroix Royal Commission in Canada, the Layton Committee Report again in Australia to name a few.

The inquiries reached similar conclusions:

1) Chiropractors are well positioned to manage musculoskeletal disorders,
2) Claims by chiropractors to be able to positively affect visceral disorders are unsupported by evidence and constitute a major obstacle to integration of chiropractic into the health care system, and
3) Chiropractic education needs to improve.

The Era of Legitimation saw chiropractic education move into government funded universities; a proliferation of chiropractic research; legislation governing the practice of chiropractic in 90 jurisdictions throughout the world and unprecedented inter-professional cooperation [45].

There was an expectation that with registration and university based education, and the removal of other obstacles, the profession would unite, embrace science and take its *legitimate* place within the health care system and that the profession's cultural authority would be enhanced.

The reality is quite different. Instead, the siege mentality of the chiropractic profession largely remains and is compounded by memory deficit disorder, whereby it seems that these important historical facts have been lost, resulting in a significant portion of the chiropractic profession steadfastly continuing to espouse the original chiropractic doctrine [46] and make "unsubstantiated claims" [47,48].

The profession's public image remains in tatters with chiropractors consistently rating towards the bottom of ethics and honesty scales [49]. The 2006 Australian Reader's Digest most trusted professions poll placed chiropractors in 13th place out of 35 professions [50]. While this is not a good result, in 2011 chiropractors do not even appear amongst the 45 professions listed, which placed real estate agents, car salesmen, politicians and tele-marketers in the last four spots [51]. While it is recognized that the Readers Digest poll is not the most scientific, this result is surely not a good sign for the chiropractic profession's cultural authority.

In the 2010 FG Roberts Memorial Lecture, Dr Reggars stated that the chiropractic profession is poised at the crossroads of marginalization and mainstream [1].

I say that the profession is at the crossroads of being relegated to the back blocks of health care provision (marginalization) or being recognized as the health care provider of choice for what bothers most of the people, most of the time.

So what is the problem?

Carl Sagan tells of a fire-breathing dragon living in his garage. When we look inside and cannot see his dragon he advises that it is invisible, and it cannot be detected with infrared because its fire is heatless; it leaves no footprints because it floats in the air and its body cannot be shown because it is incorporeal. Indeed, it cannot be detected by any known means. Sagan is the only one who knows it is there. Sagan asks what the difference is between a dragon that cannot be detected by any means and no dragon at all? If there is no way to disprove his dragon's existence, what does it mean to say that his dragon exists? The inability to invalidate his hypothesis is not at all the same thing as proving it true. Sagan advises that untestable claims and assertions incapable of disproof are worthless, even though they may excite us and fill us with wonder. To believe in Sagan's dragon in the absence of evidence is to do so on his authority alone [52].

The Association of Chiropractic Colleges defines the purpose, principles and practice of chiropractic as the finding and reduction of vertebral subluxations that "compromise neural integrity and may influence organ system function and general health". [53]. An internet search will advise that chiropractors have known about the dangers of subluxations for over one hundred years; that chiropractors are the only health professionals trained in the detection, and correction of the vertebral subluxation [54-56].

The problem is that there is no credible evidence that subluxations are any more real or dangerous [57,58] than Sagan's dragon. While Sagan may be deluding himself, he is unlikely to harm others because of his belief.

Chiropractic's problem is that subluxation based chiropractors [59] are not only deluding themselves, they are indoctrinating patients into believing in a purportedly dangerous mythical entity, and that without regular adjustments, patients will not only fail to reach their full potential, they will likely suffer serious health problems.

Some authors have suggested that this may be a threat to public health [60-62]. And this, at a time when the profession has just entered The Era of Chiropractic Opportunity.

The Era of Chiropractic Opportunity: 2000 - present

Consider the following facts regarding musculoskeletal disorders (MSD). MSD are the leading cause of pain and disability in Australia. They are the second most common cause for a visit to a general medical practitioner and the third leading cause of expenditure in the Australian health care system: $3 billion per year ($8.2 million per day). Annually, MSD are responsible for 300000 hospital admissions, 15 million general medical practitioner office visits, and 13 million prescriptions, and MSD from motor vehicle accidents account for 25% of all health care expenditure [63,64].

This is just the beginning - these figures are only going to get worse. There is an aging population that requires more care for MSD, with a shortage of health care providers who are poorly distributed [65]. The solution to this problem has been known by health economists for decades: provider substitution [66]. Until recently, governments have not had the political will to implement this major policy reform. The health care landscape has changed sufficiently so that provider substitution is not only being considered a possibility, it has been implemented, examined and found to be a viable option that results in high levels of patient satisfaction and good clinical outcomes [67,68]. In the area of MSD, in particular low back pain, chiropractic care has long been shown to be an effective and cost effective alternative to conventional medical care [69,70].

Given these circumstances, it would appear that chiropractic is favorably positioned to play a strong role in the health care delivery system, but as Dr Reggars pointed out, this seems unlikely to happen given the current chiropractic landscape [1].

The Way Forward

It seems that there are three options available to the profession:

1) Maintain the status quo.
2) Move forward as a united profession.
3) Divide the profession and let each faction fend for itself.

These options will be explored.

Option 1) While maintaining the status quo is an option, this course of action effectively prevents the profession from taking full advantage of the Era of Opportunity.

Option 2) In an ideal world, the profession would move forward in a united fashion and take its rightful place within the health care delivery system. To do this would require significant maturation on the part of the profession as demonstrated by taking the following steps:

1) Slay the one-cause (subluxation), one-cure (adjustment) sacred cow. While this may have been the original *a priori* Palmerian philosophy, in synchrony with similar concepts of the late-nineteenth century [71,72], it is not acceptable as a basis for patient care in light of today's knowledge-base [57]. Rather than bury the corpse, it should be taught as chiropractic history, warts and all. It would be a travesty to forget the profession's checkered past.
2) The profession needs to get out of the dogma-house and cease espousing Palmerian doctrine as gospel. While it was beyond distasteful to be labeled an unscientific cult that follows an exclusive dogma [3], when one considers the definitions of dogma[i] and cult[ii], the label may have been appropriate for part of the profession, and indeed may still be appropriate.

Escaping from the dogma house will require extraordinary cooperation amongst all aspects of the profession. Organizations such as the World Federation of Chiropractic and all major chiropractic associations will need to agree upon and adopt a position statement identifying the chiropractic subluxation as an historical construct that remains a hypothesis, which cannot form the basis for patient care until and unless there is a body of scientific evidence to support it. This is not dissimilar to what has occurred in the United Kingdom [73].

The position statement will need to be backed up by these organizations incorporating and enforcing appropriate statements into their ethical codes. Further, educational accrediting bodies will have to modify their standards to clearly state that subluxation is not a concept upon which to base patient care. From this, it follows that chiropractic teaching institutions will be required to restructure their curricula accordingly.

These moves will need to be reinforced by the actions of registration boards to deal harshly with misleading and deceptive advertising on the part of subluxation based chiropractors and the unconscionable conduct that typically occurs therewith. Specifically, registration boards must prohibit the common practice whereby potential clients present to a chiropractor for a musculoskeletal complaint, only to be convinced that they are in fact suffering from subluxation related disorders and require prolonged chiropractic care.

Insurance providers will need to alter their rebate guidelines to only provide payment for evidence-based care and to strike from their registers subluxation-based chiropractors.

All of this must happen and the public must be informed along the way.

Last, but by no means least, it will require each and every chiropractor to be intolerant of the nonsense that is out there.

The contract that the profession has with society and its patients is such that, in exchange for a significant degree of autonomy over education, licensing and credentialing, members of the profession are expected to maintain high standards of competence and moral responsibility and to subordinate financial gain to the higher values of responsibility to clients and the public interest [74,75].

If the profession is to gain the trust of the consuming public it must, of necessity, become truly self-policing.

Only in this way will chiropractic generate the cultural authority required for recognition as a group worthy of the title "Profession".

No longer can we cast a blind eye. By our silence we are giving consent.

Chiropractic is not about hope in a jar and philosophy is not about faith or dogma. Philosophy is about seeking truth, questioning one's beliefs and altering those beliefs in accordance with the best available evidence.

George W Bush once said:

> I know what I believe. I will continue to articulate what I believe and what I believe - I believe what I believe is right [76].

While this type of thinking may be acceptable for a United States President, faith and dogma must not be the driving forces of our profession.

According to Alvin Toffler,

> The illiterate of the 21st century will not be those who cannot read and write, but those who cannot learn, unlearn, and relearn [77].

The chiropractic profession can choose to be illiterate, but it will do so at its peril. It is realized that thinking is hard and that those who are unaccustomed to thinking may even find it unpleasant. On the other hand, thinkers have always found it rather fun and there are no confirmed reports of anyone dying or being seriously injured by thinking. Thinking may necessitate changing our minds - which may not be a bad thing. At the very least the profession owes it to its patients.

Option 3) If a unified profession is not achievable, the other path is to split the profession into clear divisions: evidence based chiropractors and subluxation based chiropractors with each division openly declaring its hand. Evidence based chiropractors will become active contributors to mainstream health care while subluxation based practitioners will "opt out" and take their chances.

Conclusion

The chiropractic profession emerged from an unregulated, unscientific era in health care. During its 116-year history, chiropractors have endured decades of prosecution and persecution and developed a siege mentality for survival. Following a protracted legal battle in the United States and a shorter non-courtroom stoush in Australia, the discriminatory anti-chiropractic behavior on the part of political medicine largely ceased. Sadly, to the detriment of the profession as a whole, some parts of the chiropractic profession remain mired in a nineteenth century mind-set. This is particularly perplexing considering the progress that the profession has made and the opportunities it now has.

This paper has explored these issues and suggested a way for the profession to proceed as a united group. This author would not be willing to wager on a unified future, but does know this: the future of the chiropractic profession is well and truly in its own hands and the time to act is now.

Endnotes

[i] Dogma: An authoritative principle, belief, or statement of ideas or opinion, especially one considered to be absolutely true.

The American Heritage Dictionary of the English Language, 4th Edition. Houghton Mifflin Company. 2009

[ii] Cult: A system for the cure of disease based on dogma set forth by its promulgator. The Merriam-Webster Online Dictionary. http://www.merriam-webster.com 2010

Competing interests

The authors declare that they have no competing interests.

References

1. Reggars J: **Chiropractic at the crossroads or are we just going around in circles?** *Chiropractic & Manual Therapies* 2011, **19**:11.
2. Linhart G: **Selling the "big idea": BJ Palmer ushers in the Golden Age, 1906-1920.** *Chiropractic History* 1988, **8**:25-30.
3. Simpson J Keith: **The Influence of Political Medicine in the Development of the Chiropractic Profession in Australia.** *PhD Dissertation* University of Queensland, Social Science; 2002.
4. King L: **Medical Sects and Their Influence.** *J Am Med Assoc* 1982, **248**:1221-1224.
5. Rothstein W: *American Physicians in the Ninetheenth Century* Baltimore: The Johns Hopkins Press; 1985.
6. Hamowy R: **The Early Development of Medical Licensing Laws in the United States, 1875-1900.** *J Libertarian Stud* 1979, **3**:73-119.
7. Mansfield C, Wilson J, Kobrinski E, Mitchell J: **Premature mortality in the United States: The roles of geographic area, October status, household type, and availability of medical care.** *Journal of Public Health* 1999, **89(6)**:893-898.
8. Rosenfield H: **Experts Are Never Right.** *Antioch Review* 1949, **9**:3-15.
9. Winkelstein W: **Lemuel Shattuck: Architect of American Public Health.** *Epidemiology* 2008, **19**:634.
10. Numbers R: **Medical Science before Scientific Medicine: Reflections on the History of Medical Geography.** *Medical History* 2000, 217-220.
11. Martin SC: **"The Only Truly Scientific Method of Healing". Chiropractic and American Science, 1895 - 1990.** *Isis* 1994, **88**:207-227.
12. Moore J: *Chiropractic in America The History of a Medical Alternative* Baltimore Maryland: The Johns Hopkins University Press; 1993.
13. Schiller F: **Spinal Irritation and osteopathy.** *Bull Hist Med* 1971, **45**:250-266.
14. Hammond WA: *Spinal Irritation* New York: D Appleton and Company; 1870.
15. Starr P: *The Social Transformation of American Medicine The rise of a sovereign profession and the making of a vast industry* Basic Books; 1982.
16. Burnham J: **American medicine's golden age: what happened to it?** *Science* 1982, **215**:1474 1479.
17. Flexner A: *Medical Education in the United States and Canada A Report to the Carnegie Foundation for the Advancement of Teaching* New York City: Carnegie Foundation; 1910.
18. Keating JC Jr: *Chiropractic History: a Primer* Davenport, Iowa. Association for the History of Chiropractic; 2004.
19. Wardwell W: *Chiropractic: History and Evolution of a New Profession* St Louis: Mosby Year Book; 1992.
20. Scotton R: *Medical Care in Australia* Adelaide: The Griffin Press, 1974.
21. Carter J: *Racketerring In Medicine The Supression of Alternatives* Norfolk VA: Hampton Roads Publishing Company Inc; 1993.
22. Jackson R: **Regretful Episodes for D.D. Palmer.** *Chiropractic Technique* 1999, **11**:33-37.
23. Kimbrough M: **Jailed Chiropractors: Those Who Blazed The Trail.** *Chiropractic History* 1998, **18**:79-100.
24. Geiger A: **Chiropractic: Its Cause and Cure.** *Medical Economics* 1942, June.
25. Wardwell W: **Chiropractors: Challengers of Medical Domination.** *Research in The Sociology of Health Care* 1981, **2**:207-250.
26. Inglis B: *Fringe Medicine* London: Faber and Faber; 1964.
27. Gibbons R: **Medical and Social Protest as Part of Hidden American History.** In *Principles and Practice of Chiropractic.*. 1 edition. Edited by: Haldeman S. New York: Appleton-Century-Crofts; 1992:.
28. Keating J: *BJ of Davenport The Early Years of Chiropractic* Davenport: Association for the History of Chiropractic; 1997.
29. Keating J: **The Age of Wonderment - Chiropractic in the early twentieth century.** In *Chiropractic: an illustrated history.* Edited by: Peterson D, Weise G. St Louis, Missouri: Mosby-Year Book Inc; 1995:.
30. Keating J: **Philosophy and science in chiropractic: essential, inseperable and misunderstood.** *European Journal of Chiropractic* 2001, **46.**
31. Peters R, Chance M: **Disasters, Discoveries, Developments and Distinction: The Year That Was 1907.** *Chiropr J Aust* 2007, **37**:145-156.
32. Wardwell W: **The Sixteen Major Events in Chiropractic History.** *Chiropractic History* 1996, **16**:66-71.
33. Keating J, Mootz R: **The Influence of Political Medicine on chiropractic dogma: implications for scientific development.** *J Manip Physiol Ther* 1989, **12**:393-398.
34. Donahue J: **Morris Fishbein, MD: The "Medical Mussolini" and Chiropractic.** *Chiropractic History* 1996, **16**:39-49.

35. Wollinsky H, Brune T: *The Serpent on the Staff The Unhealthy Politics of the American Medical Association* New York: GP Putman's Sons; 1994.
36. Simpson J Keith: **The Iowa Plan and the Activities of the Committee on Quackery.** *Chiroprac J Aust* 1997, **27**:5-12.
37. Phillips R, Triano J: **Historical perspective. Joseph Janse.** *SPINE* 1995, **20**:2349-2353.
38. Wilk C: *Medicine, Monopolies, and Malice* Garden City Park, New York: Avery Publishing; 1996.
39. Getzendanner S: **Getzendanner Decision in the United States District Court for the Northern District of Illinois Eastern Division.** 1987, No. 76 C 3777.
40. Getzendanner S: **Permanent Injunction Order Against AMA.** *J Am Med Assoc* 1988, **259**:81-82.
41. Simpson J Keith: **The Evolution of the Australian Medical Association's Exclusive Dogma Policy on Chiropractic.** *Chiropractic History* 2003, **23**:69-78.
42. Ducret A: **The AMA and chiropractic: a trade practices viewpoint.** *ACO (ACCC Journal)* 1998, **8**:27-30.
43. Gibbons R: **Evolution of Chiropractic: Medical and Social Protest in America.** In *Modern Developments in the Principles and Pracitce of Chiropractic.*. 1 edition. Edited by: Haldeman S. New York: Appleton-Century-Crofts; 1980:.
44. Gibbons R: **Chiropractic History: lost, strayed or stolen.** *J Aust Chiropractors' Assoc* 1977, **11**:19-23.
45. Chapman-Smith D: *The Chiropractic Profession. Its Education, Practice, Research and Future Directions* DeMoines, Iowa: NCMIC Group Inc; 2000.
46. Institute for Alternative Futures: *The Future of Chiropractic Revisited: 2005 -2012* Alexandria, Virginia; 2005 [http://www.altfutures.com], © the Institute for Alternative Futures. Used with permission.
47. Ernst E, Gilbey A: **Chiropractic claims in the English-speaking world.** *NZ Med J* 2010, **123**:36-44.
48. Sikorski D, Grod J: **The Unsubstantiated Web Site Claims of Chiropractic Colleges in Canada and the United States.** *The Journal of Chiropractic Education* 2003, **17**:113-119.
49. **Honesty/Ethics in Professions.** [http://www.gallup.com/poll/1654/Honesty-Ethics-Professionas.aspx].
50. **Australia's Most Trusted 2006.** [http://www.readersdigest.com.au/australias-most-trusted-2006].
51. **Australia's Most Trusted Professions 2011.** [http://www.readersdigest.com.au/australias-most-trusted-professions-2011].
52. Sagan C: *The Demon-Haunted World. Science as a candle in the dark* London: Headline Book Publishing; 1997.
53. Phillips R: **The Chiropractic Paradigm.** *The Journal of Chiropractic Education* 2001, **15**:49-52.
54. **What is a Subluxation?.** [http://www.echiropractic.net/what_is_a_subluxation.htm].
55. Roughan S: **Colquhoun's opinion versus science–a response from the New Zealand Chiropractors' Association.** *The New Zealand Medical Journal* 2008, **121**.
56. New Zealand Chiropractors Association: **Research & Literature: Examining The Evidence.**[http://www.chiropractic.org.nz/research-literature].
57. Keating J, Charlton K, Grod J, Perle S, Sikorski D, Winterstein J: **Subluxation: dogma or science?** *Chiropractic & Osteopathy* 2005, **13**:17.
58. Mirtz T, Morgan L, Wyatt L, Greene L: **An epidemiological examination of the subluxation construct using Hill's criteria of causation.** *Chiropractic & Osteopathy* 2009, **17**:13.
59. Homola S: **Real orthopaedic subluxations versus imaginary chiropractic subluxations.** *Focus on Alternative and Complementary Therapies* 2010, **15**:284-287.
60. Homola S: **Is the Chiropractic Subluxation Theory a Threat to Public Health?** *Scientific Review of Alt Med* 2001, **5**:45-53.
61. Benedetti P, MacPhail W: *Spin Doctors. The Chiropractic Industry Under Examination* Toronto: The Dundurn Group; 2002.
62. Magner G: *Chiropractic The Victim's Perspective* Amherst: Promethius Books; 1995.
63. **"Bone and Joint Decade 2000 - 2010: Australian Promotion" (video).** [http://www.bjd.org.au/files/bjd_aus.wmv].
64. **4823.0.55.001 - Musculoskeletal Conditions in Australia: A Snapshot, 2004-05.** [http://www.abs.gov.au/ausstats/abs@.nsf/mf/4823.0.55.001].
65. OECD Secretariat: **Ageing Populations: High Time for Action.** 2005 [http://www.oecd.org/dataoecd/61/50/34600619.pdf].
66. Weller G, Manga P: **The Push for Reprivatization of Health Care Services in Canada, Britain, and the United States.** *Journal of Health Politics Policy and Law* 1983, **8**:495-518.
67. Patterson E, McMurray A: **Collaborative practice between registered nurses and medical practitioners in Australian general practice: Moving from rhetoric to reality.** *Australian Journal of Advanced Nursing* 2003, **20**:43-48.
68. Laurant M, Reeves D, Hermens R, Braspenning J, Grol R, Sibbald B: **Substitution of doctors by nurses in primary care.** *Cochrane database of systematic reviews (Online)* 2004.
69. Manga P, Angus D, Papadopoulos C, Swan W: **The Effectiveness and Cost-Effectiveness of Chiropractic Management of Low-Back Pain.** 1993.
70. Manga P, Angus D, Swan W: **Effective management of low back pain: its time to accept the evidence.** *JCCA* 1993, **37**:221-229.
71. Gaucher-Peslherbe GL: *Chiropractic: Early Concepts In Their Historical Setting* Lombard, Illinois: National College of Chiropractic; 1989.
72. Gaucher-Peslherbe PL: **DD Palmer as Authentic Medical Radical.** *JNMS* 1995, **3**:175-181.
73. General Chiropractic Council UK: **Guidance on claims made for the chiropractic vertebral subluxation complex.** 2010.
74. Cruess R, Cruess S: **Expectations and Obligations. Professionalism and medicine's social contract with society.** *Perspectives in Biology and Medicine* 2008, **51**:579-598.
75. Cruess R, Cruess S, Johnston S: **Professionalism and Medicine's Social contract.** *Journal of Bone & Joint Surgery* 2000, **82**:1189-1194.
76. **The 'misunderestimated' president?.** [http://news.bbc.co.uk/go/pr/fr/-/2/hi/americas/7809160.stm].
77. **The Quotations Page.** [http://www.quotationspage.com/quote/1407.html].

Creating European guidelines for Chiropractic Incident Reporting and Learning Systems (CIRLS): relevance and structure

Martin Wangler[1*†], Ricardo Fujikawa[2†], Lise Hestbæk[3†], Tom Michielsen[4†], Timothy J Raven[5†], Haymo W Thiel[6†] and Beatrice Zaugg[7†]

Abstract

Background: In 2009, the heads of the Executive Council of the European Chiropractors' Union (ECU) and the European Academy of Chiropractic (EAC) involved in the European Committee for Standardization (CEN) process for the chiropractic profession, set out to establish European guidelines for the reporting of adverse reactions to chiropractic treatment. There were a number of reasons for this: first, to improve the overall quality of patient care by aiming to reduce the application of potentially harmful interventions and to facilitate the treatment of patients within the context of achieving maximum benefit with a minimum risk of harm; second, to inform the training objectives for the Graduate Education and Continuing Professional Development programmes of all 19 ECU member nations, regarding knowledge and skills to be acquired for maximising patient safety; and third, to develop a guideline on patient safety incident reporting as it is likely to be part of future CEN standards for ECU member nations.

Objective: To introduce patient safety incident reporting within the context of chiropractic practice in Europe and to help individual countries and their national professional associations to develop or improve reporting and learning systems.

Discussion: Providing health care of any kind, including the provision of chiropractic treatment, can be a complex and, at times, a risky activity. Safety in healthcare cannot be guaranteed, it can only be improved. One of the most important aspects of any learning and reporting system lies in the appropriate use of the data and information it gathers. Reporting should not just be seen as a vehicle for obtaining information on patient safety issues, but also be utilised as a tool to facilitate learning, advance quality improvement and to ultimately minimise the rate of the occurrence of errors linked to patient care.

Conclusions: Before a reporting and learning system can be established it has to be clear what the objectives of the system are, what resources will be required and whether the implementing organisation has the capacity to operate the system to its full advantage. Responding to adverse event reports requires the availability of experts to analyse the incidents and to provide feedback in a timely fashion. A comprehensive strategy for national implementation must be in place including, but not limited to, presentations at national meetings, the provision of written information to all practitioners and the running of workshops, so that all stakeholders fully understand the purposes of adverse event reporting. Unless this is achieved, any system runs the risk of failure, or at the very least, limited usefulness.

* Correspondence: wangler@besonet.ch
† Contributed equally
[1]European Academy of Chiropractic, academic dean and private practice, Bahnhofstrasse 15, 3400 Burgdorf, Switzerland
Full list of author information is available at the end of the article

Introduction

Incident reporting is not new. Flannagan, a psychologist, first described the "critical incident technique" in 1954 [1]. The concept originated from studies in the Aviation Psychology Program of the United States Air Force during and after the Second World War, with the aim of reducing the number of deaths of military pilots and the loss of aircraft [2,3].

The first health profession to use a critical incident technique was dentistry [4]. In 1960 the concept was introduced into medicine to identify errors in the dispensing of drugs by nurses [5]. By the 1970s the use of incident reporting became more widespread within the medical profession and was then employed as a mechanism to assess patient care given by medical specialists such as paediatricians, surgeons and obstetricians [6]. But it was not until 1978 that critical incident reporting was applied with the specific aim to improve patient safety. In the field of anaesthesia, Cooper and his colleagues [7] were the first to proactively put the emphasis of their investigations on "what could go wrong", rather than just analysing "what did go wrong" after an event had occurred. Anaesthesiology has since been regarded as the pioneer of critical incident studies in medicine. The purpose of any critical incident reporting system can be summarised as follows:

a. The occurrence of an incident should trigger the completion of a report;

b. Incident report data should then be collected and;

c. Analysed centrally to determine whether there are any trends that could represent potential problems in the delivery of care;

d. The results of the analysis must then be distributed and shared with the individuals and organisations involved [8].

In 2009, the heads of the Executive Council of the European Chiropractors' Union (ECU) and the European Academy of Chiropractic (EAC) involved in the European Committee for Standardization (CEN) process for the chiropractic profession set about establishing Chiropractic European Guidelines for Adverse Reactions (CEGAR) for a number of reasons: 1) to improve the overall quality of patient care, by aiming to reduce the application of potentially harmful interventions, and to facilitate the treatment of patients within the context of achieving maximum benefit with a minimum risk of harm; 2) to inform training objectives for the Graduate Education and Continuing Professional Development programmes of all 19 ECU member nations; and 3) to develop a guideline on patient safety standards since it is likely to become part of future CEN standards for ECU member nations.

The proposed guidelines herein are the result of a collaborative effort, involving not only members of a commission but also representatives of ECU member nations and chiropractic patients. They are based on a synthesis of the best available evidence and relevant published literature. The commission named the guidelines the European Guidelines for Chiropractic Incident Reporting and Learning Systems (EG-CIRLS) to emphasise the reporting and learning aspects. The main purpose of EG-CIRLS is to facilitate the introduction of an incident reporting culture within chiropractic practice in Europe, ultimately contributing to an improvement in the safety of patient care.

Review process and phases of the development of the guidelines

In March 2009, a commission for the development of the guidelines was formed, consisting of seven members. All of the commission's members are European chiropractors working in six European countries, i.e. Belgium, Denmark, Norway, Spain, Switzerland and the United Kingdom. Four of the members work in private practice, and three work at chiropractic institutions. Most of the communication and work of the guidelines commission was done via online (closed-group) discussions in order to keep additional expenditure on resources, including travel to a minimum.

The commission decided to use the WHO Draft Guidelines for Adverse Event Reporting and Learning Systems [9] as a guide, and obtained permission to adapt a number of its chapters to the needs of the profession in Europe.

The "Appraisal of Guidelines for Research & Evaluation" (AGREE) instrument [10] was used in order to guide a structured and rigorous development methodology and to ensure that EG-CIRLS would meet minimum quality criteria. The AGREE instrument consists of 23 key items organised in six domains, with each domain intended to capture a separate dimension of guideline quality (Tables 1 and 2). The AGREE instrument was first used via an electronic survey sent to all seven members of the commission for its development process and quality (Table 1). Individual ratings are available in Additional file 1. The European Patient Organisation had rated the domain "Stakeholder involvement" in advance of the guidelines review (Additional file 2). The method used for formulating the recommendations was developed through consensus by all members of the commission at a meeting in Frankfurt in 2009. The group discussed the domain applicability, potential organisational barriers and costs in applying the recommendations, as well as review and control criteria and/or audit purposes. The final draft of the guidelines was

Table 1 Percentage of agreement with AGREE domains by the commission

Standardised Domain Score (EG-CIRLS)	Max possible scores	Min possible scores	Obtained scores	Percentage of agreement
Domain 1: Scope and purpose	84	21	78	90%
Domain 2: Stakeholder involvement	112	28	99	85%
Domain 3: Rigour of development	196	49	176	86%
Domain 4: Clarity and presentation	112	28	97	87%
Domain 5: Applicability	84	21	65	70%
Doman 6: Editorial independence	56	14	48	81%

The standardised domain score was calculated by summing up all the scores of individual items (4 point Likert scale) in a domain and by standardising the total as a percentage of the maximum possible score for that domain.

again assessed by the commission members on the basis of all 23 AGREE items: first individually (n = 7), then by discussion and consensus (n = 5), and finally by individual ratings (n = 5) (Table 2). The overall development process for EG-CIRLS is summarised in Figure 1.

Discussion

Chiropractic and patient safety incidents

Providing health care of any kind, including the provision of chiropractic treatment, can be a complex and, at times, a risky activity. Safety in healthcare cannot be guaranteed, it can only be improved [11]. There will always be risks to patients, risks to practitioners and even risks to a profession as a whole. Capturing and recording information on patient safety incidents, and analysing this information, are essential steps to manage and reduce risk and, ultimately, improve patient safety.

So far, within Europe, information on patient safety incidents within the context of chiropractic treatment has been gathered in three ways: 1) data derived as a by-product of systems designed to investigate or respond to instances of poor quality care (for example, litigation for alleged medical negligence, a professional association's complaints procedure or cases referred to the national statutory regulator); 2) periodic internal or external studies and reviews [12,13] and 3) spontaneous reporting by individual chiropractors [14]. However, these sources of information can only give a haphazard and incomplete picture of the true nature and dimension of risks and adverse events associated with chiropractic treatment since they are usually based on individual cases, small studies in the population or rely on the review and interpretation of retrospective data often collected or initially reported by others.

Table 2 Percentage of agreement with AGREE domains in regard to the final draft

Standardised Domain Score[I.] (EG-CIRLS)	Max possible score	Min possible score	Obtained score	Percentage of agreement
Domain 1: Scope and purpose	60	15	45	67%
Domain 2: Stakeholder involvement	80	20	48	47%[II.]
Domain 3: Rigour of development	120	30	89	66%[III.]
Domain 4: Clarity and presentation	60	15	49	76%
Domain 5: Applicability	50	10	10	0%[IV.]
Domain 6: Editorial independence	40	10	40	100%

I. Was calculated by summing up all of the scores of the individual items (4 point Likert scale) in a domain and by standardising the total as a percentage of the maximum possible score for that domain; II. The domain "Stakeholder involvement" had been rated in advance of guidelines review by the European Patient Organisations (Additional file 2); III. Based on a previous literature review of a PhD thesis written at the University of Portsmouth. The method, used for formulating the recommendations, was developed through consensus by all members of the EG-CIRLS steering group at a meeting in Frankfurt in 2009; IV. The group discussed the domain Applicability. Potential organisational barriers and costs in applying the recommendations, as well as review and control criteria and/or audit purposes were considered. This item was judged as either being 'not applicable' or as 'strongly disagree'.

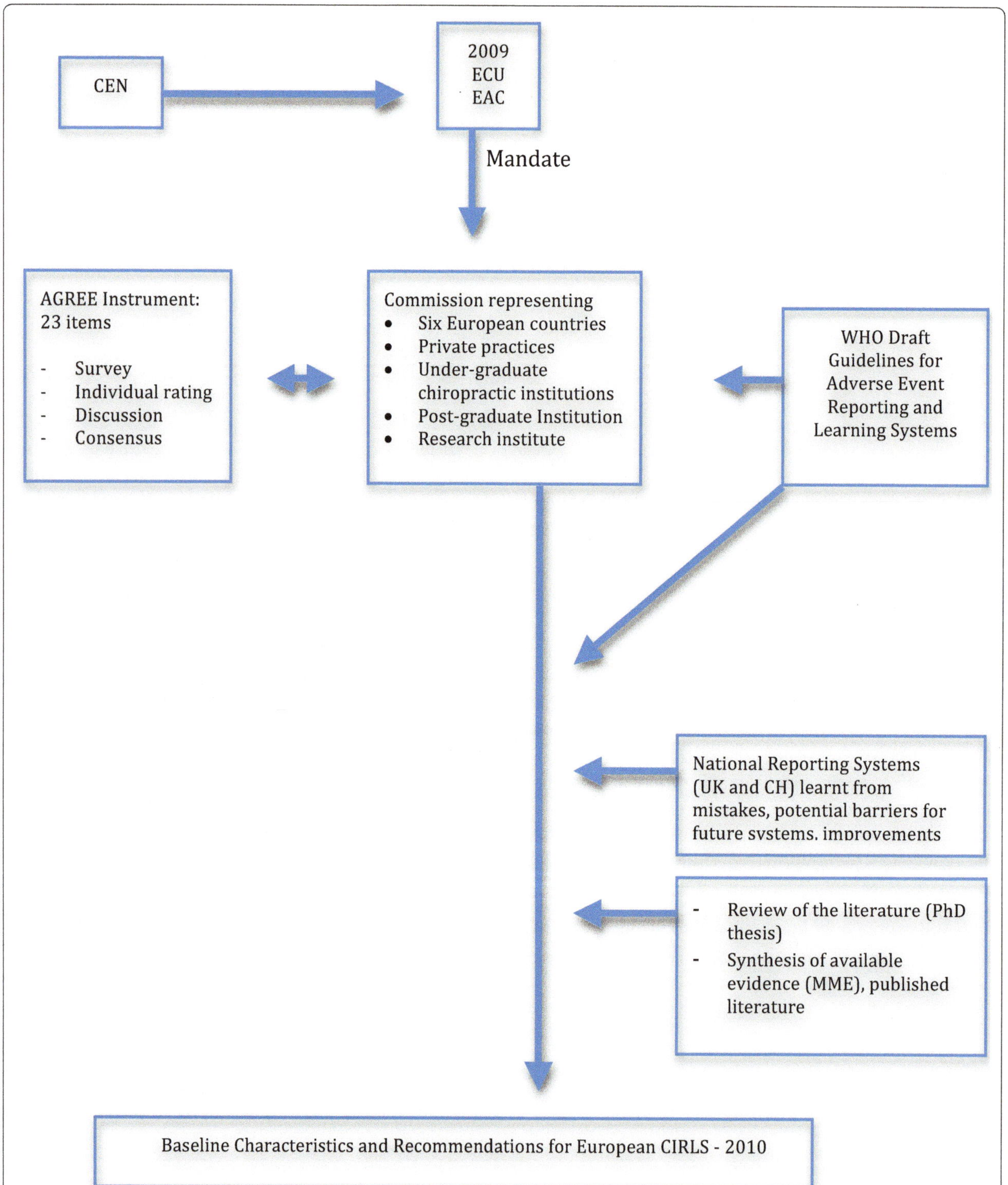

Figure 1 Flow Diagram of Guidelines Developing Process.

Furthermore, these methods are primarily reactive and strongly reflective of a blame culture, something that is not particularly conducive to individual learning or change of practice. Human error has traditionally been viewed as the factor that immediately precedes or precipitates an adverse event or serious failure. If something goes wrong at the "clinical sharp end" (that is, at the immediate practitioner-patient interface), it would seem obvious that an individual must have been responsible. However, we do know that humans are fallible and that errors are inevitable, even in the best-run organisations or systems. Errors must therefore be seen as consequences rather than causes, and as being shaped and provoked by "upstream" systemic factors. When an adverse event occurs, the crucial issue is not who caused the error but how and why the defences failed, and what factors contributed to create the conditions in which the error occurred [15]. We also know that there are often patterns and similarities in the sources of risk arising out of clinical practice, which would go undetected if incidents were not reported and analysed. Reporting is therefore the key to detect patient safety problems and can play a fundamental role in enhancing patient safety by subsequent learning from the failures and near misses that have occurred to others.

It is likely that terms such as "adverse event reporting" or "critical event audit" are likely to lead to apprehension and a feeling of intrusion amongst chiropractic clinicians and chiropractic organisations. It is therefore essential that a professional organisation encourages active learning from incidents in order to achieve an "informed culture" amongst its members. The airline industry provides evidence that "safety cultures", where open reporting and balanced analysis are encouraged in principle and by example, can have a positive and quantifiable impact on the performance of organisations [16]. Safety is therefore a strong feature of an informed culture, which has four critical components: a reporting culture; a just culture; a flexible culture; and a learning culture. These are presented in Table 3 (after Reason, 1997 [16]).

Another problem with classifying and identifying errors in healthcare is that there are so many ways of doing it. As outlined by Avery [17], one can focus on processes such as diagnosis or describe underlying systems failures. Alternatively, one can classify errors in terms of the type of disease, drug, or procedure most commonly associated with error, or in terms of the severity of outcomes. Risk and incident reporting systems are far less developed in primary care although far more patient contacts take place every year in a primary care setting. We know the therapeutic interventions and procedures are generally of a less serious nature, and nevertheless there is the potential for patients to be harmed by failures in care [15]. Almost all of the research conducted so far has concentrated on the epidemiology of medical error and its capture within hospital based secondary care largely because of a perception that this is where most serious incidents occur. The chiropractic profession, with its private primary care setting, therefore faces particular challenges in developing and maintaining an effective incident risk reporting system, not least because it is lacking some of the organisational structures, usually inherent within a national health care system, to support such systems.

Detecting and accurately recording incident errors are therefore fundamental steps in advancing clinical risk management by learning from experience. However, incident reporting should not solely focus on adverse outcomes. Not all unsafe actions, systems or situations will necessarily lead to bad outcomes all the time. The potential for an adverse outcome may exist, but for any number of reasons, for example timely detection or just sheer luck this outcome may not occur at all. This has been termed a "potential adverse event" or a "near miss" [15]. Near misses are therefore those incidents that do not result in harm and need to be clearly distinguished from adverse events and (Table 4). It is important for risk and safety management systems to collect and analyse information obtained from near miss situations since the knowledge gained as a result will proactively contribute towards the reduction of risk and prevention of harm.

Understanding the causes of adverse events

Reason [18] defines error as "the failure of planned actions to achieve their desired goal", and describes two ways in which this failure can occur (Figure 2). According to Reason [19], there are two approaches to the problem of human fallibility: the person and the system approaches. Each model gives rise to different attitudes to error management, and a basic appreciation of these differences is helpful to understand how clinical mishaps can occur. The person-centred approach focuses on the errors of individuals, blaming them for inattention, forgetfulness or carelessness. The person-centred approach is still the dominant model in medicine and healthcare at large. From an emotional perspective, the blaming of

Table 3 The critical components of an informed culture [15]

A **reporting culture**	creating an organisational climate in which individuals are prepared to report beneficial outcomes as well as adverse events or errors.
A **just culture**	not total absence of blame or disregard of individual responsibility, but an atmosphere of trust in which individuals are encouraged to provide safety related information.
A **flexible culture**	the skills and abilities of the individual are respected.
A **learning culture**	there is willingness and competence to draw the appropriate conclusions from its safety information systems, and the will to implement reforms where their need is indicated.

Table 4 Types of events defined by WHO Guidelines [9]

Types of events	Definition The definitions of the three types of events are direct quotes of WHO Guidelines[9]
Error	Error has been defined as "the failure of a planned action to be completed as intended (i.e. error of execution) or the use of a wrong plan to achieve an aim (i.e., error of planning)". Although reporting of errors, whether or not there is an injury, is sometimes done within institutions, if reporting of all errors is requested the number may be overwhelming. Therefore, some sort of threshold is usually established-such as "serious" errors, or those with the potential for causing harm (also called "near misses" or "close calls"). Establishing such a threshold for a reporting system can be difficult. Hence, most "error reporting systems" are actually "adverse events caused by errors" systems.
Adverse Event	An adverse event is an injury related to medical management, in contrast to a complication of disease. Other terms that are sometimes used are "**mishaps**", "**unanticipated events**" or "**incidents**", and "**accidents**". Most authorities caution against use of the term accident since it implies that the event was unpreventable. Adverse events are not always caused by an error. For example, one form of adverse drug event, "adverse drug reaction" is, according to the WHO definition, a complication that occurs when the medication is used as directed and in the usual dosage. Adverse drug reactions are, therefore, adverse drug events that are not caused by errors. Many adverse events are caused by errors, either of commission or omission, and do, in fact, reflects deficiencies in the systems of care. Some reporting systems require that only preventable adverse events be reported, while others solicit reports whether or not a medical error occurred. One advantage of focusing reporting on adverse events rather than on errors is that it is usually obvious when a mishap has occurred; actual events focus attention. Comment by the authors of EG-CIRLS: *An adverse event is the result of a care delivery problem related to chiropractic management, in contrast to complications of disease. Chiropractic management includes all aspects of care, including diagnosis and treatment, failure to diagnose or treat, and the systems and equipment used to deliver care. Adverse events may be preventable or non-preventable. Preventable adverse event: An adverse event caused by an error or other type of systems or equipment failure.*
Near miss or **Close call**	A near miss" or "close call" is a serious error or mishap that has the potential to cause an adverse event, but fails to do so by chance or because it was intercepted. It is assumed (though not proven) that the underlying systems failures for near misses are the same as for actual adverse events. Therefore, understanding their causes should lead to systems design changes that will improve safety. A key advantage of a near miss reporting system is that because there has been no harm the reporter is not at risk of blame or litigation. On the contrary, he or she may be deserving of praise for having intercepted an error and prevented an injury. This positive aspect of reporting of near misses, has led some to recommend near miss systems for internal reporting systems within health-care organizations or other health-care facilities where a blaming culture persists. However, any hospital [*or private chiropractic practice*] that is serious about learning will also invite reports of near misses.

individuals is arguably more satisfying and easier than targeting institutions, organisations or systems [19]. This approach treats errors as moral issues, and as such isolates unsafe acts from their context, thus making it very difficult to uncover and eliminate recurrent error traps within a system [15]. The systems approach on the other hand, takes a more holistic stance on the issue of error and failure, concentrates on the conditions under which individuals function, and relates to the defences to avert errors or to minimise their effects. It acknowledges that humans are fallible and that errors are inevitable, even in the best-run organisations or systems. Errors are seen as consequences rather than causes, and as being shaped and provoked by "upstream" systemic factors [15]. The human factor cannot be changed. However, the conditions under which people work can be altered so as to make them less error provoking (please refer to Additional file 3 and 4 for further details)[[15,18-21])].

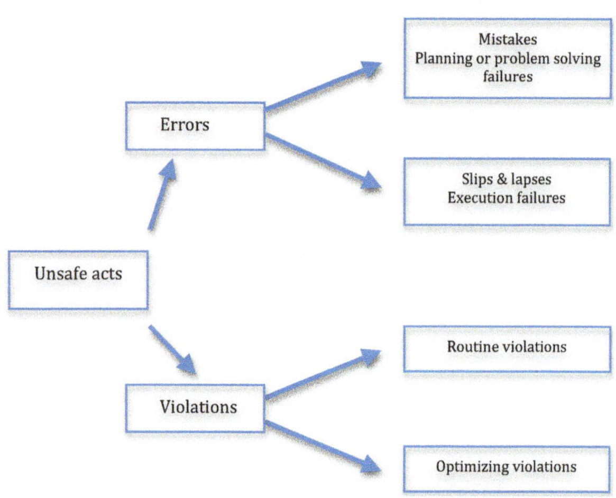

Figure 2 Unsafe Acts: adapted from Reason, 1995 [20].

Current national chiropractic reporting systems in Europe

Early efforts linked to the management of clinical risks within health care, including chiropractic, were primarily related to the setting up of processes in an attempt to control litigation and to reduce associated costs. Due to the increasing move in the late twentieth century towards documenting and learning from patient safety incidents, individuals within the chiropractic profession realised that it was paramount to become part of this developing safety culture. With this in mind, separate chiropractic patient incident reporting systems were developed in the United Kingdom and in Switzerland where chiropractors are committed to gathering all data relative to risks.

In 2005, the Anglo-European College of Chiropractic (AECC), in conjunction with the British Chiropractic Association (BCA), introduced the 'Chiropractic Reporting and Learning System' (CRLS) to collect patient safety incident data from BCA members [22]. It was taken up by the student clinics at AECC and, in modified form, at the Welsh Institute of Chiropractic, and subsequently rolled out to members of the Scottish Chiropractic Association. Although available to approximately 1600 of the UK's chiropractors, the initial take-up had been low [23]. Lack of awareness of the system and the types of incident that should be reported as well as fear and confusion regarding anonymity and the medico-legal implications of submitting reports were identified as key in explaining this underutilisation [22]. A second system known as the Patient Incident Reporting and Learning System (PIRLS) was developed at the McTimoney College of Chiropractic during 2007 [24]. PIRLS was launched by the McTimoney Chiropractic Association ensuring incident reporting was available to a further 600 UK chiropractors. In order to unify the process of safety incident reporting in the UK and to facilitate participation among all 2500 UK chiropractors, the College of Chiropractors, the three UK chiropractic educational institutions, and the four UK professional associations combined their experiences in a joint project to develop a new online reporting system known as the Chiropractic Patient Incident Reporting and Learning System (CPiRLS).

The CPiRLS project aims to enhance the learning element and improve the ease and accessibility of incident reporting, to help educate chiropractors about the types of incidents they should report and to reassure chiropractors that the administration of incident reporting is independent, secure and anonymous such that they have nothing to fear by sharing their experiences. The project forms part of a wider initiative to further enhance the culture of safety within the UK chiropractic profession. The CPiRLS website[http://www.cpirls.org] informs all visitors of the purpose and nature of incident reporting and learning but, in its initial form, is set up such that only chiropractors can submit and read reports. This is ensured through secure access with a universal password available only to chiropractors via the membership areas of their association websites. The universal nature of the password and design of the website database mean that individuals submitting reports cannot be identified by anybody, including those administering the system. This was felt to be essential if chiropractors are to feel comfortable and secure in submitting and sharing reports without fear of legal retribution. The CPiRLS online reporting form is provided in three versions according to whether the incident under report has either happened, nearly happened (near miss) or has been identified as an incident waiting to happen (following identification of an error or discrepancy of process for example).

Users start by choosing between these three types of incident and then progress through the form explaining what happened, why it happened and what actions were taken. Drop-down lists and radio buttons assist simple and rapid completion of the form. Submitted reports are published in outline form on the website. Users who are logged in to the site can read these reports and submit comments. This sharing of information and interaction among peers is designed to maximise the learning aspect of CPiRLS. All submitted material is monitored by CPiRLS team members who can edit inappropriate matter and access/download all data for future thematic analysis. The CPiRLS initiative is actively addressing the current underutilisation of incident reporting as a learning tool and will lead to the regular publication, by the CPiRLS team, of alerts and detailed guidance to assist chiropractors in managing risk more effectively.

It is primarily legislation (Swiss Sickness and Accident Insurance and the Swiss

Law on Medical Professions) that drives quality management for patient safety in chiropractic practice in Switzerland. The increasing awareness and political commitment to improve safety affects all health care sectors including the chiropractic profession. The need for health professionals to continually improve quality and enhance patient safety is omnipresent. Unfortunately, the majority of well developed critical incident reporting systems are implemented in clinical inpatient and hospital settings, almost none of them in private medical or chiropractic practices. These facts and the low reporting rate cited in the UK study conducted by Thiel and Bolton [22] encouraged the Swiss Chiropractic Association to further investigate chiropractic incident reporting, its promotion and implementation. A first reporting and learning project, the Swiss Critical Reporting and Learning System (CRLS) was launched in September 2007 by Wangler and Zaugg [25].

Regular patient safety training is not yet established in chiropractic. In order to promote a change in attitudes towards greater patient safety, information and education should be part of the training of future chiropractors. With the help of a literature synthesis [26], 10 factors developed by Bland and co-workers [27] were adapted for successful promotion of patient safety competence in private practice, i.e. reporting and learning from adverse events in chiropractic care. The annual National Continuing Education Convention (2007) was considered to be the ideal environment to introduce and promote this first reporting and learning project. A survey on chiropractors' readiness and capacity for patient safety attitude change using the

Safety Attitude Questionnaire (SAQ) [28,29] for ambulatory care was conducted to assess the competencies of Swiss chiropractors in relation to patient safety issues.

The project consisted of a number of instructional approaches, such as providing written documentation, holding platform presentations and facilitating large and small group discussions incorporating feedback by experts.

Qualitative analysis [25] indicated that the biggest challenge seemed to be the culture shift from blame to trust. Lecturing is convenient, but it did not change behaviour in practice. As with clinical reasoning, reporting cannot occur in a vacuum, but must be built into daily practice. Reporting and learning skills have first to be developed and practised. An online discussion forum between experts and practitioners could facilitate the development of such skills. Active support by leaders of the national association was minimal. Finally, safety and quality have to be integrated into continuing professional development.

The Swiss CRLS website http://www.crls-chiro.ch informs on the purpose and scope of incident reporting and learning. As with the UK CPiRLS, only chiropractors can submit and read reports on the password-protected website. Reports and discussions are kept totally anonymous. The password-secured forum is user-friendly and the reporting procedure is clear. Different to the CPiRLS system in the UK, the Swiss chiropractor describes the incident with first reflection and without categorisation. This means the user simply analyses what went wrong and what action should be taken. Regular, timely and effective feedback by experts regarding this proposed action is essential.

Approximately six months after the start of the reporting and learning project the frequency with which reports were submitted diminished significantly. Therefore another pilot project, dealing with structured and systematic analysis of real-life adverse events in chiropractic care, was initiated [30]. The London Protocol [31] was chosen as the analysis method.

WHO Draft Guidelines for Adverse Event Reporting and Learning Systems

Of utmost importance for a reporting system is the appropriate use of the information it produces. Reporting is a tool for obtaining safety information and to advance quality improvement and error prevention. According to the WHO Draft Guidelines for Adverse Event Reporting and Learning Systems [9], successful patient safety reporting systems have the following characteristics: (1) Reporting must be safe for the individuals who report; (2) reporting leads to a constructive response; (3) reporting is only of value if it leads to meaningful analysis; and (4) learning requires expertise and adequate financial resources i.e. the agency that receives reports must be capable of disseminating information and making recommendations for changes, and informing the development of solutions.

The WHO has produced Draft Guidelines for Adverse Event Reporting and Learning Systems [9] that are derived from experiences both in healthcare and in other industries, particularly aviation. Table 5 lists the characteristics and Table 6 the requirements that have been identified by various authors as essential to the success of any reporting systems concerned with patient safety in these guidelines.

Characteristics and Recommendations for European CIRLS

A reporting system needs to have a clear purpose and clear objectives. It must be obvious to the user who should report and what must be reported. It must allow users to understand the purpose of reporting and assure them that there will not be any retaliation or punitive measures taken as a result of their reporting. The mechanisms for receiving reports and managing the data must guarantee protection for the patient, the reporter and any institution involved. Once the data have been obtained, experts must be available to analyse the specific situation, circumstances and any contributing factors related to the reported incidents. All facts need to be accumulated in an integrated fashion, thus generating manageable information. Timing is of utmost importance so that the information resulting from this process is distributed efficiently through the right channels and amongst those parties who need to access it within an appropriate time span. This measure means that serious hazards, once identified, are prioritised quickly. Information needs to be converted into recommendations that will promote changes that go beyond individual performance, and target systems and operational structures. Agencies receiving the reports need to

Table 5 Characteristics of Successful Reporting Systems [9]*

Non-punitive	Reporters are free from fear of retaliation against themselves or punishment of others as a result of reporting.
Confidential	The identities of the patient, reporter, and institution are never revealed.
Independent	The reporting system is independent of any authority with power to punish the reporter or the organization.
Expert analysis	Reports are evaluated by experts who understand the clinical circumstances and are trained to recognize underlying system causes
Timely	Reports are analyzed promptly and recommendations are rapidly disseminated to those who need to know especially when serious hazards are identified.
System-oriented	Recommendations focus on changes in systems, processes, or products, rather than being targeted at individual performance.
Responsive	The agency that receives reports is capable of disseminating recommendations. Participating organizations commit to implementing recommendations whenever possible.

*Reproduced with permission of WHO Press http://www.who.int/about/licensing/en.

Table 6 Requirements of Successful Reporting Systems [9]*

Key Messages Capacity to respond to reports	
Clear objectives	Capacity to respond to reports
Clarity about who should report	A method for classifying and making sense of reported events
Clarity about what gets reported	The capacity to disseminate findings
Mechanisms for receiving reports and managing data	Technical infrastructure and data security
Expertise for analysis	

*Reproduced with permission of WHO Press http://www.who.int/about/licensing/en.

develop a technical infrastructure that will allow them to receive data, process the information and generate recommendations for the purpose of providing a learning experience for the reporter and organisations alike. This will achieve an improved safety environment for patients, where prevention is one of the cornerstones.

The commission members deliberated on the characteristics and recommendations for European Chiropractic Incident Reporting and Learning Systems and arrived at a number of criteria and requirements for successful reporting of, and learning from incidents. These are outlined in Table 7. Most recommendations were derived from the WHO draft guidelines [9].

Conclusions

Before a reporting and learning system can be established it has to be clear what the objectives of the system are, what resources will be required and whether the organisation responsible for implementation has the capacity to respond to reports. This requires the availability of experts to analyse the incidents and to provide feedback in a timely fashion. A comprehensive strategy for national implementation must be in place including, but not limited to, presentations at national meetings, written information to all practitioners and workshops to ensure standardised reporting. Training and support must be available for both experts and reporting clinicians. Patterns and similarities in the sources of risk arising out of clinical practice must be disseminated to individual practitioners and appropriate organisations and institutions. Anonymity and confidentiality for patients and practitioners must be guaranteed at any time.

When implementing a national CIRLS in Europe, special consideration must be given to cultural differences, legal obligations, available human and financial resources, as well as the commitment of an organisation's leadership to such a project as evidenced by the two existing systems in the UK and in Switzerland.

Table 7 Recommendations for European Chiropractic Incident Reporting and Learning Systems, developed by the commission (2010)

Criteria for success	Requirements for success
Clear purpose	Strategy to communicate the purpose of learning to improve patient safety in practice
Clear strategy	Specific instructions for reporters (e.g., chiropractors and staff) on incidents to be reported
Anonymity	Safe IT-systems and procedures to guarantee anonymity/confidentiality for patients, practitioners and institutions
Risk free	Administrators and experts involved in managing the system without authority for punishment and retaliation
Feedback to the reporting individual	Experts must analyse the incidents and give timely feedback. Focus should be on improving the clinical setting and/or avoiding similar incidents in the future
Feedback to organizations	If serious hazards are identified, information - after being made anonymous - should be distributed to organisations and/or the individual through pre-determined channels without delay
Accumulation of knowledge	Received data should be collated in a structured fashion to allow meaningful analyses
Formulation of guidelines	An expert panel should be appointed to transform the aggregated analyses into clinically meaningful guidelines, targeting systems and operational procedures as well as individual performance
Implementation	A comprehensive strategy for national implementation must be in place for the individual countries, including (but not limited to) presentation at national meetings, workshops and making available written information for clinicians

Considerations for the Future

A number of European patient safety incident reporting systems offer the possibility for patients or members of the public to report directly, either via a separate pathway designed for public and patient reporting (e.g., http://www.nrls.npsa.nhs.uk/report-a-patient-safety-incident) or by allowing anyone to access and utilise the same reporting format (e.g., http://www.jeder-fehler-zaehlt.de). We foresee a future mechanism whereby chiropractic patients could report incidents directly and independently. However, in order to achieve a change of culture within the profession (feel secure to report), a password-protected system, restricted to chiropractors only, is likely to be the immediate way forward.

Additional material

Additional file 1: Percentage of agreement with the AGREE domains by members of the commission (n = 5).

Additional file 2: The European Patient Organizations' review.

Additional file 3: Summary on person and system approach.

Additional file 4: The "Swiss Cheese Model" of accident causation [16].

Acknowledgements

The members of the commission would like to acknowledge the financial support provided by the European Chiropractors Union to cover meeting expenses.

Author details

[1]European Academy of Chiropractic, academic dean and private practice, Bahnhofstrasse 15, 3400 Burgdorf, Switzerland. [2]Real Centro Universitario Maria Cristina-College of Chiropractic, Paseo de los Alamillos 2, 28200 San Lorenzo de El Escorial, Spain. [3]Nordisk Institut for Kiropraktik og Klinisk Biomekanik Forskerparken 10, 5230 Odense M, Denmark. [4]European Academy of Chiropractic, Department of Research and private practice, St. Paulusstraat 15, 2400 Mol-Belgium. [5]European Council on Chiropractic Education and private practice, Kiropraktorklinikken Strandgården, Havnegt. 1, 4790 Lillesand, Norway. [6]Anglo-European College of Chiropractic, 13-15 Parkwood Road, Bournemouth BH5 2DF, UK. [7]Swiss Academy of Chiropractic and private practice, Johann-Verresius-Str. 18 2502 Biel, Switzerland.

Authors' contributions

MW was responsible for: the methodology used to collect and to summarise the evidence, leading the online discussions, organising and participating in the analysis of the collected data, formulating recommendations and conclusions, and drafting and finalising the manuscript.
HT and BZ were responsible for: the literature review, the methodology used to collect and to summarise the evidence, participating in the analysis of the collected data, formulating recommendations and conclusions, and reviewing and finalising the manuscript.
TM, RF, LH, and TJR were responsible for: summarising the evidence, participating in the analysis of the collected data, formulating recommendations and conclusions, and reviewing the manuscript.
All authors have read and approved the final abstract and manuscript.

Competing interests

The authors declare that they have no competing interests.

References

1. Flannagan J: **The critical incident technique.** *Psychological Bull* 1954, 327-357.
2. Banks IC, Tackley RM: **A standard set of terms for critical incident recording?** *Br J Anaesth* 1994, **73**:703-70.
3. Webb RK, Currie M, Morgan CA, Williamson JA, Mackay P, Russell WJ, *et al*: **The Australian Incident Monitoring Study: an analysis of 2000 incident reports.** *Anaesth Intensive Care* 1993, **21**:520-528.
4. O'Donnell R: **The development and evaluation of a test for predicting dental student performance.** [49] University Pittsburgh Bulletin; 1953, 240-245.
5. Williamson JA, Mackay P: **Incident reporting.** *Med J Aust* 1991, **155**:340-344.
6. Secker-Walker JT-AS: **Clinical incident reporting.** In *Clinical risk management Enhancing patient safety.* Edited by: Vincent C. London: BMJ Publishing Group; 2001:419-438.
7. Cooper JB, Newbower RS, Long CD, McPeek B: **Preventable anesthesia mishaps: a study of human factors.** *Anesthesiology* 1978, **49**:399-406.
8. Van Liew D: **Using information systems to support risk management.** In *Clinical risk modification A route to clinical governance.* Edited by: Wilson J, Tingle, J. Oxford: Butterworth Heinemann; 1999:66-85.
9. **WHO Draft Guidelines for Adverse Event Reporting and Learning Systems.** [http://www.who.int/patientsafety/events/05/Reporting_Guidelines.pdf].
10. **The Appraisal of Guidelines for Research & Evaluation (AGREE) Instrument.** [http://www.agreetrust.org].
11. Court D: **Quest for patient safety in a challenging environment.** *Aust N Z J Obstet Gynaecol* 2003, **43**:97-100.
12. Barrett A, Breen A: **Adverse events of spinal manipulation.** *JRSM* 2000, 258-259[http://www.ncbi.nlm.nih.gov/pmc/articles/PMC1298004/].
13. Stevinson C, Ernst E: **Risks associated with spinal manipulation.** *Am J Med* 2002, **112**:566-571.
14. Osborne N, Thiel H, Kusiar W: **Post-manipulative stroke: a study of two cases.** *The British Journal of Chiropractic* 2000, 6-11.
15. Department of Health: *An organisation with a memory* London: Sationery Office; 2000 [http://www.dh.gov.uk/en/Publicationsandstatistics/Publications/PublicationsPolicyAndGuidance/DH_4065083].
16. Reason J: *Managing the risks of organisational accidents* Aldershot: Ashgate; 1997 [http://catalogue.nla.gov.au/Record/1758678].
17. Avery AJ: **Classifying and identifying errors.** *Qual Saf Health Care* 2003, **12**:404.
18. Reason J: **Understanding adverse events: human factors.** *Qual Health Care* 1995, **4**:80-9.
19. Reason J: **Human error: models and management.** *BMJ* 2000, **320**:768-770.
20. Eagle CJ, Davies JM, Reason J: **Accident analysis of large-scale technological disasters applied to an anaesthetic complication.** *Can J Anaesth* 1992, **39**:118-122.
21. Hudson P: **Applying the lessons of high risk industries to health care.** *Qual Saf Health Care* 2003, **12(Suppl 1)**:i7-12.
22. Thiel H, Bolton JE: **The Reporting of Patient Safety Incidents-First Experiences with the Chiropractic Reporting and Learning System (CRLS): A pilot study.** *Clinical Chiropractic* 2006, **9**:139-149.
23. Gunn SJ, Thiel HW, Bolton JE: **British Chiropractic Association members' attitudes towards the Chiropractic Reporting and Learning System: A qualitative study.** *Clinical Chiropractic* 2008, 63-69.
24. Cunliffe C, Johnson IJ, Selby J: **Safety incidents, treatment complications and reactions recorded in a student teaching clinic: A retrospective analysis.** *Proceedings of the Association of Chiropractic Colleges Research Agenda Conference (ACC-RAC). Las Vegas* 2009.
25. Wangler M, Zaugg B: **Promotion of Patient Safety Competence among Licensed Chiropractors: Four Instructional Approaches.** *Master thesis* University of Berne, Switzerland; MME Department; 2008 [http://www.mme-alumni.uzh.ch/masterthesen/thesen_anzeige.php?ID=70&sprache=de].
26. Zaugg B, Wangler M: **A Model Framework for Patient Safety Training in Chiropractic: A Literature Synthesis.** *J Manipulative Physiol Ther* 2009, **32**:493-9.
27. Bland CJ, Starnaman S, Wersal L, Moorehead-Rosenberg L, Zonia S, Henry R: **Curricular change in medical schools: how to succeed.** *Acad Med* 2000, **75**:575-594.
28. Modak I, Sexton JB, Lux TR, Helmreich RL, Thomas EJ: **Measuring safety culture in the ambulatory setting: the safety attitudes questionnaire–ambulatory version.** *J Gen Intern Med* 2007, **22**:1-5.
29. Sexton JB, Helmreich RL, Neilands TB, Rowan K, Vella K, Boyden J, *et al*: **The Safety Attitudes Questionnaire: psychometric properties, bench-marking data, and emerging research.** *BMC Health Serv Res* 2006, **6**:44.
30. Wangler M: **Lernen aus Behandlungsfehlern Analyse gemäss Methode ERA.**[http://www.reportingandlearning.ch].
31. Taylor-Adam S, Vincent C: **Systems analysis of clinical incidents: the London protocol.** *Clinical Risk* 2004, **10**:211-220.

12

The treatment experience of patients with low back pain during pregnancy and their chiropractors: a qualitative study

Shabnam Sadr, Neda Pourkiani-Allah-Abad and Kent Jason Stuber*

Abstract

Background: Chiropractors regularly treat pregnant patients for low back pain during their pregnancy. An increasing amount of literature on this topic supports this form of treatment; however the experience of the pregnant patient with low back pain and their chiropractor has not yet been explored. The objective of this study is to explore the experience of chiropractic treatment for pregnant women with low back pain, and their chiropractors.

Methods: This qualitative study employed semi-structured interviews of pregnant patients in their second or third trimester, with low back pain during their pregnancy, and their treating chiropractors in separate interviews. Participants consisted of 11 patients and 12 chiropractors. The interviews consisted of 10 open-ended questions for patients, and eight open-ended questions for chiropractors, asking about their treatment experience or impressions of treating pregnant patients with LBP, respectively. All interviews were audio-recorded, transcribed verbatim, and reviewed independently by the investigators to develop codes, super-codes and themes. Thematic saturation was reached after the eleventh chiropractor and ninth patient interviews. All interviews were analyzed using the qualitative analysis software N-Vivo 9.

Results: Five themes emerged out of the chiropractor and patient interviews. The themes consisted of Treatment and Effectiveness; Chiropractor-Patient Communication; Pregnant Patient Presentation and the Chiropractic Approach to Pregnancy Care; Safety Considerations; and Self-Care.

Conclusions: Chiropractors approach pregnant patients with low back pain from a patient-centered standpoint, and the pregnant patients interviewed in this study who sought chiropractic care appeared to find this approach helpful for managing their back pain symptoms.

Keywords: Pregnancy, Chiropractic, Qualitative, Exercise, Spinal manipulative therapy, Nutrition, Adverse effects

Background

Low back pain (LBP) during pregnancy is reported by approximately 50% to 80% of pregnant women [1-3]. The structural, postural, or hormonal changes that occur during pregnancy, or any combination thereof, may lead to LBP during pregnancy [3]. Treatment options include a range of therapies, such as exercise programs, massage therapy, acupuncture, and chiropractic [4,5]. Chiropractic care may include spinal manipulative therapy (SMT), mobilizations and soft tissue therapy, as well as exercise prescription [3]. Previous studies and systematic reviews of the literature have indicated the relative safety and effectiveness of chiropractic treatment for LBP during pregnancy [3,5-7].

To date, no study has explored the treatment experience of the pregnant population seeking care for their back pain, whether that treatment is from a chiropractor or any other health care provider, nor has any study assessed the experience of chiropractors providing treatment for their pregnant patients with LBP. The qualities of the care provided by the treating chiropractor and that received by the pregnant patient may impact the outcomes of chiropractic care for women with LBP

* Correspondence: kstuber@cmcc.ca
Canadian Memorial Chiropractic College, 6100 Leslie Street, Toronto, Ontario M2H 3J1, Canada

during pregnancy. As such, the objective of this study was to explore the experience of chiropractic treatment for pregnant women who have LBP, as well as their chiropractors in providing care for such patients.

Methods

This was a qualitative study utilizing semi-structured in-person and telephone interviews conducted in Toronto, Canada. The study was approved by the Canadian Memorial Chiropractic College Research Ethics Board prior to commencement.

Participants

Participants consisted of 11 patients and 12 chiropractors. The inclusion criteria for pregnant patients in the study consisted of adults (18 years or greater), in their second or third trimester with uncomplicated pregnancies (i.e. absence of pre-eclampsia, gestational diabetes, multiple pregnancies, etc.), who were experiencing LBP during their pregnancy and were seeking treatment for relief of their low back pain symptoms from a chiropractor at the time. Chiropractors included in the study were either male or female adults of any age, who were actively seeing at least one pregnant patient with LBP and agreed to participate in the study both by referring at least one patient and by completing their own semi-structured interview. Signed informed consent was obtained from all participants prior to being interviewed. All transcribed interview records were kept confidential, with only the investigators having access to the information provided. For referencing and analysis purposes a subject identification code was assigned to the each participant based on being a patient (PT) or Doctor of Chiropractic (DC), the numerical order in which they were interviewed for their particular participant category and the date of their interview. For example, the first chiropractor interviewed on August 7, 2011 was coded as: DC01-080711.

Participant recruitment

Chiropractors were recruited through convenience sampling using chiropractors known to the study team or recommended by other participating chiropractors. The inclusion criteria for patients were explained to the chiropractors who agreed to participate, and they were asked to recruit any of their patients who they determined would meet the inclusion criteria. As such, any pregnant women who met the inclusion criteria were initially asked by their treating chiropractor if they were interested in participating in this study, and were then referred to the investigators to confirm their interest, eligibility for inclusion, and availability for an interview. Most of the chiropractors recruited were practicing in Southern Ontario, while a few were based in Calgary, Alberta.

Data collection

Semi-structured interviews were carried out in-person for those participants who were available on the CMCC campus clinic or lived within the Greater Toronto Area. Telephone interviews were conducted with those who lived or practiced outside of the Greater Toronto Area. The patient interviews lasted between 15 and 20 minutes and consisted of ten open-ended questions, asking them about their pregnancy and their chiropractic treatment experience for their LBP during the pregnancy. The chiropractor interviews lasted between ten and fifteen minutes and consisted of eight open-ended questions, asking about their experience and impressions of treating pregnant patients with LBP. Two investigators were present at all times for the duration of each interview, and questions were asked by the same investigator for consistency. Question sequencing was flexible, allowing participants to elaborate on their experiences and for questions to be posed at the most appropriate time of a given interview as determined by the investigator. All interviews were conducted between the months of June and November, 2011.

Data analysis

All of the interviews were audio-recorded using two digital devices, subsequently transcribed verbatim by one of the investigators, and later reviewed independently by the two remaining investigators for completeness and accuracy. Using a grounded theory approach, two investigators independently coded each interview, and all three investigators developed super-codes based on the initial codes, and developed themes from there. Investigator meetings were held where emergent themes, patterns and connections were discussed and reviewed by each investigator to ensure accuracy. During these investigator meetings, it was discussed as to whether or not thematic saturation had been reached. In particular after the eighth chiropractor and eighth patient interviews the three investigators discussed whether or not thematic saturation had been reached and it was felt that it had not yet been met. Subsequently all of the investigators concurred that thematic saturation was reached after the eleventh DC and ninth PT interviews. The remaining interviews allowed for elaboration of the themes. All interviews were imported, organized into themes and analyzed using the qualitative analysis N-Vivo 9 software.

Results

The 11 included patients were between the ages of 24 and 36 years and the timing of their pregnancies ranged from 17 to 38 weeks. The 12 included chiropractors were in practice between three and 38 years. During analysis five themes emerged from the DC and PT interviews. The themes identified were: Treatment and Effectiveness; Chiropractor-Patient Communication; Pregnant Patient Presentation and the Chiropractic Approach to Pregnancy Care; Safety Considerations; and Self-Care.

Treatment and effectiveness

Nearly all of the chiropractors indicated that chiropractic treatment was effective in relieving the LBP of pregnant patients. Most of them indicated that they saw positive results in their pregnant patients, for instance: (DC02) "*their symptoms seem to improve with the treatment, and also objectively I find that the joint restrictions improve as well.*" One chiropractor spoke of some of the important outcomes of care for pregnant patients:

> DC10: "*The impact for the pregnant patient is usually profound, as being able to reduce pain and increase function and getting them back into exercise, which is all important for the outcomes of the pregnancy.*"

In terms of treatment procedures, most of the chiropractors indicated employing the Diversified technique, previously reported by 86% of surveyed Canadian chiropractors, [8,9] employing high-velocity, low-amplitude spinal manipulation maneuvers [10], as well as soft tissue therapy and exercise prescription. One particular chiropractor, among the most experienced of those interviewed, said that her treatment plan depended on the patient:

> DC09: "*depends on what the patient comes in with, and it also depends on what time they're at in their pregnancy, which month. So there are a few variables to consider. We can say essentially Diversified, but again I modify it according to the presenting symptoms and the spinal configuration of the patient.*"

A few of the chiropractors used instrumented techniques for spinal manipulation, such as the Activator® [9,11] or the Integrator™ [9] when working on any sensitive areas towards the latter parts of the pregnancy. Two of the chiropractors used the Webster technique [12]:

> DC05: "*The second component of the Webster technique just requires some soft tissue work for the round ligament. I find that works quite well, people respond really well to it.*"

All of the interviewed patients reported that they found chiropractic treatment to be effective and that it helped relieve them of their LBP and associated symptoms. Patients reported that chiropractic treatment had improved their daily living activities and their mobility, while it decreased their overall pain and discomfort:

> PT01: "*I can walk longer periods of time. So that's excellent. I can go standing for four to five hours. Because prior to that I'd be standing 40 minutes to do the dishes and I'd be in agony. even the basic things, like picking things up off the floor, you'd get stuck in that position, I haven't experienced that yet [in this pregnancy]. Or just sitting for long periods of time, because I do work an office job from home, so I do sit long periods of time. I know for most people [they] have to get up and stretch for a couple minutes, even in doing that I've been doing okay.*"

> PT02: "*The pain is gone. but I do feel like I have more energy and I can do more activities. The pain doesn't prevent me anymore.*"

> PT05: "*It really allowed me to function. I could barely walk before or stand, the pain was intense, but after I went to the chiropractor. I found I could function day to day, I could walk from the bus stop to work, I could do these things, so that was pretty significant. It's just helping me function. It's just teaching me how to pick up my daughter so I don't hurt myself. To still function, to still play with my daughter and be able to go to the grocery store and do all these things without really hurting myself. As well as it allows me to sleep at night.*"

> PT06: "*I found within five days I had greater mobility in terms of twisting and turning. I'm a drama teacher so I'm constantly up on my feet and I need to be able to lean down, jump over, so I need to have a full range of motion, and I found that my range of motion had been very limited and I was getting cranky because I was in pain. I think after the treatment, it was decreased pain and increased sense of mobility, increased range of motion and decreased sense of frustration and grumpiness.*"

> PT11: "*that's the whole reason I go, [for] the pain relief, especially now that I'm a stay-at-home mom, and picking up a 30-pound, 19 month-old all day long. So seeing a chiropractor really helps because it's not ideal to be lifting a child all day long when you're in a lot of pain, just the pain relief and the effect that it has on making your daily life easier.*"

Chiropractor-patient communication

The chiropractors generally emphasized communicating well with their patients as part of providing care and outlining the outcomes to expect. A few of the chiropractors placed great emphasis on patient education about pregnancy, particularly with respect to the changes that are taking place in the patient's body as they are going through their pregnancy, or the various reasons behind their LBP symptoms. For instance, with respect to doing yoga, DC09 said: *"I encourage that if there are no contraindications, and I give them simple postural advice and things they can do at their workplace."*

One chiropractor said educating his patients is 50% of what he does, and that it is (DC11) *"a great component initially"*:

> DC11: *"I think the more knowledge they have, the better they are... the woman who is going through the first pregnancy is very scared, hesitant, anxious and wants that kind of knowledge, and wants the practitioner to know what they're going through and set their mind at ease."*

Chiropractors were generally open to referring their patients to other professionals if necessary. DC12 said when a patient comes in with a concern *"that is a bit out of my scope,"* he encourages her to contact her midwife or OB-GYN.

One pattern that emerged from the interviews was that communication between chiropractors and patients depended on the knowledge level of both parties. Only a few of the patients seemed to be very knowledgeable about their pregnancy and asked questions or challenged their chiropractors about various techniques or treatments:

> PT06: *"I think we sort of have more of a dialogue about what treatment options to pursue, I think I'm more assertive in terms of asking 'why' or 'how come' or 'is this a good option' and 'what else could we do'."*

The approach of one chiropractor in particular was shown to help her patients emotionally regarding the changes going on in their bodies. While educating the patient, the chiropractor also eased their mind simply with her communication skills, as explained by her patient:

> PT06: *"It's been emotionally helpful because at the same time I'm getting advice beyond... there's been explanations of 'physiologically this is what's happening to your body' and 'this is why your ligaments are pulling,' 'this is why you're compensating with the extra weight at the front,' 'this is why your posture is changing'... and things like that."*

Pregnant patient presentation and the chiropractic approach to pregnancy care

Each chiropractor's approach to treatment depended on their knowledge and experience with pregnant patients. A few of the chiropractors had more preventive maintenance and wellness-based practices where they provided a long-term treatment plan for their pregnant patients. For instance, patients went for regular visits and adjustments, regardless of having any pain or symptoms. One pattern that emerged among the chiropractors, was that most of the pregnant patients they saw and treated were previous "on-going" patients who later became pregnant, and then continued with modified care throughout their pregnancies. In terms of their specific approach to treatment, one chiropractor said:

> DC05: *"I definitely take a very holistic approach with my health history and my assessment. I want to get a good sense of what their pregnancy has been like, from the overall standpoint. What type of stressors have been in their world, physical stressors, chemical stressors, the foods that they eat, nutrition is a big piece, activity is a big piece, any mental or emotional concerns or fears going into labor, birth or even pregnancy in general. It can be an emotional time for some women."*

Another chiropractor (DC06) who frequently treated pregnant women in his practice had a "protocol" that he used with them, and believed that chiropractic care is a great "adjunct" to treating these patients, as part of their larger health care team.

Pregnant patients present differently in terms of their LBP symptoms, its onset, location and duration. The chiropractor's approach depended on the patient's presentation, and most of them had a patient-centered approach:

> (DC03) *"Some will respond differently than others and obviously not every pregnant patient with back pain has exactly the same issues as well. So, we obviously tailor those situations to patients."*

This was emphasized by another chiropractor:

> DC09: *"There are a variety of pregnant patients that come in, some who are 'die-hard' chiropractic patients who really don't care or ask you anything. They just know they are going to feel well, so they just want to be there to continue. Then there are the others who kind of want to try it to see where they're at, so the first trimester patient in that sense can be particular. The second trimester patient will probably ask more questions because they've heard more about*

> *chiropractic, so they know it can be beneficial in terms of their delivery especially. they are there for a reason and want to know how often they can come."*

DC09 further added, *"The bio-psycho-social model is very relevant too. Because they are not all coming to me from nice family units... I've got single moms, I've got pregnancies that have gone particularly bad... that has a huge impact on the pregnancy as well."* One chiropractor simply said: (DC12) *"It depends on what trimester they start at and how far along they are and what stresses they have on their body."*

Many of the patients had received chiropractic treatment prior to their pregnancy. Depending on their symptom presentation and background (in terms of previous pregnancies), some patients received chiropractic treatment when they felt the need, or when they felt their symptoms were flaring up. One patient said: (PT05) *"We don't really have a treatment plan. It's more like, 'when it hurts, come back'. So I've just been keeping tabs on how I'm feeling and when it hurts I go back."*

A few patients received long-term spinal care from their chiropractors who had more of a preventive maintenance and wellness-based approach to therapy, where they received treatment on regular visits for the duration of their pregnancy, even when no symptoms were present, while others were receiving treatment for other conditions and continued on with the care when the low back pain during their pregnancy came on:

> PT03: *"I've seen chiropractors over the years. I started seeing chiropractors when I was 17, I had low back problems by then and yeah, with the pregnancies it was just getting worse."*

> PT01: *"prior to the pregnancy I used to see the chiropractor for my mid back section and my neck for headaches, so that's how it all started."*

Several patients chose chiropractic care for their back pain because they had found results from their first pregnancy:

> PT11: *"it worked so well the first time, I'd even come away from the appointment feeling better. It was almost an immediate fix. So because of my positive experience the first time, there was no question that I was going to use chiropractic care for the second pregnancy."*

Generally, most of the chiropractors were knowledgeable about treating pregnant patients and had either some kind of formal post-graduate training, or had attended seminars or workshops. A few of them said they kept up-to-date with the research on pregnancy, although they admitted, (DC09) *"there is not much"* or (DC12) *"there is not a lot out there."*

Safety considerations

All of the treating chiropractors directly stated in their interviews that they believed chiropractic treatment for their pregnant patients was safe, and they had seen no adverse effects. For instance, one chiropractor said: (DC03) *"I primarily do Diversified adjusting in my practice and I consider that to be safe"* This was further emphasized by saying: (DC08) *"in pregnant patients the ligaments are very loose and require very little force to adjust, which I feel makes it much more safe, because you don't have to do a whole lot to get the response you want."* With respect to the Webster technique, it was said: (DC05) *"the method of assessment and adjustment is very safe. The patient is very comfortable lying prone on the table with the use of pregnancy pillows"*.

In terms of any contraindications to treatment, most of the chiropractors said that they would not use any electrical modalities on their pregnant patients. One said he would not do much treatment in the first trimester (DC06), whereas two said they wouldn't start their patient on a new exercise program in the last trimester. One chiropractor said he would not use any SMT on a pregnant patient if he knew that she had a miscarriage before (DC04), or if she had early dilation of the cervix (DC09).

All of the patients directly stated in their interviews that they believed chiropractic treatment was safe and they had not experienced any adverse events after any treatment, which has been reported in previous studies [13]: (PT07) *"I wouldn't say I've ever had any side effects."* Patients also described their comfort levels changing with particular treatments throughout the pregnancy, while their chiropractors generally modified the treatments to make their patients feel safe and comfortable:

> PT11: *"I'm always very aware of what he's doing to me and where the position of the baby is. I can't say I'm 100% comfortable, I know it works, and I've read quite a number of articles about it. I haven't experienced any problems, but it's always in the back of my mind [safety of my baby], especially in the very beginning, not so much right now, because I'm really big now and it has to be done differently. Now the reservations are there but they're very small, and I think that's the case with anything in pregnancy. You just want to make sure you're doing the right thing for your body and the baby."*

> PT11: *"I was on my back for a couple of the adjustments, and now because I'm so big, I can't lay*

too long on my back so comfortably and I can't lay on my front. He's given me a cushion but it's not very comfortable, and so the last adjustment I had was primarily on my side and on my back for a short period of time and nothing on my front."

Self-care

All 12 chiropractors discussed advising exercises or encouraging their patients to follow an exercise program before, during or after their pregnancy. Generally, they emphasized exercise throughout the pregnancy: (DC01) *"I do a lot of exercise therapy with my pregnant patients. It could alleviate some of their aches and pain if they worked out on a regular basis with someone who knows what they're doing and what exercises to give them."* Many of the chiropractors had a specific exercise plan or regime that they prescribed to their patients, depending on which stage of pregnancy they were in. For instance:

> DC03: *"What we're recommending are often core-strengthening exercises, and a lot more women these days are much more aware of getting ahead of the game in terms of fitness training during their pregnancy. If we have the opportunity to work with someone earlier in their pregnancy we'd be working harder to get them moving. Once they're in the latter half of their pregnancy, really what we're trying to do is maintaining and making sure we're not adding anything more than their body can handle at that point and time."*

Almost all the chiropractors who included exercise in their treatment said that they would not start a new exercise program if the patient was not exercising before pregnancy, and they would not introduce anything new later in the pregnancy: (DC04) *"If there is developing low back pain, I would give them... cat-camel, or basic yoga style stretching."*; (DC05) *"I walk patients through the type of exercises that I recommend to them. Show them and ask them to do it."*; "(DC06) *Yoga and Pilates is the only thing that I recommend. I try to keep [their] heart rate low."*; (DC08) *"I avoid extension exercises, but I still give them some pelvic tilts, of course get them to work on their kegels. Again it depends on the stage of pregnancy and assuming there is no complications or risks."*; (DC12) *"I'm only suggesting very low impact things, and they all seem to do fine and I haven't had anyone have a hard time with it."*

One patient said that her chiropractor did not give her any exercises to do, but generally most of the patients were given some sort of exercise regimen to follow, or were encouraged to do yoga, stretches and/or walking. One patient said: (PT07) *"She's given me a sheet of stretching exercises that are specifically for pregnancy."* Patients believed that this active component of their treatment empowered them to take care of themselves when in pain: (PT05) *"he gave [me] some stretches to do... I do them as needed... So when my back is particularly sore but I know I'm not going to the chiropractor for a few days, then I'll do those stretches and go from there."*

Discussion

One of the most common symptoms experienced during pregnancy is low back pain, as over half of the pregnant patient population experience LBP during their pregnancy [1,14]. Chiropractic is the third most common type of Complementary and Alternative Medicine (CAM) treatment sought by pregnant patients [15]. This study investigated the chiropractic treatment experience of pregnant patients with LBP, as well as their chiropractors. The comments of the patients and chiropractors lend some support to previous reports in the literature of positive outcomes of chiropractic care for LBP during pregnancy and provide insight as to how or why those outcomes may be achieved [5,15].

The chiropractors in this study emphasized communication with their patients [16,17] and educated them about pregnancy-related changes that they were experiencing and how the chiropractic treatments could be helpful. Pregnant patients often present differently in terms of their low back pain and symptoms, and the chiropractors in this study employed a patient-centered approach [18], where each patient's treatment plan was tailored to their specific needs and particular timing in their pregnancy. Knowledge and experience of both patients and their chiropractors played an important role in enhancing the doctor-patient relationship, as well as potentially contributing to a more positive therapeutic outcome.

The chiropractors in this study demonstrated concern regarding patient safety and were vigilant in evaluating for the presence of any contraindications to spinal manipulation. The safety of chiropractic treatments, and specifically spinal manipulation for pregnant patients has been evaluated in a previous survey of chiropractors [6] as well as a critical literature review [7]. These studies indicate that chiropractors feel that their treatments are safe for pregnant patients [6] and report that side effects may be rare, although further research is clearly needed [7].

It has been reported that women who exercise during pregnancy are likely to have more energy, fewer mood swings, better able to manage stress, and get more sleep compared with sedentary pregnant women [19,20]. Exercise prescription appears to be an important component of the treatment program as described by the participants in our study. Most of the chiropractors advised specific stretches or exercises for their patients, depending on how far along they were in their pregnancy. Moderate exercise during pregnancy has been shown to improve overall maternal well-being [19,20]. This was also reflected in the responses of the patients, who indicated that their chiropractor gave them some form of exercise to do at home. Those patients who adhered to their exercise program regularly indicated positive results and improved outcomes in their functioning and activities of daily living.

Future research into chiropractic treatment of pregnant patients with low back pain is warranted and the next step should likely involve a larger scale clinical trial at a higher level of evidence such as a randomized controlled trial [3,5,7]. Any future studies should employ well-defined inclusion and exclusion criteria and evaluate commonly used treatments such as those described by the participants in this study. It will also be necessary to utilize validated outcome measures for pain and disability due to low back pain, and track adverse events, while observing a suitable follow-up period.

Limitations

As this was a qualitative study that employed convenience sampling as opposed to purposive sampling [21], our sample is not necessarily representative of the experience of all pregnant patients who might have low back pain in their second or third trimester, nor of chiropractors who treat pregnant patients. Since only pregnant patients actively under chiropractic care were included, this study did not consider patient responses prior to receiving chiropractic treatment for their low back pain during pregnancy or after their delivery or conclusion of chiropractic care. Using clinicians to refer patients to the study team may have over-emphasized those patients with a particularly strong relationship with their chiropractors or who strongly value chiropractic care and its effects. Furthermore the clinicians may have only referred those patients that they knew or felt had good outcomes and may be more likely to express satisfaction with care, and thus the voices of those who may not have been satisfied with chiropractic care for low back pain during pregnancy may have been underrepresented. These factors could limit the transferability of our findings. However, our data has potential for transferability to a wider population, in this case other chiropractors and their pregnant patients with low back pain, as chiropractors and patients from two different jurisdictions (both Ontario and Alberta) were interviewed and the chiropractors involved had a wide range of practice experience. Furthermore, there was a wide age and gestational period range among the patients interviewed. In future qualitative evaluations of this topic, more purposive sampling of both chiropractors and patients would be beneficial, in particular by seeking out pregnant patients independent of referrals from their chiropractors.

Qualitative research inevitably suffers from issues of bias as the researchers invariably have an effect on the participants and potentially the results of a qualitative study through the concept of reflexivity [21]. However several steps were taken to account for potential bias and reduce the influence of reflexivity as our data was triangulated as we interviewed two groups, pregnant women and their chiropractors, again potentially aiding transferability. The presence of multiple team members at each interview and multiple reviewers to evaluate transcripts and generate codes and themes should further enhance the validity and aid the credibility of our findings. Determining the point of thematic saturation is another particular instance where bias could be introduced and the validity of the findings questioned, particularly if the saturation point was chosen too early, but to reduce this possibility multiple meetings were held among the investigators to help ensure that a suitable and agreed upon thematic saturation point was found and that no new themes emerged in subsequent interviews, which were used to elaborate upon the existing themes.

Conclusions

Our study was aimed at two subgroups that have not been explored together previously using qualitative research methods, thus it provides new information that can contribute to the current literature on pregnancy and chiropractic treatment. The transferability of the findings of this study may be limited to the group evaluated, particularly owing to possible selection bias as the chiropractors selected patients to refer for interviews with the study team. However, based on the comments of the participating patients and chiropractors, it could be suggested that these particular pregnant women with low-risk or uncomplicated pregnancies, who experienced low back pain, appear to have benefited from chiropractic treatment, including spinal manipulation, soft tissue therapy and exercise therapy. No adverse events were reported by the pregnant patients or their chiropractors in response to spinal manipulation received from their chiropractors. The patients involved reported that they were generally satisfied with the chiropractic care they received during their pregnancy, and had positive outcomes in terms of reduction in their low back pain symptoms, and improved range of motion and overall function. Future research into the effectiveness and safety of chiropractic care for LBP during pregnancy is still needed, potentially including mixed methods research and larger scale clinical trials.

Competing interests

The authors declare that they have no competing interest.

Authors' contributions

SS participated in study design and coordination, data collection and analysis, and helped to draft the manuscript. NPAA participated in study design and coordination, data collection and analysis, and helped to draft the manuscript. KJS conceived the study, participated in its design and coordination, data analysis, and helped to draft the manuscript. "All authors read and approved the final manuscript."

References

1. Diakow PRP, Gadsby TA, Gadsby JB, Gleddie JG, Leprich DJ, Scales AM: **Back pain during pregnancy and labor.** *J Manipulative Physiol Ther* 1991, **14**:116–8.
2. Berg G, Hammar M, Moller-Nielsen J, Linden U, Thorblad J: **Low back pain during pregnancy.** *Obstet Gynecol* 1988, **71**:71–5.
3. Khorsan R, Hawk C, Lisi AJ, Kizhakkeveettil A: **Manipulative therapy for pregnancy and related conditions: A systematic review.** *Obstet Gynecol* 2009, **64**:416–427.
4. Perkins J, Hammer RL, Loubert PV: **Identification and management of pregnancy-related low back pain.** *J Nurs Midwifery* 1998, **43**:331–40.
5. Stuber KJ, Smith DL: **Chiropractic treatment of pregnancy-related low back pain: A systematic review of the evidence.** *J Manipulative Physiol Ther* 2008, **31**:447–454.
6. Stuber KJ: **The safety of chiropractic during pregnancy: A pilot email survey of chiropractors' opinions.** *Clin Chiropr* 2007, **10**:24–35.
7. Stuber KJ, Wynd S, Weis CA: **Adverse events from spinal manipulation in the pregnant and postpartum periods: a critical review of the literature.** *Chiropr Man Ther* 2012, **20**:8.
8. Mykietiuk C, Wambolt M, Pillipo T, Malla C, Gleberzon BJ: **Technique Systems used by post-1980 graduates of the Canadian Memorial Chiropractic College practicing in five Canadian provinces: A preliminary survey.** *J Can Chiropr Assoc* 2009, **53**:32–39.
9. Gleberzon BJ: **Name techniques in Canada: current trends in utilization rates and recommendations for their inclusion at the Canadian Memorial Chiropractic College.** *J Can Chiropr Assoc* 2000, **44**:157–168.
10. Downie AS, Vemulpad S, Bull PW: **Quantifying the high-velocity, low-amplitude spinal manipulative thrust: A systematic review.** *J Manipulative Physiol Ther* 2010, **33**:542–553.
11. Huggins T, Boras AL, Gleberzon BJ, Popescu M, Bahry LA: **Clinical effectiveness of the activator adjusting instrument in the management of musculoskeletal disorders: A systematic review of the literature.** *J Can Chiropr Assoc* 2012, **56**:49–57.
12. Pistolese RA: **The Webster Technique: a chiropractic technique with obstetric implications.** *J Manip Physiol Ther* 2002, **25**:e1–e9.
13. Lisi AJ: **Chiropractic spinal manipulation for low back pain of pregnancy: A retrospective case series.** *J Midwifery Women Health* 2006, **51**:e7–e10.
14. Phillips CJ, Meyer JJ: **Chiropractic care, including craniosacral therapy, during pregnancy: a static-group comparison of obstetric interventions during labor and delivery.** *J Manipulative Physiol Ther* 1995, **18**:525–529.
15. Wang SM, DeZinno P, Fermo L, Williams K, Caldwell-Andrews AA, Kain ZN: **Complementary and alternative medicine for low-back pain in pregnancy: a cross-sectional survey.** *J Altern Complement Med* 2005, **11**:459–64.
16. Marchiori DM, Henkin AB, Hawk C: **Social communication skills of chiropractors: Implications for professional practice.** *J Manipulative Physiol Ther* 2008, **31**:682–689.
17. Allen J, Richmond VP, McCroskey JC: **Communication and the chiropractic profession., part II.** *J Chiropr* 1984, **21**:46–50.
18. Gatterman MI: **A patient-centered paradigm: A model for chiropractic education and research.** *J Altern Complement Med* 1995, **1**:371–386.
19. Morris SN, Johnson NR: **Exercise during pregnancy: A critical appraisal of the literature.** *J Reprod Med* 2005, **50**:181–188.
20. Brown W: **The benefits of physical activity during pregnancy.** *J Sci Med Sport* 2002, **5**:37–45.
21. Malterud K: **Qualitative research: standards, challenges, and guidelines.** *Lancet* 2001, **358**:483–488.

13

Extending ICPC-2 PLUS terminology to develop a classification system specific for the study of chiropractic encounters

Melanie J Charity[1], Simon D French[1,2*], Kirsty Forsdike[1], Helena Britt[3], Barbara Polus[4] and Jane Gunn[1]

Abstract

Background: Typically a large amount of information is collected during healthcare research and this information needs to be organised in a way that will make it manageable and to facilitate clear reporting. The Chiropractic Observation and Analysis STudy (COAST) was a cross sectional observational study that described the clinical practices of chiropractors in Victoria, Australia. To code chiropractic encounters COAST used the International Classification of Primary Care (ICPC-2) with the PLUS general practice clinical terminology to code chiropractic encounters. This paper describes the process by which a chiropractic-profession specific terminology was developed for use in research by expanding the current ICPC-2 PLUS system.

Methods: The coder referred to the ICPC-2 PLUS system when coding chiropractor recorded encounter details (reasons for encounter, diagnoses/problems and processes of care). The coder used rules and conventions supplied by the Family Medicine Research Unit at the University of Sydney, the developers of the PLUS system. New chiropractic specific terms and codes were created when a relevant term was not available in ICPC-2 PLUS.

Results: Information was collected from 52 chiropractors who documented 4,464 chiropractor-patient encounters. During the study, 6,225 reasons for encounter and 6,491 diagnoses/problems were documented, coded and analysed; 169 new chiropractic specific terms were added to the ICPC-2 PLUS terminology list. Most new terms were allocated to diagnoses/problems, with reasons for encounter generally well covered in the original ICPC 2 PLUS terminology: 3,074 of the 6,491 (47%) diagnoses/problems and 274 of the 6,225 (4%) reasons for encounter recorded during encounters were coded to a new term. Twenty nine new terms (17%) represented chiropractic processes of care.

Conclusion: While existing ICPC-2 PLUS terminology could not fully represent chiropractic practice, adding terms specific to chiropractic enabled coding of a large number of chiropractic encounters at the desired level. Further, the new system attempted to record the diversity among chiropractic encounters while enabling generalisation for reporting where required. COAST is ongoing, and as such, any further encounters received from chiropractors will enable addition and refinement of ICPC-2 PLUS (Chiro). More research is needed into the diagnosis/problem descriptions used by chiropractors.

Keywords: Chiropractic, International classification of primary care, Classification, Clinical coding

* Correspondence: s.french@unimelb.edu.au
[1]General Practice and Primary Health Care Academic Centre, University of Melbourne, 200 Berkeley St, Carlton, VIC 3010, Australia
[2]Centre for Health Exercise and Sports Medicine, Melbourne School of Health Sciences, University of Melbourne, 200 Berkeley St, Carlton, VIC 3010, Australia
Full list of author information is available at the end of the article

Background

The chiropractic profession in Australia is an important component of the healthcare system. There are approximately 4,300 registered chiropractors in Australia [1] and each year it is estimated that over three million people, or 16% of the Australian population, consult a chiropractor at least once [2,3]. However, very little is known about chiropractic practice and there is a need to collect observational data about chiropractic clinical practice.

Classification of information in clinical practice is useful for both clinical and research purposes. In clinical situations, classification is a way of organising information and can act as a common language between health professionals [4]. In research, classification allows the information collected to be organised in a way that will make it manageable for researchers and to facilitate clear reporting. In complex cases, such as clinical healthcare research, classification involves a specialised structure of codes to link, for example, similar symptoms or similar diagnoses. In addition to organising data, classification overcomes the variance in terms used across different health disciplines and between practitioners.

The International Classification of Primary Care (ICPC) is widely used for classification in general medical practice. The first version (ICPC Version 1) [5] was published in 1987 with the second (ICPC-2) published by the World Organization of Family Doctors (WONCA) in 1997 [6]. The Family Medicine Research Centre, University of Sydney, developed an interface terminology with each term classified according to ICPC Version 1 [7]. The resultant interface terminology, ICPC-2 PLUS, is a list of terms classified to ICPC-2. ICPC-2 PLUS continues to be used, and updated, in the well-established Australian national survey of general practitioner (GP) clinical activity, the Bettering the Evaluation And Care of Health (BEACH) project, to code and classify general practice reasons for encounter, diagnoses and processes of care in Australia [8].

In addition to general medical practice, ICPC has also been used for classification in areas such as pharmacy, nutrition and traditional Chinese medicine. Van Mil et al. (1998) created a pharmacy sub-set of ICPC codes for use by community pharmacists to document complaints/diagnoses of clients when providing pharmaceutical care [9]. Van Binsbergen and Drenthen (1999) developed a system linking ICPC codes to specific nutritional information for patients. When ICPC codes were assigned to diagnoses at the time of consultation, such as heart failure with diabetes, a particular set of nutritional information was given to the patient [10]. In relation to consultations at a university traditional Chinese medicine clinic, Meier and Rogers (2006) used ICPC classification for reporting the reason for encounter and diagnosis [11].

ICPC-2 and ICPC-2 PLUS

ICPC-2 uses three character alpha-numeric codes to classify symptoms/complaints, problems/diagnoses or processes of care. For each ICPC-2 code, the alpha component represents a chapter, or body system (such as Musculoskeletal, Cardiovascular or Neurological), and the two digit numeric component represents a concept within the body system (a symptom/complaint, problem/diagnosis or process of care). This three character code is called a rubric [6].

To allow for greater detail and specificity to be recorded in Australian general practice, the ICPC-2 PLUS terminology was developed by The Family Medicine Research Centre, University of Sydney. Each PLUS term is classified to ICPC-2. ICPC-2 PLUS uses a six character term identifier by adding a three digit number to the ICPC-2 rubric to which the term has been classified [8]. New ICPC-2 PLUS codes are created by aligning the specific problem/diagnosis, or type of care, with the most appropriate ICPC-2 rubric and then assigning the next available three digit code. As such the final three digits of the six character ICPC-2 PLUS code simply serve to identify the specific term within the rubric and do not have any other meaning. For example, the three character ICPC-2 code L01 represents 'Neck Symptom or Complaint'. In ICPC-2 PLUS there are 11 neck-related terms in the L01 rubric that are regularly used by GPs in Australia to describe patient problems. For example 'Pain;neck' and 'Stiffness;neck' are represented in ICPC-2 PLUS as L01 004 and L01 010 respectively [8].

In research situations such as BEACH, secondary coding of collected clinical data is performed to allocate an ICPC-2 PLUS term to each reason for encounter, diagnosis/problem, and process of care. To do this, coders search an extensive keyword list with keywords linking by logic to the ICPC-2 PLUS six character codes. On selecting a keyword, the coder is presented with all available associated terms. The coder then selects the term that is considered to most closely reflect the practitioner documentation [8].

To ensure consistent coding by different researchers, the BEACH program (using ICPC-2 PLUS) has developed a set of 'coding rules'. These rules cover situations such as coding a patient's history of disease and coding when no reason for encounter (or diagnosis) has been documented [8]. Another rule dictates how to code when an underlying morbidity is recorded in conjunction with a secondary (associated) condition; the rule is that the underlying condition is coded rather than the secondary condition. For example, if a GP documents 'weakness secondary to leukaemia,' the leukaemia (the primary or underlying condition) is coded rather than the weakness.

In addition to allowing coding of clinical information to a specific PLUS term, the PLUS terminology enables standardised grouping of similar concepts (or groups of concepts). This assists in the organisation of data collected for research reporting purposes. Grouping using the three digit ICPC-2 rubric provides internationally comparable data at the ICPC-2 level. However, BEACH also allows grouping using individual terms separate from any other terms within their rubric. For example, individual osteoarthritis terms from different rubrics are grouped together for reporting 'Osteoarthritis-all'.

This coding and grouping of practice generated data enables reporting at different levels depending on the audience; reporting the body system involved (chapter), a specific condition, or a grouping of similar concepts [8]. For example, all chronic conditions can be grouped together or a specific condition (such as uncomplicated hypertension) or body system (Circulatory) can be reported.

Aim

While the ICPC-2 classification and its associated ICPC-2 PLUS terminology are extensive, there is currently no classification system specifically designed for researching the clinical activities of the chiropractic profession. The aim of this study was to develop a research tool ICPC-2 PLUS (Chiro) by extending the current PLUS terminology with additional relevant terms for the chiropractic profession. This paper describes the process of development of a chiropractic specific terminology and classification system for use in research. This included the creation of new terms, codes and reporting groups to accurately represent chiropractic encounters.

Methods

Summary of Methods

The Chiropractic Observation and Analysis STudy (COAST) was a cross sectional, prospective, observational study that aimed to describe chiropractic clinical activity in Victoria, Australia. Chiropractors were trained over the telephone to complete data collection forms and recorded anonymous patient encounter data on hand written paper encounter recording forms in free text and with the use of check boxes. COAST used the ICPC-2 PLUS terminology to secondarily code free text information from chiropractor-patient encounters, but new terms were required to describe chiropractic clinical practice. In developing the chiropractic specific ICPC-2 PLUS (Chiro), researchers followed the BEACH coding rules. Upon receipt of completed COAST chiropractic clinical encounter forms, one researcher coded each form. Where necessary, and in consultation with a second researcher, new chiropractic specific terms were added to the current ICPC-2 PLUS term list. At the completion of data collection and data entry, these new terms were allocated to an ICPC-2 rubric and then grouped via these rubrics for reporting purposes. See Table 1 for the definition of a number of terms relevant to this paper.

Term allocation and creation

The BEACH coding rules (using ICPC-2 PLUS) were used to guide the coding of the chiropractic terms handwritten on the encounter forms. A maximum of three reasons for encounter and three diagnoses/problems could be documented at each chiropractic-patient encounter. When more than three reasons for encounter or diagnoses/problems were provided on the encounter form, the first three recorded were used. When a reason for encounter or diagnosis/problem was repeated on an encounter form, it was only recorded once.

Where a reason for encounter, problem, or process of care was documented that had no corresponding ICPC-2 PLUS term, a new term (and code) was created. In line with the ICPC-2 PLUS structured format, each new code contained two parts. The first three characters of each new code were 'J99' to identify it as a new code not yet classified to ICPC-2 and the last three digits provided a unique numeric identifier. Using 'J99' ensured these new codes could not be mistaken for existing codes as there is no 'J' chapter in ICPC-2. See Figure 1 for an overview of the coding procedure.

Two methods were used to create new terms for reasons for encounter, diagnoses/problems and processes of care. First, a list of anticipated terms were generated by the research team. When a reason for encounter or diagnosis/problem was common in chiropractic practice, but was not represented in ICPC-2 PLUS (such as 'chiropractic subluxation'), a 'J-code' was generated *before* data entry and coding. In these cases, the research team created a list of chiropractic specific diagnosis/problem terms (and related codes) that they anticipated would be recorded during the COAST encounters. These new terms represented a chiropractic specific diagnosis/problem and a site. These sites were uniform across each of the new terms, so each problem would have the same site options available. For example, terms created for problems with the wrist allowed the choice of 'Chiropractic subluxation;wrist', 'Dysfunction; wrist' or 'Restriction/Fixation;wrist'.

Second, if an unanticipated reason for encounter, diagnosis/problem or process of care was identified during COAST data entry for which there was no existing ICPC-2 PLUS term, and no relevant term in the anticipated list, an additional term (and corresponding J-code) was created. This was done by the coder during data entry and later discussed with the research team at a coding meeting. In each case the research team discussed the information documented by the chiropractor on the encounter form, possible ICPC-2 PLUS term options, and whether a

Table 1 Definitions of terms used throughout this paper*

Term	Definition
International Classification of Primary Care, Version 2 (ICPC-2):	A classification developed by the World Organisation of Family Doctors (WONCA). ICPC chapters are based on body systems, following the principle that localisation has precedence over aetiology.
ICPC-2 PLUS:	An interface terminology classified to ICPC-2. ICPC-2 PLUS includes the terms used by general medical practitioners to describe three important elements of the healthcare encounter: patient reasons for encounter (RFE); problems or diagnoses managed; and process of care (such as procedures, counselling and referrals).
Chapters (ICPC-2):	The main divisions within ICPC-2. There are 17 chapters primarily representing the body systems.
Code:	In ICPC-2 this is a 3-digit alphanumeric code. In ICPC-2 PLUS this is a 6-digit alpha numeric code made up of the ICPC-2 code followed by a three digit term identifier.
Diagnosis/problem:	A statement of the healthcare provider's understanding of a health problem presented by a patient, family or community. Healthcare providers are instructed to record at the most specific level possible from the information available at the time. It may be limited to the level of symptoms.
Encounter:	Any professional interchange between a patient and a healthcare provider.
Keywords:	These are used as the links to access the term in ICPC-2 PLUS. Keywords may be terms, synonyms, acronyms, etcetera, and are linked to ICPC-2 PLUS terms to facilitate data entry. Multiple keywords can be linked to a single term.
Groups:	A collection of ICPC-2 diagnosis/problem rubrics created for reporting purposes.
Process of care:	An action the health provider carries out related to the encounter, including treatment/care provided, advice given, referral to another provider, and orders for pathology or imaging.
Reason(s) for encounter (RFEs):	The subjective reason(s) given by the patient for seeing or contacting the healthcare provider. These can be expressed in terms of a symptom, diagnosis or the need for a service.
Rubric:	The title of an individual code in ICPC-2.
Term:	In the PLUS terminology, this is a structured expression of the free text description recorded by the clinician. There are currently approximately 8,000 terms within the ICPC-2 PLUS system. Terms may represent a disease (e.g. hypertension), a symptom (e.g. cough) or a procedure (e.g. dressing).

*Adapted from General practice activity in Australia 2011–12 [12].

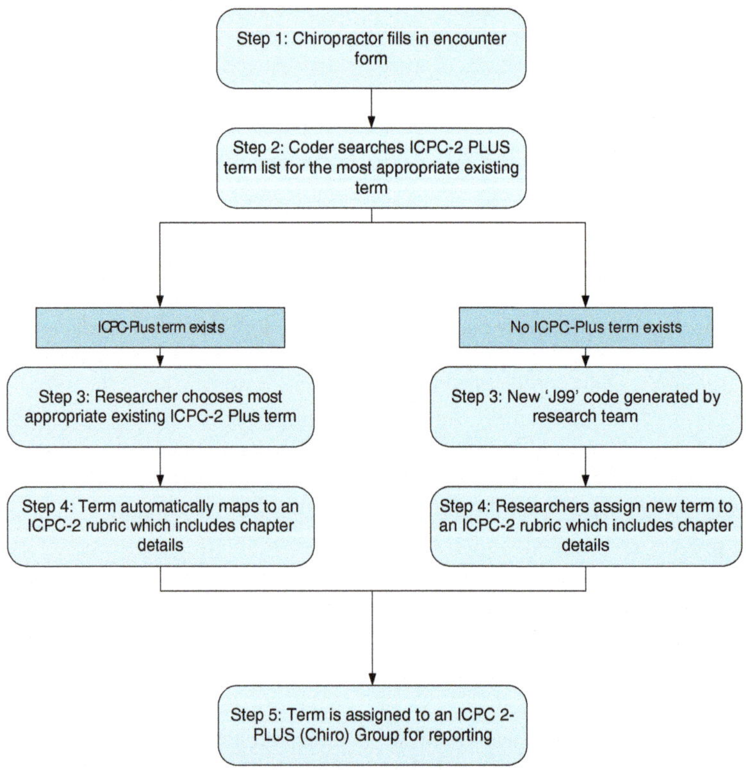

Figure 1 **An overview of the coding procedure used in this study.**

new J-code was required. Examples of terms created in this way included the reason for encounter 'Wellbeing' and the diagnosis/problem 'Piriformis Syndrome'. Because these new terms were developed to describe chiropractic practice, there was no restriction on the generation of new terms for problems/diagnoses or procedures. Further, there was no attempt to merge terms that had similar meanings, e.g. joint dysfunction and manipulable lesion, as these terms come together through their classification at a later stage at rubric level.

Any new terms generated during COAST that the research team considered to be relevant to general practice were submitted to the Family Medicine Research Centre, The University of Sydney, for consideration as additions to ICPC-2 PLUS updates.

Classifying new chiropractic terms to ICPC-2

In classifying the new chiropractic terms to ICPC-2, researchers identified the most appropriate ICPC-2 rubric for each term. ICPC-2 PLUS Keyword and Rubric Indices were searched for terms similar to the new chiropractic term. For example, the new chiropractic term 'Dysfunction;sacroiliac joint' was classified to the ICPC-2 rubric L03 (Low back symptom/complaint) using the PLUS term 'Dysfunction; joint' as a guide for chapter allocation. The term was then mapped to L03, as this rubric was more site specific than the more general L20 (Joint symptom/complaint not otherwise specified).

Grouping

The COAST research team identified that the existing ICPC-2 classes, together with the additional PLUS reporting groups, were not suited for use in reporting common reasons for encounter and diagnoses/problems in chiropractic practice. As such, entirely new COAST-specific reporting groups were devised which were based only upon data collected during the study and not ICPC-2 grouping conventions. In addition, groups were developed only at the ICPC-2 rubric level rather than using separate PLUS terms as is sometimes done in the BEACH study.

The groups were created specifically for reporting to chiropractors, and were devised in one of two ways. The first was to group problems to a site. For example, all problems related to the shoulder were grouped to 'Shoulder Problem'. The second grouping approach was to group all types of a problem (such as headache or depression) to one group. Each group was mutually exclusive, with no rubric being present in more than one group.

In this way all J99 codes could be grouped together with existing ICPC-2 PLUS terms for reporting through their link to an ICPC-2 rubric. For example, the J-code 'Spinal Subluxation Syndrome' was grouped together with ICPC-2 PLUS terms 'Dysfunction Spine' under our new group 'Spinal Problem'.

Results

Full results of COAST will be reported elsewhere. In brief, information was collected from 52 chiropractors (45% response rate) with 4,464 chiropractor-patient encounters documented, including 6,225 reasons for encounter and 6,491 diagnoses/problems, which were coded and analysed during the study. Figures 2 and 3 show worked examples of common encounter form entries by chiropractors and the subsequent coding and grouping process. Figure 2 shows the coding and grouping process of a reason for encounter recorded as back pain; Figure 3 shows the coding and grouping process of a diagnosis of sacroiliac joint dysfunction. Table 2 provides a full list of groups created during COAST. This table also details the ICPC-2 rubrics that were combined to form the groups.

In COAST, 169 new chiropractic specific terms were generated and added to the ICPC-2 PLUS term list. See the Additional file 1 for the full list of new terms. The majority of new terms were created for diagnoses/problems (140 of the 169; 83%). COAST reasons for encounter were generally well covered in the existing ICPC-2 PLUS terms with only four new terms created (2%). Other new terms represented processes of care (29 of the 169; 17%): 19 terms were generated for chiropractic methods of care and 10 terms were created for clinical advice and education given during an encounter.

The 169 new terms were used in a large proportion of the encounters recorded in COAST: 274 of the 6,225 (4%) recorded reasons for encounter, and 3,074 of the 6,491 (47%) recorded diagnoses/problems. New terms for chiropractic methods of care covered 10,855 (72%) of the total 15,179 methods of care recorded and new terms for clinical advice and education were used in coding 9% of recorded recommendations (298 of the 3,564 times a recommendation was recorded). Most (n=150, 89%) of the 169 new chiropractic terms were classified into the Musculoskeletal ICPC-2 chapter, followed by the General and Unspecified chapter (n=12, 7%).

Of the new terms generated, the most commonly used were those for techniques and care provided (e.g. 'Manual Adjustment' n= 4,250; and 'Activator Instrument' n=1,715). The most common new term for problem/diagnosis was 'Chiropractic Subluxation' (n=389). Fifty seven of the terms generated in anticipation of their use in chiropractic clinical practice were not recorded by the chiropractors in COAST. For a full list of new terms generated and their frequency of occurrence in the COAST data see the Additional file 1.

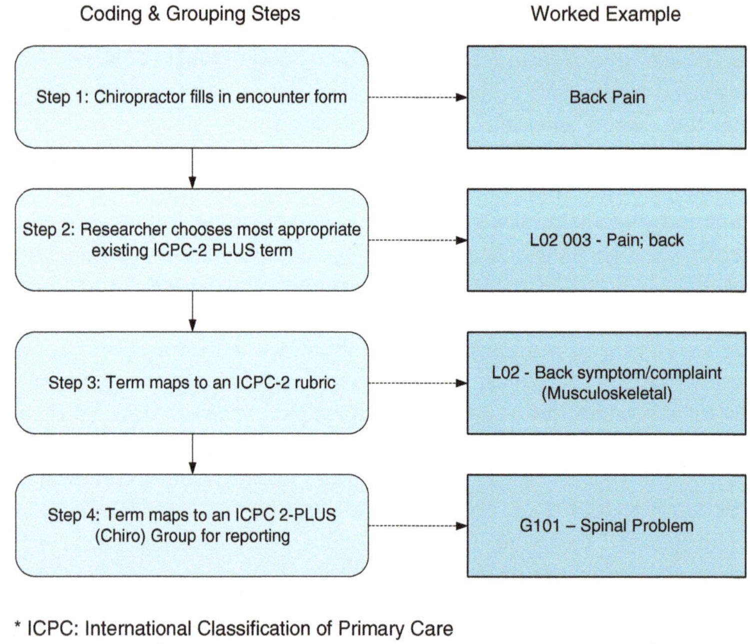

Figure 2 **Coding and Grouping process for an example of a reason for encounter (Back Pain).**

Fourteen reporting groups were generated using combinations of diagnostic terms via their rubrics. Of the 6,491 times a diagnosis was recorded by a chiropractor during COAST, 5,407 of these were grouped into one of the 14 COAST specific reporting groups. The remaining 1,084 remained as individual terms.

While the majority of terms created during COAST were chiropractic specific, some (such as 'cervicogenic headache' and 'advice about footwear') were considered to be relevant to general medical practice. Nine terms were submitted to the Family Medicine Research Centre, The University of Sydney, for consideration of addition

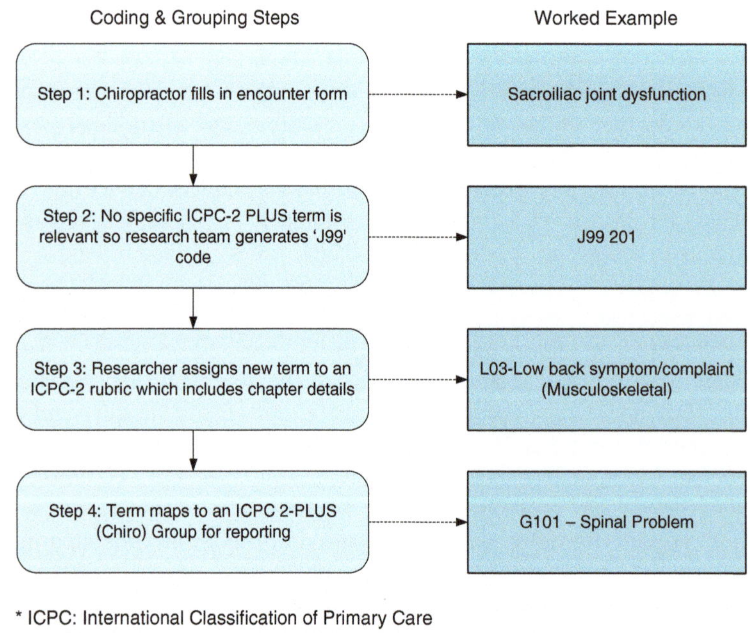

Figure 3 **Coding and Grouping process for an example of a diagnosis/problem (Sacroiliac Joint Dysfunction).**

Table 2 COAST Diagnosis/Problem groups and associated ICPC-2 rubrics of these groups

Diagnosis/Problem group	ICPC-2 rubric
CG101 - OTHER BACK PROBLEM	L02 Back symptom/complaint
	L03 Low back symptom/complaint
	L20 Joint symptom/complaint NOS
	L84 Back syndrome without radiating pain
CG102 - MUSCLE PROBLEM	L18 Pain, muscle
	L19 Muscle symptom/complaint NOS
CG103 - BACK SYNDROME WITH RADIATING PAIN	L86 Back syndrome with radiating pain
	N99 Neurological disease, other
CG104 - HEALTH MAINTENANCE/ PREVENTIVE CARE	A98 Health maintenance/preventative medicine
	A31 Check up
CG105 - HEADACHE	N01 Headache
	N95 Tension headache
CG106 - NECK PROBLEM	L01 Neck symptom/complaint
	L83 Neck syndrome
CG107 - KYPHOSIS & SCOLIOSIS	L85 Acquired deformity of spine
CG108 - SHOULDER PROBLEM	L08 Shoulder symptom/complaint
	L92 Shoulder syndrome
CG109 - ANKLE PROBLEM	L16 Ankle symptom/complaint
	L77 Sprains & strains of ankle
CG110 - DEPRESSION	P76 Depressive disorder
CG111 - NERVE RELATED PROBLEM	N94 Peripheral neuritis/neuropathy
	N29 Neurological symptom/complaint, other
CG112 - OSTEOARTHROSIS, OTHER (not spine)	L91 Osteoarthritis, other
	L89 Osteoarthritis of hip
	L90 Osteoarthritis of knee
CG113 - VERTIGO/DIZZINESS	N17 Vertigo/dizziness
	H82 Vertiginous syndromes
CG114 - FEEDING PROBLEM OR IRRITABLE INFANT/CHILD	T04 Feeding problem of infant/child
	A16 Irritable infant

to ICPC-2 PLUS. Eight of these were accepted and added to a subsequent update of ICPC-2 PLUS.

Discussion

To accurately record chiropractic encounters, the creation of a large number of new terms was required. This study has shown that by adding chiropractic specific terms to the ICPC-2 PLUS terminology, it is possible to code a large number of chiropractic encounters to enable classification and reporting of chiropractic encounters to the desired level. However this is a work in progress and further data collection will require the addition of new terms.

Although existing ICPC-2 PLUS terms mostly covered the reason for the encounters and processes of care, the PLUS terms were not as successful in representing the diagnoses/problems recorded by chiropractors. Just under half of the total diagnoses/problems recorded in COAST were coded using newly created chiropractic specific terms.

The strength of this study came from using the well-established ICPC-2 PLUS terminology as a base and then adding to this to meet chiropractic specific needs. A large number of chiropractor specific terms were added to record chiropractic encounters. General practice and chiropractic are different in their scope so this had been expected. Using the ICPC-2 PLUS process allowed the straightforward creation of these new terms and then enabled these to be grouped together for ease of reporting.

The new terms generated in this study are a reflection of terms used by chiropractors in practice to represent what occurred in their patient encounters. Having a term assigned does not mean the diagnosis/problem can be substantiated by evidence, it simply means that one or more chiropractors used the term to record their patient encounters. More research is needed into the diagnosis/problem descriptions used by chiropractors and the level of evidence that supports the existence of the condition the chiropractors labeled. This issue has been extensively examined in the general medical practice setting, including that a definitive diagnosis is not apparent in about half of general practitioners' consultations, that many patients present to general practice without a serious physical disorder, and that there is wide variance in the way general practitioners describe the diagnosis/problem under management [12].

This study highlighted the wide range of terms used in documentation of chiropractic encounters. This resulted in separate terms being created for what essentially could be considered the same diagnosis/problem. All new terms were mapped to ICPC-2 rubrics and chapters, so the inter-clinician variance in terms used in clinical practice is reduced when reported at these levels, where like terms are classified to the one rubric.

While a consultation process took place among the members of the research team to determine if a new term should be created, 169 new terms were still required. We assume that any further documentation of chiropractic encounters will require the generation of additional terms, and possible merging of the terms already generated, particularly the terms that were not used by the chiropractors in COAST. Future research in this area should include investigation into the terms used in chiropractic to distinguish synonyms from separate terms. A more extensive consultation process with members of the chiropractic profession would potentially allow synonyms to be identified and linked to one term rather than to have several separate terms. For example, Restriction/Fixation;pelvis may be linked to the PLUS term 'Dysfunction;pelvis' rather than be a separate term.

Two examples of new chiropractic terms generated in COAST highlight the different meanings of the same term used in the general medical practice profession and the chiropractic profession. First, the term 'subluxation' is already present in ICPC-2 PLUS in the L80 chapter 'Dislocation/Subluxation'. However, this term is listed under the accepted medical definition of subluxation, that is, a partial dislocation. Some chiropractors use this term in a different context hence the series of terms related to 'chiropractic subluxation' were generated (see Additional file 1) [13]. Second, in BEACH the sacroiliac joint is not considered a moving joint, like a wrist joint, and sacroiliac recordings are classified in the rubric 'L03: Low Back Symptom/Complaint', because the sacroiliac joint is regarded as part of the back. However, some chiropractors consider that the sacroiliac joint is a distinct moving joint hence a series of new codes were generated in COAST to represent this (see Additional file 1) [14].

The allocation of ICPC-2 rubrics to the new chiropractic specific terms generated in COAST was done primarily for reporting purposes. Investigators had anticipated that any terms created during COAST may be difficult to assign to a chapter, as there can be disagreement as to which body system the diagnosis/problem belongs to. In most cases rubric allocation (including chapter) was straight forward, such as allocating 'Dysfunction; joint; sacroiliac' to the Musculoskeletal chapter using 'Dysfunction; joint' as a reference guide. However, in some cases rubric selection was more subjective and investigators acknowledge that other researchers may allocate different ICPC-2 rubrics to the J99 codes.

Using the COAST grouping process made it possible to report both the distribution of individual diagnoses/problems relevant to a chiropractic audience and also to the wider health community by using broader groups. The existing groups used by BEACH are general medical practitioner focused; for example Hypertension, Neoplasm and Abdominal Pain. Although the existing groups did include musculoskeletal groups such as Osteoarthritis and Sprains/Strains, in some cases the ICPC-2 PLUS group did not include terms a chiropractor would use. For example, the ICPC-2 PLUS group 'Back Complaints (all)' did not include the rubric L20 'Joint Symptom/complaint Not Otherwise Specified' which was considered essential by the research team to include for chiropractic reporting.

Special consideration was required when assigning rubrics to COAST reporting groups, particularly as the majority of the groups were derived from newly created 'J-codes'. Great care had been taken when classifying new chiropractic terms to ICPC-2; however, with each allocation of an ICPC-2 rubric to a COAST group, a 'double check' of the rubric was made. This ensured that the 'J-code' had been classified to the most appropriate rubric and that the rubric was assigned to the most appropriate group according to the COAST data. In this way the research team produced the groups they felt were most relevant to chiropractic. For example, to better report chiropractic care, the reporting group 'Health Maintenance/Preventative Care' combined any ICPC-2 PLUS term that included 'Health Maintenance' and 'Check Up' with the J99 code of 'Wellbeing'.

It should be noted that the term 'Problem' has been used to name the COAST groups rather than 'Symptom' or 'Complaint'. Within chiropractic clinical encounters, there is often no symptom or complaint as the reason for encounter, as shown by our large number of encounters being recorded as wellbeing and health maintenance visits. The COAST research team considered that the profession would be more accepting of the alternate title for reporting of results.

Researchers who wish to use the new ICPC-2 PLUS (Chiro) need to be aware of its limitations. The chiropractic version of ICPC-2 PLUS only contains terms recorded by the 52 participants in the COAST study who recorded 4,464 chiropractor-patient encounters, including recording details of 6,225 reasons for encounter and 6,491 diagnoses. Expansion of this study to a wider group of participants would be expected to result in additional terms added to the classification system.

Further, COAST specific reporting groups are not transferable to other studies, because they only include the ICPC-2 PLUS terms used in this study, plus the newly generated chiropractic terms. This is especially true because the COAST groups were created at the rubric level rather than at the term level. For example the COAST group 'CG103-Back syndrome with radiating pain' included all terms allocated to the rubric N99 'Neurological disease, other'. In the COAST data, only the terms 'Neuralgia' (N99 014) and 'Radiculopathy' (N99 038) were present from the whole N99 rubric. In the PLUS terminology, there are currently 34 terms allocated to the N99 rubric, including terms such as 'Narcolepsy' (N99 013) and 'Encephalopathy' (N99 042) which are not relevant in the 'CG103-Back syndrome with radiating pain' group.

A comprehensive chiropractic grouping tool would require each of the ICPC-2 PLUS terms to be considered for each of the COAST groups. In some cases, this would result in individual terms within a rubric assigned to different groups. For example, neuralgia might be grouped to 'CG103-Back syndrome with radiating pain', while Narcolepsy might not be assigned to a chiropractic group. More work is needed before this grouping can be used by other research teams.

When previous studies have used ICPC in their research, the ICPC classification was used as required for each study's particular needs. The focus of Meier and Rogers' (2006) study of Traditional Chinese Medicine encounters was to develop data management and reporting guidelines [11]. While that study demonstrated the use of ICPC outside a general medical practice setting, it did not add to ICPC by producing new classes specific to Traditional Chinese Medicine. Similarly, Van Mil et al. generated a pharmacy specific classification system and provided a subset of pharmacy specific ICPC codes rather than develop a terminology that was then classified to ICPC [9].

The production of ICPC-2 PLUS (Chiro) for COAST differed in two main ways from these previous studies. COAST used ICPC-2 PLUS to develop the system rather than ICPC-2; this provided coders with a large number of chiropractic relevant terms already present within the terminology. In addition, COAST was able to create new terms specific to chiropractic rather than only using those available. By using the ICPC-2 PLUS system, researchers had a wider range of keywords to search when assigning terms to reasons for encounter, diagnoses and procedures. Although using terms specifically relevant to general practice, the ICPC-2 PLUS keyword list was suited to coding information documented at chiropractic encounters. This was shown by the low percentage of new terms that were created to accurately describe reasons for encounter.

When terms relevant only to chiropractic were not present on the ICPC-2 PLUS term list, researchers were able to add new terms. This enabled a significant number of problems identified by chiropractors to be recorded that would have otherwise been placed under a non-specific term if forced to fit into the existing system. The research team had anticipated the need for new chiropractic specific terms due to the differing styles of practice and the wide range of terminology used in the profession.

Conclusion

This is the first published chiropractic specific classification system that has been generated for reporting chiropractic clinical encounters. The research team set out to produce a system specific to chiropractic which could be used as a research tool. This is a first step in the long-term development of ICPC-2 PLUS (Chiro). COAST is ongoing, and as such, any further encounters received from chiropractors will enable addition and refinement of ICPC-2 PLUS (Chiro). We will continue to build the terminology and further develop the reporting groups as new data from a wider range of chiropractors becomes available. Development of a robust terminology and chiropractic specific classification will enable researchers to study information particular to chiropractors, using specific descriptions to accurately represent chiropractic encounters, while allowing reporting of findings to the wider health community. More research is needed into the diagnosis/problem descriptions used by chiropractors.

Additional file

Additional file 1: Full list of new chiropractic specific terms generated during COAST, their frequency in the study, and the ICPC-2 rubric and chapter they were mapped to.

Competing interests

SF is an Associate Editor with Chiropractic & Manual Therapies and had no involvement in the editorial process for this paper. Otherwise, the authors declare that they have no competing interests.

Authors' contributions

SF, MC and HB conceived the study. SF, JG and BP applied for funding for the study. SF, MC and KF participated in the study design and coordination. MC and SF drafted the manuscript, with significant input from HB. All authors read and approved the final manuscript.

Acknowledgements

This study was funded by the Chiropractors Registration Board of Victoria and the Chiropractors Association of Australia. The funding bodies provided general advice about the design of the project but had no role in the conduct of the study or in the decisions about publication of the results.

Author details
[1]General Practice and Primary Health Care Academic Centre, University of Melbourne, 200 Berkeley St, Carlton, VIC 3010, Australia. [2]Centre for Health Exercise and Sports Medicine, Melbourne School of Health Sciences, University of Melbourne, 200 Berkeley St, Carlton, VIC 3010, Australia. [3]Family Medicine Research Centre, Sydney School of Public Health, Sydney Medical School, The University of Sydney, Level 7, 16-18 Wentworth Street, Parramatta, NSW 2150, Australia. [4]Research & Innovation, RMIT University, 110 Victoria Street, Melbourne, VIC 3000, Australia.

References

1. Australian Health Practitioner Regulation Agency: 2012. Available from: www.chiropracticboard.gov.au/About-the-Board/Statistics.aspx [accessed September 2012].
2. Australian Bureau of Statistics: *National Health Survey 2004–05: Summary of Results*. Australia (cat no. 4364.0): Commonwealth of Australia; 2006.
3. Xue C, Zhang AL, Lin V, Da Costa C, Story DF: **Complementary and alternative medicine use in Australia: a national population-based survey.** *J Altern Complement Med* 2007, **13**:643–650.
4. Lewis A: **Health informatics: information and communication.** *Advances in Psychiatric Treatment* 2002, **8**:165–171.
5. Lamberts W (Ed): *ICPC: International Classification of.* Primary Care Oxford: Oxford University Press; 1987.
6. World Organisation of Family Doctors (WONCA): *ICPC-2: International Classification of Primary Care.* 2nd edition. Oxford: Oxford University Press; 1997.
7. Britt H: **A new coding tool for computerised clinical systems in primary care-ICPC plus.** *Aust Fam Physician* 1997, **26**(Suppl 2):S79–s82.
8. *ICPC-2 Plus: The BEACH coding system.* [www.sydney.edu.au/medicine/fmrc/icpc-2-plus/index.php]
9. van Mil JWF, Brenninkmeijer R, Tromp TFJ: **The ICPC coding system in pharmacy: developing a subset, ICPC-Ph.** *Pharm World Sci* 1998, **20**:38–42.
10. van Binsbergen JJ, Drenthen AJM: **ICPC-code approach of nutritional questions in general practice: a look at the future.** *Eur J Clin Nutr* 1999, **53**:S22–S24.
11. Meier PC, Rogers C: **Reporting Traditional Chinese Medicine morbidity - A University of Technology, Sydney, project with an emphasis on developing standards for testing and reporting data.** *J Altern Complement Med* 2006, **12**:529–534.
12. Britt H, Miller G, Henderson J, Charles J, Valenti L, Harrison C, Bayram C, Zhang C, Pollack AJ, O'Halloran J, Pan Y: *General practice activity in Australia 2011–12. General practice series no.31.* Sydney: Sydney University Press; 2012.
13. Mirtz TA, Perle SM: **The prevalence of the term subluxation in North American English-Language Doctor of chiropractic programs.** *Chiropr Man Ther* 2011, **19**:14.
14. Ruhe A, Bos T, Herbert A: **Pain originating from the sacroiliac joint is a common non-traumatic musculoskeletal complaint in elite inline-speedskaters - an observational study.** *Chiropr Man Ther* 2012, **20**:5.

14

Conducting practice-based projects among chiropractors: a manual

Iben Axén[1*] and Charlotte Leboeuf-Yde[2]

Abstract

Introduction: Practice-based research is a challenge as clinicians are busy with their patients and any participation in research activities will be secondary to the needs of the patients and the clinic. As a result, it is difficult to obtain high compliance among clinicians. A method to enhance compliance in multicentre practice-based research has been developed and refined for use in the chiropractic setting and possibly also by other researchers in different settings.

Method: This manual provides a stringent step-by-step approach for conducting clinic-based research. It describes the competencies and requirements of an effective working group, how to recruit participating clinicians and how to empower, encourage and support these clinicians to obtain good compliance.

Discussion: The main advantage of the method is the high compliance of participating clinicians compared to many other clinical studies. Difficulties with the method are described and suggestions for solutions are presented.

Conclusions: This manual is a description of a method that may be of use for clinical researchers in the chiropractic setting.

Keywords: Clinical study, Compliance, Multicentre

Background

Clinical research has the advantage of mimicking clinical reality. The patient population, the procedures, the decisions and the outcomes will represent what happens normally. Further, the study results are easier to implement if the studied procedures are already tested in a clinical setting.

Over the past 15 years, a number of practice-based research projects have been performed among chiropractors in the Nordic countries in which data on patients have been collected using questionnaires [1-12]. Some of these studies are summarized in Table 1. In addition, an international study has been carried out [13]. The above studies have all been multi-centre clinical studies and they have yielded high compliance rates compared to similar research [14-16].

The successful completion of these projects depended on the participation of four groups of people: 1) the professional researchers, 2) the project group members, 3) the data collecting chiropractors, and 4) the patients.

The professional researcher(s) is/are responsible for the methodological aspects of the study, data analysis and the final report. The project group together with the researcher(s) assists both in the conceptual stages and the data collection. It may also be active during analysis and report preparation. The data collecting chiropractors are responsible for the data collection and the patients provide the data needed for the study.

Over the years, we have developed procedures to optimize the involvement of all these participants. The purpose of this report is to describe our work in detail. In other words, it can be considered a manual in practice-based research for chiropractors. We explain the importance of having a dedicated project group which is responsible for personal contacts with the data collecting clinicians, how this group should be selected and instructed and how this group should organize the execution of the study. We also provide instructions for dealing with the data collecting practitioners and how these should collect data from their patients. Finally, we describe how the work after data collection could proceed.

* Correspondence: iben.axen@ki.se
[1]Karolinska Institutet, Unit of Intervention & Implementation Research, Institute of Environmental Medicine, Nobels väg 13, S-171 77 Stockholm, Sweden
Full list of author information is available at the end of the article

Table 1 Compliance rates in some studiescarried out using the herein described procedures

Study title	Country	Year	Method	Number of included patients	Compliance, chiropractors	Compliance, patients
Chiropractic in Sweden: a short description of patients and treatment.	Sweden	1997	Cross-sectional	628	78%	73%
The types and frequencies of improved nonmusculoskeletal symptoms reported after chiropractic spinal manipulative therapy.	Sweden	1999	Cross- sectional	1504	81%	86%
The nordic back pain subpopulation program: demographic and clinical predictors for outcome in patients receiving chiropractic treatment for persistent low back pain.	Norway	2004	Prospective outcome	875	56%	76%
Can patient reactions to the first chiropractic treatment predict early favorable treatment outcome in persistent low back pain?	Sweden	2002	Prospective outcome	615	74%	58%
The Nordic back pain subpopulation program: can patient reactions to the first chiropractic treatment predict early favorable treatment outcome in nonpersistent low back pain?	Sweden	2005	Prospective Outcome & predictive validity	674	86%	56%
The Nordic Back Pain Subpopulation Program: validation and improvement of a predictive model for treatment outcome in patients with low back pain receiving chiropractic treatment.	Sweden	2005	Prospective Outcome & predictive validity	1057	91%	61%

We believe that this method can be used to recruit and encourage chiropractors to participate in practice based research in other settings as well, even though it might be necessary to adapt somewhat to different cultural situations. It is likely that this procedure can be applied also to other professional groups.

Methods

The people involved

Researchers

An overview of the organisational structure is found in Figure 1. One or several researchers may recruit collaborators for a study of a predetermined topic, or a group of clinicians with an interesting research question may enlist the assistance of one or several qualified (academic) researcher(s).

The researcher will act as the intellectual anchor of the project, the guarantor of the quality of method and the final report. If several researchers are involved in the project, it would be preferable to make use of people with different areas of expertise (knowledge of the literature, methodological experience or statistical expertise, for example).

The responsible researcher should be formally appointed in the early planning stages of a research project. This person should be familiar with the topic at hand. Usually, this is the person with the research idea, the one who "owns" the project, i.e. he/she is intellectually responsible for the research project.

The researcher has the final say on each stage of the research process and must keep a close eye on people, process and progress. This person must be easily available to deal with urgent issues arising during the study process.

Project group

Research should be clinically relevant. It is possible to enlist the participation of astute clinically active practitioners only if the research project they shall help with feels clinically relevant to them.

A project group composed of clinicians helps in formulating study goals and in the planning of the project and in data collection. A dedicated and active project group is of great help in the data collection stage, as its members are needed to obtain high compliance among the data collecting clinicians, as further described below. Active participation in each stage of the study promotes ownership for the project and good collaborators which will help improve the quality of data by minimizing errors in procedures and the handling of questionnaires. If the project group participates also in the data analysis, or at least in the data interpretation, and has a say in the manuscript phase, an added benefit is that their participation will enlighten them on the rigours of research and make them knowledgeable in this particular research area. Another advantage is that if several people donate their time, the onus of the work can be divided between several persons, which will reduce the need for funding.

The participants in the project group need not be qualified in terms of research competence, but being clinicians they will provide many invaluable viewpoints when preparing a study in a clinical setting. In fact, if the research leader is not a clinician, such clinical input is vital for the successful completion of the project. Clinicians can also foresee practical issues regarding time expenditure, delegation of tasks to receptionists, willingness of colleagues to donate the necessary time and suchlike.

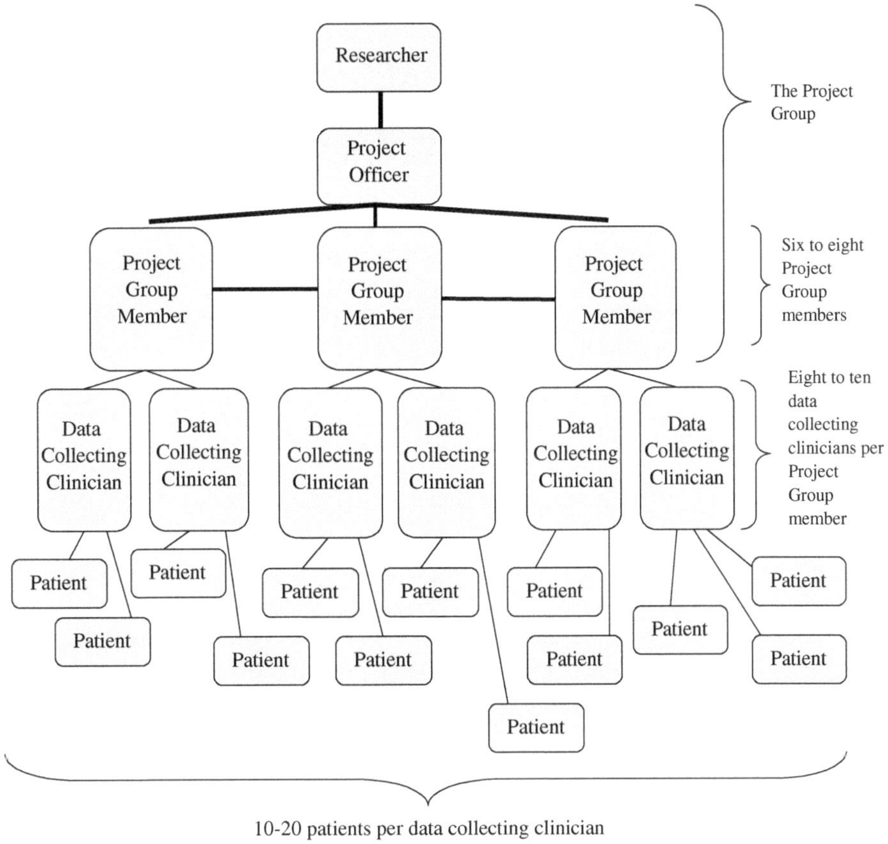

Figure 1 The organisational structure.

Only truly dedicated clinicians should be recruited as project group members. Participation should be voluntary and based on a wish to do practice based research and to search for answers to clinically important questions. A letter from the research leader explaining the need for practice-based research and asking those interested to get in touch is a good way to start out but head-hunting may be a better alternative.

An introductory meeting will make it clear who would be willing to dedicate the necessary time and effort, and the first project group can be formed. "Interested" people who cannot make it to such introduction meetings should not be included in the group, as their first difficulty in participation often is indicative of their future level of involvement.

If several projects will follow, recruitment can probably take place by word of mouth. Project group participants may vary over time. Obviously, it is an advantage if the good co-workers stay on in the group, as people who are involved in several projects in this manner get proficient, making work in the project group increasingly smooth and effective.

Practice-based projects can, of course, be carried out without the help of an active project group. This does, however, require that the researcher (or a research assistant), who is responsible for the recruitment and continued follow-up of the data collecting practitioners, will have to work more or less full time over extended periods. This is probably possible only during a Ph.D. project or for a full-time employed researcher.

It is also possible to set up specific research clinics, whose clinicians will receive training in the data collection process and who enter into a contractual position with a researcher or a research institution, with or without financial compensation for their data collection activities. Obviously, if a formal "employment" exists, the situation is different and this manual is not totally relevant for such a set up.

Project officer

The researcher may not necessarily live or work locally close to the participants of the study. If not, it is necessary to appoint a project officer from within the project group. This is the person who is responsible for the logistics of the study and the only person within the project group who communicates directly with the researcher and he/she is also the person who ensures communication within the group.

The project officer must be particularly dedicated to the project, completely trustworthy, and very methodical in his/her approach to the task at hand. He/she must be respected and liked by colleagues; kind, courteous and positive, yet firm.

If funding is available, this person should receive remuneration for some or all of his/her work, as it is quite time consuming and will sometimes have to take place during clinic hours, which will result in a loss of income.

Data collecting participants

In practice-based studies, it is important to collect data from clinicians who are typical of their professional group. It is therefore important to make such "ordinary" clinicians interested in the project. Most clinicians are interested in the future of their profession, and many will agree to participate. In our studies, these clinicians will then be asked to collect standardized information from a number of patients who fulfill some specific inclusion criteria. The number of clinicians needed for the study will depend on the number of patients needed. This in turn depends on the study design. Our experience is that most clinicians will be willing and able to collect data on 10 patients, if the patient category is one frequently seen. If also no follow-up data are required (i.e. data are only collected at one point in time), more patients per clinician can be included (e.g. 20), as the logistics for the individual clinic is easier in such studies. However, the longer time the data collection will take for each patient and the more complicated the inclusion and/or the follow-up procedure, the more difficult it will be to obtain collaboration.

A high participation rate and valid data are key components of a successful data collection. To achieve this, it will be necessary to explain the purpose of the study in such a way that the potential participants will become truly curious about the results. In other words, they must understand that the project is about finding answers that will make their clinical work easier but that the project is not about proving a preconceived idea.

There are several different ways of recruiting data collecting participants. Clinicians interested in research can sign up for participation, for instance after information is given about the project at a general assembly or a professional meeting. A letter or an e-mail can be sent out to all the members of a professional association explaining the study's aims and design, inviting those interested to sign up. Information must be short and to-the-point, including the purpose of the study, the potential benefits of the study, the tasks included for the participants, the number of patients needed and the time (number of minutes) that data collection will take per patient. This letter should be signed by the researcher and project officer, with contact addresses and telephone numbers. Recruitment can also be done by calling all the members of a target group personally and asking them if they are willing to participate, possibly after an explanatory letter has been sent out. If such calls are made, the logistics of the study can be explained during this phone conversation. If the clinicians are asked to make contact with the team to enquire more about the study, more detailed information can be provided at that point and they will not feel coerced to accept participation in the study during the conversation.

In clinics with a receptionist, the success of the data collection often depends on the involvement of the receptionist. Therefore, when the initial accept has been given by the chiropractor, the receptionist should usually be the contact person.

In order to obtain a representative sample of clinicians, it is important to give all individuals the opportunity to participate in the study. In reality, however, it will be necessary to make do with the more dedicated members of the profession

Regardless whether you attempt to recruit all registered chiropractors, all members of an association, participants at a political meeting, participants at an academic meeting or specially selected chiropractors only, it is unlikely that the data collecting chiropractors will be completely representative of the background population. It is more likely that there will be a bias towards the more academically inclined and/or those with a firm "belief", those with an interest in research, and/or those who feel that they have the time to participate in the project. Only by collecting obligatory register data would it be possible to obtain a perfectly representative group of chiropractors.

There is usually no way of knowing whether a biased selection of clinicians will have an effect on the ultimate selection of patients, treatment and outcomes. Nevertheless, it is useful to obtain some demographic information on the data collecting chiropractors in relation to known factors that can be held up against the whole population of chiropractors. The national chiropractic association or registration board may have some demographic data that can be used for such purposes, such as age, sex, area of practice, school of graduation and years in practice.

Patients

The patients involved in a research project should be representative of the patients normally seen in a clinical setting. To avoid selection bias, it is important that the patients are enrolled consecutively in the study according to the inclusion criteria. Completely random selection of study participants requires a more complex procedure and is probably not realistic. During busy periods in the clinic and prior to major holidays, it is common that suitable patients are not invited into the study.

This can be helped by selecting certain days or specific times of the day, when recruitment should take place, and allowing for some time to catch up, in case the inclusion procedure delays the usual clinic procedures somewhat.

Ideally, a record should be kept of all patients who are suitable for participation in the study and for all who were invited but declined participation. However, for practical reasons, this will probably not be feasible (as clinicians are busy). Therefore, it is primordial that clinicians are thoroughly informed of the importance of not selecting patients for inclusion in the study for some specific reason of their own but to let chance play the major role. The main reason for non-invitation into the study of an otherwise suitable study subject is acceptable if it is for administrative reasons and not for clinical reasons.

Patients should receive information about the study, both verbally and in writing, and should sign informed consent forms. This, of course, may make participation less attractive for patients who are in a hurry to get out to the parking metre or back to work. If this aspect is dealt with while the patient is waiting anyway (in the waiting room, at the reception area, in the treatment cubicle) patients in a hurry will not so easily be excluded from the study. Hopefully, this should keep non-participation to a minimum.

Planning the study

Meetings

The project group should meet with the researcher on several occasions to plan the study. These preparatory meetings could start with discussions of one or several clinical problems at hand. Clinicians are often naive about the lack of documentation for their clinical activities. At such a meeting, it might therefore be necessary to give an overview of a clinical problem and the lack of or conflicting evidence that exists, and the need for more or better knowledge could be pointed out. The study aims and objectives and the appropriate design and detailed method will then gradually take form. The researcher provides the methodological competence, whereas the project group has the knowledge needed for the practical considerations. Together, the group should be able to design a study that is relevant, methodologically sound and practically possible to perform. In addition, this process makes all the group members able to understand the study and defend the method chosen at all stages of the study process. When the preparation phase is over, the whole group should feel that it is "their" project and that the best possible study is being carried out to answer the research question at hand. Ownership is really the key issue in order to keep this group working well.

It is important that these meetings are conducted in a pleasant environment and during joyful conditions. A positive social experience will make it easier for the project group to conduct the study.

Designing and using questionnaires

During the process of planning, it will become apparent what information needs to be collected. If validated questionnaires exist, which is not always the case, it is preferable to use these. The researcher should provide advice on the available questionnaires, their validity, use and previous results. If need be, questionnaires can be designed by the project group.

Our experience with questionnaires is that if data are to be collected during the normal clinical encounter they should be short to enhance compliance. The easiest questionnaires have short and to-the-point questions with yes/no boxes to tick. It is easier to ask clinicians to collect information normally ascertained in the clinical setting than data not included in a standard consultation.

If possible, all information regarding one patient should be filled in on one piece of paper. Sometimes several questionnaires are needed (for example, one for the patient to fill in, two for the chiropractor; at baseline and another for follow up). In that case, these should be of different colours. It is easy to refer to the "blue" rather than the "inclusion" questionnaire when communicating with data collecting clinicians.

Patients' anonymity must be retained at all times also for follow-up studies or whenever multiple questionnaires are required. If information is needed from one clinical occasion only, usually no patient identification is required, but if data are collected at several occasions, the clinician must be able to identify the patient on the questionnaire whilst data are collected, in order for the data to be correctly recorded for the "right" patient. In that case, we recommend that the patient's last name and initial are written at the top or bottom of the questionnaire, at a dedicated space, to be cut off from the paper and destroyed when the data collection is complete.

When follow-up data are needed or when several questionnaires are used, it is necessary to code the questionnaires. We have used a set of three codes: one for the project group chiropractor, one for the data collecting chiropractor, and one for the patient. E.g. 010101 means project group chiropractor number 01, data collecting chiropractor number 01 and his patient number 01.

We keep the cost and effort for the data collecting clinicians to a minimum by providing them with a set of stamped and addressed return envelopes. If the patient has to fill in some information themselves, maybe of confidential type even to their treating chiropractor, also they should be provided with an individual envelope.

In order to have a good return rate on questionnaires filled out by chiropractors in relation to their patients, we have found that completing the questionnaires "in real time" (i.e. when the patient is in the clinic) is preferable. Questionnaires that patients are asked to fill in themselves should also be done whilst in the clinic. Otherwise, the patient may forget, mislay the questionnaire, or forget to return it to the clinic.

For logistic and ethical reasons, all questionnaires (at least in relation to the data collecting chiropractor) should be coded at, sent out from, and returned to the "research centre" to be handled by the project officer. This procedure minimizes errors, as all questionnaires are packed and coded the same way. The project group can assist in the packing of questionnaires and addressing envelopes. Only the project officer should have access to the "key" of codes, to ensure anonymity of the data collecting chiropractors and patients. When the project group gathers to analyse the data, no names of colleagues or patients should be available. And if, for some reason, the identity of a particular respondent becomes apparent, it must be explained to and imposed on the project group that this is highly confidential. The researchers must of course lead the way by being perfect role models in this respect.

Ethical approval and considerations

All experimental research regarding human beings (and some other forms of data collection) need approval from a regional ethics committee. Normally, if no experimental treatment is carried out, the study will be regarded as a quality assurance project and the ethics committee will return the application with this comment or no ethics application may even be necessary. However, the rules differ from country to country and can also vary over time. It will therefore be necessary to make enquiries as to whether an approval is needed. If a computerized data file is created in which individuals can be identified, it is likely that a permit is needed also for this (data protection).

Whenever individuals can be identified, for example on questionnaires, or if questionnaires are anonymous but there is a list of names that can be related to the individual questionnaires, it is important that such information is kept safely locked up and that lists of names and corresponding codes not be kept together with the coded questionnaires.

It is a useful experience for the project group members to write an ethics application. It provides an opportunity to consider the ethical aspects of the study; the routines of using codes instead of names, the integrity of the patients and the safe storage of the data collected. In any case, time should be set aside to discuss ethical aspects with the project group, to impress upon them that this is a cardinal point in research.

Pilot studies

If necessary, the project group can assist in the pilot testing of questionnaires and study routines in the clinical setting, i.e. in their own clinics. At a later stage, it will be essential for the members of this group to be able to answer questions from the data collecting clinicians regarding patients' opinions, receptionists' tasks and time spent on the study procedures. The data collecting clinicians will need information regarding time requirement before agreeing to participate, so this aspect is particularly important to settle before starting the main study.

When a new procedure or questionnaire is to be introduced, a pilot study in the clinical setting will provide the necessary measures of face validity and interpretability, and relevant changes can be made before the study commences. Pilot studies can also provide information on the feasibility of the targeted patient category, i.e. if it is common or not. This will decide the duration of the enrolment of patients in the study. Generally, we advice against collecting data on rare patient categories, as this takes too long and exhausts both project group members and clinicians.

Based on the results of the pilot study, the duration of data collection for the entire study can be estimated. However, it is a good idea to provide for more time than expected. Always estimate data collection duration by at least twice the calculated time. Various things will work against your study; clinicians go on holidays, their receptionist gets ill, their colleague quits and leaves, that particular patient type suddenly becomes rare. We also recommend that you never start a data collection period in the beginning of summer, when both clinicians and patients will soon go on holidays. Remember that also Christmas, Easter and other holidays have a tendency to disrupt routines.

Workshops

The project group should help prepare for the recruitment of data collecting clinicians and for helping them through the data collection period. This is done through targeted telephone calls. These contacts require some skills beyond that of making an ordinary telephone call. Therefore the project group members should practice the phone calls (illustrated in the appendices) with another member of the group through role play. All possible "excuse"- scenarios should be tried and all possible encouraging comments should be invented and written down. This exercise will take a couple of hours and should be done with several rotations, i.e. each member of the group gets to train with several others, until the subject is exhausted.

The data collecting chiropractors

Telephone lists

Each project group member can be assigned 8–12 participating clinicians as "theirs". The assigning is best done when the whole group is together at a planning session. If possible (easily done in a small association), friends can be assigned to each group member. This will make participation harder to refuse. People are much less willing to make up excuses when talking to a friend. Similarly, personal "enemies" should be avoided.

Each member of the project group will be responsible for making regular calls to "their" data collecting chiropractors. Thus, the same project group member will always call the same data collecting chiropractors unless later otherwise decided in conjunction with the researcher.

We suggest making telephone lists in Excel or on a similar paper version, with dates/weeks written in, so it is easy to keep track of who was called, when and what the outcome of the call was.

Telephone calls and why they are important to ensure compliance

At every new step in the data collection, human inertia is likely to work against your project. The steps participating clinicians must go through are as follows:

A. Opening the envelope with the information material.
B. Having opened the envelope, actually reading it.
C. Having read it, also having understood it and considered the implications in the clinic.
D. Starting with the first case.
E. Continuing with the rest of the cases.
F. Returning the questionnaires.

The members of the project group will have to work diligently to overcome these obstacles on the way. This is done with systematic and frequent telephone calls. These phone calls follow a special "program" explained in detail in this manual and described in the additional files. Each of the obstacles of data collection should be addressed in an explanatory phone call.

Different types of clinicians will have to be treated differently. Basically, there are three types of data collecting clinicians, in relation to understanding the purpose and process of the study: Those who understand directly, those who understand after some extra explanations, and those who understand only after detailed information.

In relation to performance, there are four different types of participants: A small group who will do what they should do without any problems, a rather large group consisting of those who do what they should do after some prodding and/or with some delay; a somewhat smaller group which needs a lot of encouragement; and a small group consisting of those who fail to perform either in silence or despite many vivid assurances of active participation. Obviously, the phone calls need to be targeted to these different types; otherwise the minority group of non-performers can grow into a very large group indeed.

The calls should all be friendly, enthusiastic, patient, encouraging and professional. Each telephone conversation must be targeted to deal with the specific hurdle at hand. There is therefore no point in simply phoning the participants and asking how they are getting on, in a non-specific manner, as the answer invariably will be "good". Then, as it becomes apparent to the participant that he is not performing, he will stop answering the phone calls and become inaccessible both by phone and e-mail.

Telephone calls

General points

The calls should be noted in the Excel sheet as: participating yes/no, next to the date called and the response to the call. If the person called is participating in the study, the date and time for the next scheduled telephone call should be noted. Similarly, all continued telephone encounters should be noted, until data have been successfully returned or the data collecting chiropractor has quit the study. Obviously, it is vital that all "appointments" for future calls are honoured. Any obstacles and the need for a new call in relation to each hurdle should be noted.

Recruitment calls

Each potential participating clinician should be approached by one of the project group members in an introductory recruitment call, approximately 1 month before the study starts. The call should be outlined as described in Additional file 1.

Complete telephone list

After this first round of telephone calls, there should be a list of who was contacted, of those refusing, those not reached and those agreeing to participate. Each project group member should receive a list of "their" data collecting chiropractors and the researcher should have the complete list of participants.

First support call; responding to the hurdles: *have you received the material, opened the letter and read it?*

One week before the study starts, all participating clinicians are contacted again by their contact person. The call is described in Additional file 2.

If the clinician did not yet open the envelope, this call has to be repeated, preferably daily, until he/she does. If the clinician has opened the envelope, but has not looked at the material, this part of the conversation should be repeated in the same manner. Most chiropractors are not making this a priority in their daily practice, and therefore it is not uncommon that they have to be called several times. All calls should be noted for future reference and so should the date and time for the agreed next phone call.

Following support calls; responding to the hurdles: *have you understood the study, have you started, are you proceeding?*

The following two or three (or as many as it takes!) weeks, each participant should be called to make sure they are proceeding as planned. If not, the call described in Additional file 2 is repeated. The important thing is to always call the clinicians back. It is fairly easy to ignore an e-mail or a letter, but a phone call (in particular from a friend) is difficult to ignore. The conversation will now concentrate on the data collection phase as described in Additional file 3.

It is, of course, everybody's right to withdraw from an engagement such as this. No negative feelings should be placed on those who do; all you can say is that you are sorry. Further; some people are procrastinators, they postpone and provide all sorts of excuses. You need to be prepared and persevere with your calls. Sadly, you will notice that some promise a lot more than they deliver.

Closing calls; responding to the hurdles: *have you finished and sent the questionnaires back to us?*

At the end of the data collection period, the participating clinicians should be reminded to collect data for the remaining patients and when this is done to send in the questionnaires. Some clinicians will not achieve the full number of patients and will have to return whatever data they have achieved at a specific deadline. This phone call is outlined in Additional file 4.

Reporting and feedback

The project officer should obtain reports from all the project group members on a regular basis, at least every week. We recommend establishing a record also of this, and since this is quite time consuming, it is a good idea to exempt the project officer from being a contact person for data collecting clinicians.

Based on the feedback information from each group member, the project officer can provide feedback on the study progress to the entire group. Further, the project officer should keep track of patients recruited to the study by means of questionnaires/informed consent-forms coming in to the research centre. This will tell whether the data collecting clinicians are performing as planned. This feedback should then be forwarded to the responsible project group member, so he knows how successful his "team" is. In the case of non-performance by one (or several) data collecting chiropractors, the project officer is responsible for discussing this with the project group member, who is responsible for the failing data collector.

As soon as it becomes obvious that a data collecting clinician does not get started, despite the relevant encouraging calls, the project officer should be informed and the case discussed. Possibly, such a participant should be removed from the list. This requires a personal contact. Of course, the failing data collector should be told this in an unemotional manner. For example: "Judging by the number of patients you have enrolled in the study, it looks like you have a busy schedule or that you may not see the right patient type for this project at the moment. This may not be the best time for you to participate in a study like this. What do you say, is it better to remove you from our list?"

Analysis and report preparation

Initial data inspection

The project group should meet with the researcher for a first inspection of the data. All the raw data should be available to the group, literally to the touch. Together, the group can count the number of questionnaires received, and complete the first data cleaning; i.e. decide which questionnaires are too incomplete to be included. These decisions should be written down for future reference and for the final report/research article.

Summative and descriptive analysis

If feasible (up to around 1000 included patients), data can be entered by hand onto large spread sheets. Each pair of project group members gets a batch of questionnaires, and is made responsible for summing up one variable at a time, each in the pair checking the quality of the data entry and counts. The estimate count for each variable obtained by this pair is then reported to an appointed "writer" for example on a board for all to see; the number of positives, negatives and missing. In this way, all the data are added up into one final estimate. This is suitable for all descriptive data and can be done also for some simple cross-tabulations. The method provides a feel for the data not otherwise provided in a computer entered analysis. Further, the members of the project group get to see all the errors possible when filling out a questionnaire, useful knowledge for future projects. These errors should also be noted for reference when designing questionnaires in future studies.

Computerized statistical analysis

Obviously, when the object of the study is to investigate associations or interactions between variables, statistical computer software needs to be used. In such a case, data can be entered by one or several members of the groups with the usual quality assurance methods (double data entry or random checks). The statistical methods can be explained to the group by the researcher or a statistician, in such a way that they understand why they are used and, in particular, how the results are interpreted.

Data interpretation

The results of the analysis should then be presented to the project group, and form the basis for discussions within the group. Are the results as expected? Why or why not? What are the clinical implications? Are any further analyses suitable? These discussions are the base for the final report or research article. It is important to include the project group at this stage, as this is when the fun starts. This is their moment of reward, after all the hard work and tedious phone calls.

Writing the research report

The project group should, after the interpretation of the results, design the crude outline of the scientific study report. Aided by the researcher, the group can decide the outline of the background, methodology, results and discussion sections. Examples from good and bad research reports can be used to make this easier. The project group can also divide the report between them, some members writing the method section, some the results, and some the discussion. The researcher or project officer will ultimately have the responsibility of putting the fragments together and editing the complete manuscript, after which the project group should proofread and comment. Their active participation during this stage will make the final report less technical and more easily understood by ordinary clinicians. This is important, because unless the research article is easily accessible to clinicians, the information it contains will not enter their conceptual world and useful information will not become generally implemented.

Management

Project group

In the beginning, it might be a good idea to include more participants in the project group than needed, as it is not uncommon that in a group of 5–8, one or two will drop out when they realize that research requires consistency and tedious tasks. Persons with the best personalities to do this type of work are those who are conscientious and socially gifted. It is always a good idea to include in the group at least one realistically critical person, who finds the weak points in the study design and in the data collection process. It is also helpful to have access to somebody who is interested in computer layout, for the successful design of questionnaires.

Individuals less well suited for this work are those who find it difficult to work together in a team and to conform. Luckily, they will soon single themselves out by their constant need to express contrary opinions. Such individuals are more comfortable working on their own and should not be convinced to stay on in the project when they start gliding out.

Sometimes one or several members of the project group do not perform according to the protocol during the crucial data collecting phase. This can take one of two forms: Phone calls are not made or phone calls are not made according to the agreed procedure. This will become apparent early in the process from the lower response rate from "their" data collection practitioners. When the project officer notices such an anomaly, it will be necessary to ask tactfully if one (or several) data collecting clinician presents a problem. In that case, it might be best to move this/these participants on to another member of the project group, who might be more successful in establishing a positive contact. It will sometimes be necessary for the project officer to take over the task of managing some or all of these data collecting chiropractors, as otherwise the whole study is jeopardized.

If however, the problem seems to lay with the project group member, the project has a problem. Either the failing group member must be made to understand that the agreed upon procedure must be followed or asked to leave the group. If this is difficult, then at least, ensure that this person is not enrolled for your next study. In the meantime the project officer must take over all or some of the failing group member's tasks.

Data collecting participants

During recruitment, we suggest that people who are consistently difficult to reach are left out of the study, as they tend to be unavailable throughout the whole study period and therefore, usually will be non-compliant.

Obviously, there are those who are less suitable participants than others, which needs to be ascertained during the recruitment phone call outlined in Additional file 1. Newly graduated chiropractors who are starting up their own clinic may not have enough patients to be able to provide the required number of study subjects. Extremely busy practitioners will not be able to carry through with their commitment, because their practice procedures usually do not allow for any flexibility.

The odd person will want to change the study protocol, and if the comments are relevant should be listened to and perhaps invited to participate in the project group. However, if the comments are uninformed and the person obviously does not trust the researcher's competence, he or she should be excluded from the data collection group, if sabotage of data seems likely

Feedback

Project group

The project group meets to discuss the results of the study and to plan the final manuscript/ publication. The final discussions should also include the issue of clinical applicability and the next possible steps forward. We have found that many times the wrap up of one study is the start of the next. The project group members' formal reward for participating is that they get their name on a scientific publication. However, the experience of doing practice based research and finding the answers to clinically relevant questions is rewarding in itself and can be a source of great joy for the group members.

Data collecting participants

Making the results of the study known to the clinicians involved in the data collection is important if their participation is wanted in future studies. In this matter, one cannot rely on clinicians reading the resulting scientific publication. We suggest that the report/ publication be sent directly to all who collected data, as well as to the members of their national association. One can include an explanatory letter (stating the results of the study in a couple of sentences) for those who are not interested in reading the full paper. Such a letter has double intentions. First the result should reach those who can implement it, i.e. the clinicians. Second, credit is given to those participating, both members of the project group and the data collecting chiropractors.

We also recommend that the researcher or project officer presents the results at a general assembly to alert all those affected by the findings. This is also an excellent opportunity to praise those donating their time and effort, and to try to awake an interest in others to participate in the next study.

To acknowledge the data collecting clinicians, after each study is completed, we provide them with a diploma. This diploma reads: "The chiropractor in this clinic is contributing to making chiropractic treatment evidence based through active participation in research". The reference of the ensuing publication could also be noted in the diploma text. The idea is that this diploma should hang in the involved clinics making patients aware that their chiropractor is involved in research. For some of our participating clinicians, the fact that they can put "participation in research" on their CV has been an advantage when applying for reimbursement plans through insurance and other funding schemes.

Scientific community

Of course, the results of any study should be made known to the scientific community as a publication in a peer reviewed journal and as presentations at scientific conferences. In fact, it would be unethical not to do so.

Discussion

To our knowledge, this is the first manual describing the procedures for conducting a multicentre clinical study in the chiropractic setting. As the method has been tried several times, we believe it to be worthwhile and it may be of value to other researchers in the clinical field.

The clinical perspective

By going through the processes outlined in this manual, clinical studies in multicentre settings are possible and it should be feasible to obtain answers to a number of research questions. In other words, we will have obtained knowledge of some clinically relevant issues that will benefit our patients.

The described procedure will enlighten the project group members as to the importance of rigours of protocol and the hard work of ensuring compliance among clinicians. Moreover, at the end of execution of a study like this, they will be knowledgeable in the methodology chosen, a valuable experience for any clinician expected to read and evaluate research articles as part of their everyday practice.

The research perspective

Because of the involvement of several "ordinary" field practitioners and patients, and because the study is taking place in the usual clinical setting, it is likely that the research conducted in this manner is not only relevant but that the study participants are representative of the "typical" clinical population and that the results are fairly generalizable. In a well conducted project one can expect the data to be trustworthy. When the various tasks are divided between many people, who are willing to donate their time to a good cause, the project will also have been cheap to conduct. The end result will, hopefully, be a clinically relevant and interesting publication, a stepping stone towards a better understanding of the clinical work carried out every day in ordinary practice.

Limitations

The procedures outlined in this manual are not scientifically tested against other procedures, they are merely empirically anchored.

Further, they are tested mainly amongst chiropractors in the Nordic countries. In these countries, the chiropractic associations are small and colleagues often know each other. Therefore, participation may be easier to achieve. Experiences from the international study [13] were that the project group members approached their task differently, some obviously not willing to follow instructions, possibly for cultural reasons, whereas others did. The response rates in the different countries reflected these differences. Hence, it is likely that cultural differences play a role in relation to this type of study set-up.

Future projects

When the study is completed, the project members will know which clinicians to contact for future studies (a convenience sample). Make a list of these! This will be a group of people who are interested in research, willing to donate the necessary time and effort, and who will be competent co-workers when you invite them in the future. Rather, they are likely to be more compliant in future studies with a need for fewer prompting calls.

Conclusions

We have described a method of conducting clinical studies in the chiropractic setting including several steps to ensure good compliance. We believe that our experience of how to set up this type of studies i.e. the organisation of collaborators, the involvement of clinicians and the procedures outlined in this manual should be made available to others as it seems to be a feasible way of obtaining high compliance and to perform relevant clinical research. This method may be expanded to other clinical fields as well.

Additional files

Additional file 1: **The recruitment call.**
Additional file 2: **The first support call.**
Additional file 3: **Following support calls.**
Additional file 4: **The closing calls.**

Competing interests

The authors declare that they have no competing interests.

Authors' contributions

Both authors have developed the method described herein, and have written and approved the final manuscript.

Author details

[1]Karolinska Institutet, Unit of Intervention & Implementation Research, Institute of Environmental Medicine, Nobels väg 13, S-171 77 Stockholm, Sweden. [2]Research Department, Spinecenter of Southern Denmark, Institute of Regional Health Research, University of Southern Denmark, Hospital Lillebælt, Østre Hougvej 55, DK-5500 Middelfart, Denmark.

References

1. Leboeuf-Yde C, Axen I, Ahlefeldt G, Lidefelt P, Rosenbaum A, Thurnherr T: **The types and frequencies of improved nonmusculoskeletal symptoms reported after chiropractic spinal manipulative therapy.** *J Manipulative Physiol Ther* 1999, **22**(9):559–564.
2. Leboeuf-Yde C, Hennius B, Rudberg E, Leufvenmark P, Thunman M: **Chiropractic in Sweden: a short description of patients and treatment.** *J Manipulative Physiol Ther* 1997, **20**(8):507–510.
3. Leboeuf-Yde C, Gronstvedt A, Borge JA, Lothe J, Magnesen E, Nilsson O, Rosok G, Stig LC, Larsen K: **The nordic back pain subpopulation program: demographic and clinical predictors for outcome in patients receiving chiropractic treatment for persistent low back pain.** *J Manipulative Physiol Ther* 2004, **27**(8):493–502.
4. Axen I, Rosenbaum A, Robech R, Wren T, Leboeuf-Yde C: **Can patient reactions to the first chiropractic treatment predict early favorable treatment outcome in persistent low back pain?** *J Manipulative Physiol Ther* 2002, **25**(7):450–454.
5. Axen I, Rosenbaum A, Robech R, Larsen K, Leboeuf-Yde C: **The Nordic back pain subpopulation program: can patient reactions to the first chiropractic treatment predict early favorable treatment outcome in nonpersistent low back pain?** *J Manipulative Physiol Ther* 2005, **28**(3):153–158.
6. Axen I, Jones JJ, Rosenbaum A, Lovgren PW, Halasz L, Larsen K, Leboeuf-Yde C: **The Nordic Back Pain Subpopulation Program: validation and improvement of a predictive model for treatment outcome in patients with low back pain receiving chiropractic treatment.** *J Manipulative Physiol Ther* 2005, **28**(6):381–385.
7. Leboeuf-Yde C, Axen I, Jones JJ, Rosenbaum A, Lovgren PW, Halasz L, Larsen K: **The Nordic back pain subpopulation program: the long-term outcome pattern in patients with low back pain treated by chiropractors in Sweden.** *J Manipulative Physiol Ther* 2005, **28**(7):472–478.
8. Leboeuf-Yde C, Gronstvedt A, Borge JA, Lothe J, Magnesen E, Nilsson O, Rosok G, Stig LC, Larsen K: **The Nordic back pain subpopulation program: a 1-year prospective multicenter study of outcomes of persistent low-back pain in chiropractic patients.** *J Manipulative Physiol Ther* 2005, **28**(2):90–96.
9. Axen I, Jensen IB, Eklund A, Halasz L, Jorgensen K, Lange F, Lovgren PW, Rosenbaum A, Leboeuf-Yde C: **The Nordic Maintenance Care Program: when do chiropractors recommend secondary and tertiary preventive care for low back pain?** *Chiropr Osteopat* 2009, **17**(Jan):1.
10. Malmqvist S, Leboeuf-Yde C, Ahola T, Andersson O, Ekstrom K, Pekkarinen H, Turpeinen M, Wedderkopp N: **The Nordic back pain subpopulation program: predicting outcome among chiropractic patients in Finland.** *Chiropr Osteopat* 2008, **16**:13.
11. Leboeuf-Yde C, Hennius B, Rudberg E, Leufvenmark P, Thunman M: **Side effects of chiropractic treatment: a prospective study.** *J Manipulative Physiol Ther* 1997, **20**(8):511–515.
12. Leboeuf-Yde C, Rosenbaum A, Axen I, Lovgren PW, Jorgensen K, Halasz L, Eklund A, Wedderkopp N: **The Nordic Subpopulation Research Programme: prediction of treatment outcome in patients with low back pain treated by chiropractors - does the psychological profile matter?** *Chiropr Osteopat* 2009, **17**(1):14.
13. Leboeuf-Yde C, Pedersen EN, Bryner P, Cosman D, Hayek R, Meeker WC, Shaik J, Terrazas O, Tucker J, Walsh M: **Self-reported nonmusculoskeletal responses to chiropractic intervention: a multination survey.** *J Manipulative Physiol Ther* 2005, **28**(5):294–302. discussion 365–296.
14. van den Hoogen HJ, Koes BW, van Eijk JT, Bouter LM, Deville W: **On the course of low back pain in general practice: a one year follow up study.** *Ann Rheum Dis* 1998, **57**(1):13–19.
15. Gheldof EL, Vinck J, Vlaeyen JW, Hidding A, Crombez G: **Development of and recovery from short- and long-term low back pain in occupational settings: a prospective cohort study.** *Eur J Pain* 2007, **11**(8):841–854.
16. Carey TS, Garrett JM, Jackman AM: **Beyond the good prognosis. Examination of an inception cohort of patients with chronic low back pain.** *Spine* 2000, **25**(1):115–120.

The United States Chiropractic Workforce: An alternative or complement to primary care?

Matthew A Davis[1*], Todd A Mackenzie[2], Ian D Coulter[3], James M Whedon[4] and William B Weeks[4]

Abstract

Background: In the United States (US) a shortage of primary care physicians has become evident. Other health care providers such as chiropractors might help address some of the nation's primary care needs simply by being located in areas of lesser primary care resources. Therefore, the purpose of this study was to examine the distribution of the chiropractic workforce across the country and compare it to that of primary care physicians.

Methods: We used nationally representative data to estimate the per 100,000 capita supply of chiropractors and primary care physicians according to the 306 predefined Hospital Referral Regions. Multiple variable Poisson regression was used to examine the influence of population characteristics on the supply of both practitioner-types.

Results: According to these data, there are 74,623 US chiropractors and the per capita supply of chiropractors varies more than 10-fold across the nation. Chiropractors practice in areas with greater supply of primary care physicians (Pearson's correlation 0.17, p-value < 0.001) and appear to be more responsive to market conditions (i.e. more heavily influenced by population characteristics) in regards to practice location than primary care physicians.

Conclusion: These findings suggest that chiropractors practice in areas of greater primary care physician supply. Therefore chiropractors may be functioning in more complementary roles to primary care as opposed to an alternative point of access.

Keywords: Chiropractic, Supply, Distribution, Health resources, Manpower

Background

In the United States (US) health care policymakers continue to be concerned about the ability of the primary care workforce to meet the future primary care needs of an aging and expanding population. Some authorities encourage increasing the general physician workforce to address the shortage [1-3]. However, others argue that, because of market forces, expansion would only perpetuate the overabundance of specialists and continue to widen the divide between high and low supply of primary care physicians [4,5]. Indeed, recent studies suggest that, after accounting for population differences, a 2- to 3-fold variation in physician supply exists across geographic regions [4]. And only primary care physician supply [4] appears to be related to improvements in population health outcomes [6].

* Correspondence: matthew.a.davis@dartmouth.edu
[1]Center for Health Policy Research, The Dartmouth Institute for Health Policy & Clinical Practice, 35 Centerra Parkway, Lebanon, NH 03766, USA
Full list of author information is available at the end of the article

To meet the nation's future primary care needs, it might be reasonable to expand the scope of practice of ancillary practitioners such as nurse practitioners and physician assistants. However, there is concern that the number of new graduates from nurse practitioner and physician assistant programs is not keeping pace with the required needs to mitigate future primary care physician shortages [7]. In addition, there is evidence that physician assistants are providing more specialty care [8,9].

Many Americans seek care for common health conditions outside the offices of primary care physicians [10,11]. More specifically, neck and lower back conditions are among the most common conditions encountered in the primary care setting [12-15]. Chiropractors in the US provide a substantial portion of satisfactory care for these complaints [16]. In this regard, chiropractors may already be offsetting primary care shortfalls (serving as an alternative) by merely being located in areas of lesser primary care supply. If chiropractors are indeed located in areas of lesser primary care physician supply, they might be serving as points of primary contact for patients, thereby improving access. On the other hand if chiropractors are located in areas of adequate primary care physicians supply, it might suggest chiropractors function in more complementary roles (i.e. treating cases that would otherwise have been treated by primary care physicians as opposed to serving as a point of primary contact). Depending on their existing role in the larger health care system, chiropractors may be positioned to play an even larger part in addressing the nation's growing health care needs.

However, little is actually known about the relationship between the chiropractic and primary care physician workforces [17-19]. We hypothesized chiropractors might be distributed across the nation in a manner, either directly or inversely, related to that of the nation's primary care physician workforce. Therefore, the purpose of our study was to examine the distribution of the chiropractic workforce and compare it to that of primary care physicians.

Methods

To examine the chiropractic workforce and compare it to that of primary care physicians, we used data from the Center for Medicare and Medicaid Service's Unique Physician Identification Number Directory, the US Census Bureau, and data on medical physician supply previously collected by the *Dartmouth Atlas of Health Care* for 2006. The *Dartmouth Atlas of Health* Care provides national information on the distribution and use of medical services across the US according to predefined geographic units.

We gathered practitioner supply and sociodemographic population data by Zone Improvement Plan (ZIP) code and aggregated all measures according to the 306 Hospital Referral Regions (HRRs) commonly used by the *Dartmouth Atlas of Health Care*. HRRs are geographic units that were initially designed based on health care utilization and have the advantage of being independent of political boundaries.

Measures

The chiropractic workforce

Estimating the national supply of chiropractors is a challenge because they can have multiple state licenses. The Unique Physician Identification Number Directory contains information on and provides a unique identification number for physicians, osteopathic physicians, and other select health care practitioners (including chiropractors) who are enrolled in the US Medicare program. Using this directory, for the years 2002 to 2008, we identified chiropractors enrolled in the Medicare program and the ZIP codes for their practice locations. In the US it is mandated that, whether they participate in billing the Centers for Medicare and Medicaid or not, chiropractors must be enrolled in Medicare in order to treat any patient over the age of 65 years. Therefore, Medicare data is likely a very complete data source for US chiropractors; albeit, it may not include the few chiropractors who, for instance, only treat children.

To confirm findings from the Medicare files, we collected data on the total number of chiropractic licenses from the Federation of Chiropractic Licensing Boards and obtained information on the total number of employed chiropractors from the National Employment Matrix (Additional file 1: Appendix 1) [20]. The National Employment Matrix is compiled biennially as part of the Employment Projections program by the US Bureau of Labor Statistics; data for the matrix comes from multiple Bureau of Labor Statistics databases including: the Occupational Employment Statistics survey (data identifying employed workforce patterns and salaries), the Current Employment Statistics Program (data on total wage in each industry), and the Current Population Survey (data on self-employed and second jobs). The dataset provides annual estimates of numbers of employed workers in specific jobs.

The primary care physician workforce

Data on the supply and practice location according to ZIP codes for medical physicians were used from the American Medical Association and American Osteopathic Association Masterfiles for 2006. These data were aggregated previously by the *Dartmouth Atlas of Health Care* and excluded physicians in graduate medical education, those working primarily in teaching, administrative, or research positions and those working less than 20 hours per week in clinical settings. The Masterfiles contain information on 406 self-designated specialties by physicians.

The Masterfiles were used to determine the relative overlap in the local supply of chiropractors and primary care physicians, operationalized as physicians who self-reported practicing internal medicine, family medicine, or general practice (note: we did not include pediatricians in our definition).

Population data

Using extrapolated 2000 US Census Bureau data we generated estimates of the number of chiropractors and primary care physicians per 100,000 adults (age $\geq$ 18 years) for 2006. We limited our analysis to the adult population age 18 and older because that population uses approximately 80 to 90 percent of all chiropractic services each year [16]. Thus we were consistent with the potential treatment population in our definition of primary care physicians. For each Dartmouth Atlas defined HRR, [21] we generated the supply of practitioners per 100,000 adult capita according to the US Census Bureau 2006 population data. We also obtained other sociodemographic data for HRRs, including age, race/ethnicity, family income, and education from the US Census Bureau.

To examine population factors that might influence the supply of practitioners, we calculated the percent of the adult population aged 65 and older, those aged 25 or older with a high school education or less, those of racial or ethnic minority, and families with a median household income < $20,000 for each HRR.

Data from Washington University's Rural Health Research Center were used to classify US ZIP codes as either urban or rural [22]. The Rural Health Research Center uses population data from the US Census Bureau as well as spatial data and commuting distances to generate rural classification scores known as Rural–urban Commuting Area codes. Rural–urban Commuting Area codes were collapsed into either urban or rural and determined the percent of the adult population that resided in rural zip codes for each HRR.

Statistical analyses

We used Pearson's correlation to compare the relationship between per adult capita supply of chiropractors to that of primary care physicians and determined the expected supply of chiropractors per HRR when accounting for population size and age. We operationally defined very high and very low chiropractic supply areas as HRRs wherein observed supply was at least 50 percent higher or lower than expected supply, respectively (observed to expected ratio of 1.5 for "Very High" and 0.5 for "Very Low"). To examine the relationship between population characteristics and the supply of the chiropractors and primary care physicians we used multiple variable Poisson regression adjusted for population size. Sandwich variance was used to generate more robust standard error estimates. We used ArcGIS version 10.0 (ESRI, Redlands, CA) for spatial analyses and Stata version 11.0 (College Station, Texas) for regression analyses.

Results

We estimated that there were 74,623 chiropractors in the US who held 87,237 state chiropractic licenses (a mean of 1.2 licenses per practitioner) in 2006. The national chiropractic workforce has been relatively stable from 2002 to 2008 (Additional file 1: Appendix 1). There were about twice as many active primary care physicians (169,843) in 2006.

The per capita supply of chiropractors ranged from 10.7 per 100,000 capita in Bryan, Texas to 126.4 per 100,000 capita in Mason City, IA, a 10.8-fold variation in supply. Although New Orleans had an even lower supply of chiropractors (6.8 per 100,000 capita) than Bryan, because the low numbers in New Orleans could have been an effect of chiropractors relocating after Hurricane Katrina in 2005, we were concerned that the New Orleans results were spurious and eliminated New Orleans from further analysis. The median supply of chiropractors was 36.6 per 100,000 capita. The supply of primary care physicians ranged from 46.0 to 123.8 per 100,000, with a median supply of 74.0 per 100,000, a considerably lower 1.7-fold variation across HRRs (Figure 1).

The supply of chiropractors and primary care physicians was correlated (Pearson correlation coefficient = 0.17, p-value < 0.01). However, the 20% of HRRs with a high supply of chiropractors per capita (defined as those greater than or equal to 50 per 100,000 capita) were roughly equally distributed across high and low primary care physician supply locales (Figure 1).

We found that variation in the supply of chiropractors across the US exhibited a specific spatial pattern (Figure 2). The Midwestern and Western regions contained considerably more chiropractors than expected after accounting for differences in population age and size — a similar but more pronounced pattern than that of the crude supply of chiropractors per 100,000 capita (Additional file 1: Appendix 2). Conversely, the Southern portion of the US had considerably fewer chiropractors than expected. Considering the high supply of medical physicians in the Northeast, we were surprised to find

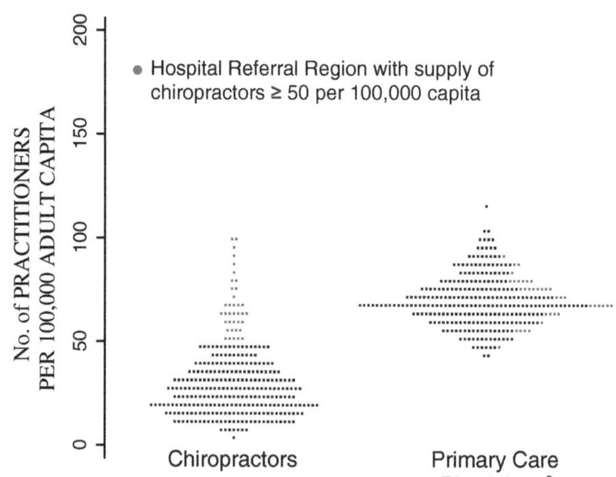

	Chiropractors	Primary Care Physicians[a]
Pearson's R:	1.0 (Reference)	0.17**
Mean:	41.2	75.3
Median:	36.6	74.0
IQR:	27.3	15.7

Figure 1 Distribution of Practitioners per United States Hospital Referral Region. Abbreviations: IQR, interquartile range. a: Primary care physicians defined as general practitioners, internal medicine, and family medicine physicians (pediatricians excluded). ** p-value < 0.01.

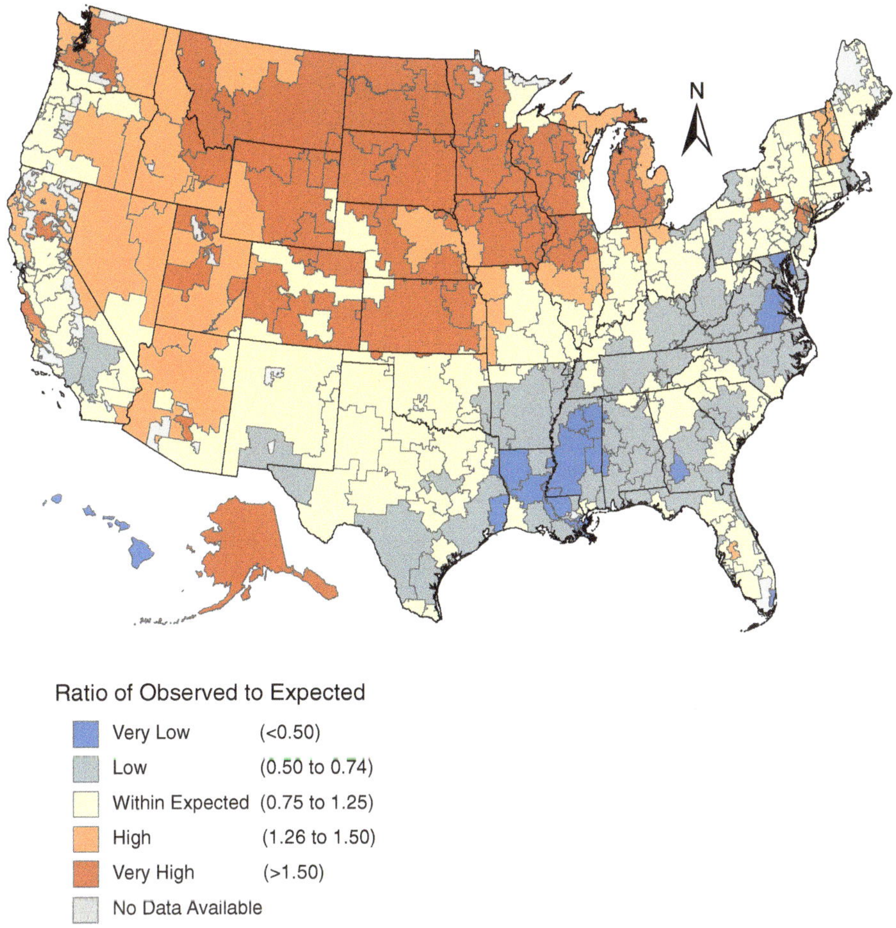

Figure 2 The Ratio of Observed to Expected[a] Supply of Chiropractors per United States Hospital Referral Region. a: Expected counts generated from Poisson regression model adjusted for total population and age.

that few HRRs in the Northeast exceeded expected supply of chiropractors. New Hampshire and Vermont Hospital Referral Areas were an exception and some of these HRRs trended towards higher concentrations of chiropractors (a ratio of 1.26 to 1.50 of observed to expected).

Population characteristics and practitioner supply

In both univariate and multiple variable Poisson regression models, population characteristics were more strongly associated with the supply of chiropractors than with that of primary care physicians (Figure 3). Population, age, and rurality were associated with higher supply of chiropractors. For instance, every 1% increase in the 65 and older population was associated with a 6.4% increase in the supply of chiropractors. Additionally, a lower proportion of minorities, those with greater than high school education, and those with income greater than $20,000 were predictive of a higher supply of chiropractors (p-value ≤ 0.001 for all three measures) (Figure 3B).

Lower population educational levels were predictive of lower chiropractor and primary care physician supply, p-value ≤ 0.001. A higher proportion of the population living in rural settings was predictive of higher supply of chiropractors in both univariate and multiple variable models (p-value < 0.001 for both) and primary care physicians in the multiple variable model.

Discussion

This is one of the few recent studies to examine the national supply of chiropractors [17,23-25] and, to our knowledge, the first to compare regional variation in the supply of chiropractors to that of primary care physicians. We estimate the total chiropractic workforce to be over 74,000 practitioners, almost half of our estimate of 169,843 *active* primary care physicians in 2006. We found greater than a 10-fold variation across the country in the supply of chiropractors, a higher concentration of chiropractic services than expected in the Midwest, and a lower one in the South which collaborates with a

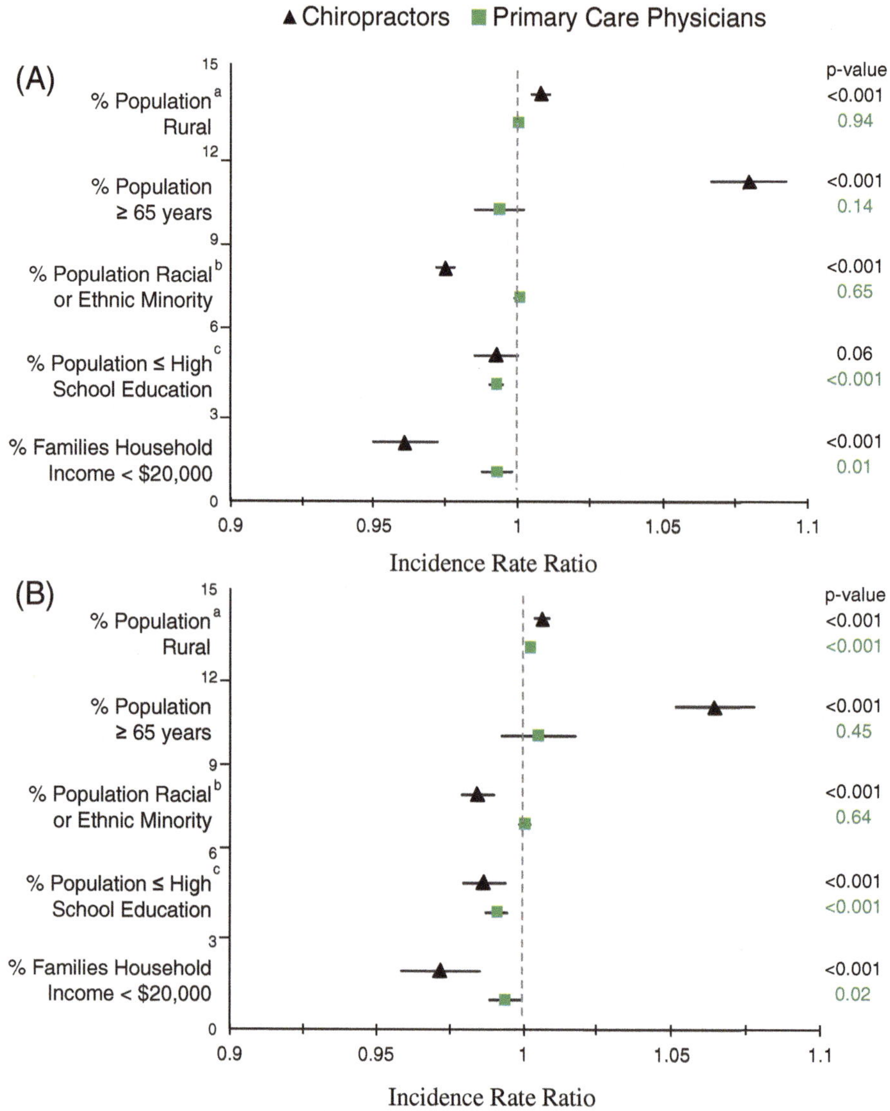

Figure 3 (A) Results of Univariate and (B) Multiple Variable Poisson Regression Models for the Association between Practitioner Supply and Population Characteristics. a: Based on urban versus rural as defined by University of Washington's Rural–urban Commuting Area Codes. b: Minority races and ethnicities include all adults that are not Non-Hispanic White. c: Among adults ≥ 25 years old (all other measures among adults ≥ 18 years).

recent report that examined the influence of supply on utilization [25]. Finally, we found a statistically significant correlation with the per capita supply of primary care physicians.

Our study suggests that chiropractors tend to establish their practices in areas that also have higher supply of primary care physicians. This is likely explained by the influence of market conditions on both groups: both are likely to locate in areas that will support their practices – however, there are many other personal and professional factors that our data did not account for. This finding may suggests that chiropractors function in a complementary role, as opposed to an alternative role, to primary care physicians. Whether that complementary role is substitutive or additive is unknown.

When chiropractors and physicians are asked independently to define the role primary care plays in population health there is significant agreement between the two professions [26]. However, chiropractors in the US remain largely considered to be neuromuscular specialists. In addition to government and private insurances designating chiropractors' as specialists in health care systems, chiropractors role as neuromuscular specialists is also is due to patients' impressions of their services – patients tend to view chiropractors as "back doctors" not as primary care providers [27]. Many within the US chiropractic profession are content with their role as neuromuscular specialists and those who wish to provide more primary care roles likely have numerous barriers to overcome [28].

Previous studies have examined the professional relationship between primary care physicians and chiropractors and uncovered an overall lack of inter-professional cooperation [29-31]. There is considerable overlap in the patient population treated by primary care physicians and chiropractors - neck and back conditions are among the most common complaints in the primary care setting [15]. This, coupled with our finding that chiropractors tend to locate in areas with higher primary care physician supply, suggests there is considerable potential for inter-professional collaboration. Health service use for neck and back conditions has risen in recent years and are attributed with substantial costs to the US economy [12,13,32]. Novel, interdisciplinary strategies are needed to address the growing needs of this population. Improved collaboration and coordinating care between chiropractors and primary care physicians has potential to help improve population health and reduce health care costs.

The relatively strong influence of population characteristics on the regional supply, of chiropractic care suggests that chiropractors are more responsive to market conditions than primary care physicians. Indeed, the chiropractic profession in the US continues to be predominately a "cottage industry", and therefore most chiropractors are also small business owners. It is likely that chiropractors establish their practices in areas of higher socioeconomic status, health care access, and overall demand for their services.

Also, there appears to be a relationship between rurality and chiropractic supply, and previous reports have explored the relationship [17,24,33]. For instance, one study found that chiropractors practicing in a Health Professional Shortage Area (which tend to be more rural) had larger patient panels than those not in Health Professional Shortage Areas, suggesting chiropractors may be playing a role in improving access to health services in certain locales [24]. Our results align with most previous reports as we found more rural areas to be predictive of a higher supply of chiropractors. Nevertheless, while chiropractors tend to be located in more rural areas (which may improve access to care in some populations), they are less likely to be located in poorer areas and areas with high proportions of racial and ethnic minorities.

These findings will inform health care policymakers as they decide how chiropractors will be part of US health care reform efforts, such as Accountable Care Organizations [34] or the potential expansion of coverage of chiropractic services. The size of the chiropractic workforce is relatively large, with higher concentrations in the Midwest, a pattern not exhibited among medical physician groups [21]. The extent to which chiropractors might be able to supplement medical care should be considered as a way to enhance the primary care workforce. Specifically, even though chiropractors might not be serving as points of primary contact role, chiropractors may be contributing to addressing the continued health care related to back and neck conditions particularly for populations residing in rural locales.

Limitations of the study

Our study has several limitations. First, we examined chiropractors who were enrolled in Medicare with the Centers for Medicare and Medicaid Services. Using data from the Centers for Medicare and Medicaid Services to estimate the national chiropractic workforce may have either underestimated the national supply (by excluding the few chiropractors not enrolled with Medicare) or overestimated it by including chiropractors working less than full-time. Nevertheless, our data regarding the chiropractic workforce appeared consistent based on other sources (Additional file 1: Appendix 1). Additionally, we used previously collected data that sought to make conservative estimates of the US primary care workforce by excluding physicians working less than 20 hours per week and those in primarily academic positions. Therefore potential underestimation of the primary care physician workforce may have affected our comparisons of the overall estimates of the two workforces exaggerating the size of the chiropractic workforce when compared to that of primary care physicians.

We used geographic units (the 306 HRRs), which were defined by regional use of specialty medical services. It is unclear whether medical services utilization patterns are comparable to those for ancillary health services such as chiropractic care. Given the size of the chiropractic workforce, HRRs are currently the only feasible geographic unit for study and does have the advantage of being independent of political borders. Lastly, because our study consisted of analyses on the ecological level, which rely on aggregate statistics and are inherently descriptive, our findings do not necessarily represent associations at the level of the individual practitioner. Despite the inherent limitations of our study design, this study provides important information regarding US chiropractic workforce and its relationship to that of the primary care physicians.

Conclusions

As the US health care system begins to recognize and reimburse more for preventive interventions, services such as chiropractic care may find more opportunities for integration with primary care. On a per visit basis, chiropractic care is inexpensive when compared to medical care [35] but larger studies are required to more thoroughly evaluate the costs associated with specific episodes of care as well as any potential indirect effects on overall cost. In light of increasing demands on an already overextended primary care workforce, it is an important time for health care policymakers to consider the direct and indirect effects of decisions regarding future coverage of chiropractic care [34]. Health care policymakers and other stakeholders should consider these findings when planning for the future health care needs of the nation.

Additional file

Additional file 1: Appendix 1. The National Supply of Chiropractors from Three Different Sources, 2002 to 2008. a: No. of State Chiropractic Licenses, Federation of Chiropractic Licensing Boards. b: No. of Chiropractors enrolled with Center for Medicare & Medicaid Services. c: No. of Chiropractors reported in the United States Bureau of Labor Statistic's Employment Matrix. Note: In 2007 and 2008 Medicare initiated replacement of the Unique Physician Identifier with the National Provider Identifier which may explain the decline in estimates. **Appendix 2** Supply of Chiropractors per United States Hospital Referral Region.

Competing interests
The authors declare that they have no competing interests.

Authors' contributions
Study concept and design: MAD and WBW. *Analysis and interpretation of data:* MAD, IDC, and TAM. *Critical revision of the manuscript for important intellectual content:* IDC, JMW, and WBW. *Statistical analysis:* MAD and TAM. *Administrative, technical, or material support:* MAD. *Study supervision:* MAD and WBW. All authors read and approved the final manuscript.

Disclaimer
The views expressed herein do not necessarily represent the official views of the National Center for Complementary & Alternative Medicine or the National Institutes of Health.

Financial disclosures and funding/support
Davis was supported by Award Number K01AT006162 from the National Center for Complementary & Alternative Medicine and Whedon was supported by Award Number K01AT005092 from the National Center for Complementary & Alternative Medicine.

Acknowledgements
The authors thank Yunjie Song, PhD at The Dartmouth Institute for his assistance with Medicare data collection and Dawn Carey, Kristopher Minsinger, and Ariannah Mirick for assistance with US Census Bureau data collection.

Author details
[1]Center for Health Policy Research, The Dartmouth Institute for Health Policy & Clinical Practice, 35 Centerra Parkway, Lebanon, NH 03766, USA. [2]Geisel School of Medicine at Dartmouth, Section of Clinical Research, HB 7505, Dartmouth Hitchcock Medical Center, One Medical Center Drive, Lebanon, NH 03766, USA. [3]University of California at Los Angeles, CA, Senior Health Policy Analyst, RAND Corporation, Santa Monica, CA 90401, USA. [4]The Dartmouth Institute for Health Policy & Clinical Practice, 35 Centerra Parkway, Lebanon, NH 03766, USA.

References

1. Cooper RA: **Weighing the evidence for expanding physician supply.** *Ann Intern Med* 2004, **141**:705–714.
2. Cooper RA: **Myth and reality underlying the needed expansion of graduate medical education.** *Gastroenterology* 2009, **136**:2045–2047.
3. Cooper RA: **Expanding physician supply - an imperative for health care reform.** *Pharos Alpha Omega Alpha Honor Med Soc* 2010, **73**:35–37.
4. Goodman DC, Grumbach K: **Does having more physicians lead to better health system performance?** *JAMA* 2008, **299**:335–337.
5. Goodman DC: *Twenty-year trends in regional variations in the U.S. physician workforce.* Suppl Variation: Health Aff (Millwood); 2004:90–97.
6. Chang CH, Stukel TA, Flood AB, Goodman DC: **Primary care physician workforce and Medicare beneficiaries' health outcomes.** *JAMA* 2011, **305**:2096–2104.
7. Cooper RA: **New directions for nurse practitioners and physician assistants in the era of physician shortages.** *Acad Med* 2007, **82**:827–828.
8. Jones PE: **Physician assistant education in the United States.** *Acad Med* 2007, **82**:882–887.
9. Jones PE, Cawley JF: **Workweek restrictions and specialty-trained physician assistants: potential opportunities.** *J Surg Educ* 2009, **66**:152–157.
10. Barnes PM, Bloom B, Nahin RL: **Complementary and alternative medicine use among adults and children: United States, 2007.** *National Health Statistics Reports* 2008, **12**:1–23.
11. Davis MA, West AN, Weeks WB, Sirovich BE: **Health behaviors and utilization among users of complementary and alternative medicine for treatment versus health promotion.** *Health Serv Res* 2011, **46**:1402–1416.
12. Martin BI, Deyo RA, Mirza SK, Turner JA, Comstock BA, Hollingworth W, Sullivan SD: **Expenditures and health status among adults with back and neck problems.** *JAMA* 2008, **299**:656–664.
13. Martin BI, Turner JA, Mirza SK, Lee MJ, Comstock BA, Deyo RA: **Trends in Health Care Expenditures, Utilization, and Health Status Among US Adults With Spine Problems, 1997-2006.** *Spine (Phila Pa 1976)* 2009, **34**:2077–2084.
14. Andersson GB: **Epidemiological features of chronic low-back pain.** *Lancet* 1999, **354**:581–585.
15. Hart LG, Deyo RA, Cherkin DC: **Physician office visits for low back pain. Frequency, clinical evaluation, and treatment patterns from a U.S. national survey.** *Spine (Phila Pa 1976)* 1995, **20**:11–19.
16. Cherkin DC, Deyo RA, Sherman KJ, Hart LG, Street JH, Hrbek A, Davis RB, Cramer E, Milliman B, Booker J, Mootz R, Barassi J, Kahn JR, Kaptchuk TJ, Eisenberg DM: **Characteristics of visits to licensed acupuncturists, chiropractors, massage therapists, and naturopathic physicians.** *J of Am Board Fam Med* 2002, **15**:463–472.
17. Smith M, Carber LA: **Chiropractors as safety net providers: first report of findings and methods from a US survey of chiropractors.** *J Manipulative Physiol Ther* 2007, **30**:718–728.
18. Smith M, Morschhauser S: *Establishing a database of U.S. chiropractic health manpower data: furthering the development of research infrastructure.* Meeting: Association for Health Services Research; 1999.
19. Davis MA, Davis AM, Luan J, Weeks WB: **The supply and demand of chiropractors in the United States from 1996 to 2005.** *Altern Ther Health Med* 2009, **15**:36–40.
20. United States Bureau of Labor Statistics: *Employment Projections: National Employment Matrix: 29-1011 Chiropractors*; 2011. Available at: http://www.bls.gov/emp/empoils.htm.
21. Goodman DC, Fisher ES, Bronner KK: *Hospital and Physician Capacity Update: A Brief Report from the Dartmouth Atlas of Health Care.* Lebanon, NH: The Dartmouth Institute for Health Policy and Clinical Practice; 2009.
22. RUCA: *Rural Health Research Center*; 2011. http://depts.washington.edu/uwruca/.
23. Cooper RA, McKee HJ: **Chiropractic in the United States: trends and issues.** *Milbank Q.* 2003, **81**:107–138.
24. Smith M, Carber L: **Chiropractic health care in health professional shortage areas in the United States.** *Am J Public Health* 2002, **92**:2001–2009.
25. Whedon JM, Song Y, Davis MA, Lurie JD: **Use of Chiropractic Spinal Manipulation in Older Adults is Strongly Correlated with Supply.** *Spine (Phila Pa 1976)* 2012, **37**:1771–7.
26. Gaumer GL, Walker A, Su S: **Chiropractic and a new taxonomy of primary care activities.** *J Manipulative Physiol Ther* 2001, **24**:239–259.

27. Teitelbaum M: **The role of chiropractic in primary care: findings of four community studies.** *J Manipulative Physiol Ther* 2000, **23:**601–609.
28. Gaumer G, Koren A, Gemmen E: **Barriers to expanding primary care roles for chiropractors: The role of chiropractic as primary care gatekeeper.** *J Manipulative Physiol Ther* 2002, **25:**427–449.
29. Greene BR, Smith M, Allareddy V, Haas M: **Referral patterns and attitudes of primary care physicians towards chiropractors.** *BMC Complement Altern Med* 2006, **6:**5.
30. Allareddy V, Greene BR, Smith M, Haas M, Liao J: **Facilitators and barriers to improving interprofessional referral relationships between primary care physicians and chiropractors.** *J Ambul Care Manage* 2007, **30:**347–354.
31. Curtis P, Bove G: **Family physicians, chiropractors, and back pain.** *J Fam Pract* 1992, **35:**551–555.
32. Davis MA, Onega T, Weeks W, Lurie J: **Where the United States Spends its Spine Dollars: Expenditures on different ambulatory services for the management of back and neck conditions.** *Spine (Phila Pa 1976)* 2012, **37:**1693–1701.
33. Cote P, Cassidy JD, Carroll L: **The treatment of neck and low back pain: who seeks care? who goes where?** *Med Care* 2001, **39:**956–967.
34. Davis MA, Whedon JM, Weeks WB: **Complementary and alternative medicine practitioners and Accountable Care Organizations: the train is leaving the station.** *J Altern Complement Med* 2011, **17:**669–674.
35. Davis MA, Sirovich BE, Weeks WB: **Utilization and expenditures on chiropractic care in the United States from 1997 to 2006.** *Health Serv Res* 2010, **45:**748–761.

Case management of chiropractic patients with cervical brachialgia: A survey of French chiropractors

Olivier Guenoun, Michel Debarle, Coralie Garnesson, Sylvie Proisl, Delphine Ray and Charlotte Leboeuf-Yde*

Abstract

Background: Not much is known about the French chiropractic profession on, for example, level of consensus on clinical issues.

Objectives: The first objective was to investigate if French chiropractors' management choices appeared reasonable for various neck problem scenarios. The second objective was to investigate if there was agreement between chiropractors on the patient management. The third objective was to see to which degree and at what stages chiropractors would consider to interact with other health-care practitioners, such as physiotherapists, general practitioners and specialists.

Method: A questionnaire was sent to a randomly selected sample of all French chiropractors known to the national chiropractic college. It consisted of an invitation to participate in the study, a brief case description, and drawings of five stages of how a case of neck pain gradually evolves into a brachialgia to end up with a compromised spinal cord. Each stage offered five management choices. Participants were asked at what stages patients would be treated solely by the chiropractor and when patients would be referred out for second opinion or other care without chiropractic treatment, plus an open ended option, resulting in a "five-by-six" table. The percentages of respondents choosing the different management strategies were identified for the different scenarios and the 95% confidence intervals were calculated. There was a pre hoc agreement on when chiropractic care would or would not be suitable. Consensus was arbitrarily defined as "moderate" when 50- 69% of respondents agreed on the same management choice and as "excellent" when 70% or more provided the same answer. It was expected that inter professional contacts would be rare.

Results: The response rate was 53% out of 254 potential participants. The first two uncomplicated cases would generally have been treated by the chiropractors. As the patient worsened, the responses tended towards external assistance and for the most severe case, the majority of respondents would have referred the patient out. There was excellent consensus for the two extreme cases (the most benign and the most severe), moderate consensus for the cases next to these two and least agreement relating to the "middle" case. Inter-professional collaboration was contemplated mainly for the severe case.

Conclusion: The French chiropractors who participated in this study seem to have a similar approach to patients with neck pain that gradually develops into a brachialgia and worsens. However, it is not known if the large group of non-participants in the study would agree with this treatment strategy.

* Correspondence: clyde@health.sdu.dk
Institute Franco-Européen de Chiropratique, 24 blv Paul Vaillant Couturier, F-94200 Ivry sur Seine, France

Background

Chiropractic is a relatively young profession in France. The first North-American educated chiropractors known to have practised in France arrived in 1920[1], and since then chiropractors could be taken to court for illegal practice of medicine. Some chiropractors probably reacted to this threat by claiming that they did not diagnose and treat diseases, similarly to how chiropractors in the US argued their defence when in the same situation in the 1920s and 1930s [2]

Chiropractic was no longer considered to be an illegal profession through a law passed in 2002 [3], and the final law text is in its final stages of completion, at the time of writing this. Compared to several other countries in Europe and elsewhere, this is a late development. Despite this difficulty, the French chiropractic profession has succeeded in establishing its own academic institution with a 6-year undergraduate program.

The number of chiropractors in France is unknown, as there is no registration board, and because not all chiropractors are members of the national chiropractic association. The number having graduated from the French chiropractic college, l'Institut Franco-Européen de Chiropratique (IFEC), between the years of 1984 to 2010 was about 500. It seems reasonable that most of these graduates would have set up their practices in France and that the vast majority of the chiropractors practising in France would be graduates from IFEC. In addition, there are some chiropractors practising in France, who graduated from other colleges elsewhere in the world, particularly before the French chiropractic college existed. In 2011 the Administration at IFEC estimated the number of actively practising chiropractors in France to be approximately 600, in a population of 65 million inhabitants.

It is possible that a small profession with such troubled history has had problems to develop its own "brand" and because the profession is so young it is understandable that it has not had the opportunity to perform research, for example, in order to establish its own demographic profile. Very little is therefore known about the French chiropractors' clinical practice. Further, being relatively isolated from the rest of the chiropractic community, because of the cultural differences and language barrier between England and France, it is possible that French chiropractors practice differently than chiropractors who were educated and/or practise in countries with a strong North-American chiropractic culture. It is therefore relevant to scrutinize the French chiropractic profession from several angles.

Students participating in a research course at IFEC were given the opportunity to perform surveys on the French chiropractic profession. One group decided to study the homogeneity of practitioners in relation to the management of brachial neuralgia emanating from the cervical spine. The cervical spine was an obvious choice for several reasons: Neck pain is a common condition in the general population [4], it is commonly treated by chiropractors [5] and, the neck being a fragile part of the spine, it requires a careful clinical approach in order not to induce injuries of various types. Further, neck pain can be very distressing, and the research team therefore suspected that it might be tempting for the chiropractor to attempt treatment also when this would be unsuitable.

Radiating pain from the neck can be very painful, indeed. An irritation or even inflammation of the nerve root would be the cause of most neck-induced arm pain. This irritation could be either directly or indirectly caused by a bulging or ruptured disc. In the early stages only localized neck pain may be present. As the condition progresses, one would expect to be able to reproduce the arm pain with certain neck movements, by compression of the nerve root within the cervical foramen or by traction of the nerve root. Eventually, if the condition worsens, nerve root signs would become obvious, and if the spinal cord were to be involved, there would also be signs of an upper motor neurone lesion.

The chiropractor is of course expected to diagnose such conditions, and should be able to decide whether manual or other conservative treatment is reasonable or not, and – in particular – to be aware of at what stage patients should be referred out for a second opinion or for other type of care. However, to refer out and ask for second opinions may be difficult for practitioners who have never been well accepted within the general health care sector.

There were three objectives of this study:

1. To investigate if French chiropractors' management choices appeared reasonable for various neck-scenarios. It was the opinion of the research team that chiropractic treatment on its own was acceptable in the early stages but more questionable as it became clear that this patient had a more serious condition with a likely disc involvement and totally out of the question when the patient showed signs of spinal cord involvement.
2. To investigate if there was consensus among the chiropractors on the patient management.
3. To ascertain to which degree and at what stages chiropractors would consider interaction with other health-care practitioners, such as physiotherapists, general practitioners and specialists.

Method

Study procedure

A team, consisting of three 4th year students and one lecturer in clinical science, was responsible for the design of the questionnaire and the analysis of data. They were assisted by three lecturers in research methodology, of which one was responsible for the logistics of the mailing out and reception of questionnaires.

A cross-sectional study was carried out between the 5th of October and 18th of November in 2009. From a list of 634 chiropractors known to practice in France at that time, a random selection was extracted consisting of 254 individuals. The remaining chiropractors were asked to participate in other surveys. The list of the targeted study population had been obtained through the membership list of the French chiropractors' association, telephone directories and the internet.

Each chiropractor in the randomly selected study sample received an envelope containing a letter of information, an addressed and pre-stamped envelope, and a questionnaire. A dead-line for answering was set and participation was voluntary and anonymous. After 10 days, a second letter was sent out with a request to respond to the questionnaire, if this had not already been done.

The Questionnaire

The questionnaire consisted of the following general information: "A 28-year old man, tennis player by profession, consults you for a right-sided intense neck pain without any radiating pain. You note an antalgic position of the head, no other musculoskeletical signs (no torticollis), no other health problems in particular, normal x-rays for his age, and no signs of alert (red flags)."

Five scenarios were thereafter presented, under the question. "In each of the cases described below, what would you do?" Each scenario consisted of a simple drawing of a mannikin showing the posterior aspect of the upper torso, arms and head, and a brief explanation of the case at the side of this mannikin. The five scenarios were as follows:

1. The mannikin was marked with a red cross in the lower cervical spine to indicate the area of pain. The text said: "Physical examination: very tense cervical musculature, no neuro-vascular problems, right C5-6 painful on palpation, pain 7/10 on a visual analogue scale".

2. The mannikin was marked with a red cross in the same spot and, in addition, an uninterrupted area of pain was drawn from the cross in the lower neck to the tip of the shoulder. The text read: "Five days later the patient comes back to you: Same clinical signs but the pain now radiates into the right shoulder".

3. The cross remained in the third drawing but the area of pain now descended all the way to the elbow. The following written information was provided: "Four days later: An MRI reveals a postero-lateral discal hernia at C5-6 which affects the C6 nerve root. There is now a neurological sign: C6 reflex diminished (1+), normal myotomes and dermatomes."

4. The pain drawing now reveals a pain from the base of the neck down the posterolateral side of the arm including the whole thumb. The accompanying text said: "Another 4 days later: The neck pain is gone. The neurological signs are obvious: C6 reflex absent (0), the C6 myotome diminished (2), C6 dermatome disturbed (reduced sensitivity)."

5. The pain drawing is the same and the accompanying text said: "Ten days later: The symptoms and signs are the same as last time but in addition the following is noted: the right leg shows hyperreflexia (3+), a positive sign of Babinski on the right and slight hypoaesthesia of the right leg."

There was a choice of 6 answers, for each of the five scenarios. These consisted of five defined management choices and one open ended question. These options were: 1. I treat the patient on my own. 2. I treat the patient with the assistance of some paramedics. 3. I treat the patient with the assistance of a general practitioner. 4. I treat the patient whilst asking the opinion of a specialist. 5. I do not treat the patient but refer him out. 6. Other, please explain on the last page.

The following three sentences were provided as footnotes: 1. In this study, kinesitherapists, ergotherapists and physiotherapists are considered to be paramedics. 2. Only neurologists, rheumatologists and surgeons are considered to be specialists. 3. If you decide to refer to some other health care professional, not mentioned here, please tick "other" and explain further on the last page.

On the last page, space was made available to write comments for each of the five scenarios, and the participants were thanked for their assistance.

Ethical considerations

Participation in the study was voluntary, anonymous, and no additional demographic data were collected, making it impossible in any way to identify the participants. The questions were innocuous and unlikely to cause any personal distress. There was no involvement of patients and no experiment was carried out. Therefore, the Ethics Committee at IFEC did not wish to review the research project and no ethics acceptance of the study was necessary.

Expectations

As a minimum, we expected that all chiropractors would prefer to treat the patient described in the first scenario (uncomplicated local neck pain) without assistance or referral and that all participants would refrain from treating the patient described in the last scenario (spinal cord signs), and instead refer out.

We also expected that the choice of treatment option would shift to the right side of the questionnaire as the condition worsened, i.e. that the chiropractors would increasingly require assistance from other health professionals, when the scenario indicated other than uncomplicated neck pain or relatively benign radiating pain.

We expected there to be high consensus in the two extreme scenarios (most benign and most serious) and moderately high consensus on the three strategies in between.

We also suspected that there would be only modest signs of collaboration with other health care practitioners.

Analysis of Data

Analysis of data was made by counting the types of response for each question. However, sometimes comments written under "other" could be placed in one of the pre-worded options. The option "other" was only retained when this box had been ticked but no other information was provided or when that information could not be used to fit the answer into any of the other options. When chiropractors provided several answers to one question, this was coded as "other".

The most frequently selected choice in each category has been highlighted in Table 1. Estimates reported in the text are accompanied by their 95% confidence intervals (CI) in order to provide an indicator of measurement error or uncertainty of estimates. Consensus was arbitrarily considered to be "moderate" when at least 50% of clinicians agreed on the treatment option and "excellent" if at least 70% agreed on a treatment strategy.

Results

Of the 254 questionnaires, 139 were returned, of which 4 were empty, giving a response rate of 135/254 (53%). In order to protect the identity of the chiropractors, no additional demographic information had been requested, thus making it impossible to perform a non-responder analysis.

As can be seen in Table 1, which provides all estimates discussed in this report, in all five scenarios, less than 10% of the respondents had given "other" suggestions to treatment options than those provided in the questionnaire. Between 0 and 7% of the five scenarios were not provided with a response.

Responsible practice pattern

In general, there was a reasonable pattern of responses, with the vast majority (87%; 95% CI 80-94) claiming that they would "treat self" the local neck pain and 57% (49-65) would do so also when the pain radiated to the tip of the shoulder.

However, when the pain radiated to the elbow with a reduced C6 reflex, 49% (CI 41-57) would treat with a generalist or specialist assistance. When obvious neurological signs appeared, 76% (69-83) would either refer out or treat with specialist assistance, and 74% (67-81) would refer out the patient with obvious signs of an upper motor neurone lesion.

There were very few respondents who showed signs of obviously inappropriate treatment behaviour. There were 2% (0-4) who would not treat but refer out the patient described in scenario 1 whereas 4% (1-7) would treat without referral or co-management the patient described in scenario 5.

Consensus between clinicians

There was excellent consensus for the first and the last two scenarios (the most benign and the most severe), moderate consensus for the two scenarios next to these

Table 1 Consensus (reported as percentages) on the choice of treatment strategy amongst 135 French chiropractors, regarding five different clinical scenarios with a choice of five clinical management options

Case scenarios	Treat self	Treat with paramedical assistance	Treat with GP assistance	Treat with specialist assistance	Do not treat but refer out	Other	No response or several answers
1.Local neck pain	87	2	6	<1	2	2	0
2.Neck pain and pain radiates to tip of shoulder	57	4	24	4	4	4	2
3.Neck pain and pain radiates to elbow, reduced C6 reflex	27	2	14	35	10	8	3
4.No neck pain. Arm pain radiates to include thumb, neurological signs C6	6	0	6	26	50	7	5
5. No neck pain. Arm pain and upper motor neurone lesion findings in lower limb.	4	0	0	12	74	3	7

The estimate with the highest percentage agreement is highlighted for each scenario.

but only 35% (27-43) consensus for the "middle" case (neck pain radiating to elbow, reduced C6 reflex).

Intention to collaborate with other health practitioners

It was very rare (0-4%) to treat with paramedical assistance. However, assistance from a general practitioner was suggested by 24% (17-31) already when the arm pain radiates to the tip of the shoulder and by 14% (8-20) when the pain radiates to the elbow with a reduced C6 reflex, but none would consider the GP for a patient with an upper motor neurone lesion. However, assistance from a specialist would be called upon as the case became more severe; 35% (27-43) would call upon help when the reflex diminished, 76% (69-83) would either seek assistance from a specialist or refer out (most likely to a specialist) when there were obvious neurological signs, and 74% (67-81) would refer out when there were upper motor neurone findings.

Discussion

Summary of findings

Patients who consult any of the chiropractors who participated in this study can expect a relatively similar overall approach to neck pain and radiating arm pain and this approach appears to be largely acceptable.

Methodological considerations

However, the response rate was low, only 53% of questionnaires were returned for the analysis, and it is not known if the 47% non-responders would have a different attitude to the treatment approach for this type of patient. Therefore, it would have been an advantage, if it were possible to make a comparison of responders and non-responders, at least on college of graduation, age, and area of work, to see, if the two groups resembled each other. However, due to privacy issues, it was decided not to collect any demographic data on the participants, as this could have been used to identify some of the clinicians. It was thought that this could help increase the participation rate, which we had anticipated to be rather low. It is not known, if this strategy worked or not.

Questionnaires are commonly tested in pilot studies. However, the present questionnaire that was designed by the research team was considered so basic and simple that no pilot study was conducted to test its user friendliness. Members of the academic staff did, however, proof-read the document for logic and absence of errors. Because of the low percentages of "no response" throughout the questionnaire we assumed that it was easy to understand and respond to.

It is our experience that clinicians sometimes claim it impossible to answer clinical questions in simple terms. There is therefore a need, in questionnaires of this type, to include the possibility to provide "other" answers. The percentages of "other" answers ranged between 2% and 8%, which is somewhat higher than in a previous similar Swedish study on management choices for low back pain, where this type of open response was selected by about 2% of the chiropractors [6]. However, the Swedish chiropractors were used to responding to questionnaires, since they had participated in a number of studies already, which might explain this difference.

Consensus

The consensus between clinicians appears fairly high although only excellent in the two extreme cases. In comparison, estimates as high as 74% and 87% were not found in the previous survey of Swedish chiropractors, who were asked about their management strategies for a number of low back pain scenarios [6]. One reason for this could be that it is easier to agree on the management of neck pain than that of low back pain. Another possible reason could be that there were more scenarios and more treatment options to choose between for the scenarios used in the Swedish study.

Clinical acceptability and collaboration with other health care professionals

Consensus is, of course, a good thing, as it unites a profession and provides it with a "brand" that is recognizable by the public. However, agreement between professionals to act irresponsibly is not desirable. The results of this study indicate that the responders of this study, on the whole, have a responsible approach to this type of neck condition.

We had expected that only a few chiropractors would use the assistance of other professional groups (paramedics, general practitioners or medical specialists), reflecting the long-term professional isolation that chiropractors have been subjected to in France. When there is a risk of prosecution for the illegal practice of medicine, the distance between the chiropractor's office and that of other practitioners can be very long. There is also no tradition in France of chiropractors working together with medical practitioners and physiotherapists in clinical teams. Nevertheless, collaboration with other health-care professionals was, at least, contemplated for the more serious situations. This does not imply that such contacts are very frequent, as such conditions would be relatively rare in primary care, and we did not study the frequency of inter-professional contacts per se.

Of concern, in the case of the obvious contra-indication to chiropractic care (signs of a spinal cord lesion, suitable for immediate referral to neurosurgeon or orthopaedic surgeon), there were 4% who would select continued care and 12% who would continue treatment albeit in collaboration with some specialist. On the other hand, it is curious that for the simplest scenario, 2% would refer the patient out of the clinic and about 7% would treat this patient in conjunction with a general practitioner or a specialist.

Conclusion

The participants in this survey agreed largely on the choice of treatment strategies for a patient with neck pain, which was described to develop increasingly severe signs and symptoms, and, in general, their strategic choices appear to be sound and safe. Collaboration with other health-care practitioners would probably mostly be contemplated for contra-indications and possible contra-indications to spinal manipulative therapy.

Acknowledgements

Funding was provided by Institute Franco-Européen de Chiropratique, France. In addition, Thierry Kuster, DC, is gratefully acknowledged for editorial assistance.

Authors' contributions

This article is based on a research project conducted as a part requirement for the chiropractic degree at the Institut Franco-Européen de Chiropratique for CG, SP and DR. All authors participated in the design of the study. On-site supervision was performed by OG and MD. CLY was responsible for the overall supervision and the final draft. All authors read and approved of the final version.

Competing interests

The authors declare that they have no competing interests.

References

1. Rouy B, Chiropractic in France: **Chiropractic in Europe.** In *An illustrated history.* Edited by: Wilson FJH. Leicester, UK: Matadour; 2007:80-3.
2. Leach RA, History of chiropractic theories: **The chiropractic theories.** In *A textbook of scientific research.* Edited by: Leach RA. Lippincott Williams 2004:13-28.
3. **Loi 2002-303 du 4 mars 2002 relative aux droits des malades et à la qualité du système de santé (article 75).** [http://www.legifrance.gouv.fr/affichTexte.do?cidTexte=JORFTEXT000000227015].
4. Hogg-Johnson S, van der Velde G, Carroll LJ, Holm LW, Cassidy JD, Guzman J, Côté P, Haldeman S, Ammendolia C, Carragee E, Hurwitz E, Nordin M, Peloso P: **The burden and determinants of neck pain in the general population: results of the Bone and Joint Decade 2000-2010 Task Force on Neck Pain and Its Associated Disorders.** *Spine* 2008, **33**(4 Suppl):S39-51.
5. Leboeuf-Yde C, Hennius B, Rudberg E, Leufvenmark P, Thunman : **Chiropractic in Sweden: A short description of patients and treatment.** *J Manipulative Physiol Ther* 1997, **20**:507-10.
6. Axén I, Rosenbaum , Eklund A, Halasz L, Jørgensen K, Lövgren PW, Lange F, Leboeuf-Yde C: **The Nordic maintenance care program. Case management of chiropractic patients with low back pain: A survey of Swedish chiropractors.** *Chiropractic & Osteopathy* 2008, **16**:6.

17

GPs opinions and perceptions of chiropractic in Sweden and Norway: a descriptive survey

Daniel Westin[1*], Tine Tandberg[2], Carol John[1] and Iben Axén[3*]

Abstract

Background: In Sweden, chiropractic is not included in mainstream health care. In Norway chiropractic is a recognized health care profession. The aim of this study was to explore the perceptions of chiropractic among Swedish and Norwegian General Practitioners (GPs).

Methods: Eight hundred surveys in each country were distributed randomly by post to Swedish and Norwegian GPs offices. The survey contained two main sections: Experiences and opinions about chiropractic and referral patterns. The data were then described and compared between the countries.

Results: In Sweden the response rate was 44.8% and in Norway 45.3%. More than half of the Swedish GPs participating in this study stated that they had poor knowledge about chiropractic, while just a tenth of Norwegian GPs stated the same. Nearly all Norwegian GPs had some experience of chiropractic treatment whilst a fairly large number of the Swedish GPs said that they had no experience at all of chiropractic. It was twice as common for GPs in Norway to refer patients to a chiropractor as compared to Sweden. However, Swedish and Norwegian GPs agreed that chiropractors were competent to treat musculo-skeletal conditions with an adequate education to be part of mainstream medicine.

Conclusions: Swedish and Norwegian GPs agree that chiropractors are competent to treat musculoskeletal conditions. However, there are many differences in GPs perceptions of chiropractic between the two countries and the overall picture indicates that chiropractic is more accepted and recognised as a health care profession in Norway.

Keywords: Chiropractic, Sweden, Norway, GP, Survey

Background

There are approximately 550 chiropractors practising in Sweden [1,2]. Two hundred of these have qualified from colleges approved by the CCEI (the Council of Chiropractic Education International), and all are members of the Swedish Chiropractic Association (SCA). The remaining 350 chiropractors have received their training at the Scandinavian College of Chiropractic in Stockholm which does not meet the demands of the CCEI (through its European member, the European Council on Chiropractic Education) and therefore has no European accreditation [1]. However, all chiropractors have full legislation from the National Board of Health and Welfare in Sweden [2], regardless of education.

In Norway, there are approximately 400 chiropractors who are all members of the Norwegian Chiropractic Association, NCA. A membership in the NCA is granted only to graduates from CCEI accredited colleges [3].

Chiropractors in Sweden are not privileged to take x-rays, refer to medical specialists or to authorise sickness absence. There is generally no financial reimbursement from the Swedish government for patients seeking chiropractic care, even though local counties may have such agreements with chiropractors and other health care professionals [4]. Furthermore, chiropractic treatment for children was not allowed until recently [2]. The Swedish National Board of Health and Welfare [5] states

* Correspondence: westind@aecc.acuk; iben.axen@ki.se
[1]Anglo European College of Chiropractic, 13-15 Parkwood Road, Bournemouth, UK
[3]Karolinska Institutet, Institute for Environmental Medicine, Unit of Intervention and Implementation Research, Nobels v 13, 171 77, Stockholm, Sweden
Full list of author information is available at the end of the article

in their guidelines that patients with chronic shoulder, neck and low back pain should be offered combination of different treatment methods including physiotherapy and Cognitive Behavioural Therapy (CBT).

In Norway chiropractors are authorised to take their own x-rays, refer to medical specialists and to refer for special imaging. In addition patients are given a greater range of treatment options in the management of musculo-skeletal problems. In 2001 the Norwegian Parliament launched a trial project; the Referral Project and lasted for two years. Nearly a million patients were involved in three Norwegian counties and the aim of the study was to improve patient satisfaction and cooperation within the health care services and to enhance socio-economic savings [6]. The participating chiropractors were given the following privileges:

- The right to issue sickness absence permits to their patients for up to 8 weeks.
- The right to refer to medical specialists when needed.
- The authority to refer for physical therapy and specialist radiological examinations.
- Patients no longer needed a GP referral in order to see a chiropractor with fee subsidisation.

The main result of the trial project was that the cost of sickness absence payments from the Labour and Welfare Service decreased by 2.4% in the three involved counties. Patients also reported that they were more satisfied with the opportunity to choose their own care [6].

As a result of the trial project new legislation was passed by the Norwegian Parliament concerning chiropractors and chiropractic treatment [7]. Hence, patients in Norway became entitled to financial compensation for up to 14 weeks per year for chiropractic treatment without GP referral. In addition chiropractors were given the right to administer sickness absence for up to 8 weeks and refer patients to medical specialists [8].

Thus, the differences regarding chiropractic care in these two neighbouring countries are substantial. Generally, General Practitioners (GPs) act as gatekeepers in the health care system and subsequently see many patients that may be suitable for chiropractic care. It is possible that their views of chiropractic influence the level of integration of chiropractic in mainstream health care as they may influence their patients' perceptions during the GP consultation.

The aim of this study was to investigate and to compare the experiences and opinions of chiropractic among Swedish and Norwegian GPs and their referral patterns to chiropractic care.

Methods

Design: A questionnaire survey. The survey is based on two Master-projects from the Anglo-European College of Chiropractic in England. In Sweden, the questionnaires were distributed in August of 2011 and in Norway in July of 2009.

The questionnaire was constructed on the basis of previous, similar surveys with the same purpose [9,10]. The questions were modified to be applicable to Swedish and Norwegian medical doctors. The questionnaire used in this study is found in Additional file 1.

There were 13 questions, all closed ended and divided into two main sections:

- Opinions and experiences about chiropractic
- Referral patterns

In the first part of the questionnaire the GPs general knowledge and opinions about chiropractors, educational standards and terminology was assessed, as well as the GP's experience of chiropractic.

In the second part of the questionnaire the GPs were asked how often they referred to chiropractors and what kinds of conditions that were commonly referred.

Furthermore, questions were asked about correspondence from chiropractors to the GPs, reasons for not referring for chiropractic care and which care provider they commonly referred to if not a chiropractor.

In addition, some demographic information regarding the respondent (gender, age, and years in practice) was collected.

As this study was directed at clinicians with little time to spare it was important that the questions were short, closed ended and easy to answer. However, based on the experiences from the Norwegian part of the survey, the GPs in Sweden were given the option to give additional comments.

As no identifying personal information was collected, merely GPs opinions, the project was deemed exempt from a formal ethical permission procedure. The questionnaire was approved by both the Swedish and Norwegian Chiropractic Associations and as undergraduate projects at the Anglo-European College of Chiropractic.

In Sweden, the addresses to the GP offices were found on the public website of each county council. In Norway, the names and addresses to the GPs were provided through the public internet pages of the Norwegian Labour and Welfare Administration.

The number of questionnaires sent to the counties was calculated in order to give a response rate roughly proportionate to the population and the number of GPs inhabiting each county. There are a total of 21 counties in Sweden, and 19 counties in Norway. In Sweden, 30 questionnaires were sent out to each county; except for

Stockholm, Västra Götaland and Skåne that received 105, 80 and 60 questionnaires respectively as these three counties are the most populated. In Norway, 41 questionnaires were sent out to each county, expect for Oslo that received 62 questionnaires according to the principle of proportion mentioned above. Thus, in each country, a total of 800 questionnaires were distributed. This accounts for 15% of the total GP population in Sweden and 20% in Norway.

In order to avoid selection bias the questionnaires were sent out to every other GP office in the order they appeared on the list from the county councils website until the quota of surveys for each county was filled. In Sweden the addresses were written by hand with the purpose of personalising the letter and thereby increasing the probability of the respondents completing the survey. In Norway the addresses were typed on the envelope.

Each envelope also contained a covering letter, found in Additional file 2, informing the GP's of the purpose of the study, and assuring them of their anonymity and the confidentiality of the study. They were also informed that by returning the questionnaire they gave their consent to take part in the study. One stamped addressed envelope for returning the questionnaire was also included in the envelope.

Results

Response rate

In Sweden, 359 questionnaires with complete answers were returned. In addition, 12 questionnaires were returned with incomplete answers and were therefore excluded from the study. Another two letters were returned unopened due to retirement. Thus, the response rate of completed questionnaires was 44.8%. In Norway, 387 questionnaires were returned, of which 376 were complete. Ten questionnaires were returned due to incorrect addresses and 1 was returned due to retirement, rendering a response rate of 45.3%.

Demographic data

The sample of Swedish GPs was slightly older than the Norwegian sample. Fifty-nine per cent of the Swedish GPs were aged 51 years or older whereas the corresponding number in Norway in this age group was 43%. Only one GP in Sweden was aged between 20 and 30, whereas in Norway, 19 GP's fitted this category. Of the Swedish GPs, 58% were male and in the Norwegian sample 64% were male.

Opinions and experiences of chiropractic

The questions and answers are summarized in Table 1.

The questionnaire started with the general question; "How would you describe your knowledge of chiropractic? Seven per cent of the Swedish GPs felt that they had good knowledge of chiropractic and 53% felt that they had poor knowledge. The remaining 40% claimed to know something about chiropractic. In Norway, 22% of the GPs felt that they had good knowledge, 12% said that they had poor knowledge and 66% claimed to know something about chiropractic.

The GPs were asked if, in their opinion, chiropractors have a satisfactory education for mainstream medicine. Forty-nine per cent of the respondents in Sweden agreed and 42% had no opinion. In Norway, the corresponding figures were 80% (satisfactory education for mainstream medicine) and 18% (no opinion). Swedish and Norwegian GPs agreed that chiropractors were competent to treat musculo-skeletal conditions (69% and 93% respectively).

The GPs were asked if they thought that chiropractors use unusual terminology, and this was agreed by 11% of the GP's in Sweden. In Norway 25% of the respondent GPs agreed.

The GPs were asked how they would describe their experiences of chiropractic treatment for their patients. Nearly half (47%) of the Swedish GPs and 66% of the GPs in Norway reported a good experience of chiropractic. Twenty per cent of the Swedish GPs reported to have a variable experience and 12% said that they had bad experience with chiropractic care for their patients. In Norway 27% of the GPs said that their experience was variable and 3% answered that they had a bad experience with chiropractic care. Furthermore, 21% of the GPs in Sweden stated that they have no experience of chiropractic. This figure in Norway was 3%.

Referrals

In Sweden, GPs cannot refer patients to a chiropractor, so for the purpose of this study the questions about referrals in reality translate to a recommendation, rather than a referral for chiropractic care. The GPs were asked if they recommend chiropractic care for their patients and if so, how many times per month?

Forty-three per cent of the GPs in Sweden recommend their patients to see a chiropractor. In Norway, the majority, 79%, refer patients to a chiropractor. The reported rate of recommendation or referral was 1–5 times per month in both countries.

The GPs were asked what types of conditions they commonly refer to a chiropractor. Acute and chronic back pain followed by disc prolapse with uncomplicated neurological symptoms were the most common conditions to refer, for both Swedish and Norwegian GPs. However, more than 20% of the Norwegian GPs referred babies with colic to the chiropractor. This was nonexistent in Sweden.

In response to the question about communication, 55% of the Swedish GPs and 67% of the Norwegian GP's

Table 1 Summary of questions in the survey and the responses from the Swedish and Norwegian GPs

Question and answer options	Sweden -%	Norway -%
My knowledge of chiropractic		
- Good	7	22
- Know something	40	66
- Poor	53	12
- Never heard of it	0	0
My experience with chiropractic care		
- Good	47	66
- Bad	12	3
- None	21	3
- Other	20	28
I agree that		
- Chiropractic education is sufficient for mainstream medicine	49	80
- Chiropractors are competent for MSK conditions	69	93
- Chiropractors are competent to treat neurologic disturbances	25	17
- Chiropractors report poorly back to GPs	55	67
- Chiropractors use unknown terminology	11	25
I refer to a chiropractor	43	79
I refer the following conditions to a chiropractor		
- Acute back pain	37	68
- Chronic back pain	30	58
- Sports trauma	13	14
- Whiplash injuries	6	17
- Disc herniation	7	14
- Prolapse with uncomplicated neurological findings	16	24
- Migraine	2	8
- Tension headaches/headaches originating from the neck	9	9
- Asthma	0.5	1
- Carpal tunnel syndrome	0.5	1
- Back and pelvic problems during pregnancy	7	22
- Lateral/medial epicondylitis	6	7
- Nerve entrapment syndromes	7	5
- Infantile Colic	0	23
- Shoulder/knee pain	14	17
- Benign paroxysmal positional vertigo	0.5	5
- Other:	0	1
I refer MSK complaints to		
Chiropractors	31	82
Manual therapists	3	75
Physiotherapists	96	95
Osteopaths	1	7
Acupuncturists	12	15
Naprapaths	26	3
Homeopaths	0	0
I do not refer to a chiropractor because		
Poor knowledge about chiropractic treatment	38	16
They charge too much	26	14
Possible side-effects of chiropractic	14	12
Not sure how effective the treatment is	25	25
No chiropractors in my area	8	6
I have had bad experiences with chiropractors	4	8

reported that there were poor levels of reporting back to the GPs from the chiropractors.

The common reasons for not referring amongst the Swedish GPs were; poor knowledge about chiropractic, not being sure of the effectiveness of chiropractic treatment and that it was too expensive for the patients. The reasons for not referring for chiropractic care in Norway were that GPs doubted the effectiveness of chiropractic care and that they had insufficient knowledge about chiropractic.

In Sweden GPs most often refer patients to physiotherapists followed by chiropractors and naprapaths. In Norway it was most common to refer patients to physiotherapists followed by chiropractors and manual therapists.

Additional comments

There were twice as many negative comments about chiropractic as there were positive comments from the GPs in Sweden. The negative comments were concerned with chiropractors having different levels of education, over-treating patients and only focussing on short term relief. Also, some of the comments were concerned with the risks associated with chiropractic manipulation. Concerning positive comments, some of the GPs stated that they wanted increased cooperation with chiropractors and that they found manipulation beneficial, especially for low back pain. Five of these GPs also stated that they had great respect for the chiropractors that were trained at the Anglo-European College of Chiropractic.

Discussion

In this questionnaire survey, the experiences and opinions of Swedish and Norwegian GPs about chiropractic were explored.

Just under half of the distributed questionnaires were returned, which is not unusual for studies of this nature [9]. As the responses were anonymous, it is not possible to perform an analysis to assess possible bias of this response rate. It is quite possible that the majority of the GPs (who did not return their questionnaires) had a totally different experience and opinion of chiropractic than what can be extracted from this study. However, the resulting picture sheds light of chiropractic's position in the two countries, and seems to be informative regarding the matters under investigation. In Sweden, the survey was sent in handwritten envelopes. However, the response rates were almost identical in the two countries, leaving the importance of this additional effort subject to doubt.

As the survey is based on two Master-projects, they were distributed two years apart which may limit the comparison of the results between the countries. However, there were no changes in the legislation concerning chiropractic during these two years in either country, thus we do not believe that the time gap has any major role in the measured perceptions and opinions. Moreover, the experience of the first survey in Norway informed the space for additional comments in the Swedish version.

The Swedish sample of GPs was older than the GPs in the Norwegian sample. The importance of this finding on the results is unknown, but one may speculate that the older practitioners have a poorer knowledge of alternative and complementary medicine in general, which may be reflected in the results.

Opinions and experiences about chiropractic

There are clear differences between the GPs in the two countries concerning their perceived knowledge about chiropractic, with the Swedish GPs reporting poorer knowledge than their Norwegian colleagues. The difference in the age distribution mentioned above may be responsible for this disparity. Perhaps the younger GPs are more aware of complementary medicine? There might also be educational differences between the younger and older GPs influencing the knowledge of chiropractic. An alternative explanation may be that in Sweden there are fewer chiropractors relative to the size of the population compared to Norway, which makes the Swedish GPs less exposed to chiropractic which could possibly be reflected in their lack of knowledge about the chiropractic profession.

About half of the GPs in Sweden thought that chiropractic education was satisfactory for mainstream medicine, and 80% of the Norwegian GPs thought so. As there are differences in the educational standards for chiropractors practising in Sweden, the profession is less homogenous which may lead to a perceived variation in the quality of care reflected in the lower Swedish score.

Chiropractic terminology and mainstream medicine terminology are different and this may potentially be problematic. However, very few (11%) of the Swedish GPs thought so, but 25% of the Norwegian GPs were aware of this potential problem. One explanation may be due to protocol differences between the countries when it comes to communication between GPs and chiropractors. In Sweden it is not mandatory for chiropractors to contact the GP after referral, whereas in Norway the chiropractor is obligated to contact the GP under such circumstances, Therefore, more communication is taking place between the chiropractors and the GPs in Norway compared to Sweden, which might explain the differences between the countries for this particular question.

In rating their experience of chiropractic, there were also marked differences between the countries. In Sweden, less than half of the GPs reported a good experience, and 21% stated that they had no experience of chiropractic care. The corresponding figures for the Norwegian GPs were two-thirds with good experience and only 3% had no experience. Again, this could reflect the before mentioned poorer exposure to chiropractic and the variable quality of chiropractic education in Sweden.

Referrals

Chiropractic in Sweden is not part of mainstream medicine and GPs cannot refer patients for chiropractic care in the same way that they refer patients for physiotherapy as chiropractic is not included in the public health care system. Therefore it is challenging to compare referral patterns between the two countries. In Norway chiropractic is accepted as a viable option for patients with musculoskeletal problems and is recommended by 79% of the GPs. This is almost twice the referral rate as in Sweden. Even if the Swedish GPs would like to refer patients to a chiropractor there are no official channels to do so and some GPs stated that they hesitate to refer patients because of the increased financial burden for the patient.

The conditions for which Swedish and Norwegian GPs refer patients to chiropractors are similar in the two countries. Acute and chronic low back pain with or without radiating leg pain were the conditions chiropractors were deemed competent to treat, which is consistent with the available evidence and for the scope of chiropractic care. The large difference in referrals for paediatric chiropractic care between the countries might be due to the fact that the ban on treating children in Sweden was only recently lifted, thus no tradition exists for this option. It may also be related to differences in recognition of the chiropractic profession in general.

There was agreement between the Swedish and Norwegian GPs that there were poor levels of reporting back to the GP. This pattern is seen in similar studies [9-11]. We speculate that an explanation for the poor levels of reporting back to the GPs might be differences in expectations of when a report is needed. Perhaps the GPs expect a report back for every patient they refer to the chiropractor and the chiropractor only reports to the GP when the patient's condition change to a non- biomechanical condition that cannot be managed by the chiropractor. This is possibly an area where the chiropractic profession has room for improvement. If chiropractors reported back to GPs more frequently, the knowledge and understanding of chiropractic care would potentially improve.

Poor knowledge and not being certain of the effectiveness of chiropractic care were the most common reasons for GPs in both Sweden and Norway for not referring to a chiropractor. It is likely that poor knowledge and doubtfulness about the benefits of chiropractic care are influenced by each other. The growing evidence base of chiropractic care being effective in the treatment of acute and chronic low back pain, [12,13] was possibly reflected in the fact that these were the most common reasons for sending patients to the chiropractor. However, there may be other reasons responsible for the fact that many GPs doubt the effectiveness of chiropractic care. As mentioned in the comments, misconceptions about risks associated with chiropractic care, economic reasons and not being up to date with the latest evidence may all play a part. However, investigating these factors further was beyond the scope of this study.

Referring patients for physiotherapy was a very common option for the majority of GPs in both Sweden and Norway. This was an expected finding as physiotherapy has been within mainstream medicine for a long time and the patients in both countries receive financial subsidisation for this type of care.

The negative comments from the Swedish GPs may offer some insight into why the referral rates in Sweden are lower than in Norway. The GPs' comments about different levels of education are justified because that is the case and a cause for concern in Sweden. To date, there are more chiropractors practicing in Sweden who are graduates from The Scandinavian College of Chiropractic than chiropractors from ECCE accredited colleges. Without a minimal level of academic quality in chiropractic education it might be difficult for the chiropractic profession to convince the medical profession that chiropractic is evidence based, effective and safe.

The comments concerning safety are linked to poor knowledge about the latest evidence. The most recent research suggests that there are very low risks associated with chiropractic manipulation [14].

Conclusions

When comparing opinions, perceptions and experience of chiropractic among Swedish and Norwegian GPs there are clearly some differences.

More than half of the Swedish GPs participating in this study stated that they had poor knowledge about chiropractic, whilst the corresponding number in Norway was just 12%. A fairly large number of the Swedish GPs said that they had no experience at all of chiropractic but most Norwegian GPs had some experience of chiropractic treatment. It is also twice as common for GPs in Norway to refer patients to a chiropractor compared to Sweden.

There seems to be agreement among Swedish and Norwegian GPs that chiropractors are competent to treat musculoskeletal conditions. Further, most GPs think that chiropractic education meets the requirements of mainstream medicine. However the overall picture indicates that chiropractic is far more accepted and recognised as a health care profession in Norway. Lack of knowledge about chiropractic education, misconceptions about the risk of treatment as well as the lack of educational accreditation may explain these differences.

Additional files

Additional file 1: The questionnaire.

Additional file 2: Covering letter in Sweden.

Competing interests

The authors declare that they have no competing interests.

Authors' contributions

DW and TT adapted, distributed and analysed the surveys in Sweden (DW) and Norway (TT). CJ supervised the projects. IA was responsible for writing the manuscript together with DW. All authors read and approved the final manuscript.

Acknowledgements

We would like to thank the GPs who answered our surveys in Sweden and Norway.

Funding to cover postal costs was received from the Swedish Chiropractic Association. The Norwegian Chiropractic Association assisted in the development of the questionnaire.

Author details

[1]Anglo European College of Chiropractic, 13-15 Parkwood Road, Bournemouth, UK. [2]Elverum Kiropraktikk & Rehabilitering, Storgata 7B 2408, Elverum, Norway. [3]Karolinska Institutet, Institute for Environmental Medicine, Unit of Intervention and Implementation Research, Nobels v 13, 171 77, Stockholm, Sweden.

References

1. The Scandinavian College of Chiropractic: *Information about chiropractic.* http://www.kiropraktik.com/hitta-kiropraktorer/.
2. The Swedish Chiropractors' Association Information about chiropractic: http://www.lkr.se/sv/kiropraktik/svensk-kiropraktorhistoria.
3. Norwegian Chiropractic Association: *The history of chiropractic in Norway;* http://www.kiropraktikk.no/?PageID=17&ItemID=10.
4. The Swedish Chiropractors' Association: *Agreements with County Councils concerning chiropractic care.* http://www.lkr.se/index.php?option=com_content&view=article&id=812:landstingsavtal&catid=121:aktuellt.
5. The Swedish National Board of Health and Welfare: *Guidelines for musculo-skeletal conditions;* 2011. http://www.socialstyrelsen.se/Lists/Artikelkatalog/Attachments/18174/2010-11-15.pdf.

6. Langworthy JM, Birkelid J: **General practice and chiropractic in Norway: how well do they communicate and what do GPs want to know?** *Journal of manipulative and physiological therapeutics* 2001, **24**(9):576–581.
7. Norwegian Government: **Ministry of Health and Care Services, 2011. Legislation regarding changes in treatment reimbursement for chiropractors and manual therapists.** In *Ot.prp nr 28.* Edited by Government N; 2005–2006. http://www.stortinget.no/no/Saker-og-publikasjoner/Vedtak/Beslutninger/Odelstinget/2005-2006/beso-200506-022/#a1.
8. Lippestad JW, Eitzen I, Harsvik T, Loeb M, Hem KG: *Norway report trial summary*; 2004. http://www.manuellterapi.no/docs/hvp/Evaluering_av_Henvisningsprosjektet.pdf.
9. Brussee WJ, Assendelft WJ, Breen AC: **Communication between general practitioners and chiropractors.** *Journal of manipulative and physiological therapeutics* 2001, **24**(1):12–16.
10. Greene BR, Smith M, Allareddy V, Haas M: **Referral patterns and attitudes of primary care physicians towards chiropractors.** *BMC Complement Altern Med* 2006, **6**:5.
11. Busse JW, Jim J, Jacobs C, Ngo T, Rodine R, Torrance D, Kulkarni AV, Petrisor B, Drew B, Bhandari M: **Attitudes towards chiropractic: an analysis of written comments from a survey of north american orthopaedic surgeons.** *Chiropr Man Therap* 2011, **19**(1):25.
12. Bronfort G, Haas M, Evans R, Leininger B, Triano J: **Effectiveness of manual therapies: the UK evidence report.** *Chiropractic & Osteopathy* 2010, **18**:3.
13. National Institute for Health and Care Exellence: *Low back pain: early management of persistent non-specific low back pain*; 2013. http://publications.nice.org.uk/low-back-pain-cg88/guidance#manual-therapy.
14. Cassidy JD, Boyle E, Cote P, He Y, Hogg-Johnson S, Silver FL, Bondy SJ: **Risk of vertebrobasilar stroke and chiropractic care: results of a population-based case–control and case-crossover study.** *Spine* 2008, **33**(4 Suppl):S176–S183.

Contemporary chiropractic practice in the UK: a field study of a chiropractor and his patients in a suburban chiropractic clinic

Bjorn J Hennius[1,2]

Abstract

Background: Two recent surveys of chiropractors in Great Britain suggest that there are discrepancies between chiropractic practice as defined in regulatory guidelines and day-to-day chiropractic clinical practice and there is in general a paucity of information regarding the characteristics of contemporary chiropractic practice in the United Kingdom. This field study describes the daily practice of a contemporary British UK-trained chiropractor.

Methods: The fieldwork took place during the spring and summer of 2008 when the author spent one day per week observing consultations and interviewing patients in a chiropractic clinic. The chiropractor was subjected to interviews on two occasions. The author also registered as a patient. Field notes were taken by the author, interviews were recorded and the transcripts were corrected and analysed by the author.

Results: A total of 25 patients took part in the study. The interaction that took place between patients and staff in reception could be considered as a prelude to consultation facilitating the transformation from individual to patient and back to individual. Coupled with the continuous physical contact between the chiropractor and each patient there was a substantial amount of verbal and non-verbal communication throughout treatment visits. The patients presented with predominantly musculo-skeletal pain and the majority had consulted the chiropractor as a result of recommendations from others in their close social environment. The majority of the interviewed patients had either an inaccurate or at best rudimentary understanding of the mechanisms of chiropractic treatment. A few of the interviewed patients indicated that they had at first experienced concerns about the nature of chiropractic treatment or getting undressed. The author was able to gain some insight into how the chiropractor's experiences, opinions and beliefs had shaped his approach to chiropractic treatment and how this formed the basis of his clinical modus operandi.

Conclusion: Although no robust conclusions should be drawn from this small scale field study it does show that the clinical chiropractic practice as carried out by this UK trained British chiropractor contains a number of elements described in earlier qualitative studies in the United States, Canada, and Australia.

Background

Contemporary complementary therapy in the western setting has been the subject of a number of surveys and reviews during the last two decades of the twentieth Century [1-11]. Chiropractic practice in particular has been studied by a number of researchers in the United States [12-14], Canada [15,16], Australia [17], and Europe [18-24]. This research has resulted in a substantial volume of predominantly quantitative data.

Ethnographers have historically taken an interest in the activities of body oriented healers using manipulative techniques in foreign cultures [25-29], but field studies that describe the characteristics of chiropractic clinical practice in western settings are rare. The first ethnography of a chiropractic clinic was carried out in the nineteen seventies in the United States and it portrayed the chiropractor as belonging to a group of "deviant" practitioners [30]. Later studies have suggested that chiropractic purists, or *straight* chiropractors, are in decline [31-34]. The most

Correspondence: bjornan@hotmail.co.uk
[1]Parkwood Chiropractic Clinic, 93, Cathedral Road, Cardiff CF11 9PG, UK
[2]Welsh Institute of Chiropractic (WIOC), University of South Wales, Treforrest, Wales, UK

comprehensive study of chiropractors and chiropractic practice took place in Canada and provided, at that time, a detailed overview of the Canadian chiropractic profession [35].

Contemporary chiropractic in the United Kingdom

There is a paucity of descriptive and qualitative information regarding the characteristics of contemporary chiropractic practice as carried out by UK trained chiropractors in the United Kingdom. Two recent questionnaire based surveys indicate that there are different approaches within the British chiropractic profession and that the beliefs, theories, and clinical rationale that underpin the practical application of chiropractic treatment vary between individual practitioners [36,37].

The surveys included questions related to treatment efficacy, scope of practice, a chiropractor's role in healthcare and within society as well as the beliefs underpinning clinical practice. A large proportion of respondents were in the age groups 31–35 years, (16.97%), and 25–35 years, (34%), respectively.

Sixty-eight per cent of respondents agreed with the statement that chiropractors are 'primary contact practitioners', and 49 per cent believed that "a chiropractor primarily treats neuro-musculoskeletal and, to some degree, visceral or organic conditions by giving adjustments and using complementary therapy modalities". Even though 55 per cent of responding practitioners believed that "Mainstream and chiropractic paradigms are compatible in practice" 30 per cent disagreed with the statement "In today's chiropractic profession science is more important than traditional chiropractic beliefs/ philosophy" [37].

The surveys further indicated that 76 per cent of respondents "strongly agreed" or "agreed" with the statement; "Traditional chiropractic beliefs (chiropractic philosophy) are an important and integral part of chiropractic" and 18 per cent "strongly agreed" that "Gastrointestinal complaints" are treatable by chiropractic methods. 17 per cent of respondents gave the same reply for the chiropractic treatment of "Menstrual disorders/ dysmenorrhoea/PMS" [36,37].

This data suggests that there may exist discrepancies between the content of regulatory guidelines on the one hand and actual day-to-day chiropractic clinical practice on the other in the British arena. This field study is an attempt to describe the daily clinical practice of a contemporary British UK-trained chiropractor through the use of participant observation, observations and recorded interviews with patients. Its specific aims are:

- To briefly describe the Chiropractic Clinic and the activities in reception;
- To describe the author's experiences as a patient during a first consultation and when undergoing chiropractic treatment;
- To describe the characteristics and structure of the treatment visits;
- To explore the reasons why patients decided to consult the chiropractor, patients' understanding of the mechanisms of treatment, and some of their concerns;
- To explore the rationale and beliefs that form the basis of the chiropractor's approach to chiropractic treatment and clinical practice.

Methodology

The study took place in the period between early April and the end of July 2008. The author, who is himself a practising chiropractor, made a conscious decision to approach a chiropractor practicing in another town in order to avoid familiarity with the setting and minimize the risk of meeting former patients. In his mid thirties and with fourteen years in clinical practice *Ken* was a suitable representative of the practicing British UK trained chiropractic population. By the end of the twentieth Century European and British chiropractors were predominantly male and of a mean age in the range 35–40 years [21]. A survey carried out on the British chiropractic population at the start of the twenty-first Century found that 55 per cent of the respondent chiropractors were males in the age range 26–45 years.

Formal consent was obtained after writing an introductory letter to the owner of the clinic, a chiropractor practicing elsewhere. It was agreed that the author could spend one afternoon per week at the Clinic. After a meeting between Ken and the author it was agreed that Wednesday afternoon suited both best. Each session at the Chiropractic Clinic lasted 3–5 hours and consisted of observations of patient treatments and in reception. Semi-structured interviews were carried out with patients in separate rooms between observations of treatments and on two occasions in June 2008 the author carried out interviews/conversations with the chiropractor. The author also consulted Ken as a patient at the Clinic and received chiropractic treatment. In addition to this the author was able to spend time observing patients and the receptionists in the reception area.

Patients attending the Clinic for treatment on Wednesday afternoons were asked by Ken in the treatment room or by the author in reception if they would agree to be observed and/or interviewed by the author. Potential interviewees were taken to a separate room after observation during treatment or straight from treatment and presented with a printed A4 sheet explaining the study, its confidentiality, and its voluntary nature, (see Additional file 1). The author found that a verbal explanation of the study was usually more effective. A maximum of 20 minutes was allocated for each interview and all were based around the following 3 questions, chosen by the author on the basis of a pilot study:

1. "How did you end up consulting [Ken] the chiropractor?"
2. "What is your understanding of what [Ken] does?"
3. "Were or are you concerned or anxious during consultations and treatment? (see Additional file 2)"

Interviews were digitally recorded and later transcribed by a medical secretary in the order that they were completed during the field study. Interviews were not formally coded and all transcriptions were checked and corrected by the author. Patients' answers to the three interview questions were often embedded in general conversation but were easily located and extracted by the author. Because of the small size of the study and the variation in individual responses to the interview questions the author did not make use of any strict method of analysis. The majority of the replies to the three questions were grouped together for use in table format in the corresponding sections of this document. A small number of responses have been integrated into the narrative of the text or used as quotes. The aim of the author has been to include all answers without exclusion in order to preserve the individuality of the responses and to provide a varied and descriptive account.

During observations in the treatment room and reception the author made field notes using pen and paper. Notes were in addition made immediately following the author's own consultation with the chiropractor. There were no specific criteria put in place by the author in relation to what to include from the notes and what to leave out when writing this document. The author did however make a conscious effort to select and include material that illustrates the personal and unique nature of the patient-clinician interaction during treatment sessions and at the same time describes the clinical routines put in place by the chiropractor.

Extracts from the field notes made in relation to the author's experiences on his first consultation with the chiropractor and the "New patient" observed in reception and during a first consultation with Ken were used to strengthen the narrative of the section of this document that describes the "First visit" to the chiropractor. Notes from 3 observed patients were used extensively in the section describing the structure of treatment visits. The 3 patients were chosen by the author as case studies on the basis of patient age, gender and main complaint. Their treatment visits are an integrated narrative of text and extracts from field notes illustrating Ken's personalized approach to his patients and his established clinical procedures.

Although there is an attempt at integration of information responses during interviews and extracts from field notes were used independently in appropriate sections of this document.

For reasons of confidentiality all patients' names, as well as those of the chiropractor and Clinic staff, have been changed. The name and exact geographic location of the Clinic have for the same reasons been omitted. Gender and age of patients have been left unaltered.

To carry out a Field study based on participant observation and recorded interviews while adopting an explorative and interpretive approach in the search for the reason for and meaning of observed phenomena would not have been possible without the pioneering efforts under the banner of *functionalism* in early anthropological field work. In broader terms this study may be considered an example of social anthropology [38]. The observation and description of the clinic as an institution and its staff-patient and patient-physician relationships does also contain elements of the *realist* style documentary approach [39].

This study has had ethical approval from the University of Brunel and is based on the data obtained during the author's research for a final dissertation in relation to an MSc Medical Anthropology.

Research findings and discussion

There are ethical and practical perils of simultaneously taking on the role both as an observer *and* as a patient in a field study. Carrying out participant observation as a fellow professional has been referred to as "housewife anthropology" [40,41], or even "anthropology at home" [42]. The risk of loss of objectivity and clouding of judgment in this field study is, in the author's opinion, counterbalanced by familiarity with clinical routines and procedures [43]. The fact that the author was the sole recorder of notes and in addition had editorial control over what material to include and what to leave out is a potential source of bias that must be taken into account in this type of study. The fact that the author had not visited the Clinic before in any capacity did enhance clarity of perception and should on the other hand, in the author's opinion, be seen as a strength of this study.

The chiropractic clinic

The Clinic, located on the ground floor of a converted bungalow, was situated in the suburban area of an industrial coastal town in western Great Britain and had been up and running for more than ten years. It was the workplace of 3 chiropractors and an herbalist, and was staffed by 3 part time receptionists working on a rota. The bungalow was situated on the corner of a main through road and had, next to the gate, a large sign visible to passing cars. Trees outside the perimeter provided shade and also functioned as a barrier to the noise of the traffic. A large part of the garden had been covered over with tarmac and another part with gravel in order to provide parking space for patients and staff.

The Clinic entrance, positioned between two bay windows, consisted of a glass door and was usually unlocked. The left bay window, that of the principal treatment room, had its blinds drawn while the right bay window was that of the reception. On entering an inner wooden door led to a dimly lit corridor where the visitor was greeted by the scent of camphor and eucalyptus. There were three treatment rooms on the ground floor and a toilet for patients at the end of the corridor. Carpeted stairs provided access to the converted attic that was now office space and staff area. The Clinic had no x-ray facilities (see Additional file 3 for a floor plan).

The reception

Immediately to the right from the corridor a wide doorway opened into the reception area, a converted front room. The walls were painted pale beige and five upright chairs were placed in lines, two along the left wall and three with their backs to the bay window. There was a potted plant by the wall to the left and a smaller one on a pedestal next to the window. A low table with magazines stood on the floor and next to it there was a box painted with a picture of Winnie-the-Pooh containing children's toys.

At the far end of the room the curved reception desk was positioned so that the receptionist was facing the entrance. A PDQ machine was placed on top of an elevated section of the desk and there was a flat computer screen next to the telephone. Another fax/telephone stood next to a tall, grey filing cabinet in the corner behind the receptionist's back. Next to the plant by the window there was a water cooler and a radio/CD player on a stand providing a background of the small talk, news and music characteristic of BBC Radio 2.

On the shelves above the reception desk there was a display of neck pillows and lumbar supports for sale to patients. A row of information brochures stood upright in a plastic holder fixed to the wall next to the reception desk. A framed poster, depicting a floating iceberg representing symptoms as its visible 'tip' and the hidden causes below the surface, hung on the wall above the brochures. Smaller framed pictures of landscapes were mounted on the wall separating the waiting room from the corridor. Two framed price lists were mounted on the wall behind the receptionist informing patients that the price of the first consultation was £45 and that subsequent treatment cost £27 per session.

In reception patient details were registered on the computer by the receptionist but patient records were handwritten, as was the Clinic diary. When patients phoned in order to book appointments the receptionists would provide information on when the three chiropractors were on site, times available for appointments, and the cost of a consultation.

The clinic management had decided to actively start selling products to patients on the condition that the item was recommended by the patient's chiropractor. Sandra, one of the receptionists, was constantly rearranging and improving the presentation of ice packs, neck pillows, lumbar supports, and other items on display.

In addition to its function as the administrative and financial hub of the Clinic the reception was a place for social interaction. Sandra chatted happily with patients and her volleys of laughter could be heard in all parts of the building. Megan, the other part time receptionist that would sometimes cover on Wednesday afternoons, was less vociferous in her approach but with her warm smile and discrete sense of humour she was equally good at making patients feel at ease. Patients in pain were always given sympathy and support, both from staff and other patients. Although not specifically a question set up as part of the interview protocol the nature of the reception area gave rise to a number of comments from patients (see Table 1).

Staff and practitioners were all on first name terms and the receptionists referred to the chiropractors by their first names when talking to patients. New patients were formally addressed as *Mr* or *Mrs/Miss* followed by their surname but after a few treatments formal tone was usually dropped. If the chiropractor was running late tea or coffee was often offered to waiting patients. Conversations in the reception were usually initiated by the receptionist and topics ranged from aches and pains to music, travel, and the youth of today. Specific details of treatment were generally not discussed although patients did at times comment on the firmness of a

Table 1 Patients' comments about the reception

Name and Age	Patient's comment with regard to the reception:
Vera, 46	*"I didn't know what to expect or as you say I hadn't been to a chiropractor. It's a very nice environment, very calm and friendly.…I only know [Ken], [chiropractor], I never had any treatment through anyone else.…The receptionists are friendly, good… Good environment."*
Ron, 30	*"It's fairly relaxed. It's not a clinical atmosphere.… You'd probably liken it to a dental practice rather (than a) hospital environment. So, it, yeah, it's fairly relaxed."*
Pat, 26	*"It looks something like a surgery because you have a reception that you need to sign into and then chairs there……and I had to sign some papers and had some general chit chat with the receptionist.… I felt quite relaxed…And quite warm colours and.…the sun was shining and lots of light coming in and… there's magazines to read. It just relaxes you before."*

chiropractor's manual techniques or how they were feeling afterwards. Most seemed pleased with their progress.

As the first point of call for anybody entering the Clinic, the reception induced a feeling of welcome and calm. It has been suggested that the layout of the reception, as well as its furniture, scent, posters, pamphlets, sounds and products for sale all have a strong symbolic function. Arriving, registering, and sitting down to wait has been described as part of a ritual with important social and psychological dimensions for the individual as an environment facilitating the transition from *ill person*, (person in pain), to *chiropractic patient* [44].

The chiropractor

Ken was a 1994 graduate of the Anglo European College of Chiropractic, (AECC), Bournemouth. As a member of the cohort that graduated in the year that the *Chiropractic Act* went through Parliament he had at first started out in another established clinic where he was able to make the transfer into clinical practice under the guidance of an experienced senior colleague. A survey in the early part of the twenty-first Century indicated that close to fifty per cent, (49.3%), of chiropractors in the UK worked alongside other chiropractors, and a third worked with other alternative or complementary practitioners. The survey further suggests that the vast majority of British chiropractors treat their patients in a clinic and only 5 per cent see their patients exclusively at home [36]. After moving on Ken had successfully built up a reputation of being a competent chiropractor who was liked by his patients. Despite the long hours, the routine of clinical procedures, and the responsibilities as a health care professional I was given the impression that Ken liked his job. I was aware that my presence in the treatment room as an observer might interfere with the patient-clinician interaction and assured Ken that I would do my utmost not to disturb. Ken said that he was happy to have me in the room as an observer provided that the patient had given consent.

Apart from my account of my consultation and treatment a total of 13 patients, 8 females and 5 males with ages ranging between 27 and 89, agreed to be observed.

The first visit to the chiropractor

I parked my car on the road outside the clinic just after 2 p.m. on a sunny Wednesday afternoon. The reception was quiet and there was only one patient, a woman in her fifties, waiting for her appointment. We were both offered a cup of tea by Sandra the receptionist and we both accepted. Sandra was busy entering data on the computer and answering the phone but had time to chat, generally about the sunny, but chilly, weather. I asked about payment and was told that it was normally taken after the consultation. Despite the music on the radio I could hear the muffled sounds of conversation in the treatment room across the corridor behind me.

A younger colleague of Ken's, a man in his late twenties, came into reception in search of a patient file. He wore a white, short-sleeved clinic jacket with the Clinic logo printed in blue on the breast pocket. Ken was running late.

When finished with the previous treatment, Ken, wearing a white clinic jacket, came into reception and shook my hand. He was given my patient records by Sandra and led me into the principal treatment room across the corridor. I was told I could bring the cup of tea with me.

The treatment room

On entering the treatment room the domiciliary nature of reception was immediately replaced by a distinct clinical atmosphere; Closed blinds ensured privacy, the light was subdued, and the scent of medicinal herbs was stronger. On a narrow office table along the far wall there was a switched off x-ray viewing box, a computer screen, and a keyboard. There were academic books on the shelves and framed diplomas hung on one of the walls. Charts showed anatomical details of the human skeleton, muscles, and the nervous system. A partly drawn circular curtain near the window concealed a stool and some folded patient gowns. Instruments for examination including a reflex hammer, a stethoscope, and a sphygmomanometer, were laid out on a small table. From a metal stand on the floor hung a life-size bone coloured plastic spine. The air was comfortably cool and there was no background music.

The space in the centre of the room was taken up by an imposing structure in leather and steel: the treatment table. Padded dark blue cushioned sections only partly concealed the complex metal machinery underneath. Electrically operated pedals, switches, and a set of levers controlled the mobility of the table sections. Thin white protective paper on a roll by the headpiece provided comfort and hygiene for patients.

Ken closed the door and I was invited to sit on the chair by the table. There was a feeling in the room of privacy. It was an environment distinctly suited to investigation, examination procedures, and treatment. Ken took up his position in his office chair and looked at my file. Sandra had assumed that I had filled out my personal details at our previous meeting. Ken was unperturbed and asked me to start filling in my personal details and medical history. While Ken left to make himself a cup of tea I proceeded with the task of revisiting my life in the light of pains, occupation, habits and lifestyle as well as past ailments, accidents, operations, and treatment.

Taking the case history

Ken read through what I had written on the form and asked questions. I explained that my general health was good. After informing me that he primarily worked as a musculoskeletal specialist and that any other health concerns affected would be a bonus not planned for, he asked me what I had come to seek help for. I explained that I had a long-standing, reoccurring left-sided neck and shoulder pain. I pointed to the area and Ken took notes. After asking about the time of onset, progress, pain patterns and any other symptoms he explained that he needed to carry out an examination. Ken seemed relaxed throughout the procedure and I had the impression that he cared about what I was saying and that he was interested in what I was telling him. Interest and compassion are both factors that have been demonstrated to have an effect on patient satisfaction [45-47].

The intelligent, sensitive, and systematic collecting of information from patients has been identified as a fundamental characteristic of the clinical encounter [48]. Arguably constituting the most important element of the first consultation, the clinical interview/case history taking also has therapeutic functions on a number of different levels. It has been suggested that taking the case history represents;

1. Communication about the condition [49];
2. A demonstration of caring and developing trust [50];
3. A narrative of the patient's experience of the condition [51,52]; and,
4. A start in the formation of a genuine relationship between the clinician and the patient [53].

Apart from the clinical importance of exploring the "archaeology of a person's past", it has also been suggested that the case history taking allows the patient to experience past memories [54]. The patient interview has even been described as a performance not unlike improvisational jazz; The experienced clinician asks questions, reacts to, and follows the patient's responses in a negotiation of *medical meaning* together [55].

Examination and treatment

Ken suggested that he would concentrate the examination on the shoulder/neck area but include a screening of my low back and lower limbs. I was asked to empty my pockets and remove all clothing apart from trousers and underpants. While undressing I fleetingly felt self conscious about the fact that although I had showered and was wearing clean clothes the car journey in the heat had made me perspire. My notes from the examination are full of detail:

> *"Examination started with me standing, facing the window. The room was cool but not cold and I was conscious of my own posture and leg stance. I was touched around the neck shoulder area, palpated, and asked to turn and tilt my head. Ken asked whether any of the procedures caused pain and I told him when I felt pain. Ken checked my toe flexibility and leg/ankle/knee alignment and I was asked to place my hands on the door and do a high stepping gait while he palpated my lower back. My finger floor distance was measured.*
>
> *Sitting tests consisted of neck range of motion, nerve stretch tests, compression and distraction. Neurological tests (reflexes) where done and I was continuously asked regarding symptoms. At certain procedures I felt very sore and achy in areas under my skull, by my left shoulder blade and on deep pressure of the neck vertebrae.*
>
> *The reflexes (upper and lower limbs) hurt as the rubber hammer hit Ken's thumb and my tendons.... Finally I was asked to lie on my back and my neck and head alignment were examined. (Deep pressure on my nerve roots from an anterior direction). I was told that my head was not sitting 'straight' (Ken asked "I don't know if anyone has said this to you before but...").*
>
> *Ken asked me to sit up again facing the desk and the x-ray box. He proceeded to outline his conclusion: "There are areas of your neck and upper thoracic spine that need treatment. Although neck range of motion is generally good there is a low (Cervico thoracic) 'dysfunction'."*

Ken explained that he proposed to treat me using manipulation of the joints and soft tissue work. He asked me if that sounded 'ok' and I said I was fine with that. This stage in the consultation has been referred to as the "Explanation to the Patient" or "The Plan of Treatment" [35]. Ken then told me to lie on my back on the treatment table. The following extract from my notes describes the first treatment:

> *"Ken proceeded to traction my neck. The stretching action was carried out with his hands firmly gripping my chin and back of the skull. The stretch was comfortable. After this Ken proceeded to do sideways rotational stretches using (his) arms elbows and hands. I told him that the stretch felt firm but that it was comfortable. A more segmental rotational stretch/mobilization was carried out after deep finger pressure on the left side of the upper vertebrae at the base of the skull...*
>
> *.....Painful – up into my head, but abating. Ken explained that he was going to 'click my neck' and*

asked if I was OK with that. I said 'Yes' and he manipulated my upper left neck. There was a slow turn to the right, then a quick turn, and another. After one or two turns there was a loud click behind and under my left ear. The point of contact in the left upper neck was sore and I had expected more pain."

Ken treated my neck on the other side and then asked me to turn over onto my stomach.

"He walked to the door and put a lubricant on his hands and then proceeded to massage, deeply, my shoulder and neck region, concentrating on the left side. The treatments were at first painful/achy but felt better as he continued the procedure.

Ken explained that I had a misalignment in the cervico thoracic junction and that he had chosen to treat the region posterior to anterior. He again asked me if I was alright with having the treatment and I said I was.

Ken asked me to inhale – then exhale. As I let the air out he applied slow pressure with his hands placed on the upper part of my back, at the thoracic spine below the base of my neck. Suddenly he pushed down, fast, and there was a moderately loud 'crunching' sound but, to my surprise, no pain."

During one of our conversations at a later date I remarked on the fact that Ken seemed to use a lot of massage prior to manipulation treatment. I recorded his answer:

"Yes, I perhaps use....I use it more judiciously now and that would, I would try and ask myself what I can do best for this patient? What will be the best thing? What will give the greatest therapeutic gain to this patient? And I think soft tissue work is part of that.... soft tissue or muscle mass represents a greater amount of mass than mere nerve endings in facet joints....And they are the work horse of the body and you need them on your side...There is going to be a protection of that area and you've got to persuade the body that it's.... what you intend to do is ok."

As treatment was completed Ken went on to assess the effect of treatment, a process sometimes termed *evaluation* [35]. My neck and shoulder area felt relaxed and warm. My notes describe the final stages of my first visit:

"My face felt hot and compressed but there was a feeling of warmth and comfort in my neck/shoulder and head. Ken proceeded to test my neck rotation and I could feel a noticeable difference in flexibility and comfort."

The first consultation had taken just over an hour. I remember that Ken's hands had felt warm, firm, and reassuring throughout the first visit. A recent survey showed that chiropractors in Great Britain spend 31–60 minutes with a patient on the first consultation, and 15–30 minutes on subsequent visits. 68 per cent of the responding chiropractors indicated that they always required the patient to undress down to their underwear on the first consultation, and 42 per cent replied that this was the case on subsequent treatment visits [36].

I was asked to dress and followed Ken into reception where I arranged my next appointment through Sandra and made a card payment of £45.

Observation of a patient visiting the chiropractor for the first time

Eric, 89, a 'New' patient

Eric sat in a chair in reception with his back to the window. I took notes:

"The 'new' patient was talking to himself and his grandson about his blood pressure and the medication taken for it (high b.p.). he continued to talk/mumble and his grandson helped clarify the questions asked on the form. The young man was embarrassed (appeared to be) about his older relative's behaviour, (talking/mumbling aloud, fussing about what to write, etc....)

.....The elderly man continued in his gravelly voice. He referred to his medication, ("The GP wants to preserve me a little longer").

Ken came out to fetch the new patient who excused himself for not 'leaping' up when standing up to shake hands.

Ken said: "That's alright, it may not be advisable".

They walked together into one of the treatment rooms, (the one at the back). The new patient brought his stick into the room."

Eric gave his permission for me to observe his consultation with Ken and I proceeded to the treatment room. The elderly man, looking remarkably fit and healthy for his age, explained that he had a severe pain in the left upper back and was unable to stand up straight. He had hurt himself gardening and then gone from bad to worse by playing golf:

> *"Ken was sitting hunched forward, (mimicking the gentleman), facing Eric.*
>
> *Ken was asking questions. Eric was describing a knee injury, that he had been on Meloxicam, then, told not to be on them for long, changed to Co-codamol.*
>
> *Ken started to ask detailed questions, ("Does it hurt when you cough?", "Have you had this before?"....) Ken was speaking loudly. He went through previous diseases, asking details. The patient commented, on his spelling, that he left school 75 years ago.*
>
> *There was lots of humour, laughter, irony. Ken asked: "Anything else I should know?".*
>
> *Eric spoke of chest x-rays – "a shadow". "I never smoked in my life", "it must be the hay".*
>
> *Ken commented: "We need to pin this down".*
>
> *Eric said he wanted to know what was wrong. (He) described how he had held on to the lawn mower. Eric said "Golf probably made it worse. Couldn't let the young ones get away with it".*
>
> *"Only 4 of us left." (Comment on his age)*
>
> *"Still bloody minded by the looks of it" said Ken.*
>
> *"Competitive" replied Eric."*

Studies have demonstrated that when clinicians use empathic and patient centred communication styles in a stress free environment this may have a positive effect on treatment outcome [56]. When Ken was satisfied that he had enough information he asked Eric to remove his top in order to prepare for the examination.

> *"Ken demonstrated Eric's stoop/antalgia (by placing him) in front of the full length mirror. Ken then asked Eric to take a seat (on the treatment table), and asked him to specify the left area of pain near the low back.*
>
> *Ken started palpating standing behind Eric on the left. Ken located a spinous process in the thoraco lumbar junction that was tender.*
>
> *Ken proceeded to percuss the spinous processes, using a reflex hammer. Eric said: "You're playing on the xylophone." Ken laughed. Ken then brought a tuning fork from next door.*
>
> *"I've got a cold piece of metal here." Ken hit his knee and placed the tuning fork 'foot' on the spinouses."*

When Eric was examined Ken took care to use a more simplified vocabulary. Ken carried out some further tests on Eric while simultaneously explaining in lay terms what the tests were for. Seeing the difficulty that Eric had in moving around Ken then arranged to swap rooms with his younger colleague in order to be able to use the *hi-lo* function on the treatment table in the principal treatment room. This mechanism allows the treatment table to rise into a near vertical position enabling elderly patients and those in severe pain to step onto a footplate and be gently lowered into the horizontal position.

Eric's treatment

I followed Ken and Eric into the principal treatment room where the elderly patient was assisted onto the footplate at the base of the vertically elevated treatment table. Ken pressed the foot pedals. There was a humming noise as the treatment table slowly lowered to a nearly horizontal position. Ken explained his findings and the proposed treatment at the same time as he was helping Eric into a comfortable position. Eric was lying on his front:

> *"Ken explained that he had concluded that (Eric) had strained a muscle in the left lower back.*
>
> *Eric asked: "Will it eventually heal?" (there was a discussion of the body's ability to repair itself and the effect of age)*
>
> *Ken explained that he was going to start working on the muscle and then (that he) would stretch it. Ken kept asking "Ok?" to get the patient to make a choice/agree.....*
>
> *.....Ken continued to work on the left muscles of the back and then raised the table up to vertical. Eric was asked to turn to his side (right side against the table). The table was lowered to horizontal and Eric was stretched in 'side posture'. He [the patient] indicated that there was some pain as Ken applied pressure. Ken was at all times close and making sure that Eric was stable."*

At this point Ken stood back and explained that this was as much as he would do on the day. It was agreed that Eric should arrange to return in 2 days. Ken instructed the patient not to play golf the following day. Eric had some questions:

> *"Eric asked about time and how many treatments would be needed. Ken explained that he would expect full recovery, but that it would take some time, albeit without numerous treatments. Eric's concerns were voiced, and Ken, although conscious of time (the next patient was waiting and he was delayed) made efforts to explain and answer questions."*

When back in reception Eric paid and made an appointment for Friday morning.

The chiropractic consultation:

It has been suggested that the chiropractic consultation consists of four separate stages:

1. Acceptance/Validation
2. Expectation/Explanation
3. Clinical Action
4. Engaging Plan [57]

Coulehan goes on to say that stage one revolves around positive regard, empathy, ("the ability to sense the patient's experience and feelings accurately, and to communicate that understanding to the patient"), and genuineness. He also states that "fulfilling expectations by using concrete, understandable explanations is the second movement in the chiropractic process" [31]. Helman [44] suggests a not dissimilar staging of the initial healthcare consultation:

1. The patient's presentation of *illness.*
2. The interpretation and translation, by the practitioner, of the presented illness into *disease.*
3. The prescription of an appropriate *plan of management,* (this could be treatment or referral), that is acceptable to both the practitioner and the patient.

Stages 2 and 3 are considered to be of particular interest to the patient and this is where the communication between the practitioner and the individual seeking help is crucial. Studies have shown that patients in general have a number of set questions that they want the answer to:

1. What is the cause of my pain?
2. Can it be treated (by you/a chiropractor)?
3. What will the treatment consist of?
4. How many treatments will I need?
5. How long will it take before I get better [44,58,59]?

In addition there may be questions such as; What will happen if I don't have treatment?; Why has this happened to me?; What will be the cost of treatment?; and, Will this happen to me again after I have finished treatment? This set of questions has been referred to as the *patient's agenda* and the *patient explanatory model* [44,60].

Kaptchuk has pointed out that the initial chiropractic consultation almost invariably results in a firm diagnosis that "matches patient perceptions" [61]. Kelner found that 84.9 percent of the chiropractors always explained the nature of the illness and 88.9 percent explained the treatment to patients [35]. A Finnish study has suggested that being told a diagnosis can in itself be a source of great relief to patients suffering from back pain [62].

Coulehan concludes that "Chiropractors 'do something'.". This includes the extensive spinal examination involving "much laying-on-of-hands" in the third stage, the *Clinical Action* [31]. Touch is generally considered a natural element in the caring for others and some authors believe that it is directly related to enjoyment and health [63,64]. It has been suggested that the prevalence of touch in the clinical encounter gives chiropractic an advantage over other forms of care where there is little or no physical contact between the clinician and the patient [54]. Kaptchuk suggests that one therapeutic advantage of chiropractic is that there is invariably an *intervention* [61]. Coulehan is of the opinion that manipulations are dramatic events:

> ".....Successful completion is indicated by a snap, click or pop audible to the patient [31]."

One of Ken's patients, Owen (aged 36), illustrated these points when I asked him about the difference between seeing his doctor and seeing the chiropractor. He replied:

> *"GPs seem to be almost reluctant to do any hands on care. They prescribe from a distance sort of thing whereas when you come here they will check you out and they will do things."*

The structure of the treatment visits

In the treatment room Ken was invariably on first name terms with his patients. Treatment visits seemed to follow a pattern starting with the greeting in reception followed by going to the treatment room. The consultation started with questions, then continued with undressing, examination, treatment, re-assessment, and advice. Treatment sessions consisted of a lot of hands on activity and were highly tactile. Ken's hands would deliver a mixture of discomfort and pain relief, always with therapeutic intent. I noted that Ken, as part of the examination, carried out *static* and *motion palpation* on all patients prior to starting treatment:

"Bjorn: "So are you checking for mobility, muscle tone (or) are you looking for alignment, or all of those?"

Ken: "Yeah, I am looking for smoothness of movement, range of movement, resistance to motion palpation if there's a muscular resistance or perhaps (an) articular or ligamentous resistance. That would make me feel like more like manipulating that area If there's a firm (feel).....If there's a sort of spongy muscular resistance, I don't think they respond quite so well to manipulation and more to massage and stretching, trigger points or manipulating those (joints) where that muscle might cross."

Ken pointed out that I would become aware of patterns in his routines, such as the fact that he nearly always started treatment with traction. At one point Ken suggested that chiropractic treatment not only involved manual procedures but an equally important element of verbal communication:

"Ken: It's hands on therapy, but you've still got to persuade each and every patient to get better and they do need encouragement. That's part of what the interview process is about, that's part of every recapping when I meet somebody...'M,' (a patient seen earlier), for example, it took me a few minutes of gauging how she was........A chat at the beginning to determine how she is feeling, what she's been doing about it, what her expectations are.....There is more communication than (barely the) physical action of doing it...So, you have to persuade people to get, and I think that might be the part of what you learn in the time. Not just that you have seen lots of cases of a certain complaint and you see the varying ways that that can respond.....Part of the experience in practice is learning how to persuade people to get better.....

...It's learning what people need from you, what interaction they need from you...physically and communicatively in conversation and the rapport...the shared experience.""

In my notes I comment on the fact that the complex interactions that take place during a consultation and treatment session are only partially visible in the patient records:

"In the patient notes I could tell that only the very skeletal aspects of treatment (subjective comments, segments treated, advice) were written. The consultation contained so much more than (just) what the S.O.A.P. notes would show."

During my sessions inside the treatment room I witnessed numerous verbal and non-verbal exchanges and interactions that were not and could not realistically be recorded by the clinician in the patient records. Jamison found that patient records consisted "largely of notations of biomechanical assessments and interventions" [33].

Observations in the treatment room

On busy days Ken would alternate between two treatment rooms so that his time could be effectively spent on treatment. The receptionist would show each patient into the vacated treatment room and then leave to let them get undressed. As I returned to the reception after observing a patient I would be told whether or not Ken's next patient had given consent for me to be in the room as an observer. The treatment sessions consisted of a series of events and interactions specifically tailored to the individual patient but always set against the framework of Ken's clinical routines. The following are three examples of patients of different ages and gender.

Brian, 32

Brian was self employed and worked with computers. He was suffering from low back pain and had been treated by Ken the previous day. When I entered the treatment room Brian was naked from the waist upwards. Ken carried out a number of orthopaedic tests checking for range of motion and pain.

"Ken:,(...as patient stands with hands on door, high step marching on the spot) "It's moving nicely, fella!" (Commenting on low back/pelvic movement)

Ken often had what may be described as conversations with the tissues that he was examining or treating. Sometimes it would seem as if the patient functioned as an interpreter and answered back.

Brian sat on the treatment table and Ken, standing behind him, palpated the low back firmly in a forward and backward motion making the patient's abdomen move with each push. There followed some orthopaedic tests with Brian lying on his back and then on his front. Ken's hands rarely left the patient' body as he talked his way through the examination, asking questions, touching the relevant parts of the body, and waiting for answers. Oths noted in her field study that there was a substantial exchange of information during examination and treatment procedures [34].

Ken went to the shelf, put massage oil on his hands, made sure his hands were well oiled up, and proceeded to massage Brian's lower back. In contrast to the first part of the visit there followed a full minute of silence before Ken spoke:

"Ken starts discussing walking [the Dog]. Ken asks what dogs Brian has.

(The patient replies:) (one Labrador – one Collie). "Crikey!" (Ken's comment)"

As Ken re-examined the low back and thoracic region he again 'talked' to the tissues:

"Ken says "Just going to ask the question of this 'glut' here"...

..... "How are you doing?" As he [Ken] presses firmly in. Brian answers ("Not too bad.")

After carrying out the re-assessment Ken made a positive comment:

"It looks heaps better than when you first came in."

After wiping excess oil off Brian's back with a tissue Ken then asked him to turn onto his right side in preparation for treatment. With the patient in this position Ken flexed Brian's left knee, placed his left hand on the patient's left shoulder, and placed his right hand on the low back. Brian was asked to breathe in and then out. Ken then carried out a *side posture* manipulation rotating the low back region and thrusting with his right hand on the lumbar spine. The procedure was repeated with Brian lying on his left side.

"With Brian supine Ken goes on to explain the healing process, ("the patient does the healing"), and explains 'his' job, (as a chiropractor).

Ken suggests that Brian should give the complaint approximately a week. Then decide (if the condition worsens) to come back.

Ken emphasized the 'nipping' in the bud. Brian asks "Your advice on how often to 'pop' in?"
Ken replies: "Young healthy bloke like yourself? Quarterly..." (Seasonally)

Ken concluded by giving advice to keep away from heavier activities."

In the reception Brian and Sandra discussed the date of his next appointment. Brian was pleased as he had responded rapidly. Oths writes:

"...treatment for long-term poorly defined problems is liable to be a discouraging and frustrating experience......The chiropractor anticipates these difficulties by providing the patient (with) a structured, supportive environment and theoretical explanations designed to take the mystery out of process and problems. This provides the patient with a greater sense of personal control. The resultant effect of the communication characterized by a high degree of information and positive affect is a strong doctor-patient relationship and a satisfied patient who continues treatment [34]."

Oths further suggests that through realigning the framework of the patient's belief structure to that of *chiropractic* the chiropractor provides an "easily understandable and culturally compatible explanation for heretofore vaguely defined health problems" [34]. Through this process the chiropractor and the patient reach a common level of understanding that should result in patient satisfaction.

Clare, 27

Clare worked in finance and was a keen horse rider in her spare time. She had been undergoing treatment with Ken for over two months. Her headaches had worsened again during the morning:

"We enter as Clare sits, in her blue gown (on the treatment table)...

Ken checks the neck range of motion and notices a 'bite' in the upper thoracic area. Clare is asked to lay supine, knees bent, and Ken starts tractioning the neck manually."

Ken sat at the head of the treatment table and applied firm finger pressure under the right side of Clare's head for several minutes. Clare, visibly in discomfort, asked questions about the muscles. Ken pointed out that although they were tiny they were the source of considerable pain. He then rocked Clare's head gently, using his left hand, turning it in right rotation. He kept the fingers of his right hand pressed firmly into her right upper neck:

"Moving the right hand down to the shoulder (right) Ken pushes into another muscle.

Clare says it's 'painful'..... describes that the pain is going to her head.
Ken: "Is it the pain that you are getting?"
Clare: "Yes..."
Ken: "Good..."

Ken retracted his statement, (*"It's not good, but..."*), explaining that he was pleased not because he was able to reproduce the symptoms of the complaint but for the fact that he had found the root of the problem. It has been suggested that the pain caused by certain treatment procedures is often experienced as positive and as a necessary part of the therapeutic process by patients [44]. During treatment Ken asked Clare about her work routines:

"Ken: "So what's the longest you'll stay at your desk?"

Clare: 3–4 hours..."
Ken: "What!?" [He] shows surprise at the length of time described by Clare."

Ken moved on to diagonal stretches, flexing the cervical spine with Clare's head resting on his forearms. Both sides were stretched. My notes describe the spinal manipulation:

"Ken moves [the] head from side to side (facing left) and says: "I'm just going to loosen this one..." He pulls/twists the head to the left, there's an audible 'click,' and Clare says: "I could feel that one..." A similar treatment is done to the right, and Clare is then sat up."

Ken went on to treat the thoracic region, with the patient lying on her back on a padded board. Clare was then asked to turn over. Ken applied massage oil to his hands:

"Before starting he unhooks the bra strap and spreads the gown to the sides. (Ken explains what he is doing).

Some joint clicking, during the massage, make Clare and Ken giggle.

Ken gets a piece of tissue and does 'rotational' manipulations along the thoracics.

Ken explains that Clare needs to 'shimmy' up 2 inches, holds Clare's shoulders and moves [her] upwards."

Clare sat up and was asked to do a shoulder stretch, mimicking Ken's demonstration. He finished by suggesting that Clare ought to do some neck stretches. We left the room and let her get dressed.

Dora, 51

Dora worked on the till in a local supermarket and kept physically active with yoga, long walks, and walking holidays. She suffered with low back pain and had first consulted Ken four months previously. Dora was receiving supportive treatment every six or seven weeks.

"Ken asked her to stand against the door, doing a high stepping gait. In the procedure, Ken examined the low back. Seated, Ken examined cervical rotation, and the patient was asked to lie supine. Dora talked about doing walks in Whitby, Yorkshire. She described the mist, the cold on the Yorkshire moors. Daily walks, 10–13 miles per day......As Ken was attempting to adjust the cervicals supine he made Dora relax by asking her to 'twiddle her fingers,' 'turn her ear to his hand,' and 'move the shoulder blades together,' to 'occupy herself' and make her relax her neck."

Dora was then asked to turn onto her front. Ken massaged the low back and shoulder area. There was talk about travel. I understood that Dora had met Ken's daughter. The patient went on to describe her yoga schedules as he treated her using *petrissage*, a gentle pummelling massage technique, in the region of the upper back.

Continuing his treatment of Dora Ken aimed his massage at the deep muscles of the left side of her lower back. Dora was concerned that her activities were the cause of her aches and pains. Ken replied:

"Ken said that the only way that muscles were kept strong and healthy was through activity, enforcing the positive benefit of training/activity."

Ken went on to treat *trigger points*, (tender points/areas of tight muscle), in the buttock region, using finger pressure. He concluded the treatment element of the visit by carrying out long lever *helicoidal* stretches with the patient lying in side posture. Using the heel of his hand he applied firm pressure along the length of the lower back muscles on each side of the spine. Dora was asked to sit up and commented that she "would probably be stiff after treatment":

"Ken finished with a seated check-up of the neck and upper back.

Dora asked: "Any do's and don'ts?"
Ken said: "Only do's."."

I thanked Dora for letting me observe her during treatment before Ken and I left the room. On entering reception I noticed for the first time a sign informing patients that the treatment fee would be increased to £28 on the 2nd of June.

The patient interviews

Of the seventeen patients that agreed to be interviewed 12 were female and 5 male. The female patients were in the age range 26 to 60 with a mean age of 42. The males were in the age range 28 to 46 with a mean age of 36.4.

Despite the modest size of the cohort age ranges reflect the data obtained in a recent survey which indicated that the majority of chiropractic patients were in the age range of 21 to 60, [36]. Interviews would last between 10 and 20 minutes. Some patients provided brief and concise answers while others gave lengthy responses to the interview questions. Only 4 patients indicated that they had concerns in relation to the treatment visits [Question 3: 'Were or are you concerned or anxious during consultations and treatment?"].

Factors that make patients seek chiropractic treatment

The processes underlying why and how people seek help are complex. There are a number of factors that influence whether individuals seek professional or complementary care, or at all. It has been suggested that although choice plays a part decisions are made by the individual interacting in social networks that provide mechanisms for learning about, understanding, and handling difficulties [58,65]. Pescosolido discusses the role of contact with others:

"[individuals] continue to ask advice and seek help from a wide variety of lay, professional, and semi-professional others until the situation is resolved or options are exhausted....Illness triggers a dynamic, social process of coping. It is through contact with others that individuals deal with situations of medical uncertainty and find ways to solve emotional and physical problems [66]."

Chiropractors are private practitioners and there is no set referral protocol linking their services to the conventional health sector. All of the patients observed and interviewed during this field study had suffered from pain or discomfort that was musculo-skeletal in origin and which had started to affect their life and daily activities. Ken's own opinion was that *pain* was what brought the majority of his patients through the door in the first place. Patients were asked about how they came to seek help at this particular Clinic (see Table 2).

Several of the patients had clearly heard about chiropractic treatment through friends or relatives but there were also other mechanisms of referral. *Kate*, 36, was a patient of the resident herbalist and consulted the chiropractor

Table 2 The reasons behind the patients' seeking a consultation with Ken the chiropractor

Name and Age	Reply to the Question: "How did you end up consulting Ken the chiropractor?"
Tanya, 54	*"I just knew that General Practitioners are not very good with bones and joints and muscles so...I can't remember how I found out about Ken....I think somebody recommended him but I can't remember exactly how now."*
Uma, 60	*"I've been to different things...I have tried one or two different things and I was talking to a neighbour and (she) recommended me to this clinic."*
Clare, 27	(Clare had suffered from headaches and seen her G.P. who had recommended her to see a chiropractor) *"The doctor said...The pain in my head was coming from my neck and a friend referred me."*
Vera, 46	(Vera was recommended by a colleague at work who was himself a patient of Ken's) *"Well, probably you noticed that I knew the gentleman in the waiting room...Ken is quite well known in our office and it was just a recommendation by somebody to come here. And it has sort of spread around the office. Most people (who) have got problems or need to see a chiropractor come here."*
Nadine, 28	*"**Bjorn:** ....Did someone recommend you...?* ***Nadine:** No, just in the phone book, the yellow pages...And just sort of rang up here...* ***B:** OK. Have you been to a chiropractor before?* ***N:** No.* ***B:** So how did you know you had to go to a chiropractor...?* ***N:** Because my mother goes to a chiropractor...."*
Pat, 26	*"I just spoke to my partner....He was fed up of seeing me clicked all the time so he said go and see someone about it, so I just did a search on the web. Chiropractors in *******. This clinic came up and then I asked around if anybody came here or if they could recommend...And a friend of mine had gone to a clinic in ***** and said that he was really good, that she (had) only one treatment and then she was really happy, so I booked an appointment."*
Sid, 46	*"It came through my aunt. She goes horse riding and she gets problems with her back and she said...Well, I use a chiropractor in *****, near where she used to live. So, I thought it's as good as any, I'll go there."*
Irene, 55	*"My husband has a slipped disc....So we were recommended by a friend to see Ken when he worked in *********. When he did so well with my husband, because he sort of hobbled in and actually walked out, I thought oh well perhaps it's worth having my back checked...So ever since then I have been coming to see Ken."*
Ron, 30	*"I live locally. Drove past this place a number of times and, speaking to Ken through the initial consultation I just thought it would be the best way to go."*
Joanne, 35	*"I was having low back pain and it was getting increasingly worse...it was affecting my daily mobility. G.P.'s aren't very good at stuff like that so I thought I'd seek an alternative treatment.... I passed daily on my way to and from work and I thought I would give him a try."*

after hurting her neck. *Liz,* also 36, had, after a serious car accident first seen an osteopath with limited success, and had then been recommended by a friend to consult Ken. For the majority of Ken's patients recommendations from others appeared to have played a substantial part in the decision making process.

Patients' understanding of the mechanisms of treatment

Chiropractors spend considerable time on explanations and instructions with their patients. Kelner suggests that there are three types of explanations:

1. An explanation of the problem itself.
2. An explanation of treatment.
3. An explanation of chiropractic [35].

Discrepancies in the understanding of common health terms between clinicians and patients are often the reasons for poor communication [67], and patients' beliefs and perceptions of treatment are factors that have been shown to influence treatment outcome [68,69]. Following on from this it has been suggested that patient-centred communication that facilitates the patient's participation in decision making in relation to treatment has health promoting effects [46,56,70].

Since the nineteen seventies the traditional chiropractic concepts of *vertebral misalignment* have been challenged. One of the more contemporary explanations for musculo skeletal pain syndromes replacing them is based around joint mobility. While observing Ken with his patients I witnessed him repeatedly explaining that a lack of joint mobility was the cause of symptoms and that treatment would involve restoring normal mobility to the joints. I wanted to explore patients' understanding of what was 'wrong' and how they interpreted the corrective mechanisms of chiropractic treatment (see Table 3).

Although some patients were clear that there were 'right' places and 'wrong' places for bones to 'be' the majority appeared to have a more fragmented understanding of the mechanisms of treatment. Vera's answer illustrates the point that as a patient she was content to leave clinical decisions in the hands of her chiropractor. The effects and importance of patient centred care, trust, informed consent, and practitioner confidence on treatment outcome has been investigated and discussed in a number of studies [61,71,72]. It has also been suggested that the technical and interpersonal skills of the chiropractor in combination with the interaction, "the personality gel", in the patient-clinician encounter in each consultation are factors that influence treatment

Table 3 Patients' understanding of the mechanism of chiropractic treatment

Name and Age	Reply to the question: "What is your understanding of what Ken does?"
Sid, 46	*"**Bjorn:** "So, what is your understanding of what Ken the chiropractor does?...."* ***Sid:** "Well, basically to put it right in alignment....You actually put the skeleton back to where it should be....."*
Uma, 60	*"I presume that he tries to manipulate things back to where they should be..."*
Liz, 36	*"I hear nice crunches, so I guess sort of things are clicking back in and....I suppose the way I think is mainly my spine is put out a little bit and it's kind of slightly off and...he's moving my bones back into place again."*
Pat, 26	*"Just getting the vertebrae back into line by clicking them, that is all I really know."*
Ron, 30	*"He said the lower muscles are quite tensed up, quite sort of fused...I need to do some exercises, where I go away and...stretch those muscles out and....I think the vertebras that need to be sort of clicked back in place...and he sort of did three clicks today on the lower back on the left hand side and he just stretched me out..."*
Mary, 50	(Mary was receiving supportive treatment for stiffness and pain in her right hip joint as well as treatment of the spine. Her understanding involved the *mobility* of the joint). *"It's releasing the things that are very, very tight....He does the gentle massage bit first but....the quick movements are like a release. That's how it feels inside me; bits that have stuck together have been opened up a bit.....I am under the impression that the spine is just sort of compacted somewhat and whatever he does sort of releases that."*
Joanne, 35	(Joanne used the term *unlocking* to describe the treatment of her lower back and pelvis) *"...Obviously the manipulation of the joints.....helps in movement in things....that don't work properly...........My pelvis was kind of locked and Ken did this manoeuvre and unlocks my pelvis so to speak."*
Dora, 51	*"I have kind of read up on things...... not that well. I'm no expert....and looked at alternative things as well and...it does make sense with the skeleton and how it works, and alignment.........Ken stretching me and clicking me and that would keep you right as opposed to if you have an injury.....you find you work yourself the wrong way."*
Clare, 27	*"From what I gather, if the joint, the muscles, the actual joints...don't they affect the muscles which can cause the pain?.......I have never really asked him as to why or what the clicking of joints does."*
Tanya, 54	*"He has said a bit about muscle and bones and shown me things....He also uses terminology that makes me laugh because I don't understand him...."*
Owen, 36	(Owen, a trainee male nurse, correlated the effects of treatment to circulation). *"The joint manipulation from what I understand is.... opening a joint up a little bit...flowing blood supply in there, crushing it all up sort of thing."*
Vera, 46	(Vera had little interest in understanding the mechanisms of treatment). *"The mechanics of it, I don't understand, no. I leave that to Ken and I am assured by what and how he is that he is doing everything correctly."*

outcome [33]. I asked Ken about his views on the traditional chiropractic concept of *spinal misalignment*:

> *Ken: "That's probably the ancient idea too isn't it? Somebody would come in antalgic and (you) say 'Your spine is crooked, I have just the thing for that' and you apply some procedure, you hear it click and you can well imagine it is your spine clicking back into place. People still believe it now, don't they?......It's a lovely metaphor and you can see why it persists."*

In spite of Ken's considerable efforts in explaining what was at fault and how it would be corrected few patients appeared to have taken the information on board. For the majority of Ken's patients the focus appeared to be on the positive outcome of treatment and many of them appeared surprised when I asked about their understanding of treatment mechanisms. Kelner writes: "Most patients adopt a pragmatic attitude toward chiropractic; they come to the practitioner because they have an ailment. For them the validity of chiropractic depends on the success that practitioners have in alleviating their miseries" [35]. *Nadine*, 28, illustrates this point in her succinct answer to my question on how the chiropractic treatment worked:

> *"I don't think I really think about it...As long as the pain goes, I don't really mind what happens."*

Patients' concerns

For most patients the first consultation with a chiropractor will involve elements that are unfamiliar and perhaps daunting. The majority of patients interviewed by me had been recommended to see Ken by someone in their immediate social environment and all patients that took part in interviews had undergone at least one treatment with him. During my observations at the Clinic it became increasingly clear that patients never doubted Ken's good intentions. I asked Ken's patients if they had been concerned or had experienced anxiety during any of their consultation and treatment visits. Although the majority of patients answered no to this question a small number had experienced some concerns (see Table 4).

It would seem that once clinical routines had been set in motion most concerns that were initially present were diminished or disappeared entirely. It has been pointed out that physical treatment such as spinal manipulation requires the development of a substantial level of trust between practitioner and patient [73]. Successful treatment in the past is another factor linked to reduced levels of anxiety in patients [74]. In the section "The Healing Encounter" Kelner writes:

> "Patients may evaluate treatment by other criteria as well as its effectiveness; for example, whether the experience is enjoyable or not. While one group of patients describes the experience as enjoyable, partly because of the physical

Table 4 Patients' concerns

Name and Age	Reply to the question: "Were or are you concerned or anxious during consultations and treatment?"
Warren, 45	*"**Warren:** ...What I like about Ken as well is that he's very....What's the word?...I'm a big guy and I am quite sort of cautious of who I take my shirt off in front of but my wife has come, and he is very sort of....I can't think of the word...Very professional and it's a case of...* ***Bjorn:** Respectful?* ***W:** Absolutely, yeah. Here's a gown for you and he's out of the room. Not so much for me because I mean I just... get on with it...* ***B:** Yes.* ***W:** ...But for like...He said to come in with the wife and so that she didn't feel like, you know what I mean.......So he was very respectful in that way."*
Ron, 30	*"**Ron:** So...so yeah, there is, I think, for a lot of people there is the embarrassment factor as well.* ***Bjorn:** Was that OK with you?* ***R:** Yeah, it was OK with me...I think sometimes if you are dealing with another male it puts you at ease a little bit....I think if you may be dealing with a female [chiropractor] then you may have in the back of your mind that you are a bit conscious about sort of taking your clothes off and things."*
Pat, 26	(Pat was anxious about undressing and the amount of physical touch. In addition to this she was concerned about the manipulative treatment of the neck). *"Yeah, I was anxious....just because I didn't really know what needed to be done, you know. Just understanding it, or telling me to strip off...how much you need to touch me and things so ...All that was completely new...but Ken reassured me and explained step by step what he was going to do and I was a bit concerned when I was lying down...He's just gonna click my neck. But he gave it 2 or 3 minutes, you know, explaining what he was doing.......This is going to be loud because it's close to your ear, and really telling exactly what was coming up."*
Vera, 46	(Vera had reacted to the imposing appearance of the treatment table). *"I think, initially, that the beds were a bit...daunting...and you do worry how...well I don't know, because I am quite confident and I am more relaxed with Ken. But you feel....I felt quite embarrassed perhaps, like moving around...The gown thing and initially. I don't have a problem with that at all now."*

contact (the laying on of the hands), and partly because of the euphoric after effects of the adjustments, there is another group who do not find it pleasant, being anxious about adjustments/manipulations......Chiropractic may also be judged in terms of patients' beliefs. There are those who treat it as a mystical or religious experience, and there are those whose attitude is pragmatic, who go strictly for the measurable results. Lastly, there are those patients who believe in chiropractic for most health problems, while others remain dubious about its capacity to help any but a narrow range related to muscular/skeletal problems [35]."

The fact that patients are usually seen by the same chiropractor for the duration of treatment is another factor that reduces anxiety levels. It would seem that most patients prefer to stay with the same practitioner for the duration of treatment, or at least within the same clinic, (personal experience and communication with other chiropractors).

The chiropractor's approach

Early chiropractic concepts included the notion that the health of the spine directly affects the health of other organs and that chiropractic treatment could be applied to all forms of ill health and disease. There is still disagreement between different schools of thought within the chiropractic profession over the effectiveness of chiropractic treatment and the appropriate scope of practice of chiropractors. Different beliefs and opinions on these matters continue to fuel divisive debates within the profession. Although a unifying idea of chiropractic has been sought since the end of the nineteenth century it has been suggested that there may in fact not exist one concept that would encompass and accommodate the entire chiropractic profession [75]. During my observations of Ken he treated patients presenting with predominantly musculo-skeletal complaints. Treatment was carried out using spinal manipulative therapy, adjunctive therapies, and in addition to this advice to patients on activity, stretches and core-stability exercises.

Although treatment outcome does ultimately depend on the therapeutic intervention it is affected by a number of other factors surrounding the treatment visit [76]. It has been suggested that the following eight elements have a therapeutic effect and that they often form part of every clinical encounter:

1. Positive verbal reinforcement
2. Encouragement
3. Developing of Trust
4. Reassurance
5. Development of a Practitioner-Patient Relationship
6. Respect of Uniqueness
7. Exploration of Values
8. Creation of ceremony [77]

During my time as an observer in the Clinic I was witness to positive verbal reinforcement, encouragement, developing of trust, reassurance, and saw evidence of the relationship between Ken and his patients. In relation to elements 6 and 7 it was evident during my observations and in my conversations with Ken that he respected each of his patient's individuality and "uniqueness", and that he did search for "common values" during interactions with his patients. "Ceremony" was very much constantly a result of the greeting, questioning, examination, and treatment routines that formed the framework of every consultation. This could even be extended to include the activities in reception before and after each consultation. Kelner writes:

"While theoretical knowledge received a great deal of attention at the college, after chiropractors have been in practice for a while, it tends to decline in importance. It is treatment therapies and the accompanying social skills that take precedence with most practicing chiropractors......While debates about the philosophy of chiropractic and the validity of its theories of illness are of strategic importance in the political arena, they prove to be of little significance in the practice [35]."

As an experienced clinician Ken was aware of the wider impact of the clinical encounter and the difficulties in precisely defining the underlying mechanisms of the health benefits that occur in relation to chiropractic treatment. In one of our conversations we discussed the nature of the therapeutic mechanisms at play in chiropractic clinical practice:

Ken: "We talk about getting people's bodies right and getting to people's 'core' to put it right and render motion right but....You transfer, effect a change in that person's wellbeing, and you try to communicate a change in that person's wellbeing and the name of that change that we practice is 'chiropractic'."

In his answer Ken had, in my opinion, made an attempt to define his own understanding of his role as a chiropractor and the *vision* or the *idea* underpinning his approach to chiropractic treatment and his clinical modus operandi. This fundamental idea of what chiropractic is and how it affects patients was probably unique to Ken. I suspect that each individual chiropractor would harbour his or her equally unique idea providing the basis for his/her understanding of and approach to chiropractic clinical practice.

Conclusions

This Field Study, based on participant observation and semi-structured interviews, has provided an insight into the nature and characteristics of the clinical practice of a UK trained chiropractor at work in a suburban chiropractic clinic in western Great Britain. Despite its limitations there is, in the author's opinion, valuable information to be extracted from this study.

The account describes the reception area suggesting its function in providing an effective and at the same time comforting prelude to the chiropractic consultation in this particular clinic. This field study has also described the initial chiropractic consultation and how the consultation room provides a private and secluded space suited to examination and treatment.

Earlier studies of chiropractic clinical practice have described the characteristics and elements that constitute the treatment visit. In this study the author was able to observe and describe the pre-treatment interview, examination, treatment, and re-assessment that form the basis of consultations at this particular clinic. This account also makes an attempt to describe the richness and nature of communication between the chiropractor and his patients in the consultation room. The author has attempted to illustrate how physical contact, both of an investigating and of a therapeutic nature, formed a substantial part of each chiropractic clinical encounter.

The patient interviews carried out by the author suggest that the majority of this chiropractor's patients presented with pain of musculo-skeletal origin and that this, in combination with recommendations from relatives, friends, and work colleagues, constituted the principal reasons for these patients when making a decision to consult the chiropractor.

The majority of interviewed patients were found to have either an inaccurate or a rudimentary understanding of the mechanisms of chiropractic treatment and some patients even made it clear that they had little interest in treatment mechanisms. Despite the efforts made by this chiropractor in explaining why a patient would experience pain and how treatment worked most of these patients showed only a limited understanding of treatment mechanisms. This difference in patient attitudes and understanding of treatment has been identified by authors in earlier studies.

Only a small number of patients in this cohort reported concerns in relation to the treatment. This study suggests that any heightened anxiety levels were reduced as a result of the actions of the chiropractor and as individuals got accustomed to clinic routines.

In the interviews and conversations with the chiropractor the author was able to gain some insight into this chiropractor's experiences, beliefs and opinions and how these provided the basis for his understanding of chiropractic treatment and his approach to chiropractic clinical practice.

This small-scale field study, despite being based on observations of a single chiropractor and a small number of his patients on one afternoon per week in one particular clinic, does suggest that the clinical chiropractic practice carried out by this particular UK trained British chiropractor contains a number of elements described in earlier qualitative studies of chiropractic clinical practice in the U.S., Canada, and Australia. Due to its size and the fact that the author is the sole observer, sole interpreter of observations and sole editor of interview transcripts, no robust conclusions can be drawn from this study. Further field work, both in depth and on a larger scale is, in the author's opinion, necessary in order to establish whether or not the findings of this field study are more broadly represented in chiropractic clinical practice in the United Kingdom.

Additional files

Additional file 1: Research Information Sheet.
Additional file 2: Patient interviews.
Additional file 3: Clinic Layout.

Competing interests
The author declares that he has no competing interests.

Acknowledgements
The author would like to thank Professor Cecil Helman and Professor Melissa Parker as well as the staff in the Department of Anthropology at Brunel University, Uxbridge, London. The author would also like to thank Professor Peter McCarthy of the Welsh Institute of Chiropractic, the University of Glamorgan, Treforrest, for his support and input and Professor Charlotte Leboeuf-Yde, Department of Chiropractic and Clinical Biomechanics, University of Southern Denmark, for her help and input.

References
1. Zollman C, Vickers A: Users and practitioners of complementary medicine. *Br Med J* 1993, **319**:836–838.
2. Sharma U: Contextualizing alternative medicine: the exotic, the marginal and the perfectly mundane. *Anthropol Today* 1993, **9**:15–18.
3. Wardwell WI: Alternative medicine in the United States. *Soc Sci Med* 1994, **38**:1061–1068.
4. Fisher P, Ward A: Complementary medicine in Europe. *Br Med J* 1994, **309**:107–110.
5. Kelner M, Wellman B: Health care and consumer choice: medical and alternative therapies. *Soc Sci Med* 1997, **45**:203–212.
6. Siahpush M: A critical review of the sociology of alternative medicine: research on users, practitioners and the orthodoxy. *Health* 1999, **4**:159–178.
7. Kaptchuk T, Eisenberg D: Varieties of healing.2: a taxonomy of unconventional healing practices. *Ann Intern Med* 2001, **135**:196–204.
8. Walker LA, Budd S: UK: the current state of regulation of complementary and alternative medicine. *Complement Ther Med* 2002, **10**:8–13.
9. Swartzman L, Harshman R, Burkell J, Lundy M: What accounts for the appeal of complementary/alternative medicine, and what makes complementary/alternative medicine 'alternative'? *Med Decis Making* 2002, **Sep-Oct**:431–450.
10. Kelner M, Wellman B, Boon H, Welsh S: The role of the state in the social inclusion of complementary and alternative medical occupations. *Complement Ther Med* 2004, **12**:79–89.
11. Quinn F, Hughes C, Baxter D: Complementary and alternative medicine in the treatment of low back pain: a systematic review. *Phys Ther Rev* 2006, **11**:107–116.
12. Cherkin D, MacCornack F: Patient evaluations of Low back pain care from family physicians and chiropractors. *West J Med* 1989, **150**:351–355.
13. Shekelle P: What role for chiropractic in health care. *N Engl J Med* 1998, **339**:1074–1075.

14. Coulter I, Hurwitz E, Adams A, Genovese B, Hays R, Shekelle P: **Patients using chiropractors in North America.** *Spine* 2002, **27**:291–298.
15. Mannington J, Moss J, Josefowitz N: **Women chiropractors: issues of career and family.** *J Manipulative Physiol Ther* 1989, **12**:434–439.
16. Kelner M, Wellman B, Welsh S, Boon H: **How far can complementary and alternative medicine go? The case of chiropractic and homeopathy.** *Soc Sci Med* 2006, **63**:2617–2627.
17. Jamison J: **The health information brochure: a useful tool for chiropractic practice?** *J Manipulative Physiol Ther* 2001, **24**:331–334.
18. Pedersen P: **The identity of chiropractic practice with special reference to Western Europe: a literature review.** *Eur J Chiropractic* 1990, **38**:41–55.
19. Pedersen P, Nøddeskou H, Wejse B: **A pilot survey of diagnoses, radiographic and laboratory procedures encountered in European chiropractic practices.** *Eur J Chiropractic* 1992, **40**:71–82.
20. Pedersen P, Kleberg P, Walker K: **A pilot survey of patients and chiropractors in European chiropractic practices: sociodemographic, anamnestic and management procedures.** *Eur J Chiropractic* 1993, **41**:5–19.
21. Pedersen P: **A survey of chiropractic practice in Europe.** *Eur J Chiropractic* 1994, **42**:3–28.
22. Bolton J: **Chiropractors' attitudes to, and perceptions of, the impact of continuing professional education on clinical practice.** *Med Educ* 2002, **36**:317–324.
23. Vinci C, Peterson C: **A pilot survey of chiropractic practice in Italy.** *Eur J Chiropractic* 2003, **47**:61–78.
24. Gkolfinopoulos V, Byfield D, McCarthy P: **A survey of low back pain patients in chiropractic practices in South Wales.** *Eur J Chiropractic* 2003, **49**:289–294.
25. Mull JD, Mull DS: **A visit with a Curandero.** *West J Med* 1983, **139**:730–736.
26. Anderson R: **The treatment of musculoskeletal disorders by a Mexican bonesetter (sobador).** *Soc Sci Med* 1987, **24**:43–46.
27. Rubel A, Hass M: **Ethnomedicine.** In *Medical Anthropology, Contemporary Theory and Method, Revised edition.* Edited by Sargent C, Johnson T. London: Praeger; 1996. Chapter 6.
28. Hinojosa S: **Bonesetting and radiography in the southern Maya highlands.** *Med Anthropol* 2004, **23**:263–293.
29. Oths K, Hinojosa S: *Healing by Hand: Manual Medicine and Bonesetting in Global perspective.* New York: Altamira Press; 2004.
30. Cowie J, Roebuck J: *An Ethnography of a Chiropractic Clinic.* New York: The Free Press, A Division of Macmillan Publishing; 1975.
31. Coulehan J: **Adjustment, the hands and healing.** *Cult Med Psychiatry* 1985, **9**:353–382.
32. Coulehan J: **Chiropractic and the clinical art.** *Soc Sci Med* 1985, **21**:383–390.
33. Jamison J: **Chiropractic holism: interactively becoming in a reductionist health care system.** *Chiropractic J Aust* 1993, **23**:98–105.
34. Oths K: **Communication in a chiropractic clinic: how a D.C. Treats his patients.** *Culture Med Psychiatry* 1994, **18**:83–113.
35. Kelner M, Hall O, Coulter I: *Chiropractors Do They Help?* Toronto: Fitzhenry & Whiteside Limited; 1980.
36. General Chiropractic Council (GCC) survey: *Consulting the Profession: A Survey of UK Chiropractors;* 2004. enquiries@gcc-uk.org and www.gcc-uk.org.
37. Pollentier A, Langworthy J: **The scope of chiropractic practice: a survey of chiropractors in the UK.** *Clin Chiropractic* 2007, **10**:147–155.
38. Kuper A: *Anthropology Anthropologists.* London: Routledge; 1996.
39. Van Maanen J: **Realist tales.** In *Tales of the Field.* 1st edition. Chicago: The university of Chicago Press; 1988.
40. O'Neill M: **Participation or observation? Some practical and ethical dilemmas.** In *Inside Organizations: Anthropologists at work.* Edited by Gellner D, Hirsch E. Oxford/New York: Berg; 2001.
41. Posner J: **Urban anthropology: fieldwork in semifamiliar settings.** In *Fieldwork Experience, Qualitative Approaches to Social Research.* Edited by Shaffir W, Stebbing R, Turowetz A. New York: St. Martin's Press; 1980.
42. Helman C: *Department of Anthropology.* Uxbridge, London: Brunel University. Personal communication August 2008.
43. Fabian J: **Ethnographic misunderstanding and the perils of context.** *Am Anthropol* 1995, **97**:41–50.
44. Helman C: *Culture, Health and Illness.* 5th edition. London: Hodder Arnold; 2007.
45. Larsen K, Smith CK: **Assessment of nonverbal communication in the patient-physician interview.** *J Fam Pract* 1981, **12**:481–488.
46. Buller MK, Buller DB: **Physicians' communication style and patient satisfaction.** *J Health Soc Behav* 1987, **28**:375–388.
47. Bensing J: **Doctor-patient communication and the quality of care.** *Soc Sci Med* 1991, **32**:1301–1310.
48. Lipkin M, Quill T, Napodano R: **The medical interview: a core curriculum for residencies in internal medicine.** *Ann Int Med* 1984, **100**:277–284.
49. Waitzkin H, Stoeckle JD: **The communication of information about illness.** *Ad Psychosom Med* 1972, **8**:180–215.
50. Semmes CE: **Developing trust; patient-practitioner encounters in natural health care.** *J Contemp Ethnography* 1991, **19**:450–470.
51. Greenhalgh T: **Narrative based medicine in an evidence based world.** *Brit Med J* 1999, **318**:323–325.
52. Hurwitz B: **Narrative and the practice of medicine.** *Lancet* 2000, **356**:2086–2089.
53. Beach MC, Inui T, The Relationship-Centered Care Research Network: **Relationship-centered care, a constructive reframing.** *J Gen Int Med* 2006, **21**:S3–S8.
54. Oths K: **Unintended therapy: psychotherapeutic aspects of chiropractic.** In *Ethnopsychiatry: The Cultural Construction of Professional and Folk Psychiatries.* Edited by Gaines AD. New York: State University of New York Press; 1992. Chapter 4.
55. Neuwirth Z, Schrader S: **Performing medical conversations: "between" physicians and patients.** *Adv Mind-Body Med* 2004, **20**:8–12.
56. Van Dulmen AM, Bensing JM: **Health promoting effects of the physician-patient encounter.** *Psychol Health Med* 2002, **7**:289–299.
57. Coulehan J: **Adjustment, the hands and healing.** *Cult Med Psychiatry* 1985, **9**:363.
58. Sirois F, Gick M: **An investigation of the health beliefs and motivations of complementary medicine clients.** *Soc Sci Med* 2002, **55**:1025–1037.
59. **Clinical experience of the author; Clinical practice in Cardiff, UK, in the period November 2002 to September 2008.**
60. Kleinman A, Eisenberg L, Good B: **Culture, illness, and care; clinical lessons from anthropologic and cross-cultural research.** *Ann Int Med* 1978, **88**:251–258.
61. Kaptchuk T: **The placebo effect in alternative medicine: can the performance of a healing ritual have clinical significance?** *Ann Int Med* 2002, **136**:817–825.
62. Lillrank A: **Back Pain and the resolution of diagnostic uncertainty in illness narratives.** *Soc Sci Med* 2003, **57**:1045–1054.
63. Van Dongen E, Elema R: **The art of touching: the culture of 'body work' in nursing.** *Anthropol Med* 2001, **8**:149–162.
64. Turp M: **Touch, enjoyment and health: in adult life.** *Eur J Psychother, Counsel Health* 2000, **3**:61–76.
65. Debacher DE Jr: **Cognitive models and health decision making.** *Med Anthropol Newslett* 1979, **10**:10–17.
66. Pescosolido BA: **Beyond rational choice: the social dynamics of How people seek help.** *Am J Soc* 1992, **97**:1096–1138.
67. Hadlow J, Pitts M: **The understanding of common health terms by doctors, nurses and patients.** *Soc Sci Med* 1991, **32**:193–196.
68. Horne R: **Patients' Beliefs about treatment: the hidden determinant of treatment outcome?** *J Psychosom Res* 1999, **47**:491–495.
69. Yardley L, Sharples K, Beech S, Lewith G: **Developing a dynamic model of treatment perceptions.** *J Health Psychol* 2001, **6**:269–282.
70. Guadagnoli E, Ward P: **Patient participation in decision-making.** *Soc Sci Med* 1998, **47**:329–339.
71. Smucker D, Konrad T, Curtis P, Carey T: **Practitioner self-confidence and patient outcomes in acute Low back pain.** *Arch Fam Med* 1998, **7**:223–228.
72. Moerman D: **Doctors and patients: the role of clinicians in the placebo effect.** *Adv Mind Body Med* 2003, **19**:14–22.
73. Meeker W, Haldeman S: **Chiropractic: a profession at the crossroads of mainstream and alternative medicine.** *Ann Intern Med* 2002, **136**:216–227.
74. Caterinicchio RP: **Testing plausible path models of interpersonal trust in patient-physician treatment relationships.** *Soc Sci Med* 1979, **13A**:81–99.
75. Martin S: **The only truly scientific method of healing: chiropractic and American science, 1895–1990.** *Isis* 1994, **85**:viii+207–227.
76. Moerman D: *Meaning, medicine, and the 'Placebo Effect'.* 1st edition. Cambridge: Cambridge University Press; 2002.
77. Barrett B, Muller D, Rakel D, Rabago D, Marchand L, Scheder J: **Placebo, meaning, and health.** *Perspect Biol Med* 2006, **49**:178–195.

Paraplegia in a chiropractic patient secondary to atraumatic dural arteriovenous fistula with perimedullary hypertension: case report

Stephen M Foreman[1*], Michael J Stahl[1] and Gary D Schultz[2]

Abstract

Intracranial dural arteriovenous fistulas are abnormal communications between higher-pressure arterial circulation and lower-pressure venous circulation. This abnormal communication can result in important and frequently misdiagnosed neurological abnormalities.

A case of rapid onset paraplegia following cervical chiropractic manipulation is reviewed. The patient's generalized spinal cord edema, lower extremity paraplegia and upper extremity weakness, were initially believed to be a complication of the cervical spinal manipulation that had occurred earlier on the day of admission. Subsequent diagnostic testing determined the patient suffered from impaired circulation of the cervical spinal cord produced by a Type V intracranial arteriovenous fistula and resultant venous hypertension in the pontomesencephalic and anterior spinal veins.

The clinical and imaging findings of an intracranial dural arteriovenous fistula with pontomesencephalic venous congestion and paraplegia are reviewed.

This case report emphasizes the importance of thorough and serial diagnostic imaging in the presence of sudden onset paraplegia and the potential for error when concluding atypical neurological presentations are the result of therapeutic misadventure.

Keywords: Chiropractic, Manipulation, Dural arteriovenous fistula, Paraplegia, Pontomesencephalic venous congestion, Complication, Stroke

Background

Dural arteriovenous fistulas (DAVF) are abnormal communications between arterial and venous circulation that may arise either spontaneously or as a result of trauma [1]. DAVFs account for 15% of all cerebrovascular malformations [2]. Previous studies have determined DAVFs occur in both sexes equally and the onset of symptoms most commonly occurs between the third and sixth decade of life [3]. The frequent association of patients with DAVF and cerebral venous sinus thrombosis [4] indicates spontaneous DAVFs may be the result of venous thrombosis and venous hypertension [5]. The symptoms and physical findings of DAVF vary greatly depending on the affected anatomy and resulting vascular changes, flow restrictions within the DAVF, the presence and size of arterial feeders and the location and direction of venous drainage. Symptoms, produced by the shunting of higher-pressure arterial flow into the lower-pressure venous system appear to depend on the direction of venous drainage [6] and this in turn determines whether the symptoms will be benign or aggressive.

Cougard [7] reviewed 258 cases of cerebral DAVFs and classified the patients into groups with aggressive and nonaggressive neurological symptoms. Aggressive neurological symptoms included "intracranial hypertension (i.e., headache, nausea or vomiting, transient visual defect or visual loss and papilledema), intracranial hemorrhage, focal deficits, seizures, altered mental status and ascending myelopathy." The nonaggressive neurological symptoms included isolated headache, bruit and all ocular symptoms not related to intracranial myelopathy.

Cougard's [7] classification of DAVF presentation, based on the drainage pattern (Table 1), helps explain

* Correspondence: smfdoc@sbcglobal.net
[1]Private practice of chiropractic, West Hills, California, USA
Full list of author information is available at the end of the article

Table 1 Classifications of intracranial dural arteriovenous fistulas

Type	Description
Type I	Drainage into a sinus without flow restriction
Type II	Drainage into a sinus with flow restriction and reflux into other sinuses or into cortical veins
Type III	Drainage into a cortical vein
Type IV	Drainage into a cortical vein with a large varix
Type V	Spinous perimedullary venous drainage

Adapted from: [7].

the variability of clinical presentation. Cougard classified the pattern of DAVF drainage into five types, with the associated neurological symptoms progressively worsening from Type I to Type V.

Type I, the most common and least aggressive form of DAVF, is based on arterial drainage into an intracranial sinus without flow restriction. Type I DAVFs are generally benign and may be asymptomatic [8]. In Type II, reflux produces intracranial hypertension in 20% of cases and hemorrhage in 10%. Intracranial hemorrhage is present in 40% of the Type III cases and in 65% of Type IV. Finally, Type V cases, with spinal perimedullary drainage, produce an ascending myelopathy in 50% of cases. The development of ascending myelopathy from perimedullary venous hypertension, first documented in 1982 [9], is rare and was only present in 2.3% (n=6) of Cougard's 258 cases [7]. The Type V pattern of drainage is the least common and produces the most aggressive and serious neurological symptoms. The ascending myelopathy associated with Type V cases may result in brainstem dysfunction manifesting as respiratory insufficiency [1]. Brainstem involvement seems to be related to involvement of the anterior pontomesencephalic and petrosal vein [10].

Case presentation

A 59-year-old male presented to a chiropractic office with a three-week history of pain in the lumbar and lower cervical spine, which began subsequent to moving boxes in his home. Physical examination findings were consistent with musculoskeletal strain and the chiropractor performed spinal manipulation in both the cervical and lumbar spine without consequence. Later that same day the patient began to experience muscular weakness in his lower extremities and loss of bladder control. These serious neurological symptoms prompted him to seek care within an emergency room. MR scans of the cervical spine and brain, with and without contrast, were performed and initially interpreted as normal. A secondary review of the cervical spine MR noted swelling of the cervical cord, without hemorrhage from C1 to C6 (Figure 1), consistent with a clinical impression of "infarction vs. contusion." Attending physicians at the ER, based on the patient's history of cervical manipulation earlier that same day, erroneously concluded the patient suffered spinal cord contusion secondary to a manipulation with excessive force.

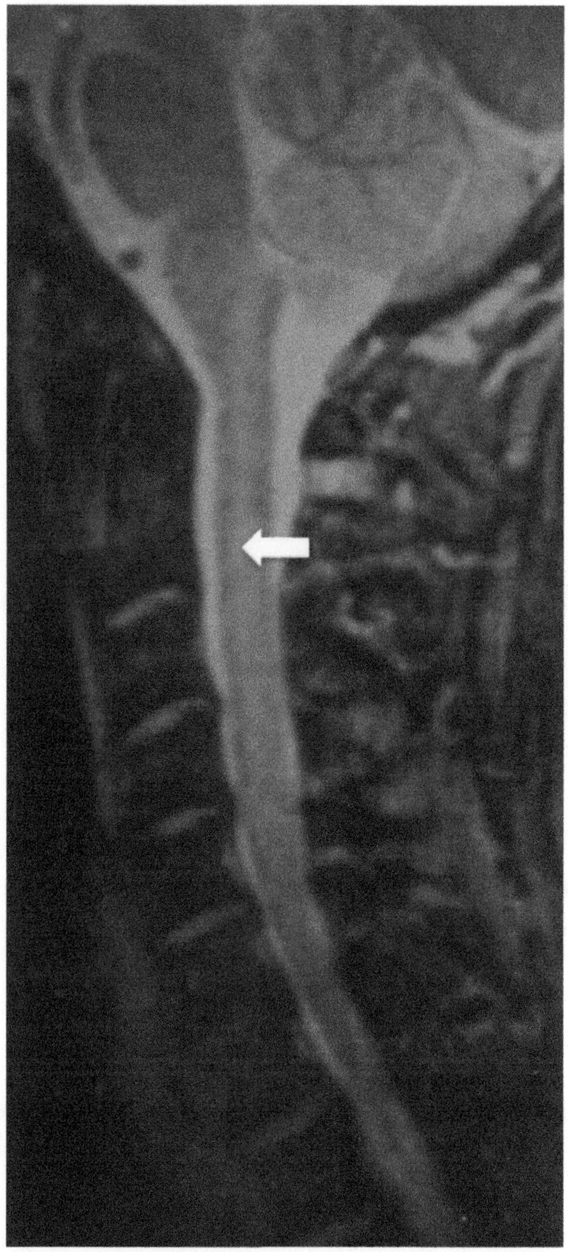

Figure 1 Initial Sagittal MR scan of cervical spine. MR scan, T2 weighted, sagittal view without contrast, reveals diffuse increased signal intensity (arrow) covering the entirety of the medulla and extending to C5-6. The high signal intensity is affecting the central portion of the spinal cord and sparing the outer (subpial) tissues. Initial review concluded the findings were consistent with "infarction vs. contusion."

The patient was hospitalized and his neurological status continued to deteriorate over the ensuing days. The continued neurological deterioration, along with the

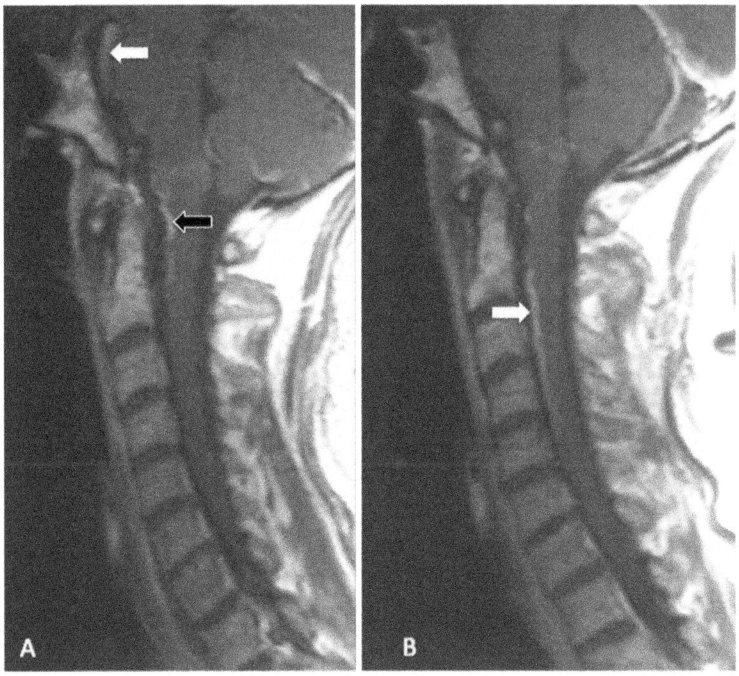

Figure 2 Follow-up Sagittal MR scan of cervical spine. (A) MR scan, T1 weighted, sagittal view without contrast, reveals increased signal intensity and size of the pontomesencephalic vein (white arrow). Increased signal intensity is also noted in the mesenecephalic vein and anterior spinal vein (black arrow), both of which are continuations of the pontomesencephalic vein. **(B)** The next image in the series provides a clearer view of the increased signal intensity in the anterior spinal vein, (white arrow) well visualized between the lower aspects of C2 to mid portion of C5.

subsequent review of the initial MR scan, called into question the initial etiological conclusions related to the chiropractic manipulation. The widespread edematous changes seen in Figure 1, extending from the medulla to C5, were inconsistent with a theory that a single manipulation directed to a specific spinal level, could produce such findings. The edematous cord changes, ascending myelopathy and quality of the initial MR, led to acquisition of a second cervical MR (Figure 2A and B).

The second cervical MR scan, performed two days after admission, revealed increased signal intensity along the path of the pontomesencephic vein anterior to the medulla and the anterior spinal vein as it continues along the anterior surface of the spinal cord. These new MR findings also revealed the possible presence of an intracranial DAVF and prompted the performance of a cerebral angiogram. The cerebral angiogram revealed a Type V DAVF draining into the perimedullary venous system. The arterial phase of the angiogram (Figure 3) revealed contrast enhancement of the anterior and posterior spinal vein. Surgical inspection, via a retrosigmoid approach, revealed a fistula between the hypophyseal-meningeal trunk, a branch off the internal carotid artery, and the pontomesencephalic vein. Arterialized blood within the pontomesencephalic vein was visualized

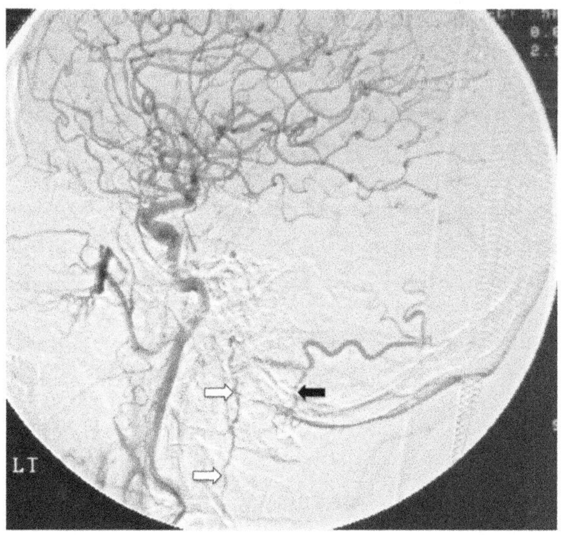

Figure 3 Digital subtraction angiogram of the cerebellum. A digital subtraction angiogram, early arterial phase, performed by injection of the left internal carotid artery. The anterior spinal vein (white arrows) was visualized during the study from C1 to C5. The posterior spinal vein (black arrow) was visualized from C1-2. No visualization of the anterior and posterior spinal vein was noted in the angiogram performed subsequent to the insertion of the neurovascular clip.

during surgery. A neurovascular clip was placed over the fistula, between the arterial and venous sides and restored the normal venous color within the pontomesencephalic vein. Surgical intervention halted the neurological deterioration. Minimal function returned with rehabilitation.

Conclusions

This case illustrates the potential difficulties in determining the etiology of rapidly developing paraplegia and ascending myelopathy. The abnormalities noted in Figure 1 were initially overlooked and only appreciated on a secondary review, when the patient's myelopathy began to ascend. The observations on the second review of Figure 1, combined with the history of chiropractic manipulation earlier on the day of admission, led to an erroneous etiological conclusion. Attending physicians initially believed the patient had experienced a rare complication from cervical manipulation, an impression that prevailed for several days, delaying proper intervention. The location and breadth of the patient's ischemia and the absence of similar cases in the literature, should have argued against chiropractic manipulation as the cause of the patient's ascending myelopathy. The admitting physician's prolonged focus on a possible complication from chiropractic manipulation may be characterized as an anchoring bias [11].

The continued deterioration of the patient's condition over the first 48 hours after admission stimulated initiation of serial diagnostic testing, including a second MR scan of the cervical spine. Increased signal intensity within the ponto/medulo/spinal venous network on the second cervical MR examination (Figure 2) raised the specter of an intracranial etiology. Angiography identified the Type V intracranial DAVF as the true cause of the ascending myelopathy.

This case also illustrates the value of multiple as well as serial advanced diagnostic imaging procedures capable of demonstrating pathology responsible for such clinical presentations. Serial studies are warranted (even when the time elapsed between studies is small) when clinical deterioration of the patient's status suggests that significant changes in the pathoanatomy have occurred. This case also illustrates how complex problems are sometimes inadequately evaluated from a single diagnostic study. The actual cause of the patient's myelopathy was only discovered after higher quality MR scans and angiography isolated the DAVF. This case also demonstrates the potential for attending clinicians to formulate inaccurate etiological opinions of causation based solely on temporal association in patients with a history of receiving chiropractic manipulation. This case further illustrates the danger of assumption, similar to other peer-reviewed papers reporting neurological complications from chiropractic manipulation [12,13], that were later shown to be inaccurate [14,15].

Consent

Written informed consent was obtained from the patient for publication of this case report and any accompanying images. A copy of the written consent is available for review by the Editor-in-Chief of this journal.

Abbreviations

DAVF: Dural arteriovenous fistula; MR: Magnetic resonance.

Competing interests

The authors declare they have no competing interests.

Authors' contributions

SMF conducted the initial review of the case and prepared the first draft of the manuscript. MJS and GDS participated in the conception of the report, the revision and coordination of the final manuscript. GDS obtained reference literature used in the manuscript. All authors read and approved of the final manuscript.

Author details

[1]Private practice of chiropractic, West Hills, California, USA. [2]University of Western States, Portland, Oregon, USA.

References

1. Herrera D, Vargas S, Dublin A: **Traumatic carotid-cavernous fistula with pontomesencephalic and cervical cord venous drainage presenting as tetraparesis.** *J Neuroimaging* 2001, **21**:73–75.
2. Gobin YP, Rogopoulos A, Avmard A, Khayata M, Reizine D, Chiras J, Merland JJ: **Endovascular treatment of intracranial dural arteriovenous fistulas with spinal medullary venous drainage.** *J Neurosurg* 1992, **77**:718–723.
3. Brenereau L, Gobin YP, Merder JF, Cognand C, Tubiana JM, Merland JJ: **Intracranial Dural artiovenous fstulas with spinal venous drainage: relation between clinical presentation and angiographic findings.** *Am J Neuroradiol* 1996, **17**:1549–1554.
4. Tsai LK, Jeng JS, Liu HM, Wang HJ, Yip PK: **Intracranial Dural arteriovenous fistulas with or without cerebral sinus thrombosis: analysis of 69 patients.** *J Neurol Neurosurg Psychiatry* 2004, **75**:1639–1641.
5. Mullan S: **Reflections upon the nature and management of intracranial and intraspinal vascular malformations and fistulae.** *J Neurosurg* 1994, **80**:606–616.
6. Lasjunias P, Ming C, Brugge KT, Tolia A, Hurth M, Bernstein M: **Neurological manifestations of intracranial dural arteriovenous malformations.** *J Neurosurg* 1986, **64**:724–730.
7. Cognard C, Gobin YP, Pierot L, Bailly AL, Houdart E, Casasco A, Chiras J, Merland JJ: **Cerebral Dural arteriovenous fistulas: clinical and angiographic correlation with a revised classification of venous drainage.** *Radiology* 1995, **194**:671–680.
8. Bernstein RA, Gress DR: *Dural arteriovenous fistulas and the neurology of venous hypertension.* Stroke: Seminars in Cerebrovascular Disease and; 2004:168–175.
9. Woimant F, Merland JJ, Riché MC, de Liège P, Bertrand HJ, Bacri D, Haguenau M, Pépin B: **Syndrome bulbo-médullaire en rapport avec une fistule arétio-veineuse méningée du sinus latéral a drainage veineux médullaire.** *Rev Neurol* 1982, **138**:559–566.
10. Lagares A, Perez-Nunez A, Alday R, *et al*: **Dural arteriovenous fistulas presenting as brainstem ischemia.** *Acta Neurochir (Wien)* 2007, **149**:965–967.
11. Croskerry P: **Achieving quality in clinical decision making: cognitive strategies and detection of bias.** *Acad Emerg Med* 2002, **9**(11):1184–1204.
12. Reuter U, Hämling M, Kavik I, Einhäupl KM, Schiekle E: **Vertebral artery dissections after chiropractic neck manipulations in Germany over three years.** *J Neurol* 2006 Jun, **253**(6):724–730.

13. Chen WL, Chern CH, Wu YL, Lee CH: **Vertebral artery dissection and cerebellar infarction following chiropractic manipulation.** *Emerg Med J* 2006, **23**:84.
14. Wenban A: **Inappropriate use of the title 'chiropractor' and the term 'chiropractic manipulation' in peer-reviewed biomedical literature.** *Chiropractic and Osteopathy* 2006, **14**:16.
15. Liu D: **Cervical manipulation causing dissection was not performed by a chiropractor.** *Emerg Med J* 2007, **24**:146.

20

A framework for chiropractic training in clinical preventive services

Cheryl Hawk[1*] and Marion Willard Evans Jr[2]

Abstract

The 2010 Patient Protection and Affordable Care Act provides incentives for both patients and providers to engage in evidence-based clinical preventive services recommended by the United States Preventive Services Task Force (USPSTF). Depending upon the application of the new health care act, Doctors of Chiropractic (DC) may be considered to be covered providers of many of these services. It is therefore essential that DCs' training prepare them to competently deliver them. The aim of this commentary is to describe a framework for training in clinical preventive services, based largely on the USPSTF recommendations, which could be readily integrated into existing DC educational programs.

Keywords: Chiropractic, Preventive health services, Health promotion

Background

The necessity for preventive care

The United States, despite spending more money on health care than any other country, has a population with shorter life expectancy and greater morbidity than any other wealthy nation [1]. The areas in which the U.S. lags behind its 16 peer nations are all lifestyle-related to a great degree [1]. Clearly this situation requires an approach that engages people in modifying their health behavior, as early as possible, rather than relying on heroic measures once conditions have become chronic and life-threatening. That approach is systematically addressed in the science of health promotion and disease prevention, often simply called "prevention" or "preventive care [2]".

With the passage of the Patient Protection and Affordable Care Act (PPACA) in 2010, the U.S. government conveyed a strong message that preventive care is essential to reverse the downward spiral of our nation's health. It also addresses the out-of-control upward spiral of medical expenditures, now more than $2.6 trillion annually [3]. The PPACA takes a number of concrete actions with respect to prevention. Among other actions, it legislates economic incentives for both patients and providers to engage in evidence-based clinical preventive services [4]. Which services are covered is determined by recommendations of the U.S. Preventive Services Task Force (USPSTF) [5].

* Correspondence: cheryl.hawk@logan.edu
[1]Logan College of Chiropractic, 1851 Schoettler Rd, 63017 Chesterfield, MO, USA
Full list of author information is available at the end of the article

Clinical preventive services

Clinical preventive services are services delivered by health care providers to prevent or detect a condition at an early stage. The USPSTF, under the Agency for Healthcare Research and Quality (AHRQ), is mandated by Public Law Section 915 to conduct evidence reviews and make recommendations on clinical preventive services [6]. The USPSTF recommendations therefore represent the "gold standard" for clinical preventive services. Most relevant to this discussion is the fact that all services that the USPSTF rates as A or B—meaning there is certainty of substantial net benefit to patients—are covered under the PPACA. Table 1 summarizes the services rated by USPSTF as A or B. Training is being conducted among primary care practitioners to be sure they are well-versed in these services, and much of this is provided by resources available from the USPSTF [7].

Chiropractic and clinical preventive services

The Council on Chiropractic Education states that "As a gatekeeper for direct access to the health delivery system, the doctor of chiropractic's responsibilities as a primary care physician include wellness promotion, health assessment, diagnosis and the chiropractic management

Table 1 USPSTF screening and counseling recommendations rated A or B*

Screening	Within scope in most states?[1]	Relevant course(s)
Abdominal aortic aneurysm (ultrasound)	no	physical diagnosis
Alcohol misuse	yes	public health/psychology
Breast cancer (mammography)	no	radiology/obstetrics/gynecology
Cervical cancer	no	obstetrics/gynecology
Colorectal cancer	yes	physical diagnosis
Depression[2]	yes	psychology
Diabetes (Type 2)	yes	physical diagnosis
Hearing loss	yes	physical diagnosis/pediatrics
Hypertension	yes	physical diagnosis
Iron deficiency anemia	yes	nutrition
Obesity	yes	nutrition
Osteoporosis	yes	nutrition/geriatrics
Tobacco use	yes	pathology/public health
Lipid disorders	yes	nutrition
Vision	yes	physical diagnosis
Counseling/interventions		
Alcohol misuse	yes	public health/psychology
Aspirin for CVD prevention[3]	no	physiology/clinical decision-making
Breastfeeding	yes	obstetrics/gynecology/pediatrics
Folic acid supplement	yes	nutrition
Iron deficiency anemia supplement	yes	nutrition
Obesity weight management[4]	yes	nutrition/psychology
Tobacco use intervention	yes	public health/psychology

* Source: USPSTF, *Guide to Clinical Preventive Services* [2]. Recommendations on screening and counseling for infectious diseases are not included.
[1] If "no," training should be included in order to enable appropriate referrals.
[2] Only if there are systems in place for diagnosis, treatment and follow-up.
[3] Only if benefits outweigh harm.
[4] Intensive behavioral intervention to facilitate sustained weight loss.

Table 2 Mandatory topics for Doctor of Chiropractic Programs (DCP)*

Topic	Topic
adjustive techniques	neurology
anatomy	nutrition/dietetics
biochemistry	obstetrics
biomechanics	orthopedics;
chiropractic principles and practice	otolaryngology
clinical decision making	pathology
dermatology	pediatrics
diagnosis (physical, clinical and laboratory)	physiology
diagnostic imaging	professional practice ethics
first aid and emergency procedures	psychology
geriatrics	public health
gynecology	research methods and procedures
microbiology	spinal analysis

*Source: Council on Chiropractic Education. *Standards for Doctor of Chiropractic Programs and Requirements for Institutional Status*, p. 18 [8].

of the patient's health care needs ([8]'p.15)." In spite of this, these concepts are not prominent in the academic standards of chiropractic training institutions. These standards have tended to emphasize conventional concepts of disease diagnosis and treatment, as exemplified in Table 2. However, in 2007 the Council on Chiropractic Education (CCE) added a set of general competencies in wellness to the requirements for chiropractic training [8,9]. In 2012, "best practices" recommendations on chiropractic care provided for the purposes of health promotion, disease prevention and wellness were published, laying out the essential components somewhat more specifically [10]. These core competencies and best practices will be discussed further in this paper.

The PPACA has a nondiscrimination clause that prohibits denial of payment for a covered service by a class of provider acting within their scope of practice, if payment is made to another class of provider for the same service [4]. Depending upon exactly how this clause is interpreted, it could mean that Doctors of Chiropractic (DC) will be able to be paid to deliver most of the USPSTF-recommended clinical preventive services. Thus it is important for DCs to be able to deliver these services in a manner consistent with USPSTF recommendations.

The purpose of this paper is to describe a framework based on the USPSTF recommendations, through which the CCE competencies and 2012 best practices can be operationalized to build a curriculum for clinical preventive services that could be integrated into both DC programs and post-graduate training.

Discussion

Current Standards in Chiropractic

The competencies in wellness from the CCE's *Standards for Doctor of Chiropractic Programs and Requirements for Institutional Status* are shown in Table 3. These specify that, in terms of knowledge, students should know the components of health promotion and the role of the doctor of chiropractic in health promotion, as well as be able to identify health promotion and wellness resources and minimum screening activities for health promotion. With respect to behavior, this document specifies that students be able to perform recommended screening

Table 3 Wellness competencies for doctor of Chiropractic Programs*

Attitudes	
•	appreciate role of lifestyle, behavior, psychological factors in health and wellness
•	appreciate multidimensionality of wellness
•	appreciate and accept active patient participation
•	explain and emphasize benefits of health promotion on response to treatment
•	appreciate community health and DCs' role in community health
•	recognize and appreciate impact of environment on patient's well being
•	appreciate social determinants of health.
Knowledge	
•	discuss basic principles and perspectives of health promotion and wellness
•	describe concepts of health promotion in the context of chiropractic health care;
•	describe components of health promotion for the needs of the patient and the public
•	describe the role of the doctor of chiropractic in health promotion
•	relate necessity of lifestyle changes to promote patients' and the public's health
•	identify health promotion and wellness resources for patients and the public
•	identify the minimum screening activities for health promotion
•	describe factors related to the leading health indicators (physical activity, overweight and obesity, tobacco, substance abuse, sexual behavior, mental health, injury and violence, environmental quality, immunization, and access to health care)
•	describe issues related to years of healthy life and health disparities.
Behavior	
•	communicate effectively with patients about dimensions of health (biological, psychological, social, and spiritual) as part of history taking
•	use appropriate techniques to encourage patient participation in his/her health
•	implement recommended preventive screening activities
•	perform screening and wellness assessments in different age groups
•	provide patient counseling for health promotion and assess its outcomes.

*Source: Council on Chiropractic Education. *Standards for Doctor of Chiropractic Programs and Requirements for Institutional Status*, p.46-48 [8].

activities and provide patient counseling on health promotion. This document also specifies the topics which must be covered in DC programs.

Furthermore, in 2013, the CCE refined the wellness competencies in their new meta-competency approach [11]. The new Meta-competency 3 is "health promotion and disease prevention". Table 4 summarizes the required components and outcomes for this meta-competency. Colleges must demonstrate to CCE where in their curriculum they achieve these outcomes. This meta-competency is basically a directive for chiropractic colleges to train students in screening for risk factors and counseling on health behavior. As shown in Table 2, there are no topics explicitly addressing the "wellness" competencies. However, it is conceivable that the necessary information could be combined with topics such as chiropractic principles and practice, public health and nutrition, for counseling, and diagnosis for screening. The Standards do not require a specific course for any topic; the institution needs to demonstrate that all the topics are included in coursework. Thus there is considerable flexibility in how preventive services training can be integrated into existing courses.

The National Board of Chiropractic Examiners (NBCE) covers the following topics on board examinations DCs must pass in order to be licensed:

Community Health and Wellness (11% of NBCE board examination, Part II score)

- Public health organizations
- Healthy People initiatives
- Screening activities for health promotion
- Tobacco, alcohol and substance abuse
- Exercise and healthy diet for obesity
- Behavior theories and lifestyle change
- Wellness counseling

Table 4 Meta-competency 3: health promotion and disease prevention*

Required components	Identify areas for health improvement (that is, screen for disease and risk factors)
	Address appropriate hygiene (that is, advise on health behavior)
	Coordinate strategies with other providers.
	Identify public health issues relevant to patients
Outcomes	Document management of health risks.
	Explain health risk factors to patients.
	Provide recommendations on patients' health status, behavior and lifestyle.
	Recommend/provide resources and instruction to assist health behavior change.
	Recommend dietary approaches to restore, maintain or improve patient's health.
	Implement appropriate hygiene practices in the clinical environment.
	Communicate strategies to other treating providers.

*Source: Council on Chiropractic Education. Accreditation Standards, Principles, Processes & Requirements for Accreditation. Scottsdale, AZ; 2013.

The "best practices" recommendations, based on the results of a formal consensus process conducted through a multidisciplinary Delphi panel, are summarized in Table 5 [10]. Obviously these recommendations are consistent with, although more detailed than, both the general CCE competencies and the more specific topics listed by the NBCE. The "best practice" recommendations operationalize some of the broader items in the CCE and NBCE documents. For example, the "best practice" recommendations state that all patients should be screened for obesity/overweight using the Body Mass Index (BMI), and that tobacco cessation advice should at least include provision of a quit line phone number [10]. This document also states that DCs should be familiar with nationally recognized recommendations on disease screening and health promotion counseling, such as those made by the USPSTF [10].

USPSTF recommendations as a framework

A pragmatic approach to integrating clinical preventive services would be to use the USPSTF recommendations as the basis for operationalizing the CCE standards and "best practices". Table 1 lists the USPSTF recommendations rated A or B (excluding infectious diseases), [2] along with whether or not they are generally within chiropractic scope of practice, and courses within which they might most readily be integrated. It should be noted that the USPSTF recommendations encompass all the current chiropractic standards—CCE competencies, "best practice" recommendations and NBCE topics.

Table 5 Summary of "best practice" recommendations for chiropractic wellness care*

General

Be familiar with nationally recognized recommendations on disease screening and health promotion counseling, such as those made by the USPSTF.

Screening for risk factors—all patients

- Obesity/overweight, as assessed by Body Mass Index (BMI)
- Physical inactivity or sedentary behaviors
- Tobacco use
- Hypertension

Other considerations

- Awareness of symptoms of depression and availability of appropriate referral system for depression or other psychological issues.
- Awareness of signs and symptoms of skin cancer and availability of appropriate referral system.

Health promotion information, advice or referral to all patients for whom screening indicates that they are at risk:

- Physical activity appropriate for the individual
- Tobacco cessation, at least through provision of quit line phone number.
- Healthy diet
- Weight management appropriate for the individual.

Other considerations

- Although immunization is not within the chiropractic scope of practice, if patients ask for information, they should be referred to or receive balanced, evidence-based information from credible resources such as the Centers for Disease Control.

*Source: Hawk C, Schneider M, Evans MW, Jr., Redwood D. Consensus process to develop a best-practice document on the role of chiropractic care in health promotion, disease prevention, and wellness. *J Manipulative Physiol Ther.* Sep 2012;35(7):556–567 [10].

Clinical experience in counseling/advising patients

Students within a doctor of chiropractic program already have opportunities to counsel patients on behavior change during their internship. For example, since the majority of U.S. adults are overweight or obese and get less than the recommended amount of physical activity, [2] it is likely that students will encounter such patients. We suggest that colleges might use the USPSTF recommendations as a framework to ensure that opportunities to counsel patients on the recommended topics be included, through use of standardized patients if necessary [12]. This would simultaneously address the CCE behavioral competencies, NBCE topics and "best practices". The standardized patient encounter could be as simple as having a patient present with chronic spinal pain and a history of cigarette smoking for several years, or the need to implement age-appropriate physical activity guidelines. In addition, at the USPSTF website there is also information on whom to contact to access information about how to test students on preventive services using a Preventive Care Objective Structured Clinical Examination (OSCE). This OSCE was developed jointly by the Indiana University School of Medicine and the Indiana Area Health Education Center (AHEC). Current use of OSCEs is common in chiropractic colleges; our suggestion is merely to extend their use to include prevention counseling.

This approach would provide assurance that DCs are trained to provide the preventive services within their scope of practice that are well-documented to have an important net benefit for patients' health. Furthermore, it would provide documentation that DCs are capable of providing the services covered by the PPACA, which would therefore help in making a case for DCs to be covered providers of these services.

Challenges to implementing the wellness competencies

In a curriculum which is already overfull with didactic coursework, many administrators and faculty may feel that it is impossible to add additional material. However, the CCE requirement to do exactly that may induce some creative thinking. Reducing some basic science material, such as microbiology or biochemistry, could make room for more material on health behavior and health education. In terms of clinical experience, it seems quite feasible to simply "get more mileage" out of existing standardized and actual patients. That is, rather than restricting the history and examination to vital signs, orthopedic, neurological, postural, or palpatory findings, simply broaden them to include BMI assessment, health habits and other lifestyle factors. In fact, many and perhaps most chiropractic colleges already do include lifestyle in the history. The next step, not uniformly taken as yet, would be to require students to counsel patients on changing risky health behaviors. These patients may be presenting for musculoskeletal complaints or, like many patients in chiropractic teaching clinics, may be presenting for "wellness care". These are opportunities to screen for health risks, particularly those which are extremely common, such as physical inactivity and overweight/obesity, and to counsel patients when the risks are present. Thus, current patients (both standardized and actual) could provide opportunities for screening and counseling at the same time that they are being treated for symptoms/conditions.

Resources for faculty

In the end, success in integrating training in clinical preventive services into chiropractic education depends upon the faculty. Since many chiropractic college faculty do not have specific training in clinical preventive services, it is essential that colleges develop faculty in-services or support selected faculty in pursuing appropriate coursework, in areas such as public health, health education, health psychology, or health/wellness coaching. The USPSTF's Pocket Guide to Clinical Preventive Services, along with other electronic resources, is available at www.USPreventiveServicesTaskForce.org.

Because of its pivotal role in the implementation of the PPACA, the USPSTF provides a wealth of teaching resources available to health professions training institutions and/or other organizations [7]. They were created to assist in the training of primary care providers in use of the recommended preventive services in practice. The American Association of the Colleges of Osteopathic Medicine's Task Force on Integrating Preventive Medicine into Medical and Health Professions Curricula created one- and two-hour PowerPoint presentations for health care professionals titled "Putting Prevention into Practice". These are case-based tutorials which serve as an introduction to use of the USPSTF recommendations.

Combining the existing USPSTF resources with books and other resources, and integrating modules into appropriate existing courses, as well as with clinical training using standardized patients and OSCEs, would not require extensive curriculum revision. Preparing faculty through a series of in-services, again using readily accessible resources, could also be integrated into existing academic schedules. Using the USPSTF recommendations as a framework for health promotion and disease prevention training could assist in operationalizing the CCE requirements for this competency. Also, since they are in broad use by all health professions, they could assist in interprofessional communications between doctors of chiropractic and other providers.

Conclusion

Combining the framework of the USPSTF recommendations with the publicly available USPSTF resources should be relatively easily adapted to different chiropractic colleges' needs and preferences. It would ensure that graduates are prepared to contribute substantively to the national effort toward disease prevention and promoting the health of all Americans.

Competing interests
The authors have recently published a book on the topic of clinical preventive services and developed a certification program with the National Wellness Institute on health promotion and wellness. The authors declare that they have no competing interests.

Authors' contributions
CH conceived of the paper and drafted the manuscript. WE contributed to the concepts and references and to writing the manuscript. Both authors read and approved the final manuscript.

Acknowledgements
The authors would like to acknowledge David Beavers, MEd, DC, MPH; Bryce Conrad, M Chir; Martha Kaeser, DC, MEd, and Daniel Redwood, DC, for the many discussions on the wellness competencies in which we engaged with them and which contributed to the refinement of the conceptual basis of this article.

Author details
[1]Logan College of Chiropractic, 1851 Schoettler Rd, 63017 Chesterfield, MO, USA. [2]University of Western States, 2900 NE 132nd Ave, 97230 Portland, OR, USA.

References

1. Woolf S, Aron L: *U.S. Health in International Perspective: Shorter Lives, Poorer Health.* Washington DC: National Academy of Sciences; 2013.
2. USPSTF: *Guide to Clinical Preventive Services.* Rockville, MD: Agency for Healthcare Research and Quality; 2012. http://www.ahrq.gov/professionals/clinicians-providers/guidelines-recommendations/guide/section2.html Accessed April 30, 2013.
3. Martin AB, Lassman D, Washington B, Catlin A, National Health Expenditure Accounts T: **Growth in US health spending remained slow in 2010; health share of gross domestic product was unchanged from 2009.** *Health Aff (Millwood)* 2012, **31**(1):208–219.
4. *Patient Protection and Affordable Care Act of 2010. H.R. 3590.* Washington DC; 2010. http://www.govtrack.us/congress/bills/111/hr3590/text **Accessed April 25, 2013.**
5. Redwood D: **Health reform, prevention and health promotion: milestone moment on a long journey.** *J Altern Complement Med* 2010, **16**(5):521–523.
6. About the USPSTF: *Introduction. U.S. Preventive Services Task Force.* 2010. http://www.uspreventiveservicestaskforce.org/intro.htm Accessed April 25, 2013.
7. *Implementing U.S. Preventive Services Task Force (USPSTF) Recommendations into Health Professions Education.* Rockville, MD: Agency for Healthcare Research and Quality; 2011. http://www.ahrq.gov/qual/kt/tfmethods/impuspstf.htm Accessed April 30, 2013.

8. Council on Chiropractic Education: *Standards for Doctor of Chiropractic Programs and Requirements for Institutional Status.* Scottsdale, AZ: Council on Chiropractic Education; 2007.
9. Evans MW Jr, Rupert R: **The Council on Chiropractic Education's new wellness standard: a call to action for the chiropractic profession.** *Chiropr Osteopat* 2006, **14**:23.
10. Hawk C, Schneider M, Evans MW Jr, Redwood D: **Consensus process to develop a best-practice document on the role of chiropractic care in health promotion, disease prevention, and wellness.** *J Manipulative Physiol Ther* 2012, **35**(7):556–567.
11. Council on Chiropractic Education: *Accreditation Standards, Principles, Processes & Requirements for Accreditation.* Scottsdale, AZ: Council on Chiropractic Education; 2013.
12. Hawk C, Kaeser MA, Beavers DV: **Feasibility of using a standardized patient encounter for training chiropractic students in tobacco cessation counseling.** *J Chiropr Educ* 2013. in press.

Review of methods used by chiropractors to determine the site for applying manipulation

John J Triano[1*†], Brian Budgell[1†], Angela Bagnulo[2], Benjamin Roffey[3], Thomas Bergmann[5], Robert Cooperstein[6], Brian Gleberzon[1], Christopher Good[7], Jacquelyn Perron[4] and Rodger Tepe[8]

Abstract

Background: With the development of increasing evidence for the use of manipulation in the management of musculoskeletal conditions, there is growing interest in identifying the appropriate indications for care. Recently, attempts have been made to develop clinical prediction rules, however the validity of these clinical prediction rules remains unclear and their impact on care delivery has yet to be established. The current study was designed to evaluate the literature on the validity and reliability of the more common methods used by doctors of chiropractic to inform the choice of the site at which to apply spinal manipulation.

Methods: Structured searches were conducted in Medline, PubMed, CINAHL and ICL, supported by hand searches of archives, to identify studies of the diagnostic reliability and validity of common methods used to identify the site of treatment application. To be included, studies were to present original data from studies of human subjects and be designed to address the region or location of care delivery. Only English language manuscripts from peer-reviewed journals were included. The quality of evidence was ranked using QUADAS for validity and QAREL for reliability, as appropriate. Data were extracted and synthesized, and were evaluated in terms of strength of evidence and the degree to which the evidence was favourable for clinical use of the method under investigation.

Results: A total of 2594 titles were screened from which 201 articles met all inclusion criteria. The spectrum of manuscript quality was quite broad, as was the degree to which the evidence favoured clinical application of the diagnostic methods reviewed. The most convincing favourable evidence was for methods which confirmed or provoked pain at a specific spinal segmental level or region. There was also high quality evidence supporting the use, with limitations, of static and motion palpation, and measures of leg length inequality. Evidence of mixed quality supported the use, with limitations, of postural evaluation. The evidence was unclear on the applicability of measures of stiffness and the use of spinal x-rays. The evidence was of mixed quality, but unfavourable for the use of manual muscle testing, skin conductance, surface electromyography and skin temperature measurement.

Conclusions: A considerable range of methods is in use for determining where in the spine to administer spinal manipulation. The currently published evidence falls across a spectrum ranging from strongly favourable to strongly unfavourable in regard to using these methods. In general, the stronger and more favourable evidence is for those procedures which take a direct measure of the presumptive site of care– methods involving pain provocation upon palpation or localized tissue examination. Procedures which involve some indirect assessment for identifying the manipulable lesion of the spine–such as skin conductance or thermography–tend not to be supported by the available evidence.

Keywords: Diagnostic accuracy, Validity, Reliability, Spinal manipulation, Chiropractic

* Correspondence: jtriano@cmcc.ca
†Equal contributors
[1]Canadian Memorial Chiropractic College, 6100 Leslie St., Toronto, Ontario, Canada
Full list of author information is available at the end of the article

Background

The primary focus of chiropractic practice is the evaluation and management of disorders of the neuromusculoskeletal system. Treatment of these disorders includes manual manipulation procedures directed toward normalizing alterations of the locomotor system [1]. With increasing evidence of clinical benefit for spinal manipulation (for example, see Gross et al. [2]; Rubinstein et al. [3]; Bronfort et al. [4]), there is growing interest in identifying the appropriate indications for localizing the site of care.

Patient evaluation can be viewed as a sequence of procedures designed to progressively narrow the focus of attention, first to region then local site and, sometimes, tissue. In the ideal circumstance, the clinical value of a test or maneuver is based more on the health consequences from using it rather than on its accuracy alone [5]. In the case of the spine, however, over 90% of complaints have been categorized as a heterogeneous grouping which might be termed "non-specific" spinal pain [6]. An additional 5% to 9% are attributed to neurological deficits referable to the spine. Currently, there is no consensus on the mechanism(s) or identity of the pain generators of non-specific spinal pain. Even the validity and impact on care delivery of recent clinical prediction rules remain uncertain [7]. Consequently, there is no gold standard for diagnosis, in the traditional sense. A more pragmatic concept, the clinically important manipulable or functional spinal lesion, has emerged that recognizes the heterogeneous clinical manifestations from local tissue strains and altered neuromotor control [8,9] seen in these patients.

As in other fields of medicine, it is the clinical presentation, rather than a gold standard diagnosis, that directs decision making [10 12]. Faced with the dilemma of an absent gold standard [10] and yet a duty to care [13], one of the options is to evaluate the consequences of the disorder being treated. For example, there currently is no means to differentiate the specific pain generator in the presence of multiple abnormalities on imaging [14]. For a patient who has radicular pain, an imaging abnormality that has the potential to produce symptoms must be concordant with the location and distribution of signs and symptoms to correctly frame the diagnosis. This is the framing of gold standard that is adopted for use within the remainder of this article.

The pathophysiologic consequences of manipulable lesions have been loosely aggregated, primarily from common clinical wisdom and collective experience, into related categories; Pain, Asymmetry, relative Range of motion, changes in Tissue temperature/texture/tone, and findings from Special tests (P.A.R.T.S.). Thus, P.A.R.T.S. is commonly viewed [15] as a required foundation for manipulation treatment and is likely the most widely utilized method to justify a treatment application site [16]. There appear to be six core and overlapping constructs underlying the P.A.R.T.S. These constructs define somatotopic relationships between the patient's signs and symptoms and biological substrates including dermatomes, sclerotomes and myotomes, as detailed below:

- Pain–P.
    - Findings from self-report and the reproduction of pain through diagnostic manoeuvres are spatially related to the local presence of pathology/dysfunction.
- Asymmetry–A.
    - Anatomical landmarks present an observable cephalo-caudal pattern, within the sagittal plane, and/or a bilateral symmetry in their location, motion and compliance/stiffness in response to challenge or perturbation.
- Range of motion–R.
    - Joints, within a linkage system, contribute a predictable proportion and path to the regional movement expressed by the linkage system as a function of task.
- Tissue temperature, texture, and tone–T.
    - Muscle, as both a sense organ and actuator, responds to pathology that is spatially related with hypertonicity, hypotonicity, hypertrophy or atrophy as a function of the primary tissue disease process present.
    - In the presence of pathology/dysfunction, a spatially consistent change in the relative ratio of fluid (edema) to cellular and acellular components is observable.
- Special tests–S.
    - In the presence of pathology/dysfunction, there is a spatially consistent neurogenic activity that demonstrates a muscular, kinematic, vascular, or secretory response that is observable.

When a course of manipulation is elected, the provider must use her/his clinical judgment, often employing the constructs above, to determine which procedures to apply and where. It is this topic that motivates the present work. To be clear, the topic of investigation was not to determine the bases for a judgement to apply manipulation, rather that once such a judgement has been made, what are the foundations to determine the site to which treatment would be directed. The purpose of this study is to identify the best available evidence as to what methods of assessment can inform the provider as to localization of treatment.

Methods

The core question on where to site the application of manipulation treatment, while simple in concept, is remarkably complex to answer. The literature involves a breadth of evidence which often has been studied using heterogeneous methods or measures and requires contextual interpretation. The approach used was a hybrid method allowing for both a consensus process, after the work of Bigos et al. [17], Haldeman, Chapman-Smith and Petersen [18] and the RAND expert panels on the appropriateness in use of manipulation [19,20], with the use of explicit and systematic tools to evaluate the quality of evidence in the manner of a systematic review [21]. Unlike the evaluation of outcome-related studies that lend themselves to use of PRISMA [21], MOOSE [22] or RAMSES [23] guidelines, studies that evaluate the "accuracy" of tests require different criteria to appropriately assess the quality of studies and the potential for bias [24].

A team of reviewers was assembled under sponsorship of the Association of Chiropractic Colleges (ACC) in conjunction with the Council on Chiropractic Guidelines and Practice Parameters (CCGPP). Two team leads (JT & BB) were identified who together held prior experience and publications in methods of literature synthesis and/or analysis. Administrative support was provided by two recent graduate clinicians (AB & BR) who tracked article reviews and team member participation. A request for nominations to the review panel was sent to constituent members of the ACC and CCGPP. The panel of reviewers consisted of 7 members (1 PhD; 2 DC, PhD; 1 DC, MSc; 3 DC) representing 5 different chiropractic institutions. One reviewer was based in private practice, 5 DCs were in part-time practice or had recently retired from full time practice. The panel conducted reviews and developed consensus for conclusions presented in this report, independently from the sponsors.

Electronic searches were conducted using EBSCO host search engine within Medline, PubMed, CINAHL and ICL through July 2010. A series of terms were searched individually and concatenated with anatomical region (i.e. spine, vertebr*, cervical spine or neck, thoracic spine or mid back, lumbar spine or low back, sacroiliac joint or pelvis) and/or treatment type (i.e. manip* or mobilis* or mobiliz*) and/or discipline (e.g. chiropract*). The terms list was inclusive of the following: applied kinesiology, arm fossa test, current perception threshold, diagnos*/assessment, electromyography/electromyograph*/emg, joint play/challenge, leg length inequality/asymmetry, muscle testing/manual muscle test*, neurocalometer/neurocalomet*, orthopedic/orthopedic test, pain/pain provocation, palpation–static and motion, PARTS (pain, asymmetry, range of motion, tone and texture and special tests)', physical examination, posture, radiography/radiograph*/x-ray, range of motion/rom.

Hand searches of publication references and of archives were also conducted. References retained for review by the team had to meet five prospective inclusion criteria: 1) topics focused on diagnostic validity and/or reliability for methods of patient evaluation used to identify the site of care by manual treatment, 2) articles were primary source research reports containing original data obtained from humans, 3) examiners were experienced providers or health sciences students, 4) for validity studies, at least some of the subjects must have been symptomatic or have had a known anatomical anomaly, and 5) publication was in the indexed and peer reviewed English language literature. No limits were placed on the date of publication.

In addition to searching for studies pertaining to individual assessment procedures, studies that investigated clusters of tests were also retrieved. Search topics were informed by the background focus on spinal manipulation and the P.A.R.T.S. constructs. Searching was assisted and full text copies of papers were made available for administrative review through the services of the Cleveland Chiropractic College and Canadian Memorial Chiropractic College Libraries.

The administrative screening confirmed eligibility of the paper according to the prescribed inclusion criteria checklist. Subsequently, each eligible paper was assigned to one of two research assistants who worked independently of the reviewers and who extracted data which was placed in an evidence table. In addition to manuscript metadata (author, journal etc.), the evidence table recorded the spinal region investigated, the reference standard ('gold standard'), disease spectrum of patients/subjects, whether the manuscript referred to intra-rater reliability, inter-rater reliability or validity, a summary of the experimental design, the statistics/outcome measures reported, and any limitations to be taken into consideration in interpreting the findings.

Each article then was assigned, on a rotating basis, to two reviewers. Within the two classes of studies, validity and reliability, papers were scored independently by each reviewer based on their content using the QUADAS [25,26] and QAREL [27] instruments, respectively. Some validity studies contained nested reliability studies for specific aspects of the methods under investigation. These minor reliability exercises were not scored independently. Each member of the team participated in training with respect to use of the two instruments under supervision of an experienced user (BB). Exercises consisting of review and scoring of validity and reliability studies were conducted using literature unrelated to the purpose of this study. Scored checklists were returned to the research assistants, who were not part of the review team, and results were recorded. If there was disagreement between reviewers on any element of the QUADAS or QAREL ratings, communication over the point of disagreement was facilitated by the research assistant to attempt reconciliation. For any disagreement not reconciled between reviewers, the topic was set aside for the full review panel meeting and discussion.

Item response theory was used to weight QUADAS and QAREL items based on the inverse of their prevalence among the papers reviewed (see Nakayama and Budgell 2009) [28]. A separate manuscript, under preparation, describes the validation of this approach for QUADAS and QAREL. In brief, however, papers were not simply awarded 1 point for each criterion which they satisfied. Rather, criteria were weighted and their ability to discriminate between papers of higher and lower quality was confirmed. These scores only indicate relative quality within the cohort of papers reviewed and only based on the QUADAS and QAREL checklists. The full listing of scores by primary author and date may be found in Tables 1 and 2. Question level data for each paper scored with QUADAS and QAREL may be found in Additional files 1 and 2, respectively.

The full team met to review scores and to summarize the evidence. Seed definitions for quality of evidence, prepared in advance of the team meeting by the project

Table 1 Rankings of validity studies per QUADAS scores

Article ID	Percentile	Rank	Article ID	Percentile	Rank
Abbott_2003	78	19	King_2007	77	20
Abbott_2005	92	6	Knutson_2002	77	21
Abbott_2006	100	1	Landel_2008	90	8
Beattie_1990	83	14	Laslet_2003	73	28
Bierma-Zeinstra_2001	90	8	Laslet_2005	94	2
Brismee_2006	41	40	Leach_1993	91	7
Bryner_1994	64	31	Lebeouf_1990	75	26
Caruso_2000	27	44	Leboeuf-Yde_2000	93	3
Chafetz_1988	76	24	Leboeuf-Yde_2002	100	1
Chakraverty_2007	85	10	Lehman_2002	77	23
Cibulka 1999	35	41	Levanqie_1999	92	5
Cooperstein_2003	59	35	McCulloch_1993	100	1
Cooperstein_2004	84	11	Montgomery_1995	55	37
Dankaerts_2006	78	18	Nansel_1988	64	32
Diakow_1988	48	38	Ogince_2007	78	17
Erikson_1996	32	43	Osterbauer_1996	33	42
Fernandez-de-las-Pinas _2005	57	36	Peterson_2008	77	22
Fortin_1997	45	39	Petrone_2003	93	4
Fritz_2011	83	12	Phillips_1996	100	1
Fryer_2010	69	29	Pollard_2006	84	11
Haas&Peterson_1992	75	25	Roy_2008	87	9
Harlick_2007	79	16	Sandmark_1995	90	8
Harrison_1998	64	33	Taylor_1990	83	13
Harrison_2003	92	5	Viitanen_2000	83	12
Harrison_2004	62	34	Yamashita_2002	67	30
Humphreys_2004	84	11	Zaproudina_2006	74	27
Imoto_2007	83	15			
Jende_1997	92	6			
Jull_1988	100	1			

Summary scores (not shown) were generated using weightings of QUADAS checklist items, where weights of individual items were based on the inverse of their prevalence within this cohort of articles. Subsequently, articles were ranked according to their normalized (Percentile) score and their relative position (Rank) within this cohort of articles.

Table 2 Rankings of reliability studies per QAREL scores

Article ID	Percentile	Rank	Article ID	Percentile	Rank	Article ID	Percentile	Rank
Agarwal_2005	26	73	Danneels_2001	18	82	Herzog_1989	37	56
Amiri_2003	24	79	Degenhardt_2005	30	65	Hicks_2003	60	31
Antos_1990	38	53	Degenhardt_2010	66	16	Hinson_1998	22	80
Arab_2009	62	26	Diakow_1988	17	83	Holmgren_2008	85	6
Bergstrom_1986	11	87	Downey_2003	77	9	Holt_2009	32	60
Bertilson_2003	61	28	Fjelhner_1999	69	13	Hoppenbrouwer_2006	48	41
Binkley_1995	47	43	Fortin 1997	13	86	Horneij_2002	46	46
Bo_1997	29	67	French_2000	41	50	Hsieh_1990	16	85
Bockenhauer_2007	22	80	Fryer_2005	78	8	Hubka_1994	33	59
Boline_1988	41	49	Fryer_2006	53	37	Hungerford_2007	32	61
Boline_1993	38	53	Fuhr_1989	16	85	Hunt_2001	22	80
Breum_1995	32	60	Gemmell_1990	46	47	Jackson_1993	64	19
Brismee_2005	46	47	Ghoukssian_2001	17	84	Jackson_1998	26	70
Brismee_2006	64	18	Gibbons_2002	26	72	Jende_1997	40	51
Byfield_1992	29	67	Gross_1998	24	76	Johansson_2006	77	9
Calderon_1994	38	55	Haas_1990	37	57	Keating_1990	61	28
Carmichael_1987	39	52	Haas_1992	72	11	Kilpikoski_2002	46	47
Chakraverty_2007	30	66	Haas_1993	100	1	Kim_2007	22	80
Chiarello_1993	32	61	Haas_1995	100	1	Kmita_2008	100	1
Christensen_2002	77	9	Hall_2004	61	30	Kokmeyer_2002	63	21
Cibulka_1999	24	78	Hanada_2001	24	77	Laslett_1994	46	47
Clare_2004	53	36	Hanten_2002	35	58	Latimer_1998	10	88
Clare_2005	31	64	Harrison_2003	26	73	Leach_2003	69	12
Cleland_2006	46	47	Hart_2007	53	39	Leard_2009	63	23
Comeaux_2001	61	30	Haswell_2004	68	14	Lee_2002	31	64
Cook_2004	37	56	Hawk_1999	29	67	Love_1987	68	15
Cooperstein_2010	61	27	Haynes_2002	22	80	Ludtke_2001	47	45
Cowherd_1992	0	91	Heiderscheit_2008	22	80	Lundberg_1999	46	47
Croft_1994	68	14	Heiss_2004	37	56	Maher_1994	46	47
Article ID	**Percentile**	**Rank**	**Article ID**	**Percentile**	**Rank**	**Article ID**	**Percentile**	**Rank**
Maigne_2009	76	10	Plaugher_1991 #67	62	24	Vikai_Juntura_1987	63	22
Marcotte_2002	29	67	Plaugher_1993	22	80	Vincent-Smith_1999	32	60
Marcotte_2005	6	89	Pool_2004	46	47	Weiner_2006	24	78
Mayer_2004	20	81	Potter_2006	61	29	Woodfield_2011	46	47
McCombe_1989	31	64	Qvistgraad_2007	92	4	Younquist_1989	84	7
McKenzie_1997	53	38	Razmjou_2000	46	47			
McPartland_1996	46	47	Rhodes_1995	54	34			
Meijne_1999	32	63	Rhudy_1988	46	47			
Mior_1985	48	40	Riddle_2002	31	64			
Mootz_1989	32	62	Robinson_2007	94	3			
Moran_2001	48	42	Robinson_2009	54	35			
Nansel_1989	48	42	Rouwmaat_1998	92	5			
Nguyen_1999	62	26	Roy_2006	18	82			

Table 2 Rankings of reliability studies per QAREL scores *(Continued)*

Normand_2007	22	80	Schneider_2007	25	74
O'Haire_2000	38	54	Schneider_2008	77	9
Olson_1998	24	79	Seay_2007	28	68
Olson_2009	42	48	Smedmark_2000	46	47
Owens_2000	17	83	Solinger_2000	24	75
Owens_2004	27	69	Strender_1997 (160)	46	47
Owens_2007	26	71	Strender_1997 (167)	38	53
Paatelma_2010	38	53	Sweat_1988	5	90
Paulet_2009	47	44	Tong_2006	30	66
Paydar_1994	26	72	Tousignant_2001	29	67
Peterson_2004	55	33	Toussaint_1999	65	17
Petrone_2003	37	56	Troke_1998	62	25
Phillips_1986	63	20	Troke_2007	55	32
Piva_2003	46	47	Troyanovich_1999	94	2
Piva_2006	94	2	Van Dillen_1998	40	51
Plaugher_1991 #107	100	1	VanSuijlekoma_2000	24	78

Summary scores (not shown) were generated using weightings of QAREL checklist items, where weights of individual items were based on the inverse of their prevalence within this cohort of articles. Subsequently, articles were ranked according to their normalized (Percentile) score and their relative position (Rank) within this cohort of articles.

support staff, were derived from the earlier work by Bronfort et al. [4]. Final definitions for consensus were adopted by vote at the outset of the meeting. Each reviewer presented summary overviews on up to 3 of the patient assessment methods, discussing the quality and content of each paper and the overall quality and content of the body of literature on the topic. Discussion was conducted following presentation of each summary, using a facilitated round-robin method [29,30]. Thus, after each reviewer had made their presentation, each participant was addressed, in turn, with the opportunity to comment with respect to a topic and to ask questions until he/she was satisfied. Following one round, a second round was conducted where each member was offered a further opportunity to emphasize or introduce comments. Summary notes on comments were maintained electronically and on a white-board. Then, by consensus vote, the group ranked the quality of the body of literature on each topic and the degree to which the literature supported the use of the modality in question. Consensus summary scores for each paper served to rank the quality of each article as a percentile within its cohort of reliability or validity papers. Where both intra- and inter-examiner reliability was assessed, we chose to weight only the latter as it speaks more to the generalizability of use. Similarly, where papers reviewing literature on reliability and/or validity were used to establish topic background and context, the precursor studies were not independently rated.

A mechanism for a minority opinion report was prospectively designed for the circumstance where a consensus by simple majority could not be achieved. Final recommendations on whether or not the diagnostic tool should be utilized in practice came from the consensus rankings.

Results

The interprofessional relevance of the literature retrieved will be immediately evident. Not unexpectedly, while the search strategies were narrowed to those topics arising from or related to the PARTS concepts and the discipline focus, work from authors of various disciplines were represented and suggests that the findings reported herein have broader application than to the chiropractic discipline alone.

A total of 2577 titles identified through the electronic literature search were screened, and, from these, 184 articles met all inclusion criteria and were accepted into this study. In the course of the project, an additional 17 articles were brought forward by reviewers, determined to meet the inclusion criteria and were incorporated into the analysis. Hence, the great majority of studies identified in our initial literature search were excluded from analysis. The most common reasons were that the studies were not directed towards identifying the site of care, region or segment, to be treated, and that the study involved subjects who were, in the main or entirely, healthy (Figure 1). Topic areas were aggregated following the P.A.R.T.S. constructs with the number of studies at each level of evidence listed with the section title. Some papers were included in more than one section if they

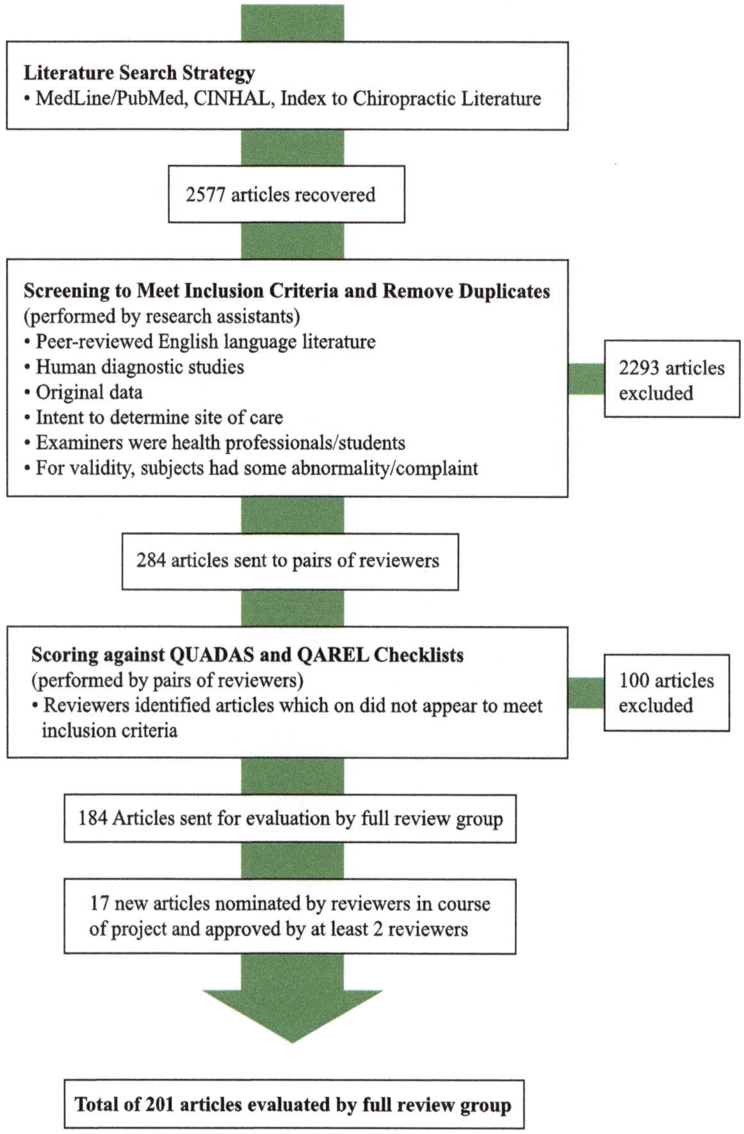

Figure 1 Literature search strategy.

investigated more than one assessment modality. A summary of the literature representative of the breadth of quality scores is provided under each heading with panel recommendations and ratings of the evidence. No conflicts on QUADAS or QAREL scores remained between reviewer pairs for the consensus meeting agenda. Similarly, no minority reports resulted from the consensus rankings.

Consensus and levels of evidence

Consensus was defined as an agreement of greater than or equal to 70% by panel vote. Following the reviewer ranking according to QUADAS and/or QAREL scores, each paper was considered as providing a 'high' level of evidence if it achieved a quality score ≥ 70%, a 'moderate' level of evidence if its score ranged between 40% and 69%, and a "low" level of evidence if the score was ≤ 39% (see Table 3, Column 2). These criteria were set based on what appeared, early in the study, to be natural clusterings of scores.

Table 3 Levels of evidence defined by quality scores of individual papers

Level	Quality scores for individual papers	Quality definition for topic/procedure
High	≥ 70%	Two high or one high AND two moderate scores
Moderate	≥ 40% < 70%	One high OR two moderate scores
Low	< 40%	Everything else

Table 4 Definitions of levels of agreement for reliability study scores

Kappa		Intra-class correlation	
Range	Definition	Range	Definition
< 0	Less than chance	< 0.4	Poor
0.01–0.20	Slight	0.4-0.75	Moderate
0.21– 0.40	Moderate	0.75-0.9	Good
0.61–0.80	Substantial	> 0.9	Excellent
0.81–0.99	Near perfect		

Interpretations of reliability Kappa (κ) scores follow the work of Viera and Garrett [31] and for intra-class correlations (ICC) that of Fleiss [32]. Definitions relating score value with levels of agreement are provided, for convenience, in Table 4.

A summary of recommendations, themselves reported at the end of each section below, can be found in Tables 5 and 6. Table 5 provides a description of each of the five possible types of recommendation while Table 6 gives a summary of recommendations for each category of evaluation method. It should be emphasized for clarity that there were a significant number of the studies that offered evidence on more than one assessment approach. The definitions for rating of evidence (Table 3) were based on the number of papers for which the QUADAS or QAREL scoring met or exceeded the threshold level.

Pain

[Quality scores: Validity 0 low, 1 moderate, 11 high; Reliability 12 low, 17 moderate, 1 high].

Provocative manoeuvres, evoking relief or aggravation of familiar pain, augmented by historical factors, have been used to localize the suspected pain generator throughout the spine [33-67].

Pain history

[Quality scores: Reliability 0 low, 5 moderate, 0 high].

In general, reliability of evaluations suffers unless pain provocation or pain history associated with the physical examination are taken into account [34-39]. In work on the cervical spine by Bertilson et al. [37], the awareness of complaint history enhanced reliability, measured by kappa, from 0.57 to 0.67 for evaluation of dermatomal sensitivity to pain, and from 0.4 to 0.49 for tenderness assessment. Cleland et al. [39] conducted a wide ranging study of reliability for history and physical findings related to neck pain. Categorical variables from the history that resulted in very good to excellent reliability ($0.72 \leq \kappa \leq 1.0$) included mode of onset, nature of symptoms, prior episodes, downward or upward looking, and sleeping postures aggravating symptoms. The inter-rater reliability of patient classification ranged from $0.68 \leq \kappa \leq 0.88$, with judgments made strictly from recorded data on forms showing the lower reliability [38]. Fortin [35], in a low quality study, looked at the validity of patients pointing and thereby localizing symptoms to the sacroiliac joint. Sixteen subjects received provocative joint injections. All were positive for local pain. A subset of 10 subjects was further evaluated for comorbid discogenic or zygapophyseal joint pain generators with negative results for these conditions.

Recommendation: Favourable, based on moderate quality evidence, for use of pain history to increase reliability of symptom provoking findings during the assessment of site to apply treatment.

Pain on provocation–tenderness

[Quality scores: Validity 0 low, 0 moderate, 5 high; Reliability 5 low, 7 moderate, 2 high].

The finding of tenderness connotes an unusual or increased sensitivity to pressure on palpation that localizes to the area examined. Where possible, the sensitivity of a site is evaluated by comparison to its contralateral asymptomatic counterpart. Twenty-two papers dealing with pain/tenderness on palpation were reviewed [33,40-50]. Bryner [43] used patient self-report of painful region as a reference standard to evaluate validity of examiner marked pain drawings for areas of tenderness to palpation. Sensitivity (0.73) and specificity (0.98) were excellent between the examiner and patient reports with respective positive (0.78) and negative (0.96) predictive values. Tenderness of the cervical articular pillars was evaluated

Table 5 Definitions for each of the possible types of recommendation

Recommendation	Description
Favourable	Favourable for general use by clinicians to determine site of care
Favourable with limitations	Favourable for determining site of care although limits exist such as number and quality of studies, limited generalizability, etc.
Unclear	Based on the evidence available, it is unclear whether or not this procedure should be recommended for use
Unfavourable with exceptions	Procedure is not recommended for general use but may be used in limited circumstances (e.g. other techniques unavailable.)
Unfavourable	Procedure is not recommended for use (limited number of studies, significant flaws in methods, not generalizable, high quality evidence against validity and/or reliability)

Table 6 Summary of recommendations for each category of evaluation method

Evaluation method			Summary	Quality of evidence	Recommendation
Complaint History			Gives context to the complaint and increases the reliability of the interpretation of physical findings.	Moderate	Favourable
Pain provocation					
		Tenderness	Localizes region/tissues of involvement	High	Favourable
		Orthopedic manoeuver	Pain with movement localizes region/tissue of involvement	High	Favourable
Asymmetry					
		Posture	Antalgia, kyphosis, lordosis, scoliosis	High	Favourable
			Localizing to site of care	High	Unfavourable
	Stiffness	Palpatory manual	Passive physiologic/accessory motion, joint springing, overpressure testing	High	Unclear
		Instrumented	Questions of generalizability	Low	Favourable with limitations
	Palpation	Static	Identifying major anatomical landmarks	High	Favourable with limitations
			Localizing to site of care	High	Unclear
		Motion	Enhanced if pain provocation present	High	Favourable with limitations
Leg Length Inequality			Pelvic assessment; method dependent	High	Favourable with limitations
Manual Muscle Testing			Strength grading to localize root involvement.	Moderate	Favourable
			Non-pathologic altered function	Moderate	Unfavourable
Range of motion			Localization to region	High	Favourable
Tissue temperature, texture, tone			Thermography/thermometry of the lower limb in confirming frank sciatica	High	Favourable
			Paraspinal skin temperature to locate site of care	High	Unfavourable
			Texture-skin rolling	Moderate	Favourable
Specialized Tests		Current Perception Threshold	Frank neuropathy with sensory deficit	High	Favourable
		Galvanic skin response	Localizing to site of care	Moderate	Unfavourable
		Surface EMG	Flexion-relaxation phenomenon to target lumbar region	High	Favourable
			Localizing to site of care	Moderate	Unfavourable
		Radiographic imaging	Localizing to site of care	High	Unfavourable
Integrated P.A.R.T.S. Montages			Localizing to site of care beyond individual component contributions	Moderate	Unclear

in patients with neck pain and in healthy controls by Sandmark and Nissel 1995 [45]. High sensitivity (0.82) and specificity (0.79), with moderate positive (0.62) and high negative (0.91) predictive values were found. Leboeuf-Yde et al. [48], in a high quality study, looked at tenderness of the spinous processes on percussion, finding tenderness to have low sensitivity (0.39) and positive predictive (0.41) values with high specificity (0.78) and negative predictive (0.78) values. Lundberg and Gerdle [47] found substantial agreement between abnormal passive mobility tests of the lower lumbar spine and segmental pain provocation tests at L4/5 (κ=0.71) and L5/S1 (κ=0.67), somewhat better than the results reported by Hicks et al. (2003) [57]. Inter-rater reliability was substantial (κ=0.68) among seven examiners of neck pain patients in the report by Hubka and Phelan [44]. For the thoracic spinal region [50,51] and rib cage, substantial ($0.62 \leq \kappa \leq 0.70$) and almost perfect ($\kappa$=0.88) inter-rater reliability were reported for tenderness to pressure on the spinous and transverse processes, respectively. Tender points in the anterior and posterior soft tissue compartments of the upper neck [46] showed moderate inter-rater agreement (κ = 0.45).

King et al. [52] investigated the validity of palpation for cervical facet joint pain using response to medial branch nerve blockade as the reference standard. Whereas preliminary work by Jull et al. [53] reported 100% sensitivity and near 100% specificity, King et al. reported that manual palpation provided high sensitivities (0.88–0.89) and low specificities (0.39–0.50) but with low likelihood ratios of 1.4 to 1.8. The most common joint involvements in this study were C2-3 and C5-6. The high prevalence of C2-3 and C5-6 lesions, consistent with other reports, erodes the sensitivity values, drawing into question the ability to localize pain to the zygapophyseal joint itself [47].

The study by Viikari-Juntura et al. [33] evaluated inter-rater reliability of examination findings in 52 neck pain patients referred for myelography. Pain response to pin prick had moderate agreement ($0.41 \leq \kappa \leq 0.51$), with change in light touch ($0.1 \leq \kappa \leq 0.6$) and palpatory tenderness ($0.24 \leq \kappa \leq 0.56$) rating only fair to moderate. The inter-rater reliability of localizing pain to the upper, mid and lower cervical spine gave moderate (κ=0.53) agreement in the report by Maigne et al. [54]. A positive, but low, correlation (r=0.35, p<0.007) was noted between the number of areas of tenderness and the patient's neck disability questionnaire scores. Agreement [54] for tenderness over neck muscle insertions ranged from fair (κ=0.33) to substantial (κ=0.62). Boline et al. [40,55] reported that pain on palpation over spinal/paraspinal osseous and soft tissue structures showed inter-rater reliability ($0.48 < \kappa < 0.90$) that was moderate to almost perfect in agreement.

Recommendation: Favourable, based on high quality evidence for validity and reliability of using tenderness to localize treatment.

Pain provocation by orthopedic maneouvres

[Quality scores: Validity 1 low, 0 moderate, 2 high; Reliability 11 low, 15 moderate, 5 high].

In terms of the quality of the evidence, two studies [48,56] evaluating validity were of high quality, while one was of low quality [57]. Eleven reliability studies [41,57-66] were ranked as being of low quality, fifteen were ranked as moderate quality [33,34,36,37,39,67-76] and five, three of which contained nested reliability studies, were ranked as high quality [54,77-80].

Leboeuf et al. [48], using low back pain symptom history as a gold standard, evaluated the validity of provocation of pain by movement and seated forced extension with added manual pressure. Ranges of sensitivity (0.22–0.44), specificity (0.98–1.0), and positive (0.86–1.0) and negative (0.77–0.82) predictive values were found, depending on the direction of movement. Forced extension was sensitive at 0.78 with specificity at 0.71, a positive predictive value of 0.52 and a negative predictive value at 0.89. Hicks et al. [74] found moderate to near perfect reliability for the findings considered to be related to instability, including i) a painful arc in flexion ($0.42 < \kappa < 0.77$) pain on return to upright posture ($0.42 < \kappa < 0.63$) and the prone instability test ($0.74 < \kappa < 1.00$).

Van Dillen et al. [36], in a reliability study using 5 examiners, looked at symptom behavior during various postural tasks involving standing, sitting, supine and prone recumbency, hook lying and quadraped kneeling. For all 28 items, kappa values for inter-examiner reliability were ≥ 0.75 when symptom response was included, but reduced to ≥ 0.40 without them. Maher and Adams [34] found similar results when 3 pairs of examiners assessed spinal segment stiffness manually. Intra-class correlation coefficients were higher ($0.67 \leq ICC \leq 0.72$) when pain provocation was considered, but dropped dramatically ($0.03 \leq ICC \leq 0.37$) when it was not. Symptom provoking movement assessments, in the work of Haswell et al. [56], showed a hierarchy of reliability with movements which they termed side-bending (κ = 0.6), flexion-side-bend rotation (κ = 0.39), side-bend rotation (κ = 0.29), extension side-bend rotation (κ = 0.29) and rotation (κ = 0.17). Inter-rater reliability between two examiners was assessed by McCombe et al. [41] for straight leg raising, in two separate groups of low back pain patients using a correlation model. The angular position of pain onset and the maximum tolerated pain both correlated strongly ($0.68 < r < 0.86$). Maigne et al. [54] found good inter-examiner reliability for pain with cervical flexion (κ = 0.71) and extension (κ = 0.76).

A series of studies has examined the validity and inter-rater reliability of provocative postural manoeuvres to classify patients into categories of mechanical versus non-mechanical back pain.

Laslett et al. [79] used provocative discography as a gold standard to evaluate the classification of patients by "centralization" of pain during the examination. Sensitivity, specificity, and positive likelihood ratios for centralization were 40%, 94%, and 6.9 respectively. Clare et al. [81] studied the construct validity of the predicted response of extension in groups classified by provocative maneouvre as mechanical derangement versus non-derangement. The global perceived effect was significantly higher ($p < 0.001$) after treatment in the derangement group.

Inter-rater agreement for classification of low back patients into the subgroups of mechanical back pain, overall, has been good. Razmjou et al. [75] found very good agreement on derangement subsyndromes with κ = 0.96. Inter-rater agreement for presence of lateral shift, relevance of lateral shift, relevance of lateral component, and deformity in the sagittal plane were κ = 0.52, 0.85, 0.95, and 1.00, respectively. Kilpikoski et al. [76] found that agreement on centralization and direction of preference for helpful movements were substantial ($0.7 < \kappa < 0.9$). Clare et al. [82] found nearly perfect reliability for classifying both low back patients (κ = 0.89) and neck pain patients (κ = 0.84).

Laslett et al. [78] and Laslett et al. [79,80] used criterion validity to evaluate a cluster of orthopedic manoeuvres for pain which was considered to arise from the sacro-iliac joint, contrasting these manoeuvres against pain relief from intra-articular joint anesthesia. The choice of manoeuvres was based on earlier literature [67]; Kokmeyer et al. [69] citing "acceptable" inter-rater reliability for iliac distraction, thigh thrust, Gaenslen's test, lateral recumbent iliac compression and prone sacral thrust. Using ROC curves they determined that, as a cluster, Gaenslen's tests did not contribute to increased accuracy. With two or more of the remaining tests positive, the cluster sensitivity was reported at 0.94 with a specificity of 0.78 and predictive values positive at 0.68 and negative at 0.96.

Leboeuf-Yde et al. [48] evaluated the "stork" (a.k.a. Gillet) test for sacroiliac motion during the standing leg lift maneuver with generally poor results (sensitivity = 0.41, specificity = 0.75, positive predictive value = 0.39 and negative predictive value = 0.56). Levangie [56], in a high quality study, assessed the relationship between four clinical tests for sacroiliac function (Gillet, standing flexion test, sitting flexion test, and the supine-to-sit test) and both objectively measured pelvic torsion and low back pain. She found very little concordance with each other in any of the tests or with low back pain with the exception of the Gillet test (likelihood ratio 4.57). However all four tests had low to moderate sensitivity (range, 0.08 to 0.44) and moderate to high specificity (range, 0.64 to 0.93) with only moderate predictive values (range, 0.28 to 0.78).

The study by Viikari-Juntura et al. [33], rated a moderate quality study, evaluated inter-rater reliability of examination findings in 52 neck pain patients referred for myelography. Neck compression orthopedic testing varied in reliability ($0.28 \leq \kappa \leq 0.77$) according to head position at the time of axial compression. The reliability of brachial plexus tension tests was fair ($\kappa = 0.35$) while that of shoulder abduction relief was slight to fair ($0.21 \leq \kappa \leq 0.40$) and reliability of relief of symptoms by cervical traction was moderate ($\kappa = 0.50$). McCombe et al. [41] found provocation with movement to be variable in reliability depending on the direction of movement ($0.1 \leq \kappa \leq 0.56$).

Recommendation: Favourable, with high quality evidence for both validity and reliability in use of orthopedic manoeuvres to narrow the region of interest for applying treatment. Evidence supports seated forced extension; pain on lumbar motion (side-bending > flexion side-bending rotation > side-bend rotation > extension side-bend-rotation > rotation); three or more sacroiliac manoeuvres (iliac distraction, thigh thrust, lateral recumbent iliac compression and prone sacral thrust); cervical compression and traction tests; and McKenzie manoeuvres including lateral shift, relevance of lateral shift, relevance of lateral component, and deformity in the sagittal plane. A painful arc in flexion and/or on return to upright posture and the prone instability test may suggest local instability.

Asymmetry

The assumptions of bilateral symmetry and some sort of structural and physiological axial pattern are common to a number of modes of patient examination. Absence of symmetry in some cases (e.g. scoliosis) is sufficient to result in a distinct diagnosis. In the majority of cases, however, it is the comparison from side-to-side or axially that is considered meaningful. In terms of assessment for localizing treatment to a specific site, the forms of examination involving symmetry include postural evaluation, palpation for stiffness of tissues/segments, static palpation of landmarks, segmental motion palpation, bilateral leg length measurement and manual muscle testing.

Postural assessment

[Quality scores: Validity 0 low, 0 moderate, 1 high; Reliability 5 low, 4 moderate, 0 high].

Examiners inspect the relative positions of body segments/landmarks with respect to each other and with respect to an idealized configuration. Methods include visual inspection, photography, radiography and palpation of surface landmarks with or without aids. Deviations are noted and tend to direct further investigation. Nine articles which satisfied the inclusion criteria addressed postural assessment [39,41,48,68,83-87].

In the report by Lebouef-Yde et al. [48], validity of antalgic posture was assessed through the capture of data on subjects with known histories of back pain ranging from none in their life time to one or more episodes across preceding intervals up to one year. Antalgia was low in sensitivity (0.11) and positive predictive value (0.18) but high in specificity (0.80) and negative predictive value (0.69). Lordosis measurement, as the distance from the point of maximum thoracic kyphosis to maximum sacral kyphosis, was assessed by McCombe et al. [41]. Pearson correlations were calculated on measures taken by two examiners ($0.67 < r < 0.7$) from two sets of low back pain patients. Cleland et al. [39] found that the inter-rater reliability for evaluation of hyperkyphosis above T6 was better ($0.69 < \kappa < 0.79$) than for hypokyphosis ($\kappa = 0.58$). Photographic assessment of body surface landmarks [87] determined by palpation through tight fitting clothing resulted in poor reliability for judgment of kyphosis ($\kappa = 0.441$) and lordosis ($\kappa = 0.327$), but good reliability for scoliosis ($\kappa = 0.769$). In the work by Normand et al. [86], three examiners used palpation independently to locate surface landmarks and to place reflective markers. ICCs were calculated with both a conservative and liberal approach. Three landmarks from different angles served as input to a commercial computer program (PosturePrint®) which evaluated displacements of the head, rib cage, and pelvis (in degrees of rotation or millimeters of translation) from a normal upright stance. Depending on the vagaries of ICC analysis, results ranged from good to excellent ($0.51 < ICC < 0.97$).

Leard et al. [87] assessed the reliability of 22 clinical measures related to posture, including some manoeuvres that would be regarded as orthopedic tests. Intra-class correlations were reported for quantitative measures and weighted kappas for qualitative measures. Two clinicians, using a palpation meter (PALMeter™), produced ICCs ≥ 0.997 in measuring intra-rater reliability for sagittal pelvic inclination and ≥ 0.9661 for inter-rater reliability. Frontal plane inclination, however, had very low inter-rater reliability, with ICCs of approximately zero. Piva et al. [85] also looked at the iliac crest level in the frontal plane (i.e., pelvic obliquity) using a caliper mounted inclinometer. ICCs in their study were much higher than those of Leard et al. [87] 0.80 and 0.73 for standing and sitting, respectively.

French et al. [68] monitored the reliability of 5 examiners with respect to their conclusions as to the necessity to treat at a given site. A cluster of exam methods included postural inspection, patient self-report of pain characteristics, leg length assessment, motion and static palpation of the spine, as well as neurologic and orthopedic tests chosen at their discretion. Unfortunately, no breakdown of the analysis was reported by examination method. The yield in pooled reliability, for the cluster as a whole across the extent of the spinal column was only fair ($\kappa = 0.27$).

Cowherd et al. [83] attempted a criterion related validity study of common postural indices from digitized surface landmarks during erect stance using a triaxial, digitizing goniometer (Metrecom™). Results were compared to radiographs taken without changing position. While a stronger analysis would use an ICC, correlation of measures between the postural analysis and the radiographs showed only a weak association with significant ($p<0.001$) differences suggesting large offsets between the measures.

Recommendation: High quality evidence is favorable with limitations to the specificity of antalgia and reliability of postural assessment for kyphosis, lordosis and scoliosis. The evidence is unfavourable for the use of postural analysis to determine the local site of care.

Palpatory stiffness

During the process of tissue palpation, the examiner attempts to assess the relative stiffness (conversely, compliance) to postural or applied load to a segment. Recent work in biomechanics has shown that the paraspinal soft tissues, particularly the multifidus muscles, differ in transverse stiffness based on patient posture and clinical state. Using the effective Young's modulus, a direct measure of stiffness of the muscle estimated by force-deformation data from ultrasound elastography, Chan et al. [88] found a 50% to 300% increase ($p<0.001$) in elastic modulus depending on posture (prone, standing, 25° and 45° flexion). Similarly, with the exception of prone recumbency, chronic back pain patients showed a higher modulus than healthy subjects. The difference decreases with increased flexion, ranging from 30% to 14% in the mean. Effective spinal stiffness was similarly evaluated by Fritz et al. [89] before and after manipulation therapy. Improvements in self-reported disability correlated with decreases in stiffness ($0.01 \leq p \leq 0.025$). In parallel work [90], multifidus thickening was observed. Their results raise a question as to the interpretation of multifidus thickness, since 53.4% of subjects increased muscle dimension while 46.6% decreased after treatment.

The challenge that paraspinal stiffness poses to the clinician is finding evaluation methods that are able to discern these changes across the spectrum of disease and across the multiple spinal regions beyond the low back. Studies meeting the inclusion criteria fell into two categories, those that used manually applied forces and those using instrumentation.

Stiffness- manual assessment

[Quality scores: Validity 0 low, 1 moderate, 3 high; Reliability 1 low, 8 moderate, 1 high].

Thirteen studies used manual assessment to evaluate segmental stiffness/mobility. The works of Abbott and Mercer [77], a high quality study, and Fernandez-de-las-Pinas et al. [91], a moderate quality study, both examined the validity of assessing hypomobility. Two high quality [42,92] studies and five moderate quality studies [34,39,93-95] and one low quality study [96] evaluated PA pressure or springing tests in the thoracic/lumbar spine, while evidence from two moderate quality studies [46,97] and one low quality study addressed the neck region [49].

Patients and healthy subjects were evaluated by four examiners using observation of active and abnormal ranges of motion, and motion palpation manoeuvres to assess for passive physiological intervertebral motion (PPIVM) and passive accessory intervertebral motion (PAIVM). Sensitivity ranged from 42% to 75%, while sensitivity was 35% to 89% [77]. Radiographic measures of segmental displacement on flexion/extension x-rays of the same subjects revealed that the number of segments falling more than 2 standard deviations below the mean of normal subjects is much higher in low back pain subjects than expected ($\chi2$, $p<0.001$). Fernandez-de-las-Pinas et al.

[91] evaluated manual lateral glide stiffness compared to intervertebral radiological motion in lateral bending. Radiologically visualized intervertebral motion on the hypomobile side (mean 19.1 mm, SD 2.1 mm) was 3.44 mm ± 1.9 mm less than on the contralateral side (mean 22.6 mm, SD 2.5 mm) with $p = .002$ by Wilcoxon rank test.

Taylor et al. [42] evaluated prone joint springing for fixation in the thoracic spine and found a moderate agreement ($\kappa = 0.48$) with tenderness on skin rolling to determine spinal joint dysfunction within one vertebrae above or below the level of the tender point. In a report by Downey et al. [92], three pairs of examiners attempted to identify the symptomatic segment through posterior-to-anterior pressures. While examiners showed fair agreement ($\kappa = 0.37$) in locating segments (± 1 segment), they were less reliable in agreeing on the name of the segment ($\kappa = 0.09$), introducing an alternative source of error. Agreement of thoracic springing with provocation of pain was fair to moderate in the work of Cleland et al. [39], depending on spinal level. Similarly, inter-rater reliability ranged from fair to substantial [39,94], with symptomatic subjects producing more reliable responses ($\kappa \geq 0.6$) [95]. Maher and Adams [34] found manual spinal segment stiffness intra-class correlation coefficients higher ($0.67 \leq ICC \leq 0.72$) when pain provocation was considered, but dropped dramatically ($0.03 \leq ICC \leq 0.37$) without pain provocation.

Studies of palpation of the cervical spine are less common. The work by Hanten et al. [49], a lower quality study, used subjects who met the International Headache Society criteria for cervicogenic headache. A panel of 15 cervical mobility and palpation tests was studied for reliability using two examiners. The inter-rater agreement for tests that exceeded $\kappa > 0.50$ included: cervical protraction and retraction, both with and without overpressure, and pressure sensitivity paraspinally at C1 and C2. The mean number of positive findings per subject was 3.50, with a Spearman rho =0.943 over two days of testing. However, mixed results were described for overpressure testing ($-0.09 \leq \kappa \leq 0.46$) by others [97]. Comeaux et al. [93] and McPartland and Goodridge [46] found cervical stiffness testing to have fair to moderate in reliability.

Recommendation: Unclear–high quality evidence suggests moderate validity for the concept of intersegmental restrictions. There is a mix of studies reporting low to substantial reliability for manually locating a site within one segment.

Stiffness- instrumented

[Quality scores: Validity 0 low, 0 moderate, 0 high; Reliability 2 low, 1 moderate, 0 high].

Few mechanized methods for evaluation of stiffness are accessible in general practice. Three studies [98-100] investigated the usefulness of identifying joint stiffness by instrumentation to locate the site of care. The work of Latimer et al. [100], with a laboratory based instrument, is notable as it observes that the level of stiffness detected is a function of magnitude of the application force. Similarly, the more stable measures of effective stiffness arise from applied forces above 50 N (11.25 lbs).

Leach et al. [98], in a study ranked as being of moderate quality, measured inter- and intra-examiner reliability using a commercially available instrument (Pulstar™) which provides impulse force to the spine above the 50 N threshold for stable measures. Two examiners evaluated 18 healthy 20-to-25 year old subjects for patterns of stiffness along the spine. Good agreement was observed in the pattern of stiffness measures along the length of the spinal column. Inter-examiner ICC=0.87 while intra-examiner findings were 0.78 and 0.89 yielding good to excellent results for reliability.

The work of Owens et al. [99] was rated as low quality evidence. Using a custom built device, posterior-to-anterior spinal stiffness of the lumbar spinal segments was assessed by 9 examiners in low back pain patients. The ICC for inter-rater reliability was very good at 0.79. A quantitative stiffness value of 11.2 N/mm (±3.5) was found, although no differences between segments or comparisons with healthy subjects were available.

Recommendation: Favorable with limitations based on low quality evidence. Limitations are based on instrument availability and uncertainty concerning the generalizability of results to the broader population.

Static palpation

[Quality scores: Validity 0 low, 0 moderate, 2 high; Reliability 4 low, 7 moderate, 4 high].

The identification and evaluation of relative position of topographical or percutaneous landmarks has long been a part of health care practice. Of the six high quality studies, two evaluated validity [101,102] and four assessed reliability [103-106]. Seven more moderate quality studies [94,107-112] and four low quality studies [113-116] also addressed reliability.

The work of Jende and Peterson [101] utilized what may be termed a 'proof-by-contradiction' approach to evaluate seated palpation of C1. Posing an alternative explanation for palpatory prominence as originating from osseous asymmetry (±2 mm), the authors compared the lateral prominence of C1 on palpation in 47 patients against radiographic measures. The ICC for repeated measure of atlas transverse length on x-ray was 0.93. In 57% of cases with laterality on palpation, radiographic measures were equal or more prominent on the opposite side, suggesting that palpatory laterality was not due to an anatomical variant. Unfortunately, no clinical information was reported.

The validity and reliability of locating spinal levels and pelvic landmarks have been reported in six studies [102,108,109,111,112,116] using various means including radiographs to quantify site identification error. Examiners differed in localization of landmarks across a range from 0.5 cm to 2.5 cm, ($0.28 \le \kappa \le 0.98$), often reporting findings from adjacent segments.

Fryer et al. [104] evaluated the intra-examiner and inter-examiner reliability of trained and untrained osteopathic students palpating symmetry in anatomical landmarks (anterior and posterior superior iliac spines (ASIS and PSIS), medial malleoli, sacral inferior lateral angle (SILA) and performing the seated flexion test (SFL). Inter-examiner agreements (kappa scores) for the trained versus untrained examiners were: medial malleoli, 0.31 vs 0.28; ASIS, 0.24 vs –0.01; SFT, 0.14 vs 0.07; PSIS 0.08 vs 0.15; SILA 0.04 vs –0.01. Others [106,115] have followed similar protocols with essentially the same results. Holmgren and Waling [105] and Binkley et al. [107] explored inter-examiner reliability for identifying segmental levels ($-0.03 \le \kappa \le 0.69$, across studies), with comparable results. The prone posture was shown as the more reliable patient positioning for locating spinous processes (inter-examiner agreement $69 < \kappa < 81$) by Byfield and Humphreys [114].

Special cases of static palpatory findings have been studied by others [94,103,110]. In a high quality study, intra-examiner agreement on skin fold thickness and compliance were mixed ($-.41 \le \kappa \le .23$; $0.25 \le ICC \le 0.28$) [96]. Similar results were found by Moran and Gibbons [110] in evaluating ICCs for cranial rhythmic impulses. Conversely, agreement on the identification of the piriformis muscle and iliolumbar ligaments has been reported as substantial ($0.61 < \kappa < 0.87$).

Recommendation: Based on high quality evidence, the validity of palpation for localizing the site of care is unclear. A recommendation of favorable with limitations, depending upon the target structure, is made for reliability in localizing common anatomical landmarks.

Motion palpation

[Quality scores: Validity 1 low, 0 moderate, 8 high; Reliability 8 low, 9 moderate, 11 high].

The underlying premise of motion palpation, particularly with segmental dysfunction of the spine, is that there may be abnormal patterns in relative motion. That the response to manipulation may be related to the degree to which segments are more or less stiff has been shown by Fritz et al. [89]. Motion palpation uses examiner guided motions to manually monitor the relative displacement of bony landmarks through the skin surface. Motions are categorized as being limited/restricted; excessive/unstable or aberrant, suggesting a deviation in path at some point within the range of motion.

Nine studies have assessed validity of motion palpation alone [89,117-121], twenty-five studies have assessed reliability alone [47,50,72,74,104,107,122-139], and three studies have assessed both reliability and validity [140-142].

Humphreys et al. [120] evaluated motion palpation in asymptomatic volunteers with congenital block vertebrae (C2-3 or C5-6) in the cervical spine. Substantial overall agreement (C2-3, $\kappa = 0.65$; C5-6, $\kappa = 0.76$) was found for identification of the site of greatest hypomobility. Sensitivity ranged from 55% to 78%, greater for the C2-3 level, with specificity that was high (91–98%) for both. Ogince et al. [121] assessed cervicogenic headache patients and asymptomatic controls for C1/2 dysfunction using seated flexion-rotation tests. Blinded examiners identified dysfunction with 91% sensitivity and 90% specificity. Abbott et al. [118] tested the validity of passive physiologic intervertebral motion (PPIVM) of the lumbar spine in recurrent/chronic low back pain patients. Flexion/extension movement of vertebral segments, induced by flexion of the thigh on the pelvis in a side-lying posture, was compared to flexion/extension radiographs. Abnormal motion was defined as a range of normalized movement (segment range/region range) beyond 2 standard deviations (+/–) for a given level in comparison to a sample of healthy subjects. Inter-rater reliability of the radiographic measures, to set the gold standard, ranged between $0.83 \le ICC \le 0.99$). Motion palpation was highly specific (99.5%) for increased translation but was very poor for sensitivity (5%). Likelihood ratios (7.1) for low back pain were significant only for translation in extension.

Landel et al. [119] evaluated a slow application of posterior-to-anterior force to the lumbar spine under MRI imaging, and separately by two examiners, attempting to localize the least and most flexible segments. The study reported substantial and fair inter-examiner reliability of the least ($\kappa = 0.71$) and most ($\kappa = 0.29$) mobile segments, respectively. Similarly, Abbott et al. [118] looked at posterior-to-anterior translation in response to pressure, with flexion and extension x-rays as the gold standard. Translation was found to be significantly associated with recurrent/chronic low back pain ($p < 0.05$), with specificity of 89% but poor sensitivity of 29%. Subjects with a positive test had a likelihood ratio of 2.52. The opposite conclusion was found for flexion where specificity was high (99.5%) but sensitivity was low (5%).

Using lateral recumbent patient posture during tests for passive intersegmental motion, the agreement between abnormal flexibilities and pain provocation at the same level was substantial ($0.67 < \kappa < 0.71$) for Lundberg and Gerdle [47]. Inter-rater reliability for abnormal motions alone was moderate to substantial ($0.59 < \kappa < 0.75$). Phillips and Twomey [142], rated as high quality evidence, compared analysis of lumbar passive segmental movement, coupled with pain provocation response, and results from anesthetic blocks obtained retrospectively in one group and prospectively in another. Sensitivity was 60%, with specificity of 100% in the retrospective group, and 94% sensitivity with 100% specificity in the prospective group. Others have had much less promising results.

Reliability results for motion palpation, absent a gold standard, have been inconsistent. Three studies reported moderate agreement ($\kappa \geq 0.40$) and three reported fair agreement ($\kappa < 0.40$). Haas et al. [126] evaluated manual end-play palpation of the thoracic spine and found a moderate intra-examiner reliability ($\kappa = 0.5$) but only slight inter-examiner reliability ($\kappa = 0.14$). Christensen et al. [50], Brismee et al. [132,140] and Smedmark et al. [129] reported fair ($0.22 \leq \kappa \leq 0.24$) [50] to substantial agreement ($\kappa \leq 0.65$) [132,140]. Others [74,107,117,132,141] have had less impressive outcomes, with mixed agreements on passive segmental flexibility ($-0.02 \leq \kappa \leq 0.26$, across studies) in the prone position. In asymptomatic subjects [125] agreement between examiners of the cervical spine has been no greater than chance.

Qvistgaard et al. [136] assessed both the intra and inter-examiner reliability of two experts using the stork test, pelvic girdle rotation, and the lumbar spring test to identify dysfunctional lumbar spinal levels. The study considered two definitions of reliability; perfect match (PER) defined as positive results on the same segmental level, and acceptable match (ACC) defined as positive results within one segmental level. The study found moderate and substantial levels of intra-examiner reliability (PER, $\kappa = 0.60$; ACC, $\kappa = 0.70$) with fair and moderate levels of inter-examiner reliability (PER, $\kappa = 0.21$; ACC, $\kappa = 0.57$). The work of Love [123] and Mootz et al. [124] indicated only chance agreement.

Robinson et al. [137] found near perfect inter-examiner reliability among expert examiners assessing passive sacroiliac joint play ($0.78 \leq \kappa \leq 0.88$). Similar results were obtained by Hungerford et al. [135] ($0.67 \leq \kappa \leq 0.77$). In contrast, Schneider et al. [138] reported mixed results ($-0.17 \leq \kappa \leq 0.17$) for two experts utilizing a segmental mobility test to assess normal or restricted mobility across the lumbar spine and sacroiliac joints. Fryer et al. [104] looked at the seated flexion test for sacroiliac fixation finding slight levels of inter-examiner reliability ($\kappa = 0.14$). Vincent-Smith and Gibbons [128] had better results with the standing flexion test ($\kappa = 0.052$). Arab et al. [72] constructed composite tests from motion palpation (standing flexion, seated flexion, Gillet, prone knee flexion test, leg length) and provocation manoeuvres (Patrick-Fabre, thigh thrust, resisted abduction). With positive findings on three or more of the palpation tests and two or more of the provocation manoeuvres, the inter-examiner agreement was substantial to excellent (prevalence-adjusted and bias-adjusted kappa; $0.52 \leq \kappa \leq 0.92$). Meijne et al. [127], Tong et al. [133] and Carmichael [122] found the same manoeuvres individually less reliable ($-0.32 \leq \kappa \leq 0.27$, across studies).

A few investigators have attempted to identify procedural characteristics that improve inter-rater reliability. Marcotte et al. [130] suggest that the orientation of the examination input force, but not amplitude of force [131] may increase reliability (from $\kappa = 0.34$ to $\kappa = 0.68$). Cooperstein et al. [139] found that high examiner confidence raises agreement to $\kappa = 0.82$.

Recommendation: Favorable with limitations (region of the spine, direction of movement and method employed), based on high quality evidence for both validity and reliability for use in localizing the site of care.

Leg length inequality (LLI)

[Quality scores: Validity 1 low, 1 moderate, 4 high; Reliability 6 low, 4 moderate, 6 high].

Much attention has been given to the question of relative leg length and change in apparent relative leg length as an indicator for site of treatment. Six articles pertaining to the validity of measures of LLI [143-148] and fourteen articles pertaining to the reliability of LLI assessment [106,108,148-159] were retrieved and reviewed. Most of the studies assessed LLI with the subject in the prone position, but some had subjects in the standing or supine position.

The construct validity for an etiological role of LLI in lower quadrant and low back dysfunction is controversial. Motion, alignment and muscular endurance of the low back and pelvis are altered in the presence of leg length differences [160], yet cross-sectional studies [160-162] fail to show a relationship between LBP and LLI alone. At the same time, in a 4 year prospective study of 136 students, Twellaar et al. [161] found pelvic obliquity to be associated with injury rates including backache. Knutson [146] measured leg length inequality among selected volunteers who were partitioned according to their history of recurring low back pain. Pain scales were higher ($p < 0.001$) in subjects with length asymmetry, with sensitivity of 87% and specificity of 84%.

Petrone et al. [148] found similar validity and reliability of standing evaluations using the PALM™ assessment of iliac crest level using a gold standard of standing pelvic radiographs with the central ray at the level of the femoral heads. The ICC for inter-rater reliability was 0.97. The agreement between tape measure assessment (ASIS to the medial malleoli and scanogram) fared less well with $0.359 \leq ICC \leq 0.770$.

Hinson et al. [152], Woodfield et al. [159], Kmita and Lucas [106], and Fryer [156] found supine visual leg checks to show varying degrees of inter-examiner reliability. Cooperstein et al. [163] evaluated the validity and reliability of prone compressive leg length assessment using standardized foot wear containing shims of various thicknesses in one shoe. Artificial leg length differences over 3.7 mm were reliably identified with an intra-examiner ICC of 0.85. Fuhr and Osterbauer [149], Nguyen et al. [153], Schneider et al. [157], and Holt et al. [158] used prone compressive leg length estimates of volunteers, finding substantial reliability ($0.65 \leq \kappa \leq. 0.70$).

Some clinicians follow prone compressive leg length checks with knee flexion to 90 degrees in order to reveal change in relative length. Schneider et al. [157] found this maneuver to result in a high prevalence (95%) of increased length on the short leg side, confounding calculation of the kappa statistic. Holt et al. [158] were able to define reliability with knee flexion at $\kappa = 0.65$. Low level evidence from Eriksen [145] examined change in leg length with specific challenge to a vertebral level on an unspecified number of subjects. Of 18 variables, only one had a notable concordance ($\kappa < 0.40$) between the change in LLI and x-ray findings.

Blocking methods insert varying sized blocks/lifts under the feet to level the standing pelvis or to simulate LLI. The method investigated by Gross et al. [151] was less accurate (±0.46 cm) and of lower inter-rater reliability (ICC=0.77) than prone compression or the PALM™ method. Hanada et al. 2001 [154] found nearly identical results, comparing block height with scanogram measures. Gibbons et al. [155] assessed the ability of examiners to palpate the iliac crest levels on subjects who had an artificially created asymmetry in standing leg length, finding that they were unable to reliably detect discrepancies of 1 cm or less.

Three reports were identified which met the inclusion criteria and specifically addressed the question of leg length as an indicator for the site of care. Montgomery et al. [144], in a low quality validity study, reported substantial agreement ($\kappa = 0.664$) between palpatory findings of unilateral sacral prominence suggestive of pelvic torsion and radiographic findings of leg length difference. Using variants in positioning of the extremities and head, leg length has been offered as a means to identify the site for necessary care. Younqvist et al. [150] evaluated this maneuver for the C1 segment, reporting a $\kappa = 0.52$. In contrast, Schneider et al. [157] evaluated head positioning in subjects with leg length difference ≤ 0.25 inch with mixed, but poor reliability ($-0.02 \leq \kappa \leq 0.04$).

Recommendation: Favorable with limitations for assessing the pelvis, based on high quality studies. Validity for relationship to symptoms has not been demonstrated. Reliability appears method-dependent.

Manual muscle testing

[Quality scores: Validity 1 low, 0 moderate, 1 high; Reliability 3 low, 3 moderate, 1 high].

Manual examination of the capacity to produce powerful contraction by muscle is a classical part of the examination for neuromotor control. Traditionally, it has been used as a graded system [164] of testing individual or isolated groups of muscles related to a specific function (e.g. deltoid for abduction). In this role, muscle testing may provide information consistent with the myotomal connections, potentially indicating nerve root involvement. Its use has been extended from assessing frank neuromuscular pathology to determination altered function which is not necessarily pathological [165-167].

Nine papers were identified within the inclusion criteria [33,39,41,165,167-171].

Used to grade strength, McCombe et al. [41] found inter-rater reliability for motor power in the lower extremities was substantial to perfect ($0.65 \leq \kappa \leq 1.0$) for one pair of examiners, but only poor to moderate ($0.02 \leq \kappa \leq 0.35$) for another pair. The study by Viikari-Juntura et al. [33] in neck pain patients, found agreement on muscle atrophy was fair to substantial ($0.35 \leq \kappa \leq 0.81$) while reliability for grading muscle strength was moderate to substantial ($0.40 \leq \kappa \leq 0.64$). Cleland et al. [39], in a limited sample of muscle tests, found inter-rater agreement to vary depending on the muscle being tested, with overall agreement ranging from 41% to 91%.

Used as an indicator of altered function, not necessarily pathological, the validity of muscle testing was evaluated by Ludtke et al. [170] in a double blind study with 4 examiners using 7 volunteers with confirmed allergy (IgE production) to wasp venom. The venom or a saline solution vial was randomly placed below the umbilicus, and change in muscle strength (anterior deltoid) was evaluated. The correct assessments of placebo versus allergen were 60% and 40%, respectively. Inter-rater reliability overall was $\kappa = -0.01$, suggesting less than chance agreement. Calderon and Lawson [165] found a highly mixed inter-rater reliability, based on which muscle was being isolated for testing ($-0.07 < \kappa < 0.90$). The same data was replicated (for purposes of this report, scored only once) in a publication under Lawson and Calderon [166]. Patient initiated strength by dynamometry [168] has been shown to have substantial reliability ($\kappa = 0.96$–0.99) whereas doctor initiated testing showed lower reliability ($\kappa = 0.55$–0.76). Haas et al. [169] evaluated the reliability of muscle testing in response to a provocative challenge attempting to localize the vertebral site needing treatment in both symptomatic and asymptomatic subjects. A 5 kg force directed to produce rotational stress was applied to thoracic spinous processes, preceded and followed by a manual muscle test of the strength in the piriformis muscle. Inter-rater reliability approached zero ($\kappa = -0.04$, symptomatic; $\kappa = -0.02$, asymptomatic) indicating agreement by chance alone. Caruso and Leisman [171], in a low quality study, suggest that accuracy in functional muscle testing improves with years of clinical experience. While reliability was claimed, no kappa or ICC values were presented.

Pollard et al. [167] took a novel approach asking whether a change in muscle strength (deltoid) following identification of palpatory tenderness over the lower right quadrant (ileocecal valve/McBurney's point) may be related to the presence of low back pain. While one cell of the 2x2 table was underpopulated, the authors calculated a sensitivity of 0.86 and specificity of 0.97.

Recommendation: Favorable, with a moderate level of evidence, for strength grading to localize nerve/nerve root levels. Unfavorable as a diagnostic indicator of non-pathological altered function leading to localizing site of care.

Range of motion

[Quality scores: Validity 1 low, 0 moderate, 3 high; Reliability 12 low, 8 moderate, 2 high].

Many studies have investigated range of motion in healthy and unhealthy subjects. Five high quality studies [54,172-175], eight moderate quality studies [33,39,97,111,176-179] and twelve low quality studies [41,180-190] which met the inclusion criteria for this review were identified. Four assessed validity [48,172,175,182] and the others assessed reliability.

The construct validity of reduced range of motion in painful disorders has been examined by several groups. Viitanen et al. [172] correlated different spinal ranges of motion (ROM) and the results of 17 repeated tests with spinal radiological changes in 52 male patients with ankylosing spondylitis. Inter-rater reliability on motion measures was good to excellent ($0.84 \le ICC \le 0.98$). Osterbauer et al. [182] measured kinematic parameters of head motion during tracking tasks (flexion, extension, etc.), and cervical ROM was measured via a head mounted optoelectronic inclinometer. Pain and disability were assessed via the neck disability index questionnaire and visual analog pain scale. A scoring system of kinematic abnormalities was created ranging from 0 to 3. A cutoff of ≥ 0.5 correctly identified the greatest number of subjects and minimized false positives (sensitivity 77%, specificity 82%, likelihood ratio 4.5). ROM performed similarly well at a cutoff of 1 SD below the normative mean (sensitivity 77%, specificity 84%, likelihood ratio 3.9). Hall and Robinson [177] also found a strong correlation ($r = 0.8$) between severity of headache and restriction, with excellent reliability ($0.92 \le ICC \le 0.99$) in measuring neck motion. Mayer et al. [182] examined reliability and responsiveness of inclinometric measures of rigidity at intervertebral levels during lumbar flexion/extension and lateral bending in seventy chronic low back pain patients. Four had measurable rigidity at one level, thirty-six at two, and thirty at three levels. Repeatability was assessed, with high correlation in flexion/extension ($0.90 < r < 0.97$, $p < 0.01$) and moderate correlation for lateral bending ($0.65 < r < 0.95$, $p < 0.05$). Patients were assigned to one of two treatment groups: exercise only, or exercise with localized joint anesthesia. Pain intensity (VAS) and ROM improved with treatment and patients who received joint anesthesia showed greater improvements in ROM. Leboeuf-Yde and colleagues [48] evaluated the range of motion in 166 individuals, 46 of whom had never had low back pain, 18 of whom had pain on the day of examination, the remainder having had a history of pain sometime within the past year. Sensitivity for "low back pain today" was low, ranging from 22% to 44% in a hierarchy of rotation < flexion < side bending < extension. Specificity fared better (range 98% to 100%) with side bending < extension = flexion = rotation. All tests reported high levels of positive predictive value (range= 86%-100%) and negative predictive value (range= 77%-90%). A novel description of the quality of movement, "gearbox flexion" denoting an uneven path of motion, was evaluated. This type of movement was highly specific (1.0), with strong positive (1.0) and negative (0.73) predictive values, although the finding had very low prevalence.

Goniometric devices of several kinds have been studied [111,175,180,182-186,188,190]. These devices include gravity and electronic goniometers, optoelectronic monitoring of body markers and tape measure approaches. In general, the reliability of measures has been good to excellent ($0.72 \le ICC \le 0.995$). Several special circumstances have been noted with range of motion measures. Haynes et al. [186] observed degradation in repeated measures with forward head tilt of up to 10 degrees. Lateral neck flexion was only fair in agreement for Hoppenbrouwers et al. [178]. Using a tape measure [41,172,190] to monitor landmark displacements is comparable to goniometry in reliability. Whether active or passive neck ROM is measured, extension may be more reliable ($\kappa \ge 0.85$) than flexion ($\kappa \ge 0.33$). Piva et al. 2006 [85] found substantial and almost perfect levels of inter-examiner reliability ($0.78 \le \kappa \le 0.94$) in examining the neck, while Viikari-Juntura et al. [33] reported lower levels of reliability ($0.40 \le \kappa \le 0.56$). Also for the neck, Cleland et al. [39] showed good reliability ($0.57 < ICC < 0.78$) for measuring range of motion, and moderate to substantial kappa agreement in eliciting self-report of symptom aggravation with specific motions. Maigne et al. [54] found moderate agreement ($\kappa = 0.57$) when examiners classified patients as being slightly, moderately or severely restricted.

Recommendation: Favourable for use to localize the site of treatment within a spinal region, based on high quality evidence for validity and reliability.

Tissue temperature, texture, and tone

[Quality scores: Validity 0 low, 0 moderate, 5 high; Reliability 5 low, 4 moderate, 4 high].

Modern thermography uses infrared sensing devices to evaluate the relative levels of heat emitted through the skin, while thermometry uses direct skin contact via thermocouples. The temperature of tissues is determined by a number of factors, including metabolic activity, perfusion and environmental temperature. Two papers [191,192] suggest that while thermometry may provide valid measures of skin temperature, stringent environmental control is necessary to achieve stable readings. Readings are perturbed by the skin contact accompanying spinal manipulation, at least with instrumented methods, and the responses to manipulation are multiphasic, confounding interpretation.

Four additional studies met the inclusion criteria for examining the validity of skin temperature [193-196] to identify the site for application of treatment. Chafetz et al. [193] evaluated a small sample of patients with confirmed L4/5, L5/S1 root distortion on CT scans versus healthy controls. The authors reported specificity of 60% and sensitivity of 100% in thermographic results. McCulloch et al. [194], in somewhat larger groups, reported sensitivities for two examiners at 60% and 50%, and specificities at 45% and 48%, using patients with clinical sciatica, and CT or MRI results as the gold standard. More recently, Zaproudina et al. [196] evaluated the side-to-side differences in temperature of the plantar surface in chronic low back pain patients. Differences were observed between patients with low back pain only versus those with referred leg pain (Mann–Whitney test $p < 0.05$). The severity of Oswestry scores for current LBP disability level correlated with the magnitude of temperature differences with coefficients of correlation of 0.502 ($p = .000$). There were also correlations between magnitude of temperature asymmetry and both straight leg raise ($p < 0.005$) and side bending motion ($p < 0.05$). A study which was ranked as providing low quality evidence [195] reported poor to moderate correlation between thermography and palpatory findings of segmental restrictions, defined by tenderness, positive skin rolling and motion palpation.

Plaugher et al. [197] which was ranked as providing high quality evidence, reported inter-examiner reliability ranging from slight to substantial ($0.03 \leq \kappa \leq 0.65$) and fair to substantial intra-examiner reliability ($0.03 \leq \kappa \leq 0.66$,) depending upon the region of spine. Two other studies, ranked respectively as of moderate [40] and low quality [55] found slight to moderate agreement ($0.0 < \kappa < 0.63$) of paraspinal skin temperature measures. Hart et al. [198] attempted reliability testing with 10 minute intervals between samples with good ICCs of > 0.75, while Owens et al. [199] reported excellent ICCs using a handheld thermographic device ($0.918 < ICC < 0.975$). The inter-rater reliability of mastoid fossa temperature measurement was also good ($0.671 < ICC < 0.748$) [200]. Finally, Owens et al. [199] were able to obtain excellent reliability when repeated measures were obtained over 3 minute intervals.

Five papers evaluated tissue texture assessment. Differences in response to skin rolling have been claimed to be a function of surface/subsurface texture (e.g. Diakow et al. [195]). Tests using skin rolling, however, do not have any independent measure of texture. In a variation of classical palpation, a high quality paper compared pain production on skin rolling with pressure algometry readings. A highly significant ($p < 0.0005$) decrease in pain threshold tolerance at the level of tenderness on skin rolling was found in comparison to non-tender control points in the thoracic spine [42]. Degenhardt et al. [201] defined a positive test for tissue texture as the presence of localized edema or fibrotic changes. After an interval of consensus training for 2 examiners, agreement on tissue texture was moderate (κ=0.45). McPartland and Goodridge [46] used palpatory sense of 'fullness' over articulations of the upper cervical spine, rated on a 10 point scale, with only slight agreement (κ =0.19) but had a low prevalence which may have artificially reduced the kappa score. A more clear definition of texture was given by Paulet and Fryer [202] as an abnormal hardness, bogginess, or ropiness of the underlying paraspinal muscles. Inter-examiner agreement for the site with the most marked tissue texture changes was fair (k = 0.26).

Recommendation: The evidence from studies with high validity and reliability is favorable for the use of thermography/thermometry of the lower limb in confirming frank sciatica. The evidence from high quality studies is unfavourable toward the use of paraspinal skin temperature measures to locate the site of care, due to limited reliability. Evidence of moderate quality is favourable toward the use of skin rolling and palpatory assessment of tissue texture, although the relationship of skin rolling to tissue texture is uncertain.

Specialized tests

Current perception threshold

[Quality scores: Validity 0 low, 1 moderate, 2 high; Reliability 0 low, 2 moderate, 0 high].

Current perception threshold (CPT) is a measure of peripheral sensory nerve sensitivity to surface electrical stimulation and was introduced by Rendell et al. [203] in the management of diabetic sensory neuropathy. Segmental specificity of CPT for lumbar radiculopathy was validated by Yamashita et al. [204] and Imoto et al. [205]. Tests demonstrated significant differences ($p<0.01$) in sensory function between healthy volunteers and patients with unilateral disc herniation confirmed by magnetic resonance imaging and pain within the distribution of the corresponding lumbar nerve root (L5 or S1). Attesting to the validity of CPT in identifying the level of neuropathy, Imoto et al. [205] demonstrated that following microdiscectomy, 66% of cases showed significant improvement in CPT ($p<0.05$), along with symptomatic improvement. Patients who did not show improvement in symptomatology, as a cohort, did not show any significant change in CPT.

Recommendation: High quality evidence is favourable for the validity of using CPT to identify the segmental level of frank neuropathy. No evidence which met our inclusion criteria addresses the validity or reliability of CPT in otherwise localizing the site for manual treatment.

Galvanic skin response

[Quality scores: Validity 0 low, 1 moderate, 0 high; Reliability 1 low, 0 moderate, 0 high]

Galvanic skin response (GSR) is the measure of electrical conductance of the skin and in the short term is most strongly influenced by the rate of sweat secretion, since higher moisture content improves electrical conductance. Because sweat secretion is modulated by the sympathetic nervous system, GSR has sometimes been used as an indirect measure of changes in sympathetic nervous system activity, as for example occurs in some instances of psychological or physiological stress. Two articles concerning GSR satisfied the inclusion criteria [206,207].

Nansel and Jansen [206] were unable to validate GSR changes by examining concordance with findings on manual palpation. While they did not publish their kappa values, reliability was low. Plaugher et al. [207] reported moderate to substantial interexaminer reliability in a study which was rated as low quality.

Recommendation: The evidence from a small number of studies of low to moderate quality is unfavorable, in terms of both validity and reliability, for the use of GSR in determining the site of care.

Surface electromyography (SEMG]

[Quality scores: Validity 0 low, 1 moderate, 3 high; Reliability 2 low, 1 moderate, 1 high].

Three recent reviews of the literature have evaluated the validity [208,209] and reliability Danneels et al. [210] of SEMG as a tool for identifying subjects with back pain. SEMG results vary widely [208,209] based on test methodology. Multiple technical factors complicate the interpretation of results including the choice of electrodes, the variation in skin impedance from site-to-site, the site of electrodes in relation to muscle motor points, the signal normalization method, the temperature of the muscle and skin, the fat layer thickness and the presence of postural support. While SEMG does not reliably isolate the activity of a specific muscle [208], the results of intramuscular EMG and SEMG seem correlated with each other [209].

Geisser et al. [208] conducted a meta-analysis of studies evaluating SEMG in static posture, isometric tasks, and myoelectric response to expected or unexpected sudden loads. Five studies showed no difference between healthy and unhealthy subjects in upright posture, including no difference in side-to-side asymmetry, except during forward flexion. Another five showed higher SEMG amplitudes for static upright postures in low back pain patients than in controls. Patients with disc disorders had higher amplitudes during seated SEMG tasks than normals and other LBP patients. No group differences were observed when SEMG was measured while subjects were lying prone or sitting unsupported. Studies consistently found a lower flexion-relaxation response among subjects with LBP with a large effect size, and good sensitivity (88.8%), specificity (81.3%) and responsiveness to treatment.

Within the context of the present study, only six additional studies met the inclusion criteria for examining the validity and reliability of using SEMG to target sites for spinal manipulation. Dankaerts et al. [211], found differences between healthy subjects and subgroups of chronic low back pain patients ($p<0.001$). However, the myoelectric differences were dependent upon clinical pre-classification into groups according to postural habits. Fryer et al. [212] demonstrated resting paraspinal muscle variation in the thoracic spine with poor to moderate repeatability using either intramuscular ($0.55 \leq ICC \leq 0.94$) or surface ($0.35 \leq ICC \leq 0.69$) electrodes. Under conditions of maximal voluntary contraction, however, both methods of measure had increased reliability ($\kappa \geq 0.91$). When EMG measures were partitioned between sites considered by two experienced clinicians as being normal to palpation versus sites with local abnormality in tissue texture and tenderness, no statistical differences were found for either intramuscular ($F_{1,14}=3.18$, P=.10) or for SEMG electrodes ($F_{1,18}=1.53$, P=.76). A study ranked as high quality [213], examined the reliability and validity of surface EMG in identifying the laterality and segmental level of dysfunction in patients with low back pain. Repeatability of measures was acceptable over several days in pain free subjects (ICC > 0.75). However, static tests showed no ability to identify the laterality or segmental levels of tenderness to palpation in subjects with back pain. A study rated of low quality found that inter-examiner agreement was mixed ($0.20 < ICC < 0.55$; $-0.13 \leq \kappa \leq 0.59$) and unacceptable for clinical application [55].

Leach et al. [214], in a study consistent with the review by Geissler et al. [208], examined a small sample of acute LBP patients and control subjects without neurological deficit. Robust group differences were seen in flexion-relaxation between groups, negatively correlated ($-0.74 < r < -0.50$) with straight leg raising, and were responsive to treatment, improving in terms of disability as measured by the Oswestry scale (r = .42).

Recommendation: The current evidence, which is of high quality, is favorable with limitations towards the validity and reliability of using SEMG to identify cohorts of patients with abnormal neuromuscular control, such as an altered flexion-relaxation response. However, evidence of moderate quality is unfavourable toward the use of SEMG in localizing treatment to a specific site.

Radiographic imaging

[Quality scores: Validity 1 low, 1 moderate, 5 high; Reliability 5 low, 5 moderate, 1 high].

The validity of computer modeling for differentiating normal from symptomatic cases based on x-ray digitization of the lumbar and cervical lordoses has been studied by the Harrison group [215,216]. X-ray digitization itself has shown inter-examiner reliability for three examiners ranging from 0.71 to 0.99, depending on the measure [217,218]. Differences in ellipse parameters fit to spinal curvature and some standard radiographic measures demonstrated significant (lumbar, $0.0001 \leq p \leq 0.0113$; cervical, $0.0001 \leq p \leq 0.05$) differences between groups of healthy and unhealthy subjects. Careful repeated positioning of patients for x-ray can be achieved [219] with no significant difference in measures. Radiographic measures of sacral angle show poor correlation with measures taken by an inclinometer placed externally over the sacrum [220]. However, none of these measures have been shown to have predictive value for assessing individual patients.

Abbott et al. [118], examined the hypothesis that palpable intersegmental hypermobility correlated with hypermobility revealed in lateral flexion-extension radiographic studies in chronic low back pain patients. The authors concluded that, overall, the clinical examination procedures displayed moderate validity in comparison to radiography, with palpation of translation in the sagittal plane faring better than rotation. Continuing on this theme, Abbott and colleagues [221] looked at the prevalence of radiographic movement disorders related to low back symptom status. Using flexion-extension lateral radiographs from cohorts of healthy and chronic/recurrent low back patients, the relative contribution of each segment's motion to the regional motion was computed. Lumbar segmental movement disorder was defined by 2 methods: i) motion beyond 2 standard deviations from the mean of a healthy, control cohort and ii) a normalized, within subject measure of segmental motion beyond 2 standard deviations from the mean of the relative contributions of each lumbar segment. The latter measure was more sensitive, but both identified significantly more instances of lumbar segmental movement disorder in the low back pain patients than in the health controls. Lumbar spine translational rigidity (as opposed to rigidity in rotation or instability in general) was associated with higher disability scores (p=0.010) Again, the predictive value for individual patients has not been determined.

Independent radiologists [118] have evaluated the concurrent validity and reliability of manual tracings and computer generated measures of sagittal rotation (ICC = 0.98) and translation (ICC=0.98). Harrison et al. [222] repeated x-rays of subjects at intervals of 3 to 12 months. Follow-up measures in control subjects were similar in the mean to baseline measures; however, no reliability statistics were performed. Jende and Peterson [101], in a high quality validity study with a small nested intra-examiner reliability study took bone geometry measures from the same radiographs on separate occasions, giving an ICC = 0.93. Similarly, two examiners digitized x-ray landmarks twice [215], obtaining ICCs for intra-examiner and inter-examiner that were described as "high" with standard error of measure < 2%.

Reliability of radiographic markings from the Gonstead system of analysis was tested by Plaugher and Hendricks [223]. Examiners were independent and, for the study of intra-examiner reliability, blinded on their second evaluation with respect to findings on their first evaluation. Intra-examiner scores ($0.846<ICC<0.999$) tended to be minimally higher than inter-examiner scores ($0.812<ICC<0.995$). Antos et al. [224], in a paper ranked as of low quality found strong reliability (κ =0.80) for assessing flexion of C4/5, by videofluoroscopy, as the increase in spinolaminar distance between segments. Higher concordance was found for radiologists more experienced in fluoroscopic interpretation [225].

The extensive work of Jackson et al. [84,226] attempted to evaluate the reliability of various measures of alignment in lateral x-rays of the spine, including anterior head translation, atlas plane to horizontal, Ruth Jackson's cervical stress lines, and five relative intersegmental rotation angles for the neck. Inter-rater reliabilities were substantial to near perfect in the cervical spine ($0.74 \le \kappa \le 0.99$). Phillips et al. [227] evaluated 56 radiographic variables demonstrating a high inter-observer reliability for interpretations by chiropractors, but not for medical physicians. Most notably, findings related to disc space narrowing were the few statistically associated with back or leg complaints ($P = 0.025$).

Lumbar patterns of vertebral displacement on lateral bending films, following the definitions attributed to Grice [228], measuring lateral tilt combined with rotation have been studied for reliability. In this low quality study, inter-rater concordance for lateral tilt was moderate ($0.49 < \kappa < 0.65$) for L1 to L4 but fair ($0.23 < \kappa < 0.24$) for L5. Reliability for rotation was varied over a broader range ($0.19 < \kappa < 0.60$) for all spinal levels depending on pairing of examiners. The ability to predict aberrant lateral bending of a vertebral segment from x-rays taken in the neutral orientation of the segment was studied by Haas and Petersen [229]. Healthy and low back pain subjects were examined. In this high quality study, a moderate negative correlation ($-0.39 < r < -0.16$) was found between the amount of neutral lateral tilt of the vertebrae and its tendency to increase that tilt when lateral bending to the opposite side. Both symptomatic and asymptomatic subjects revealed the same behaviour.

Olson et al. [230] hypothesized a difference in motion in lateral bending of the upper cervical spine based on different standardized starting postures: neutral or minimally flexed. However, in this low quality reliability study, no difference was observed ($p > 0.05$).

Rhudy et al. [231] examined agreement on the decision of lesion site based on systems of analysis. Two of those systems, full spine radiography listings and Gonstead, use full spine x-rays, although the Gonstead approach adds information from skin temperature readings. No details of the system analyses were included and comparison of systems in this fashion has little meaning.

Recommendation: Evidence of high quality supports the use of static and motion studies to identify hypermobile segments but not hypomobile segments. Thus, in terms of validity, the high quality evidence available at this time is unfavourable for use of x-rays to determine the site of care.

Integrated P.A.R.T.S. Studies

[Quality scores: Validity 0 low, 0 moderate, 1 high; Reliability 3 low, 7 moderate ,1 high].

Several reports have utilized a montage or large panel of examination techniques in order to localize the target of care to a region or within a narrow anatomical limit, such as an individual articulation. Ten of these studies [48,68,136,201,232-234] attempted to combine results into a form of summary score to guide the decision to provide care. Two studies [33,71] evaluated neurological tests designed to localize pathology according to sclerotome or dermatome, and orthopedic tests localizing to specific regions/articulations. Results from separate tests were not analyzed statistically to determine their individual contributions to a global decision to treat. Where in fact integrated PARTS studies did analyze the individual contributions of specific tests, these results have been discussed within the appropriate preceding sections.

Leboeuf-Yde et al. [48], in a high quality study, asked examiners to categorize subjects into groups of "low back pain today" and "low back pain never" after using a panel of tests for posture, motion and pain provocation. The accuracy rates were 78% and 67%, respectively.

An early study by Rhudy et al. [231] focused on the tools used to identify the site of care. The inter-examiner agreement findings of three examiners who analyzed full spine x-ray films were compared with their motion palpation findings and each of these were also compared with their Gonstead style analysis of neurocalometer readings on a small sample of fourteen symptomatic patients. The investigators reported almost perfect/substantial correlation only 19% of time, fair/moderate correlation 21% of time and poor/nil correlation 60% of the time. Hawk et al. [232], bundled assessment of segmental hypomobility/hypermobility, tissue texture, palpable temperature, and tenderness elicited on palpation to identify the site of treatment. Agreement was slight, at best.

An inter-examiner reliability study by Keating et al. [235] attempted to correlate eight different tools common in chiropractic practice: i) palpatory pain over osseous structures and ii) paraspinal soft tissues, iii) temperature differences between adjacent segments as measured by the dermothermograph, iv) visual inspection for segmental abnormality, v) active and vi) passive motion palpation, vii) muscle tension palpation, and viii) misalignment palpation. Scores were combined to form a composite joint abnormality index, with osseous pain and soft tissue pain, temperature and visual observation giving the strongest correlations ($0.34 < r < 0.65$). In a follow-up study that was also rated as moderate quality, Boline et al. [55] assessed the composite from visual inspection, palpation for pain over osseous and soft tissue structures, surface EMG and the dermothermograph. Reliability of the combined scores was mixed ($-0.3 < \kappa < 0.56$) and judged unacceptable for clinical application. They again reported that palpation for pain over osseous and soft tissue structures and visual observation of posture produced good to excellent inter-examiner agreement. Results from visual postural analysis, pain description by the patient, plain static erect x-ray films, leg length discrepancy, neurological tests, motion palpation, static palpation and orthopedic tests were evaluated by French et al. [68]. Overall, the measures were not reproducible and the decision to treat, either by different examiners on the same occasion or the same examiner on different occasions, was not reproducible.

Petersen et al. [71] linked a systematic partitioning of patients according to suspected pathoanatomical site of pain production based on pain distribution, response to postural movements and orthopedic maneuver. Inter-rater kappa scores ranged from $0.44 \leq \kappa \leq 1.00$ for assignment of patients in groups for discogenic, radicular, zygapophyseal, sacroiliac and myofascial categories.

Qvistgaard et al. [136] focused on identifying abnormal spinal segments (± 1 segment) as the most pronounced dysfunction in the lumbar spine. Testing combined standing (trunk side bending, flexion, 'stork test'), supine pelvic girdle clockwise/counter clockwise rotation, prone lumbar springing, and side-lying multifidus tension manoeuvres. Kappa values were: segmental diagnosis, 0.57; multifidus test, 0.48; side flexion, 0.45; and ventral flexion 0.44. A similar approach to the thoracic spine was used by Potter et al. [233]. Combining inspection of posture, voluntary movement, passive movement and static palpation, identification of a dysfunctional joint in the thoracic spine showed moderate to poor reliability (ICC = 0.70, C.I. 0.27–0.90). For the lumbar spine, the results were better: ICC = 0.96 (95% CI, 0.87 to 0.99). Toussaint et al. [236] examined the sacroiliac joint with a combination of the standing flexion test, spine test (Gillet), and iliac springing test. Agreement on side, based on a positive result combined for any two tests, was moderate to substantial ($0.483 \leq \kappa \leq 0.677$).

Degenhardt et al. [201,234] evaluated a consensus training method to enhance the inter-rater reliability of a panel of tests. After training intervention [234] for 12 groups of 3 examiners, agreement on tenderness rose from κ =0.32 to κ =0.68 and that for tissue texture improved from κ =0.12 to κ =0.45. In the separate study [201], training was able to produce increased agreement in static palpation asymmetry (κ =0.18 to 0.59), tissue texture (κ = −0.01 to 0.45), anterior springing (κ =0.29 to 0.44) and palpatory tenderness (κ = 0.32 to 0.65). Retention of the improved skill has not been reported.

Recommendation: Unclear, based on moderate quality evidence, for examination montages contributing any more than their component elements to the decision to localize treatment.

Discussion

The work of this report represents the most comprehensive review of the literature, to date, in relation to the diagnostic methods used for locating the site of care at which to apply manipulation treatment methods. Despite a number of studies addressing the questions of validity and reliability over the years, the research community's sense of what constitutes a good study of diagnostic accuracy appears to be evolving. Guidelines for evaluating the strength of evidence are relatively recent in comparison to guidelines for studies of treatment. The first broadly accepted sets of standards for the design of studies of diagnostic accuracy, Standards for Reporting of Diagnostic Accuracy (STARD) and the Quality Assessment of Diagnostic Accuracy Studies (QUADAS), were published in 2003 [25,26,237,238]. The Quality Appraisal tool for Studies of Diagnostic Reliability (QAREL) only appeared in 2010 [27].

Applying these tools to the literature found high quality evidence for the majority of the P.A.R.T.S. constructs. Constrained by the current understandings of manipulation treatment methods and the patients to whom they are applied, better practices, if not best, for practitioners are evident and summarized in Table 3. Very few methods can be used in isolation. Taken as a whole, the literature continues to support the fundamental principles of clinical differential diagnosis [10]. The physical examination should be contextualized by the patient's history and presenting complaint to progressively narrow the focus of attention, first to region then local site and, sometimes, tissue. The body of evidence seems to support more direct, mechanical methods of assessing and identifying the site of care, and in general is not supportive of less direct methods such as manual muscle testing for nonpathological states, thermography, surface electromyography and measures of electrodermal activity. Fixed examination montages are no more helpful than information derived from the individual components. Manoeuvres that replicate the patient's familiar pain may be the most consistent sources for diagnostic information. A number of assessment methods were judged to be useful for patient screening or for narrowing the topographical focus of examination. These included postural assessment, orthopedic testing in general, and range of motion testing, as well as assessment of leg length inequality. While there is favourable evidence for a number of palpation methods, there are significant limitations. The inability to locate anatomical landmarks likely is a common underlying feature. When the error in accuracy is taken into account by enfolding those errors (e.g. ± one vertebral segment) into the decision criteria, inter-rater reliability increases substantially.

Examining this error construct in light of more recent work may be instructive. Is the error a result of limitations in communicating what is being perceived by the examiner? May it be a result of the variation in clinical presentations in patients that are believed to respond to manipulation treatments? Future diagnostic studies are likely to benefit from studies on mechanisms of the examination and of the underlying clinical state. For example, the work of Degenhardt et al. [201,234] strives to understand the elements of examiner perceptions and to train examiners to reliably locate them and convey their interpretations. Fritz and colleagues [74,89,90,221] are attempting to tease apart the objective static and dynamic features of spinal function in relation to examination findings and responses to treatment.

The ambiguity of the clinical state of the underlying lesion or lesions treated with manipulation is a constraint on the literature and this constraint cannot be effectively controlled by research methodologies. At present, there is no ideal gold standard of comparison. In response, a pragmatic approach has been taken in this, consistent with the practitioner's experience, and accepts forms of concurrent, construct and face validity for the necessity of care as derived from the patient's clinical presentation.

Limitations

- Although every effort was made to perform an exhaustive and complete search, the abundance of relevant literature, coupled with the fact that some authors did not choose useful indexing terms, guarantees that some literature was missed.
- A number of studies used examiners of doubtful ability–commonly students–and this seems incongruous when investigating what may be complex psychomotor skills, as suggested by the work of Degenhardt et al. [201,234].
- Rules that are used to rate the strength of evidence are by definition arbitrary and thus subject to discussion.
- A number of authors utilized suboptimal methods of data analysis (e.g. correlation analysis) particularly for addressing inter-rater reliability. Found usually in the lower ranked articles, correlation analysis may yield a high value for correlation between measures where the accuracy may be meaningfully in question.
- This review, having examined the evidence on the reliability and validity of research on the site of care, by design did not address the larger question as to the clinical value of identifying a putative appropriate site of care. We cannot rule out the possibility that the clinical consequences of the manipulation treatment are to some extent site-independent.
- While it is generally recognized that using checklists to generate summary quality scores may be problematic (for example, see Whiting et al. [25,26,238]), especially when the weighting of items is arbitrary, the method which we used–employing item response theory to weight items based on the inverse of their prevalence with a set of papers, has been used previously for STARD [239] and validated for the CONSORT statement for papers within manual medicine [28].
- Systematic use of QUADAS and QAREL independently address only metrics of validity and reliability within the context of each study. It is important to bear in mind that neither characteristic necessarily implies the other. That is, an assessment may be valid but unreliable, and the obverse, reliable but not valid. The implication of either alone or both together is insufficient to define clinical utility.
- An important deficiency in the literature is the absence of significant discussion on the clinical utility of the various assessment methods.

Conclusion

The broad search which was conducted has likely resulted in a corpus of literature which is generally representative of the current state of research in this area. Thus, where high levels of evidence were available and collective findings coherent–either favourable or unfavourable towards the use of a particular method–individual new studies are unlikely to affect the results presented herein. On the other hand, where the level of available evidence was relatively low or the findings of different studies incoherent, then new studies may well lead to new conclusions. Furthermore, the technologies themselves evolve. Thus, for example, while this review found coherent, moderate or high quality evidence which was not supportive of the use of methods that indirectly assess the tissues, technical improvements could see the future clinical validation of such methods.

Finally, while there is a need for more and better research into the underlying functional and/or pathological states that respond to manipulation, future diagnostic studies ought to focus beyond the metrics of accuracy. As posited by Bossuyt et al. [240], the value of diagnostic tests/maneuvers ought to rely on their clinical utility and capacity to change health outcomes.

Additional files

Additional file 1: QUADAS question level data.
Additional file 2: QAREL question level data.

Competing interests
The authors declare that they have no competing interests.

Authors' contributions
JT and BB designed the study. AB and BR completed the literature searches and data extraction. JT, BB, TB, RC, BG, CG, JP and RT performed the data analysis and contributed to the writing of the manuscript. All authors read and approved the final manuscript.

Acknowledgements
The Association of Chiropractic Colleges in conjunction with the Council on Chiropractic Guidelines and Practice Parameters provided support for communications and face-to-face meetings of team members. Special appreciation is extended to Dr. Carl Cleveland III who acted as liaison between the ACC, the CCGPP and the review team.

Author details
[1]Canadian Memorial Chiropractic College, 6100 Leslie St., Toronto, Ontario, Canada. [2]Private Practice of Chiropractic, Burlington, Canada. [3]Private Practice of Chiropractic, Toronto, Canada. [4]Private Practice of Chiropractic, Calgary, Canada. [5]Northwestern Health Sciences University, Bloomington, MN, USA. [6]Palmer College of Chiropractic, San Jose, CA, USA. [7]University of Bridgeport College of Chiropractic, Bridgeport, CT, USA. [8]Logan College of Chiropractic, Chesterfield, MO, USA.

References

1. Hurwitz EL: **Epidemiology: spinal manipulation utilization.** *J Electromyogr Kinesiol* 2012, **22:**648–654.
2. Gross A, Miller J, D'Sylva J, Burnie SJ, Goldsmith CH, Graham N, *et al*: **Manipulation or mobilisation for neck pain: a Cochrane review.** *Man Ther* 2010, **15:**315–333.
3. Rubinstein SM, van MM, Assendelft WJ, de Boer MR, van Tulder MW: **Spinal manipulative therapy for chronic low-back pain.** *Cochrane Database Syst Rev* 2011, **2:**CD008112.
4. Bronfort G, Haas M, Evans R, Leininger B, Triano J: **Effectiveness of manual therapies: the UK evidence report.** *Chiropr Osteopat* 2010, **18:**3–18.
5. di RL F, Hyde CJ, McCaffery KJ, Bossuyt PM, Deeks JJ: **Assessing the value of diagnostic tests: a framework for designing and evaluating trials.** *BMJ* 2012, **344:**e686.
6. Haldeman S, Kopansky-Giles D, Hurwitz EL, Hoy D, Mark EW, Dagenais S, *et al*: **Advancements in the management of spine disorders.** *Best Pract Res Clin Rheumatol* 2012, **26:**263–280.
7. Stanton TR, Hancock MJ, Maher CG, Koes BW: **Critical appraisal of clinical prediction rules that aim to optimize treatment selection for musculoskeletal conditions.** *Phys Ther* 2010, **90:**843–854.
8. Triano JJ: **Biomechanics of spinal manipulative therapy.** *Spine J* 2001, **1:**121–130.
9. Triano J: **Survey of mechanotransduction disorders.** In *The science and clinical application of manual therapy.* Edited by King HH, Janig W, Patterson MM. Edinburgh: Churchill Livingstone Elsevier Publishing; 2011:97–103.
10. Sackett DL, Haynes RB, Guyatt GH, Tugwell P: *Clinical epidemiology: a basic science for clinical medicine.* Toronto: Little Brown and Company; 1991:53–57.
11. Straus SE, McAlister FA, Sackett DL, Deeks JJ: **The accuracy of patient history, wheezing, and laryngeal measurements in diagnosing obstructive airway disease. CARE-COAD1 group. Clinical assessment of the reliability of the examination-chronic obstructive airways disease.** *JAMA* 2000, **283:**1853–1857.
12. Poddubnyy D, Vahldiek J, Spiller I, Buss B, Listing J, Rudwaleit M, *et al*: **Evaluation of 2 screening strategies for early identification of patients with axial spondyloarthritis in primary care.** *J Rheumatol* 2011, **38:**2452–2460.
13. Hancock MJ, Maher CG, Laslett M, Hay E, Koes B: **Discussion paper: what happened to the 'bio' in the bio-psycho-social model of low back pain?** *Eur Spine J* 2011, **20:**2105–2110.
14. Boden SD, Davis DO, Dina TS, Patronas NJ, Wiesel SW: **Abnormal magnetic-resonance scans of the lumbar spine in asymptomatic subjects. A prospective investigation.** *J Bone Joint Surg Am* 1990, **72:**403–408.
15. Bergman T, Courtis G: **Joint assessment–P.A.R.T.S.** *Top Clin Chiropract* 2000, **7:**1–10.
16. Christensen MG: *Practice analysis of chiropractic 2010.* Greeley, Colorado: National Board of Chiropractic Examiners; 2010.
17. Bigos S, Bower O, Braen G, Brown K, Deyo R, Halderman S, *et al*: *Acute Low back problems in adults*, [14]. Rockville, MD: Agency for Health Care Policy and Research, Public Health Service. Clinical Practice Guidelines; 1994.
18. Haldeman S, Chapman-Smith D, Petersen DM: *Guidelines for chiropractic quality assurance and practice parameters.* Gaithersburg, Maryland: Aspen Publishers; 1993.
19. Shekelle P, Adams A, Chassin M, Hurwitz E, Phillips R, Brook R: *The appropriateness of spinal manipulation for low-back pain. Indications and ratings by a multidisciplinary expert panel.* Santa Monica, CA: RAND Corporation; 1991.
20. Coulter I, Hurwitz E, Adams A, Meeker W, Hansen D, Mootz R, *et al*: *The appropriateness of manipulation and mobilization of the cervical spine.* Santa Monica, CA: RAND Corporation; 1996.
21. Moher D, Liberati A, Tetzlaff J, Altman D: **Preferred reporting items for systematic reviews and meta-analyses: the PRISMA statement.** *PLoS Med* 2009, **6:**e1000097.
22. Stroup DF, Berlin JA, Morton SC, Olkin I, Williamson GD, Rennie D, *et al*: **Meta-analysis of observational studies in epidemiology: a proposal for reporting. Meta-analysis of observational studies in epidemiology (MOOSE) group.** *JAMA* 2000, **283:**2008–2012.
23. Wong G, Greenhalgh T, Westhorp G, Buckingham J, Pawson R: **RAMESES publication standards: realist syntheses.** *BMC Med* 2013, **11:**11–21.
24. Deeks JJ: **Systematic reviews in health care: systematic reviews of evaluations of diagnostic and screening tests.** *BMJ* 2001, **323:**157–162.
25. Whiting P, Rutjes AW, Reitsma JB, Bossuyt PM, Kleijnen J: **The development of QUADAS: a tool for the quality assessment of studies of diagnostic accuracy included in systematic reviews.** *BMC Med Res Methodol* 2003, **3:**25.
26. Whiting PF, Weswood ME, Rutjes AW, Reitsma JB, Bossuyt PN, Kleijnen J: **Evaluation of QUADAS, a tool for the quality assessment of diagnostic accuracy studies.** *BMC Med Res Methodol* 2006, **6:**9.
27. Lucas NP, Macaskill P, Irwig L, Bogduk N: **The development of a quality appraisal tool for studies of diagnostic reliability (QAREL).** *J Clin Epidemiol* 2010, **63:**854–861.
28. Nakayama T, Budgell B: *The application of item response theory to manuscript rating scales.* Vancouver, Canada: International Congress on Peer Review and Biomedical Publication; 2009.
29. Jones J, Hunter D: **Consensus methods for medical and health services research.** *BMJ* 1995, **311:**376–380.
30. Triano JJ, Goertz C, Weeks J, Murphy DR, Kranz KC, McClelland GC, *et al*: **Chiropractic in north America: toward a strategic plan for professional renewal--outcomes from the 2006 chiropractic strategic planning conference.** *J Manipulative Physiol Ther* 2010, **33:**395–405.
31. Viera AJ, Garrett JM: **Understanding interobserver agreement: the kappa statistic.** *Fam Med* 2005, **37:**360–363.
32. Fleiss JL: *The design and analysis of clinical experiment.* New York: John Wiley & Sons Inc; 1986:1–32.
33. Viikari-Juntura E: **Interexaminer reliability of observations in physical examinations of the neck.** *Phys Ther* 1987, **67:**1526–1532.
34. Maher C, Adams R: **Reliability of pain and stiffness assessments in clinical manual lumbar spine examination.** *Phys Ther* 1994, **74:**801–809.
35. Fortin JD, Falco FJ: **The Fortin finger test: an indicator of sacroiliac pain.** *Am J Orthop (Belle Mead NJ)* 1997, **26:**477–480.
36. Van Dillen LR, Sahrmann SA, Norton BJ, Caldwell CA, Fleming DA, McDonnell MK, *et al*: **Reliability of physical examination items used for classification of patients with low back pain.** *Phys Ther* 1998, **78:**979–988.
37. Bertilson BC, Grunnesjo M, Strender LE: **Reliability of clinical tests in the assessment of patients with neck/shoulder problems-impact of history.** *Spine (Phila Pa)* 2003, **28:**2222–2231.
38. Clare HA, Adams R, Maher CG: **Reliabilityof the McKenzie spinal pain classification using patient sassessment forms.** *Physiotherapy* 2004, **90:**114–119.
39. Cleland JA, Childs JD, Fritz JM, Whitman JM: **Interrater reliability of the history and physical examination in patients with mechanical neck pain.** *Arch Phys Med Rehabil* 2006, **87:**1388–1395.
40. Boline P, Keating JC, Brist J, Denver G: **Interexaminer reliability of palpatory evaluations of the lumbar spine.** *Am J Chiropractic Med* 1988, **1:**5–11.

41. McCombe PF, Fairbank JC, Cockersole BC, Pynsent PB: **1989 Volvo award in clinical sciences. Reproducibility of physical signs in low-back pain.** *Spine (Phila Pa)* 1989, **14**:908–918.
42. Taylor P, Tole G, Vernon H: **Skin rolling technique as an indicator of spinal joint dysfunction.** *J Can Chiropract Assoc* 1990, **34**:82–86.
43. Bryner P: **Tenderness distribution: a pilot study.** *Chiropract Tech* 1994, **6**:37–43.
44. Hubka MJ, Phelan SP: **Interexaminer reliability of palpation for cervical spine tenderness.** *J Manipulative Physiol Ther* 1994, **17**:591–595.
45. Sandmark H, Nisell R: **Validity of five common manual neck pain provoking tests.** *Scand J Rehabil Med* 1995, **27**:131–136.
46. McPartland JM, Goodridge JP: **Counterstrain and traditional osteopathic examination of the cervical spine compared.** *J Bodyw Mov Ther* 1997, **1**:173–178.
47. Lundberg G, Gerdle B: **The relationships between spinal sagittal configuration, joint mobility, general low back mobility and segmental mobility in female homecare personnel.** *Scand J Rehabil Med* 1999, **31**:197–206.
48. Leboeuf-Yde C, Kyvik KO: **Is it possible to differentiate people with or without low-back pain on the basis of test of lumbopelvic dysfunction?** *J Manipulative Physiol Ther* 2000, **23**:160–167.
49. Hanten WP, Olson SL, Ludwig GM: **Reliability of manual mobility testing of the upper cervical spine in subjects with cervicogenic headache.** *J Man Manip Ther* 2002, **10**:76–82.
50. Christensen HW, Vach W, Vach K, Manniche C, Haghfelt T, Hartvigsen L, *et al*: **Palpation of the upper thoracic spine: an observer reliability study.** *J Manipulative Physiol Ther* 2002, **25**:285–292.
51. Heiderscheit B, Boissonnault W: **Reliability of joint mobility and pain assessment of the thoracic spine and rib cage in asymptomatic individuals.** *J Man Manip Ther* 2008, **16**:210–216.
52. King W, Lau P, Lees R, Bogduk N: **The validity of manual examination in assessing patients with neck pain.** *Spine J* 2007, **7**:22–26.
53. Jull G, Bogduk N, Marsland A: **The accuracy of manual diagnosis for cervical zygapophysial joint pain syndromes.** *Med J Aust* 1988, **148**:233–236.
54. Maigne JY, Chantelot F, Chatellier G: **Interexaminer agreement of clinical examination of the neck in manual medicine.** *Ann Phys Rehabil Med* 2009, **52**:41–48.
55. Boline PD, Haas M, Meyer JJ, Kassak K, Nelson C, Keating JC Jr: **Interexaminer reliability of eight evaluative dimensions of lumbar segmental abnormality: part II.** *J Manipulative Physiol Ther* 1993, **16**:363–374.
56. Levangie PK: **Four clinical tests of sacroiliac joint dysfunction: the association of test results with innominate torsion among patients with and without low back pain.** *Phys Ther* 1999, **79**:1043–1057.
57. Cibulka MT, Koldehoff R: **Clinical usefulness of a cluster of sacroiliac joint tests in patients with and without low back pain.** *J Orthop Sports Phys Ther* 1999, **29**:83–89.
58. Strender LE, Lundin M, Nell K: **Interexaminer reliability in physical examination of the neck.** *J Manipulative Physiol Ther* 1997, **20**:516–520.
59. Van Suijlekom HA, de Vet HC, Van Den Berg SG, Weber WE: **Interobserver reliability in physical examination of the cervical spine in patients with headache.** *Headache* 2000, **40**:581–586.
60. Hunt DG, Zuberbier OA, Kozlowski AJ, Robinson J, Berkowitz J, Schultz IZ, *et al*: **Reliability of the lumbar flexion, lumbar extension, and passive straight leg raise test in normal populations embedded within a complete physical examination.** *Spine (Phila Pa)* 2001, **26**:2714–2718.
61. Riddle DL, Freburger JK: **Evaluation of the presence of sacroiliac joint region dysfunction using a combination of tests: a multicenter intertester reliability study.** *Phys Ther* 2002, **82**:772–781.
62. Cook C, Stickley L, Akram N, Benavides Y, Renz C, Ramey K: **Inter-rater reliability of coupling pattern observations of the pathological lumbar spine: a pilot study.** *J Man Manip Ther* 2013, **12**:192–198.
63. Clare HA, Adams R, Maher CG: **Reliability of McKenzie classification of patients with cervical or lumbar pain.** *J Manipulative Physiol Ther* 2005, **28**:122–127.
64. Heiss DG, Fitch DS, Fritz JM, Sanchez WJ, Roberts KE, Buford JA: **The interrater reliability among physical therapists newly trained in a classification system for acute low back pain.** *J Orthop Sports Phys Ther* 2004, **34**:430–439.
65. Weiner DK, Sakamoto S, Perera S, Breuer P: **Chronic low back pain in older adults: prevalence, reliability, and validity of physical examination findings.** *J Am Geriatr Soc* 2006, **54**:11–20.
66. Paatelma M, Karvonen E, Heinonen A: **Inter- and intra-tester reliability of selected clinical tests in examining patients with early phase lumbar spine and sacroiliac joint pain and dysfunction.** *Adv Physiother* 2010, **12**:74–80.
67. Laslett M, Williams M: **The reliability of selected pain provocation tests for sacroiliac joint pathology.** *Spine (Phila Pa)* 1994, **19**:1243–1249.
68. French SD, Green S, Forbes A: **Reliability of chiropractic methods commonly used to detect manipulable lesions in patients with chronic low-back pain.** *J Manipulative Physiol Ther* 2000, **23**:231–238.
69. Kokmeyer DJ, der WP V, Aufdemkampe G, Fickenscher TC: **The reliability of multitest regimens with sacroiliac pain provocation tests.** *J Manipulative Physiol Ther* 2002, **25**:42–48.
70. Haswell K, Williams M, Hing W: **Reliability of symptom-provoking active sidebend, rotation and combined movement assessments of patients with Low back pain.** *J Man Manip Ther* 2004, **12**:11–20.
71. Petersen T, Olsen S, Laslett M, Thorsen H, Manniche C, Ekdahl C, *et al*: **Inter-tester reliability of a new diagnostic classification system for patients with non-specific low back pain.** *Aust J Physiother* 2004, **50**:85–94.
72. Arab AM, Abdollahi I, Joghataei MT, Golafshani Z, Kazemnejad A: **Inter- and intra-examiner reliability of single and composites of selected motion palpation and pain provocation tests for sacroiliac joint.** *Man Ther* 2009, **14**:213–221.
73. Strender LE, Sjoblom A, Sundell K, Ludwig R, Taube A: **Interexaminer reliability in physical examination of patients with low back pain.** *Spine (Phila Pa)* 1997, **22**:814–820.
74. Hicks GE, Fritz JM, Delitto A, Mishock J: **Interrater reliability of clinical examination measures for identification of lumbar segmental instability.** *Arch Phys Med Rehabil* 2003, **84**:1858–1864.
75. Razmjou H, Kramer JF, Yamada R: **Intertester reliability of the McKenzie evaluation in assessing patients with mechanical low-back pain.** *J Orthop Sports Phys Ther* 2000, **30**:368–383.
76. Kilpikoski S, Airaksinen O, Kankaanpaa M, Leminen P, Videman T, Alen M: **Interexaminer reliability of low back pain assessment using the McKenzie method.** *Spine (Phila Pa)* 2002, **27**:E207–E214.
77. Abbott JH, Mercer SR: **Lumbar segmental hypomobility: criterion-related validity of clinical examination items (a pilot study).** *New Zeal J Physiother* 2003, **31**:3–9.
78. Laslett M, Young SB, Aprill CN, McDonald B: **Diagnosing painful sacroiliac joints: a validity study of a McKenzie evaluation and sacroiliac provocation tests.** *Aust J Physiother* 2003, **49**:89–97.
79. Laslett M, Oberg B, Aprill CN, McDonald B: **Centralization as a predictor of provocation discography results in chronic low back pain, and the influence of disability and distress on diagnostic power.** *Spine J* 2005, **5**:370–380.
80. Laslett M, Aprill CN, McDonald B, Young SB: **Diagnosis of sacroiliac joint pain: validity of individual provocation tests and composites of tests.** *Man Ther* 2005, **10**:207–218.
81. Clare HA, Adams R, Maher CG: **Construct validity of lumbar extension measures in McKenzie's derangement syndrome.** *Man Ther* 2007, **12**:328–334.
82. Clare HA, Adams R, Maher CG: **Reliability of the McKenzie classification of patients with cervical or lumbar pain.** *J Manipulative Physiol Ther* 2003, **90**:122–127.
83. Cowherd GP, Gringmuth R, Nolet PA: **A comparison of the metrecom skeletal analysis system vs plain film radiography in the measurement of sacral base angle and lumbar lordosis.** *J Can Chiropract Assoc* 1992, **36**:156–160.
84. Jackson RP, Peterson MD, McManus AC, Hales C: **Compensatory spinopelvic balance over the hip axis and better reliability in measuring lordosis to the pelvic radius on standing lateral radiographs of adult volunteers and patients.** *Spine (Phila Pa)* 1998, **23**:1750–1767.
85. Piva SR, Erhard RE, Childs JD, Hicks G, Al-Abdulmohsin H: **Reliability of measuring iliac crest level in the standing and sitting position using a new measurement device.** *J Manipulative Physiol Ther* 2003, **26**:437–441.
86. Normand MC, Descarreaux M, Harrison DD, Harrison DE, Perron DL, Ferrantelli JR, *et al*: **Three dimensional evaluation of posture in standing with the PosturePrint: an intra- and inter-examiner reliability study.** *Chiropr Osteopat* 2007, **15**:15.
87. Leard JS, Crane BA, Ball KA: **Intrarater and interrater reliability of 22 clinical measures associated with lower quarter malalignment.** *J Manipulative Physiol Ther* 2009, **32**:270–276.
88. Chan ST, Fung PK, Ng NY, Ngan TL, Chong MY, Tang CN, *et al*: **Dynamic changes of elasticity, cross-sectional area, and fat infiltration of multifidus at

different postures in men with chronic low back pain. *Spine J* 2012, **12**:381–388.
89. Fritz JM, Koppenhaver SL, Kawchuk GN, Teyhen DS, Hebert JJ, Childs JD: **Preliminary investigation of the mechanisms underlying the effects of manipulation: exploration of a multivariate model including spinal stiffness, multifidus recruitment, and clinical findings.** *Spine (Phila Pa)* 2011, **36**:1772–1781.
90. Koppenhaver SL, Fritz JM, Hebert JJ, Kawchuk GN, Parent EC, Gill NW, *et al*: **Association between history and physical examination factors and change in lumbar multifidus muscle thickness after spinal manipulation in patients with low back pain.** *J Electromyogr Kinesiol* 2012, **22**:724–731.
91. Fernandez-de-las-Pinas C, Downey C, Miangolarra-Page JC: **Validity of the lateral gliding test as tool for the diagnosis of intervertebral joint dysfunction in the lower C-spine.** *J Manipulative Physiol Ther* 2005, **28**:610–616.
92. Downey B, Taylor N, Niere K: **Can manipulative physiotherapists agree on which lumbar level to treat based on palpation?** *Physiotherapy* 2003, **80**:74–81.
93. Comeaux Z, Eland D, Chila A, Pheley A: **Measurement challenges in physical diagnosis: refining inter-rater palpation, perception and communication.** *J Bodyw Mov Ther* 2001, **5**:245–253.
94. Horneij E, Hemborg B, Johnsson B, Ekdahl C: **Clinical tests on impairment level related to low back pain: a study of test reliability.** *J Rehabil Med* 2002, **34**:176–182.
95. Fjellner A, Bexander C, Faleij R, Strender LE: **Interexaminer reliability in physical examination of the cervical spine.** *J Manipulative Physiol Ther* 1999, **22**:511–516.
96. Ghoukssian M, Nicholls B, McLaghlin P: **Inter-examiner reliability of the Johnson and Friedman percussion scan of the thoracic spine.** *J Osteopath Med* 2013, **4**:15–20.
97. Pool JJ, Hoving JL, de Vet HC, van MH, Bouter LM: **The interexaminer reproducibility of physical examination of the cervical spine.** *J Manipulative Physiol Ther* 2004, **27**:84–90.
98. Leach RA, Parker PL, Veal PS: **PulStar differential compliance spinal instrument: a randomized interexaminer and intraexaminer reliability study.** *J Manipulative Physiol Ther* 2003, **26**:493–501.
99. Owens EF Jr, DeVocht JW, Wilder DG, Gudavalli MR, Meeker WC: **The reliability of a posterior-to-anterior spinal stiffness measuring system in a population of patients with low back pain.** *J Manipulative Physiol Ther* 2007, **30**:116–123.
100. Latimer J, Lee M, Adams RD: **The effects of high and low loading forces on measured values of lumbar stiffness.** *J Manipulative Physiol Ther* 1998, **21**:157–163.
101. Jende A, Peterson CK: **Validity of static palpation as an indicator of atlas transverse process asymmetry.** *Eur J Chiropract* 1997, **45**:35–42.
102. Harlick JC, Milosavljevic S, Milburn PD: **Palpation identification of spinous processes in the lumbar spine.** *Man Ther* 2007, **12**:56–62.
103. Rouwmaat PH, Everaert D, Stappaerts KH, Aufdemkampe G: **Reliability of manual skinfold tests in a healthy male population.** *J Manipulative Physiol Ther* 1998, **21**:327–332.
104. Fryer G, McPherson HC, O'Keefe P: **The effect of training on the inter-examiner and intra-examiner reliability of the seated flexion test and assessment of pelvic anatomical landmarks with palpation.** *Int J Osteopath Med* 2005, **8**:131–138.
105. Holmgren U, Waling K: **Inter-examiner reliability of four static palpation tests used for assessing pelvic dysfunction.** *Man Ther* 2008, **13**:50–56.
106. Kmita A, Lucas NP: **Reliability of physical examination to assess asymmetry of anatomical landmarks indicative of pelvic somatic dysfunction in subjects with and without Low back pain.** *Int J Osteopath Med* 2008, **11**:16–18.
107. Binkley J, Stratford PW, Gill C: **Interrater reliability of lumbar accessory motion mobility testing.** *Phys Ther* 1995, **75**:786–792.
108. Rhodes DW, Mansfield ER, Bishop PA, Smith JF: **The validity of the prone leg check as an estimate of standing leg length inequality measured by X-ray.** *J Manipulative Physiol Ther* 1995, **18**:343–346.
109. McKenzie AM, Taylor NF: **Can physiotherapists locate lumbar spinal levels by palpation?** *Physiotherapy* 1997, **83**:235–239.
110. Moran RW, Gibbons P: **Intraexaminer and interexaminer reliability for palpation of the cranial rhythmic impulse at the head and sacrum.** *J Manipulative Physiol Ther* 2001, **24**:183–190.
111. Troke M, Schuit D, Petersen CM: **Reliability of lumbar spinal palpation, range of motion, and determination of position.** *BMC Musculoskelet Disord* 2007, **8**:103.
112. Robinson R, Robinson HS, Bjorke G, Kvale A: **Reliability and validity of a palpation technique for identifying the spinous processes of C7 and L5.** *Man Ther* 2009, **14**:409–414.
113. Herzog W, Read LJ, Conway PJ, Shaw LD, McEwen MC: **Reliability of motion palpation procedures to detect sacroiliac joint fixations.** *J Manipulative Physiol Ther* 1989, **12**:86–92.
114. Byfield D, Humphreys BK: **Intra- and inter-examiner reliability of bony landmark identification in the lumbar spine.** *Eur J Chiropract* 1992, **40**:13–17.
115. O'Haire C, Gibbons P: **Inter-examiner and intra-examiner agreement for assessing sacroiliac anatomical landmarks using palpation and observation: pilot study.** *Man Ther* 2000, **5**:13–20.
116. Kim HW, Ko YJ, Rhee WI, Lee JS, Lim JE, Lee SJ, *et al*: **Interexaminer reliability and accuracy of posterior superior iliac spine and iliac crest palpation for spinal level estimations.** *J Manipulative Physiol Ther* 2007, **30**:386–389.
117. Leboeuf-Yde C, van DJ, Franz C, Hustad SA, Olsen D, Pihl T, *et al*: **Motion palpation findings and self-reported low back pain in a population-based study sample.** *J Manipulative Physiol Ther* 2002, **25**:80–87.
118. Abbott JH, McCane B, Herbison P, Moginie G, Chapple C, Hogarty T: **Lumbar segmental instability: a criterion-related validity study of manual therapy assessment.** *BMC Musculoskelet Disord* 2005, **6**:56.
119. Landel R, Kulig K, Fredericson M, Li B, Powers CM: **Intertester reliability and validity of motion assessments during lumbar spine accessory motion testing.** *Phys Ther* 2008, **88**:43–49.
120. Humphreys BK, Delahaye M, Peterson CK: **An investigation into the validity of cervical spine motion palpation using subjects with congenital block vertebrae as a 'gold standard'.** *BMC Musculoskelet Disord* 2004, **5**:19.
121. Ogince M, Hall T, Robinson K, Blackmore AM: **The diagnostic validity of the cervical flexion-rotation test in C1/2-related cervicogenic headache.** *Man Ther* 2007, **12**:256–262.
122. Carmichael JP: **Inter- and intra-examiner reliability of palpation for sacroiliac joint dysfunction.** *J Manipulative Physiol Ther* 1987, **10**:164–171.
123. Love RM, Brodeur RR: **Inter- and intra-examiner reliability of motion palpation for the thoracolumbar spine.** *J Manipulative Physiol Ther* 1987, **10**:1–4.
124. Mootz RD, Keating JC Jr, Kontz HP, Milus TB, Jacobs GE: **Intra- and interobserver reliability of passive motion palpation of the lumbar spine.** *J Manipulative Physiol Ther* 1989, **12**:440–445.
125. Nansel DD, Peneff AL, Jansen RD, Cooperstein R: **Interexaminer concordance in detecting joint-play asymmetries in the cervical spines of otherwise asymptomatic subjects.** *J Manipulative Physiol Ther* 1989, **12**:428–433.
126. Haas M, Raphael R, Panzer D, Peterson D: **Reliability of manual End-play palpation of the thoracic spine.** *Chiropract Tech* 1995, **7**:120–124.
127. Meijne W, van Neerbos K, Aufdemkampe G, van der Wurff P: **Intraexaminer and interexaminer reliability of the gillet test.** *J Manipulative Physiol Ther* 1999, **22**:4–9.
128. Vincent-Smith B, Gibbons P: **Inter-examiner and intra-examiner reliability of the standing flexion test.** *Man Ther* 1999, **4**:87–93.
129. Smedmark V, Wallin M, Arvidsson I: **Inter-examiner reliability in assessing passive intervertebral motion of the cervical spine.** *Man Ther* 2000, **5**:97–101.
130. Marcotte J, Normand MC, Black P: **The kinematics of motion palpation and its effect on the reliability for cervical spine rotation.** *J Manipulative Physiol Ther* 2002, **25**:E7.
131. Marcotte J, Normand MC, Black P: **Measurement of the pressure applied during motion palpation and reliability for cervical spine rotation.** *J Manipulative Physiol Ther* 2005, **28**:591–596.
132. Brismee JM, Atwood K, Fain M, Hodges J, Sperle A, Swaney M, *et al*: **Inter-rater reliability of palpation of three-dimensional segmental motion of the lumbar spine.** *J Man Manip Ther* 2005, **13**:215–220.
133. Tong HC, Heyman OG, Lado DA, Isser MM: **Interexaminer reliability of three methods of combining test results to determine side of sacral restriction, sacral base position, and innominate bone position.** *J Am Osteopath Assoc* 2006, **106**:464–468.
134. Johansson F: **Interexaminer reliability of lumbar segmental mobility tests.** *Man Ther* 2006, **11**:331–336.
135. Hungerford BA, Gilleard W, Moran M, Emmerson C: **Evaluation of the ability of physical therapists to palpate intrapelvic motion with the stork test on the support side.** *Phys Ther* 2007, **87**:879–887.
136. Qvistgaard E, Rasmussen J, Laetgaard J, Hecksher-Sorensen S, Bliddal H: **Intra-observer and inter-observer agreement of the manual examination of the lumbar spine in chronic low-back pain.** *Eur Spine J* 2007, **16**:277–282.

137. Robinson HS, Brox JI, Robinson R, Bjelland E, Solem S, Telje T: **The reliability of selected motion- and pain provocation tests for the sacroiliac joint.** *Man Ther* 2007, **12**:72–79.
138. Schneider M, Erhard R, Brach J, Tellin W, Imbarlina F, Delitto A: **Spinal palpation for lumbar segmental mobility and pain provocation: an interexaminer reliability study.** *J Manipulative Physiol Ther* 2008, **31**:465–473.
139. Cooperstein R, Haneline M, Young M: **Interexaminer reliability of thoracic motion palpation using confidence ratings and continuous analysis.** *J Chiropr Med* 2010, **9**:99–106.
140. Brismee JM, Gipson D, Ivie D, Lopez A, Moore M, Matthijs O, *et al*: **Interrater reliability of a passive physiological intervertebral motion test in the mid-thoracic spine.** *J Manipulative Physiol Ther* 2006, **29**:368–373.
141. Chakraverty RC, Pynsent PB, Westwood A, Chakraverty JK: **Identification of the correct lumbar level using passive intersegmental motion testing.** *Anaesthesia* 2007, **62**:1121–1125.
142. Phillips DR, Twomey LT: **A comparison of manual diagnosis with a diagnosis established by a uni-level lumbar spinal block procedure.** *Man Ther* 1996, **1**:82–87.
143. Beattie P, Isaacson K, Riddle DL, Rothstein JM: **Validity of derived measurements of leg-length differences obtained by use of a tape measure.** *Phys Ther* 1990, **70**:150–157.
144. Montgomery DM, Egan IF, Pollard HP: **Palpable unilateral sacral prominence as a clinical sign of lower limb anisomelia: a pilot study.** *J Manipulative Physiol Ther* 1995, **18**:353–356.
145. Eriksen K: **Comparison between upper cervical X-ray listings and technique analysis utilizing a computerized database.** *Chiropr Res J* 1996, **3**:13–24.
146. Knutson GA: **Incidence of foot rotation, pelvic crest unleveling, and supine leg length alignment asymmetry and their relationship to self-reported back pain.** *J Manipulative Physiol Ther* 2002, **25**:110E.
147. Cooperstein R, Morschhauser E, Lisi AJ: **Cross-sectional validity study of compressive leg checking in measuring artificially created leg length inequality.** *J Chiropr Med* 2004, **3**:91–95.
148. Petrone MR, Guinn J, Reddin A, Sutlive TG, Flynn TW, Garber MP: **The accuracy of the palpation meter (PALM) for measuring pelvic crest height difference and leg length discrepancy.** *J Orthop Sports Phys Ther* 2003, **33**:319–325.
149. Fuhr AW, Osterbauer PJ: **Interexaminer reliability of relative Leg-length evaluations in the prone, extended position.** *Chiropract Tech* 1989, **1**:13–18.
150. Youngquist MW, Fuhr AW, Osterbauer PJ: **Interexaminer reliability of an isolation test for the identification of cervical subluxation.** *J Manipulative Physiol Ther* 1989, **12**:93–97.
151. Gross MT, Burns CB, Chapman SW, Hudson CJ, Curtis HS, Lehmann JR, *et al*: **Reliability and validity of rigid lift and pelvic leveling device method in assessing functional leg length inequality.** *J Orthop Sports Phys Ther* 1998, **27**:285–294.
152. Hinson R, Brown SH: **Supine Leg length differential estimation: an inter- and intra-examiner reliability study.** *Chiropr Res J* 1998, **5**:17–22.
153. Nguyen HT, Resnick DN, Caldwell SG, Elston EW Jr, Bishop BB, Steinhouser JB, *et al*: **Interexaminer reliability of activator methods' relative leg-length evaluation in the prone extended position.** *J Manipulative Physiol Ther* 1999, **22**:565–569.
154. Hanada E, Kirby RL, Mitchell M, Swuste JM: **Measuring leg-length discrepancy by the "iliac crest palpation and book correction" method: reliability and validity.** *Arch Phys Med Rehabil* 2001, **82**:938–942.
155. Gibbons P, Dumper C, Gosling C: **Inter-examiner and intra-examiner agreement for assessing simulated leg length inequality using palpation and observation during a standing assessment.** *J Osteopath Med* 2002, **5**:53–58.
156. Fryer G: **Factors affecting the intra-examiner and inter-examiner reliability of palpation for supine medial malleoli asymmetry.** *Int J Osteopath Med* 2006, **9**:58–65.
157. Schneider M, Homonai R, Moreland B, Delitto A: **Interexaminer reliability of the prone leg length analysis procedure.** *J Manipulative Physiol Ther* 2007, **30**:514–521.
158. Holt KR, Russell DG, Hoffmann NJ, Bruce BI, Bushell PM, Taylor HH: **Interexaminer reliability of a leg length analysis procedure among novice and experienced practitioners.** *J Manipulative Physiol Ther* 2009, **32**:216–222.
159. Woodfield HC, Gerstman BB, Olaisen RH, Johnson DF: **Interexaminer reliability of supine leg checks for discriminating leg-length inequality.** *J Manipulative Physiol Ther* 2011, **34**:239–246.
160. Papaioannou T, Stokes I, Kenwright J: **Scoliosis associated with limb-length inequality.** *J Bone Joint Surg Am* 1982, **64**:59–62.
161. Twellaar M, Verstappen FT, Huson A, van MW: **Physical characteristics as risk factors for sports injuries: a four year prospective study.** *Int J Sports Med* 1997, **18**:66–71.
162. Nourbakhsh MR, Arab AM: **Relationship between mechanical factors and incidence of low back pain.** *J Orthop Sports Phys Ther* 2002, **32**:447–460.
163. Cooperstein R, Morschhauser E, Lisi A, Nick TG: **Validity of compressive leg checking in measuring artificial leg-length inequality.** *J Manipulative Physiol Ther* 2003, **26**:557–566.
164. Schmeir AA: **Research work on a more precise method of determining muscle strength in poliomyelitis patients.** *J Bone Joint Surg* 1945, **27**:317–326.
165. Calderon L, Lawson AP: **Interexaminer reliability of applied kinesiology manual muscle testing.** *Chiropract Sports Med* 1994, **8**:148–152.
166. Lawson A, Calderon L: **Interexaminer agreement for applied kinesiology manual muscle testing.** *Percept Mot Skills* 1997, **84**:539–546.
167. Pollard HP, Bablis P, Bonello R: **Can the ileocecal valve point predict Low back pain using manual muscle testing?** *Chiropract J Aust* 2006, **36**:58–62.
168. Hsieh CY, Phillips RB: **Reliability of manual muscle testing with a computerized dynamometer.** *J Manipulative Physiol Ther* 1990, **13**:72–82.
169. Haas M, Peterson D, Hayr D, Ross G: **The reliability of muscle testing response to a provocative vertebral challenge.** *Chiropract Tech* 1993, **6**:95–100.
170. Ludtke R, Kunz B, Seeber N, Ring J: **Test-retest-reliability and validity of the kinesiology muscle test.** *Complement Ther Med* 2001, **9**:141–145.
171. Caruso W, Leisman G: **A force/displacement analysis of muscle testing.** *Percept Mot Skills* 2000, **91**:683–692.
172. Viitanen JV, Heikkila S, Kokko ML, Kautiainen H: **Clinical assessment of spinal mobility measurements in ankylosing spondylitis: a compact set for follow-up and trials?** *Clin Rheumatol* 2000, **19**:131–137.
173. Hestbaek L, Leboeuf-Yde C: **Are chiropractic tests for the lumbo-pelvic spine reliable and valid? a systematic critical literature review.** *J Manipulative Physiol Ther* 2000, **23**:258–275.
174. Piva SR, Erhard RE, Childs JD, Browder DA: **Inter-tester reliability of passive intervertebral and active movements of the cervical spine.** *Man Ther* 2006, **11**:321–330.
175. Petersen CM, Schuit D, Johnson RD, Knecht H, Levine P: **Agreement of measures obtained radiographically and by the OSI CA-6000 spine motion analyzer for cervical spinal motion.** *Man Ther* 2008, **13**:200–205.
176. Troke M, Moore AP, Cheek E: **Reliability of the OSI CA 6000 spine motion analyzer with a new skin fixation system when used on the thoracic spine.** *Man Ther* 1998, **3**:27–33.
177. Hall T, Robinson K: **The flexion-rotation test and active cervical mobility–a comparative measurement study in cervicogenic headache.** *Man Ther* 2004, **9**:197–202.
178. Hoppenbrouwers M, Eckhardt MM, Verkerk K, Verhagen A: **Reproducibility of the measurement of active and passive cervical range of motion.** *J Manipulative Physiol Ther* 2006, **29**:363–367.
179. Olson KA, Goehring MT: **Intra and inter-rater reliability of a goniometric lower trunk rotation measurement.** *J Back Musculoskelet Rehabil* 2009, **22**:157–164.
180. Chiarello CM, Savidge R: **Interrater reliability of the cybex EDI-320 and fluid goniometer in normals and patients with low back pain.** *Arch Phys Med Rehabil* 1993, **74**:32–37.
181. Breum J, Wiberg J, Bolton JE: **Reliability and concurrent validity of the BROM II for measuring lumbar mobility.** *J Manipulative Physiol Ther* 1995, **18**:497–502.
182. Osterbauer PJ, Long K, Ribaudo TA, Petermann EA, Fuhr AW, Bigos SJ, *et al*: **Three-dimensional head kinematics and cervical range of motion in the diagnosis of patients with neck trauma.** *J Manipulative Physiol Ther* 1996, **19**:231–237.
183. Bo K, Hilde G, Storheim K: **Intra- and interobserver reproducibility of cybex EDI 320 measuring spinal mobility.** *Scand J Med Sci Sports* 1997, **7**:140–143.
184. Solinger AB, Chen J, Lantz CA: **Standardized initial head position in cervical range-of-motion assessment: reliability and error analysis.** *J Manipulative Physiol Ther* 2000, **23**:20–26.
185. Tousignant M, Boucher N, Bourbonnais J, Gravelle T, Quesnel M, Brosseau L: **Intratester and intertester reliability of the cybex electronic digital inclinometer (EDI-320) for measurement of active neck flexion and extension in healthy subjects.** *Man Ther* 2001, **6**:235–241.

186. Haynes MJ, Edmondston S: **Accuracy and reliability of a new, protractor-based neck goniometer.** *J Manipulative Physiol Ther* 2002, **25:**579–586.
187. Lee SW, Wong KW, Chan MK, Yeung HM, Chiu JL, Leong JC: **Development and validation of a new technique for assessing lumbar spine motion.** *Spine (Phila Pa)* 2002, **27:**E215–E220.
188. Mayer TG, Gatchel RJ, Keeley J, McGeary D, Dersh J, Anagnostis C: **A randomized clinical trial of treatment for lumbar segmental rigidity.** *Spine (Phila Pa)* 2004, **29:**2199–2205.
189. Agarwal S, Allison GT, Singer KP: **Reliability of the spin-T cervical goniometer in measuring cervical range of motion in an asymptomatic Indian population.** *J Manipulative Physiol Ther* 2005, **28:**487–492.
190. Bockenhauer SE, Chen H, Julliard KN, Weedon J: **Measuring thoracic excursion: reliability of the cloth tape measure technique.** *J Am Osteopath Assoc* 2007, **107:**191–196.
191. Roy R, Boucher JP, Comtois AS: **Validity of infrared thermal measurements of segmental paraspinal skin surface temperature.** *J Manipulative Physiol Ther* 2006, **29:**150–155.
192. Roy RA, Boucher JP, Comtois AS: **Effects of a manually assisted mechanical force on cutaneous temperature.** *J Manipulative Physiol Ther* 2008, **31:**230–236.
193. Chafetz N, Wexler CE, Kaiser JA: **Neuromuscular thermography of the lumbar spine with CT correlation.** *Spine (Phila Pa)* 1988, **13:**922–925.
194. McCulloch J, Frymoyer J, Steurer P, Riaz G, Hurst F: **Thermography as a diagnostic aid in sciatica.** *J Spinal Disord* 1993, **6:**427–431.
195. Diakow PRP, Ouellet S, Lee S, Blackmore EJ: **Correlation of thermography with spinal dysfunction: preliminary results.** *J Can Chiropract Assoc* 1988, **32:**77–80.
196. Zaproudina N, Ming Z, Hanninen OO: **Plantar infrared thermography measurements and low back pain intensity.** *J Manipulative Physiol Ther* 2006, **29:**219–223.
197. Plaugher G, Lopes MA, Melch PE, Cremata EE: **The inter- and intraexaminer reliability of a paraspinal skin temperature differential instrument.** *J Manipulative Physiol Ther* 1991, **14:**361–367.
198. Hart JH, Omolo B, Boone WR, Brown C, Ashton A: **Reliability of three methods of computer-aided thermal pattern analysis.** *J Can Chiropract Assoc* 2007, **51:**175–185.
199. Owens EF Jr, Hart JF, Donofrio JJ, Haralambous J, Mierzejewski E: **Paraspinal skin temperature patterns: an interexaminer and intraexaminer reliability study.** *J Manipulative Physiol Ther* 2004, **27:**155–159.
200. Seay C, Gibbon C, Hart J: **Intraexaminer and interexaminer reliability of mastoid fossa readings using a temporal artery thermometer.** *J Chiropr Med* 2007, **6:**66–69.
201. Degenhardt BF, Johnson JC, Snider KT, Snider EJ: **Maintenance and improvement of interobserver reliability of osteopathic palpatory tests over a 4-month period.** *J Am Osteopath Assoc* 2010, **110:**579–586.
202. Paulet T, Fryer G: **Inter-examiner reliability of palpation for tissue texture abnormality in the thoracic paraspinal region.** *Int J Osteopath Med* 2009, **12:**92–96.
203. Rendell MS, Dovgan DJ, Bergman TF, O'Donnell GP, Drobny EP, Katims JJ: **Mapping diabetic sensory neuropathy by current perception threshold testing.** *Diabetes Care* 1989, **12:**636–640.
204. Yamashita T, Kanaya K, Sekine M, Takebayashi T, Kawaguchi S, Katahira G: **A quantitative analysis of sensory function in lumbar radiculopathy using current perception threshold testing.** *Spine (Phila Pa)* 2002, **27:**1567–1570.
205. Imoto K, Takebayashi T, Kanaya K, Kawaguchi S, Katahira G, Yamashita T: **Quantitative analysis of sensory functions after lumbar discectomy using current perception threshold testing.** *Eur Spine J* 2007, **16:**971–975.
206. Nansel DD, Jansen RD: **Concordance between galvanic skin response and spinal palpation findings in pain-free males.** *J Manipulative Physiol Ther* 1988, **11:**267–272.
207. Plaugher G, Haas M, Doble RW Jr, Lopes MA, Cremata EE, Lantz C: **The interexaminer reliability of a galvanic skin response instrument.** *J Manipulative Physiol Ther* 1993, **16:**453–459.
208. Geisser ME, Ranavaya M, Haig AJ, Roth RS, Zucker R, Ambroz C, *et al*: **A meta-analytic review of surface electromyography among persons with low back pain and normal, healthy controls.** *J Pain* 2005, **6:**711–726.
209. Demoulin C, Crielaard JM, Vanderthommen M: **Spinal muscle evaluation in healthy individuals and low-back-pain patients: a literature review.** *Joint Bone Spine* 2007, **74:**9–13.
210. Danneels LA, Cagnie BJ, Cools AM, Vanderstraeten GG, Cambier DC, Witvrouw EE, *et al*: **Intra-operator and inter-operator reliability of surface electromyography in the clinical evaluation of back muscles.** *Man Ther* 2001, **6:**145–153.
211. Dankaerts W, O'Sullivan P, Burnett A, Straker L: **Altered patterns of superficial trunk muscle activation during sitting in nonspecific chronic low back pain patients: importance of subclassification.** *Spine (Phila Pa)* 1976, **31:**2017–2023.
212. Fryer G, Bird M, Robbins B, Fossum C, Johnson JC: **Resting electromyographic activity of deep thoracic transversospinalis muscles identified as abnormal with palpation.** *J Am Osteopath Assoc* 2010, **110:**61–68.
213. Lehman GJ: **Clinical considerations in the use of surface electromyography: three experimental studies.** *J Manipulative Physiol Ther* 2002, **25:**293–299.
214. Leach RA, Owens EF Jr, Giesen JM: **Correlates of myoelectric asymmetry detected in low back pain patients using hand-held post-style surface electromyography.** *J Manipulative Physiol Ther* 1993, **16:**140–149.
215. Harrison DD, Cailliet R, Janik TJ, Troyanovich SJ, Harrison DE, Holland B: **Elliptical modeling of the sagittal lumbar lordosis and segmental rotation angles as a method to discriminate between normal and low back pain subjects.** *J Spinal Disord* 1998, **11:**430–439.
216. Harrison DD, Harrison DE, Janik TJ, Cailliet R, Ferrantelli JR, Haas JW, *et al*: **Modeling of the sagittal cervical spine as a method to discriminate hypolordosis: results of elliptical and circular modeling in 72 asymptomatic subjects, 52 acute neck pain subjects, and 70 chronic neck pain subjects.** *Spine (Phila Pa)* 2004, **29:**2485–2492.
217. Troyanovich SJ, Harrison SO, Harrison DD, Harrison DE, Payne MR, Janik TJ, *et al*: **Chiropractic biophysics digitized radiographic mensuration analysis of the anteroposterior lumbopelvic view: a reliability study.** *J Manipulative Physiol Ther* 1999, **22:**309–315.
218. Troyanovich SJ, Harrison D, Harrison DD, Harrison SO, Janik T, Holland B: **Chiropractic biophysics digitized radiographic mensuration analysis of the anteroposterior cervicothoracic view: a reliability study.** *J Manipulative Physiol Ther* 2000, **23:**476–482.
219. Plaugher G, Hendricks AH, Doble RW Jr, Bachman TR, Araghi HJ, Hoffart VM: **The reliability of patient positioning for evaluating static radiologic parameters of the human pelvis.** *J Manipulative Physiol Ther* 1993, **16:**517–522.
220. Bierma-Zeinstra SM, van Gool JJ, Bernsen RM, Njoo KH: **Measuring the sacral inclination angle in clinical practice: is there an alternative to radiographs?** *J Manipulative Physiol Ther* 2001, **24:**505–508.
221. Abbott JH, Fritz JM, McCane B, Shultz B, Herbison P, Lyons B, *et al*: **Lumbar segmental mobility disorders: comparison of two methods of defining abnormal displacement kinematics in a cohort of patients with non specific mechanical low back pain.** *BMC Musculoskelet Disord* 2006, **7:**45.
222. Harrison DE, Harrison DD, Colloca CJ, Betz J, Janik TJ, Holland B: **Repeatability over time of posture, radiograph positioning, and radiograph line drawing: an analysis of six control groups.** *J Manipulative Physiol Ther* 2003, **26:**87–98.
223. Plaugher G, Hendricks AH: **The inter- and intraexaminer reliability of the gonstead pelvic marking system.** *J Manipulative Physiol Ther* 1991, **14:**503–508.
224. Antos JC, Robinson K, Keating JC, Jacobs GE: **Inter-rater reliability of fluoroscopic detection of fixation in the Mid cervical spine.** *Chiropract Tech* 1990, **2:**53–55.
225. Croft AC, Krage JS, Pate D, Young DN: **Videofluoroscopy in cervical spine trauma: an interinterpreter reliability study.** *J Manipulative Physiol Ther* 1994, **17:**20–24.
226. Jackson BL, Harrison DD, Robertson GA, Barker WF: **Chiropractic biophysics lateral cervical film analysis reliability.** *J Manipulative Physiol Ther* 1993, **16:**384–391.
227. Phillips RB, Frymoyer JW, Mac Pherson BV, Newburg AH: **Low back pain: a radiographic enigma.** *J Manipulative Physiol Ther* 1986, **9:**183–187.
228. Haas M, Nyiendo J, Peterson C, Thiel H, Sellers T, Cassidy D, *et al*: **Interrater reliability of roentgenological evaluation of the lumbar spine in lateral bending.** *J Manipulative Physiol Ther* 1990, **13:**179–189.
229. Haas M, Peterson D: **A roentgenological evaluation of the relationship between segmental motion and malalignment in lateral bending.** *J Manipulative Physiol Ther* 1992, **15:**350–360.
230. Olson KA, Paris SV, Spohr C: **Radiographic assessment and reliability study of the craniovertebral sidebending.** *J Manipulative Physiol Ther* 1998, **6:**87–96.
231. Rhudy T, Sandefur M, Burk J: **Interexaminer/intertechnique reliability in spinal subluxation assessment: a multifactorial approach.** *Am J Chiropractic Med* 1988, **1:**111–114.
232. Hawk C, Phongphua C, Bleecker J, Swank L, Lopez D, Rubley T: **Preliminary study of the reliability of assessment procedures for indications for chiropractic adjustments of the lumbar spine.** *J Manipulative Physiol Ther* 1999, **22:**382–389.

233. Potter L, McCarthy C, Oldham J: **Intraexaminer reliability of identifying a dysfunctional segment in the thoracic and lumbar spine.** *J Manipulative Physiol Ther* 2006, **29**:203–207.
234. Degenhardt BF, Snider KT, Snider EJ, Johnson JC: **Interobserver reliability of osteopathic palpatory diagnostic tests of the lumbar spine: improvements from consensus training.** *J Am Osteopath Assoc* 2005, **105**:465–473.
235. Keating JC Jr, Bergmann TF, Jacobs GE, Finer BA, Larson K: **Interexaminer reliability of eight evaluative dimensions of lumbar segmental abnormality.** *J Manipulative Physiol Ther* 1990, **13**:463–470.
236. Toussaint R, Gawlik CS, Rehder U, Ruther W: **Sacroiliac joint diagnostics in the Hamburg construction workers study.** *J Manipulative Physiol Ther* 1999, **22**:139–143.
237. Bossuyt PM, Reitsma JB, Bruns DE, Gatsonis CA, Glasziou PP, Irwig LM, *et al*: **The STARD statement for reporting studies of diagnostic accuracy: explanation and elaboration.** *Ann Intern Med* 2003, **138**:W1–W12.
238. Whiting PF, Rutjes AW, Westwood ME, Mallett S, Deeks JJ, Reitsma JB, *et al*: **QUADAS-2: a revised tool for the quality assessment of diagnostic accuracy studies.** *Ann Intern Med* 2011, **155**:529–536.
239. Budgell B: *The use of surface electromyography in the assessment of functional biomechanical disorders of the spine.* Victoria, Australia: Chiropractors Registration Board of Victoria; 2007.
240. Bossuyt PM, Reitsma JB, Linnet K, Moons KG: **Beyond diagnostic accuracy: the clinical utility of diagnostic tests.** *Clin Chem* 2012, **58**:1636–1643.

Essential literature for the chiropractic profession: a survey of chiropractic research leaders

Barbara A Mansholt[1*], John S Stites[2], Dustin C Derby[3], Ron J Boesch[4] and Stacie A Salsbury[5]

Abstract

Background: Evidence-based clinical practice (EBCP) is an accepted practice for informed clinical decision making in mainstream health care professions. EBCP augments clinical experience and can have far reaching effects in education, policy, reimbursement and clinical management. The proliferation of published research can be overwhelming—finding a mechanism to identify literature that is essential for practitioners and students is desirable. The purpose of this study was to survey leaders in the chiropractic profession on their opinions of essential literature for doctors of chiropractic, faculty, and students to read or reference.

Methods: Deployment of an IRB exempted survey occurred with 68 academic and research leaders using SurveyMonkey®. Individuals were solicited via e-mail in August of 2011; the study closed in October of 2011. Collected data were checked for citation accuracy and compiled to determine multiple responses. A secondary analysis assessed the scholarly impact and Internet accessibility of the recommended literature.

Results: Forty-three (43) individuals consented to participate; seventeen (17) contributed at least one article of importance. A total of 41 unique articles were reported. Of the six articles contributed more than once, one article was reported 6 times, and 5 were reported twice.

Conclusions: A manageable list of relevant literature was created. Shortcomings of methods were identified, and improvements for continued implementation are suggested. A wide variety of articles were reported as "essential" knowledge, annual or bi-annual surveys would be helpful for the profession.

Keywords: Evidence-based practice, Evidence-based health care, Chiropractic, Web-based survey, Publications, Professional education

Background

Evidence based clinical practice (EBCP) may be defined as "the conscientious and judicious use of clinical expertise, patient values, and current best evidence" [1]. Each component of EBCP may assume greater or lesser importance depending upon such factors as the doctor-patient relationship or the patient's presenting condition and preferences, and assert varying emphases within different healthcare environments or health service delivery contexts [2] (Figure 1). While definitions may vary, evidence within an EBCP framework refers to published, peer-reviewed, scientific research [1]. Thus, EBCP requires that clinicians are knowledgeable of current scientific evidence and best practices based upon published research [3].

The chiropractic profession has maintained its position as the largest alternative or non-traditional approach to healthcare [4-6]. At the same time, the profession seeks wider mainstream acceptance by both the public and its healthcare peers [7-16]. In response, many chiropractic colleges now teach EBCP approaches to chiropractic care [17-20]. Used appropriately, EBCP gives chiropractic professionals of all stages of experience insight beyond their own clinical expertise to guide clinical decision making and helps patients make educated, informed choices [21]. However, recent studies suggest chiropractors and chiropractic students may not yet possess the attitudes, knowledge, reading habits or critical appraisal skills needed to implement EBCP in educational or practice settings [19,22-24].

One issue in EBCP consistently identified by chiropractic students and clinicians is the process of searching,

* Correspondence: barbara.mansholt@palmer.edu
[1]Technique Department, Palmer College of Chiropractic, 1000 Brady St, Davenport, IA 52803, USA
Full list of author information is available at the end of the article

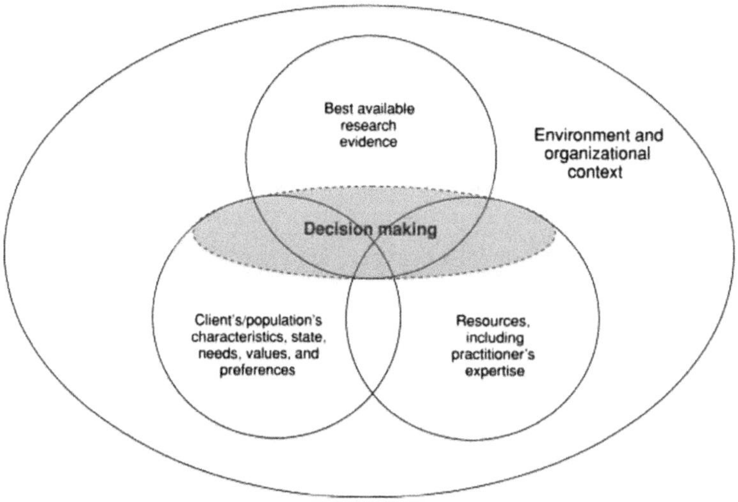

Figure 1 Evidence based clinical decision making Venn diagram[2].

reading, and appraising the scientific literature to apply this evidence to clinical practice [22-26]. At the same time, published research in the chiropractic profession is increasing in quality and quantity at a rapid pace [27-30]. Clinicians in all stages of practice might benefit from compiled resources that identify key studies and other evidence to support chiropractic practice. Chiropractic researchers frequently review and appraise the scholarly literature related to the field of chiropractic and might provide input into which articles would be most important to doctors of chiropractic [28]. Our goal in this study was to compile a list of the most important published research germane to the field of chiropractic—articles every doctor of chiropractic, students, or faculty should read, reference, and put into EBCP.

Methods

The Palmer College of Chiropractic Institutional Review Board (IRB) Human Protections Administrator exempted this survey from full IRB review, and the study was approved as submitted. The authors compiled a list of potential survey respondents that included the research department directors at 18 chiropractic colleges in North America, editors of 17 chiropractic journals, and respected leaders within the profession based upon their current involvement in research and/or regard as a prominent research author. We identified an initial list of 68 chiropractic research leaders.

We developed a web-based survey using Survey Monkey® software and pre-tested it among the authors. Recipients received the survey link via e-mail and cover letter with a short explanation regarding the purpose and methods of the study. Upon linking to the survey, recipients were informed that no personal benefit would be gained through their response and that their response was anonymous. Checking a box "yes" to advance into the survey served as informed consent and was stated as such in the dialogue box. Survey deployment occurred between August and October 2011. Respondents received up to four automated reminder messages, depending on their response status within the software. Demographic data collected included respondents' age, gender, highest degree earned, primary academic assignment (e.g., research, faculty, clinician, administration), and area of focus.

The survey used qualitative data collection methods as presenting respondents with an exhaustive list of research studies germane to the field of chiropractic in a checklist format was not feasible. Instead, respondents listed the author, title, journal, and year of an article the respondent considered important and one "that every doctor of chiropractic should read". Respondents then categorized the article as education, research, health care policy, patient education, or other. Each respondent also wrote a short statement indicating why the recommended article was important for the field. Each respondent could list up to six research studies. Quality control checks assured citation accuracy. Citation recommendations were analyzed thematically according to Bogdan and Biklen's "subjects" ways of thinking about people and objects" [31]. In other words, we were interested in knowing which objects (e.g., published research) the respondent believed were the most critical for chiropractic practitioners and students (e.g., their thoughts on importance).

We performed a secondary analysis to characterize the scholarly impact and accessibility of each recommended article to assist chiropractic professionals in the process of selecting high-quality evidence from among the scholarly literature. Scholarly impact refers to the relative importance of a publication within its field and across disciplines. Google Scholar was selected as the literature search engine over alternate scientific and academic literature repositories (e.g., PubMed, Index of Chiropractic Literature, Scopus, Web of Science) for its no-cost public access, breadth of coverage across disciplines, ability to search multiple databases simultaneously, embedded links to recent and full-text articles, and literature citation metrics. We estimated scholarly impact by counts of the number of times other researchers had cited each article.

Practitioners' access to scholarly literature is a known barrier to implementation of EBCP across disciplines with many clinicians reporting little to no access to electronic resources in their workplaces [25,32-34]. Article accessibility was assessed through the 'All Versions' feature of Google Scholar. We characterized each article as fully accessible if it was available without cost through open access sources (e.g., PubMed Central [PMC] or the journal/publisher website), limitedly accessible if an article required purchase from the publisher for on-line access, and inaccessible if no link to an on-line source or purchase options was identified.

Statement on ethics

This study was submitted to the Palmer College of Chiropractic Human Protections Administrator in June of 2011, determined exempt according to 45 CFR 46.101 (b)(2), and conducted from August of 2011 through October or 2011. A signed copy of IRB assurance # X2011-2-1-S is available upon request.

Results

Response rates and respondent demographics

Although 43 of 68 potential respondents agreed to participate in the study (63%), only 17 respondents contributed at least one article of importance, for a response rate of 25%. Of the final respondents, six were between 41–50 years of age, ten were between 51 and 60, and one was 61 or older. In addition to possessing a clinical doctorate, nine held academic doctorates, six master's degrees, and twelve bachelor's degrees. Demographic characteristics of survey respondents are presented in Table 1.

Table 1 Respondent demographics of essential literature study

Characteristic	n = 17
Age	
41-50	6
51-60	10
61 or older	1
Gender	
Female	1
Male	16
Degrees earned (mark all that apply)	
BS	12
MS	6
Clinical doctorate (DC, DO, MD)	17
Academic doctorate (PhD or EdD)	9
Primary involvement in chiropractic profession	
Research	8
Teaching (full-time)	2
Faculty Clinician	1
Practicing clinician (non-academic)	3
Administration	2
Other	1
Area of focus	
Health care policy	1
Patient care	2
Education	3
Research	9
Other	2

Article citation data

Respondents contributed 50 pieces of evidence (PE). Forty-one PE were mentioned at least once, with six articles mentioned by two or more respondents. Respondents categorized 26 as research, six as education, six as health care policy, and the remaining three as other. Additionally, forty were published within journals and one was a book. Recommended articles were published most often in the *Journal of Manipulative and Physiological Therapeutics* and *The Spine Journal* (Figure 2). Publications years for the recommended PE ranged from 1995 to 2011, with an emphasis on recently published journal articles. Seventeen (17) PE were published in 2005–2009 and 11 PE between 2010–2011 (Figure 3).

Table 2 reports the 41 recommended PE. Citations are listed first by the number of recommendations by survey respondents and then by number of Google Scholar citations. Each PE also includes information about its accessibility. Lastly, a quotation from the recommending respondent is provided demonstrating the importance of the article for chiropractic professionals.

Articles with multiple recommendations

Six distinct articles were recommended by more than one respondent. Six respondents recommended the article, "Effectiveness of manual therapies: the UK evidence report", by Bronfort et al. [35]. A majority of the respondents noted the comprehensive nature of this systematic review of randomized clinical trials of spinal manipulation, mobilization and massage. This article addresses varying levels of evidence and cites 322 articles on spinal

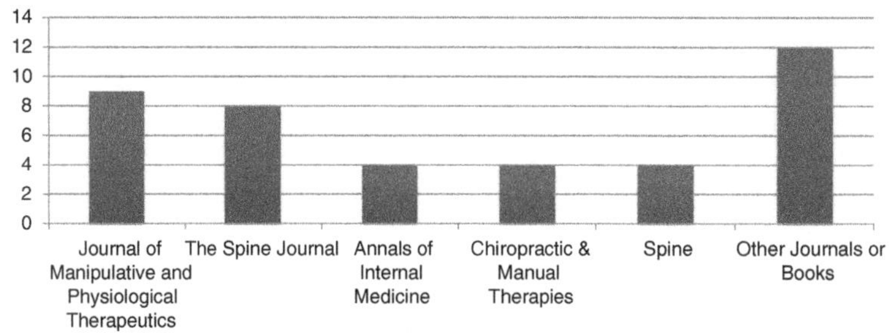

Figure 2 Recommended citations by journal.

manipulation and other manual therapies as treatments for musculoskeletal, headache and non-musculoskeletal conditions in an organized and easily readable manner. One respondent wrote, "This is the most comprehensive systematic review of the literature pertinent to DCs for both musculoskeletal (MSK) and non-MSK conditions".

Two respondents each recommended five additional studies [8,36-39]. An article published in 2002 by Pickar [36], "Neurophysiological effects of spinal manipulation", is one of the earliest publications making the list, confirming the author's early attention to identifying the basic mechanisms of action underlying spinal manipulation and the relevance of the topic for doctors of chiropractic. One respondent wrote, "[the article] provides evidence based scientific rationale for the effects of spinal manipulation".

Another basic science article, this one by Ianuzzi and Khalsa [39], "Comparison of human lumbar facet joint capsule strains during simulated high-velocity, low-amplitude spinal manipulation versus physiological motions," was similarly recommended by respondents: "an important paper for mechanisms of action of spinal manipulation" and "demonstrated intrinsic biomechanical safety of lumbar spinal manipulation".

The large population-based study by Cassidy et al. [37] "Risk of vertebrobasilar stroke and chiropractic care: results of a population-based case–control and case-crossover study", demonstrated vertebrobasilar stroke as a very rare adverse event. This article is a relevant reference for chiropractic professionals who educate their patients, other healthcare providers and the media about the risks of chiropractic care. One respondent commented, *"This presents the best evidence about the risk of stroke after cervical manipulation"*.

A Cochrane Collaboration systematic review published by Walker and colleagues [38], "Combined chiropractic interventions for low back pain", represented a rigorous, international, and interdisciplinary evaluation of the merits combined chiropractic therapies over spinal manipulation alone for pain and disability. Of this article, one respondent wrote, *"This systematic review shows that usual chiropractic care is as effective as many other therapies for acute or sub acute low back pain"*.

An article by Murphy et al. [8], "The establishment of a primary spine care practitioner and its benefits to health care reform in the United States," presented a cogent health policy rationale for changing the role of chiropractors in the U.S. health care delivery system based on research evidence. Individuals interested in the evolution of the chiropractic profession should be familiar with this document, as a respondent commented, *"This article outlines the need for a primary spine care clinician in the health care system, and highlights the qualifications of DCs to fill this niche"*.

Literature with single recommendations

Of the 41 unique PEs, 34 were unduplicated articles or books mentioned by a single respondent. Six singly recommended articles address interdisciplinary clinical

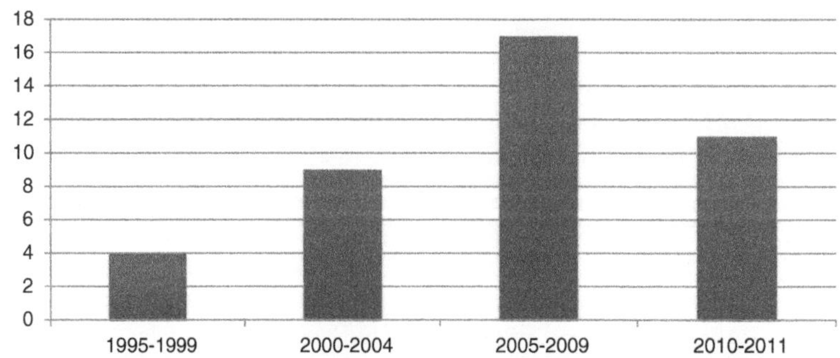

Figure 3 Recommended citations by publication year.

Table 2 Essential literature for the chiropractic profession: articles submitted, number of recommendations and justification, Google scholar citation frequency, and accessibility

Citation	Survey votes	Google scholar citations	Open access available	*Recommendation quote*
Bronfort G, et al [35]	6	134	PMC	*"This is the most comprehensive systematic review of the literature pertinent to DCs for both musculoskeletal (MSK) and non-MSK conditions."*
Pickar JG [36]	2	183	Purchase Un/author	*"provides evidence based scientific rationale for the effects of spinal manipulation."*
Cassidy JD, et al [37]	2	174	PMC	*"This presents the best evidence about the risk of stroke after cervical manipulation."*
Walker BF, et al [38]	2	32	Purchase	*"This systematic review shows that usual chiropractic care is as effective as many other therapies for acute or sub acute low back pain."*
Ianuzzi A, et al [39]	2	24	PMC	*"An important paper for mechanisms of action of spinal manipulation." "Demonstrated intrinsic biomechanical safety of lumbar spinal manipulation."*
Murphy DR, et al [8]	2	6	Journal	*"This article outlines the need for a primary spine care clinician in the health care system, and highlights the qualifications of DCs to fill this niche."*
Chou R, et al [40]	1	753	Journal	*"Excellent summary of 7 recommendations related to the diagnosis and treatment of low back pain."*
Childs JD, et al [41]	1	435	Journal	*"...published by PTs and is cited as the first clinical prediction rule (CPR) for spinal manipulation. Although as DCs we feel "underwhelmed" by the simplistic nature of this CPR, we must recognize that this paper has catapulted the PT profession's image within the spine care world."*
Chou R, et al [42]	1	389	Journal	*"clinical practice guidelines for primary care physicians for treatment of low back pain that includes spinal manipulation"*
UK BEAM Trial Team [43]	1	245	PMC	*"largest effectiveness trial to date of benefits of spinal manipulation for low back pain"*
Senstad O, et al [44]	1	209	Purchase	*"Chiropractors need to know that there are side effects to SMT and that not all patients have a positive experience or outcome."*
Hurwitz EL, et al [45]	1	207	Purchase Un/author	*"The authors assess the evidence base for spinal manipulation and other conservative therapies for the treatment of neck-related disorders."*
Nelson CF, et al [46]	1	154	Purchase	*"showed long term benefits of manipulation over most commonly used medication for migraine headaches."*
Olafsdottir E, et al [47]	1	141	Journal	*"This paper demonstrates that the benefit of chiropractic for infantile colic is the same as a placebo."*
Skyba DA, et al [48]	1	88	PMC	*"This paper presents the best neurophysiological evidence regarding post manipulative analgesia."*
Haldeman S, et al [49]	1	79	PMC	*"good summary of status of neck pain research relevant to chiropractors; would recommend all papers in that series"*
Dagenais S, et al [50]	1	76	Purchase Un/author	*"important to understand the current evidence and its implication for practice."*
Legorreta AP, et al [51]	1	59	Journal	*"excellent paper assessing cost benefits to chiropractic care"*
Cramer GD, et al [52]	1	56	Purchase Un/author	*"mechanisms of action of spinal manipulation"*
Haas M, et al [53]	1	50	Purchase Un/author	*"Dose studies of manipulation are extremely important. This one showing that more care [is] better than less..."*
Carroll LJ, et al [54]	1	44	PMC	*"The authors assess the evidence base for spinal manipulation and other conservative therapies for the treatment of neck-related disorders."*
Bogduk N, et al [55]	1	37	No online access	"This would give chiropractors a clear insight into and synthesis of the evidence available for the treatment and management of neck pain"
Pickar JG, et al [56]	1	37	Purchase	*"important paper for mechanism of action of spinal manipulation"*
Haas M, et al [57]	1	34	Purchase Un/author	*"provides evidence that the frequency of effective manipulative care may not be what is generally thought in clinical practice"*
Reggars JW, et al [58]	1	33	Purchase	*"it demonstrates which joints cavitate in the neck when the head is rotated left or right."*

Table 2 Essential literature for the chiropractic profession: articles submitted, number of recommendations and justification, Google scholar citation frequency, and accessibility *(Continued)*

Murphy DR, et al [59]	1	32	Journal	*"This paper is the first in a series to present a rationale for and the details of a rational evidence based approach to the management of patients with spinal pain."*
Bishop PB, et al [60]	1	27	Purchase Un/author	*"demonstrates practical application of EBM to clinical care"*
Little JS, et al [61]	1	26	Purchase	*"demonstrated that vertebral motion unit fixation (aka subluxation) creates abnormal facet joint capsule strain patterns"*
Pickar JG, et al [62]	1	23	PMC	*"demonstrated [that] spinal manipulation induces paraspinal muscle afferent response"*
Herzog W [63]	1	19	Purchase Un/author	*"reviews the current evidence related to adjusting"*
Haas M, et al [30]	1	18	Purchase	*"provides a historical summary"*
Murphy DR, et al [59]	1	15	Journal	*"2nd in the series by Murphy et al. that presents the evidence for the model presented earlier on a chiropractic management approach to spinal pain"*
Ianuzzi A, et al [64]	1	14	Purchase	*"determined unique biomechanics created by spinal manipulation"*
Hartman SE [65]	1	13	PMC Journal	*"helps explain why our belief in clinical effectiveness may not jibe with the research"*
Henderson CN, et al [66]	1	13	Purchase Un/author	*"establishes animal model for studying mechanisms of action of spinal manipulation"*
McGinn T, et al [67]	1	11	PMC	*"teaches CPRs in applying evidence"*
Cramer GD, et al [68]	1	10	Purchase	*"mechanism of action of spinal manipulation"*
Chevan J, et al [69]	1	8	Journal	*"This article written by PTs cites survey research showing that more LBP patients seek DC services (28%) compared to PT services (11%). Their discussion about the disparities between DCs and PTs is quite revealing."*
Villanueva-Russell Y [14]	1	6	Purchase	*"helps create professional identity"*
Bogduk N [70]	1	3	No online access	*"This article provides the reader with the [simple] tools to determine if a manuscript provides the necessary information to identify the reliability and validity of diagnostic tests. Chiropractors often adopt tests that they do not determine these characteristics for and need to know how to do this…"*
Haneline M [71]	1	0	Purchase	*"informs the practitioner of what is and what is not evidence-based practice"*

PMC = Article available through open access on PubMed Central.
Journal = Article available through open access on journal homepage.
Purchase = Article available for purchase from journal.
Un/Author = Unauthorized posting on Internet website.

decision-making for the care of patients with low back pain [40-42,50,59,72], while two texts highlight treatment approaches to neck pain and related conditions [45,55]. Five articles report findings from clinical trials of manual therapies or spinal manipulation [43,46,53,57,60], while three other papers discuss either ineffective applications, [47,65] or common side effects of manipulation [44]. Lastly, nine articles demonstrate chiropractic research priorities [30,73,74], analyze health policy issues for the chiropractic profession [14,51,69], or discuss evidence-based practice concepts for doctors and students of chiropractic [67,70,71]. That only one respondent mentioned each of these studies should not undermine their potential relevance to the chiropractic profession. Instead, many unduplicated references are important references on key concepts, evidence or issues for practicing doctors of chiropractic. For example, 10 recommended articles provide theoretical rationale or basic science evidence on the mechanisms of action of spinal or joint manipulation [48,52,56,58,61-64,66,68].

Scholarly impact

The secondary analysis of the scholarly impact of the recommended PEs revealed interesting patterns that may further assist doctors of chiropractic in selecting from among this list of essential literature for the profession (Table 2). The Google Scholar citation analysis identified some articles as highly referenced within the field of chiropractic and in associated disciplines. Researchers have cited some chiropractic research articles more than 100 times including work by Senstad et al. [44], Hurwitz et al. [45], Pickar [36], Cassidy et al. [37], Nelson et al. [46], Bronfort et al. [35] and Olafsdottir and colleagues [47]. Several articles in fields related to chiropractic, specifically regarding the interdisciplinary care of persons with back pain, also demonstrated very high citation rates [40-43]. These articles have clearly influenced how other researchers view the field. Other articles recommended as essential literature have received much less attention from researchers. This analysis of scholarly impact does not necessarily indicate the possible influence of any article among chiropractic educators, clinicians or students.

Article accessibility

The accessibility of scholarly articles also is an important factor for the dissemination, uptake, and clinical application of scientific knowledge. Many of the most highly cited articles were freely available as full-text articles on the Internet, either from the journal publisher or through the U.S. National Library of Medicine (NLM) and its PubMed Central (PMC) database of biomedical and life sciences literatures. For example, the articles with the broadest uptake by other authors were the low back pain clinical practice guidelines and the clinical prediction rule for identifying responders to spinal manipulation, three freely accessible articles published in *Annals of Internal Medicine* (Table 2). In contrast, articles published in *Spine*, *The Spine Journal*, and *Journal of Manipulative and Physiologic Therapeutics* were available only by subscription or direct purchase, at a cost of about $30 US per article. Perhaps not surprisingly, these articles also had lower overall citation rates from papers published in open access journals or those available from PMC. Of note, several of these articles were available on websites from individuals or institutions in possible violation of article copyright agreements.

Discussion

This survey of chiropractic research leaders sought to identify essential literature that every doctor of chiropractic and chiropractic student should read and reference to inform evidence-based clinical practice. Survey respondents identified 41 unique articles or books they considered key readings within the field of chiropractic or related disciplines. Essential literature included basic science and clinical research, health policy statements, education-based articles, and other types of evidence for the chiropractic profession. The majority of the recommended articles (n = 34) were published in the past 10 years, with no citations prior to 1995 offered by respondents. Two or more respondents recommended six journal articles as key pieces of evidence for doctors of chiropractic and chiropractic students [8,35-39]. These articles offered evidence on the effectiveness of manual therapies [35,38], the physiological underpinnings of spinal manipulation [36,39], risks related to chiropractic care [37], and arguments for an expanded role for chiropractors within the health care system [8], all timely and important topics for the chiropractic profession. Thirty-four additional citations on a topics ranging from low back pain and neck pain, chiropractic side effects, biomechanical and physiological effects of chiropractic adjustments, research priorities, costs and access for chiropractic therapy, and evidence-based clinical practice also were identified.

Many articles selected by respondents as essential literature had achieved some degree of scholarly impact in that they were referenced by many researchers in multiple publications [35-37,40-42,46,49,50,53,54]. While the selection of scholarly literature is dependent upon the specific goals and interests of the reader, an argument is made that articles cited more often both within the profession and in disciplines with a shared scope are more essential for the chiropractic professional than articles not as widely referenced. A shared knowledge base will assist doctors of chiropractic to communicate with one another, our patients, and other healthcare professionals about the evidence underpinning various treatment approaches.

The scholarly impact and clinical importance of this essential literature for the chiropractic profession also may be influenced by the access clinicians have to scientific articles [25,32-34]. Our secondary analysis found that articles published in open access journals generally had higher citation rates than journals where article access was limited to subscribers or by purchase. Clinicians may be prevented from accessing articles recommended as essential literature by costly fees, a concern identified in previous research [75]. Editors and publishers of chiropractic and spine-related journals may wish to reconsider their access policies in order to increase use of their articles by researchers and practicing clinicians.

Limitations

Extremely low response rate, high rate of attrition, coverage and non-response survey errors, and self-report bias are limitations of this study. This extremely low response rate and high attrition rate were problematic. While 43 of 68 potential respondents agreed to participate, only 25% completed the survey. Of these 17 respondents, eight contributed only one piece of evidence, six contributed 2–5 references, and only three contributed more than five citations. This response rate is low by survey standards [76], including among surveys of doctors of chiropractic, which average about 53% for postal surveys [77]. The reasons for the sharp decline between respondents agreeing to participate in the study and their actual participation are unknown. While only four e-mails were returned undeliverable, it is unknown how many potential respondents may have not have received the initial e-mail due to spam filters. Future studies could be designed using a multi-modal approach. The attrition rate was high as respondents could re-enter the survey at any time during deployment if they left the session after agreeing to participate. Both of these issues potentially affect the quality of data, specifically coverage and non-response error. Coverage and non-response errors result from all members of a population not having a known, nonzero chance of being included in the sample and by non-respondents potentially differing from respondents [76]. The high attrition, both in terms of starting the survey and stopping after submitting only one recommendation might be attributed to recall bias and or source amnesia (e.g., inability to remember where, when or how one has learned prior information while retaining its factual knowledge) [78]. Respondents also performed mental work to complete this short-answer survey rather than answering discrete categorical questions, which also can result in increased attrition [76]. And yet, this survey was web-based. Respondents were not asked to recall references from memory nor were they restricted from using on-line databases to identify essential literature, which might suggest either low familiarity with the chiropractic literature or a disinterest in the survey topic among respondents. Varying degrees of self-report bias also are possible. Respondents may have entered socially desired responses (i.e., often-cited references or citations from well-known researchers) or responses that might benefit themselves or their colleagues (i.e., referencing articles that either they or their colleagues have published). An additional limitation is the potential geographic bias in the survey as the potential respondents for this study were recruited from North American institutions. Future surveys should include chiropractic colleges and programs internationally. It is suspected that the philosophy and scope of chiropractic education, research, and practice differs between regions and, consequently, affect (or enhance) survey responses. Lastly, in such a rapidly progressing subject, new impactful articles have undoubtedly been published that should be included as "essential," prior to actual publication of this study. We should disseminate thoroughly yet quickly when compiling and distributing future study results. In spite of these limitations, we consider these responses a fruitful start to this initial investigation into a previously unexplored subject, essential literature for the chiropractic profession.

Relevance/future research

Now that a preliminary list of essential literature for doctors of chiropractic exists, a future researcher may consider surveying practicing doctors of chiropractic or chiropractic students and faculty to determine their awareness of this essential literature and to expand the key articles from the perspective of non-researchers.

Conclusions

This survey of chiropractic research leaders resulted in a manageable list of essential literature for chiropractic students and practitioners. A variety of perspectives and values are evident when looking at the outcomes of the survey. The recommended literature might be broken down into three major categories:

1. Foundational understanding of the pathophysiology underlying chiropractic concepts and practices.
2. Importance of practitioner awareness of the state of the evidence for patient care and clinical practice.
3. Potential societal impact fostering improved integration or acceptance.

The actual impact is limited to the perspectives of the responding research leaders. Regular annual or biannual surveys could be of benefit to many in the profession.

Abbreviations

EBCP: Evidence-based clinical practice; PE: Pieces of evidence; DC: Doctor of chiropractic; NLM: United States National Library of Medicine; PMC: PubMed Central.

Competing interests

The authors declare that this paper is original and has not been published nor is being considered elsewhere for publication. The authors, individually and collectively, declare no conflicts of interests.

Authors' contributions

The corresponding author, BM, planned the design, was involved in supervision, data collection/processing, analysis/interpretation, literature search, writing, and critical review of this manuscript. JS was responsible for concept development, supervision, writing, and critical review. DD was integral for design, supervision, data collection, and writing. RB was involved in writing and supervision. SS completed the secondary analysis and assisted in interpretation, writing, and critical review of this manuscript. All authors read and approved the final manuscript.

Authors' information

Barbara A. Mansholt, D.C., M.S., Assistant Professor, Technique Department, Palmer College of Chiropractic, 1000 Brady St., Davenport, IA 52803, USA.
John S. Stites, D.C., Director, Community Clinics, Palmer College of Chiropractic, 2001 52nd Ave. , Moline, IL 61265, USA.
Dustin C. Derby, Ed.D., Senior Director, Institutional Planning & Research, Palmer College of Chiropractic, 723 Brady St., Davenport, IA 52803, USA.
Ronald J. Boesch, D.C., Dean of Clinics, Palmer Davenport Clinical Affairs, Palmer College of Chiropractic, 1000 Brady St., Davenport, IA 52803, USA.
Stacie A. Salsbury, Ph.D., R.N., Clinical Project Manager, Palmer Center for Chiropractic Research, Palmer College of Chiropractic, 741 Brady St., Davenport, IA 52803, USA.

Author details

[1]Technique Department, Palmer College of Chiropractic, 1000 Brady St, Davenport, IA 52803, USA. [2]Community Clinics, Palmer College of

Chiropractic, 2001 52nd Ave, Moline, IL 61265, USA. [3]Institutional Planning & Research, Palmer College of Chiropractic, 723 Brady St, Davenport, IA 52803, USA. [4]Palmer Davenport Clinical Affairs, Palmer College of Chiropractic, 1000 Brady St, Davenport, IA 52803, USA. [5]Palmer Center for Chiropractic Research, Palmer College of Chiropractic, 741 Brady St, Davenport, IA 52803, USA.

References

1. Sackett DL, Rosenberg WM, Gray JA, Haynes RB, Richardson WS: **Evidence based medicine: what it is and what it isn't.** *BMJ* 1996, **312**:71–72.
2. Satterfield JM, Spring B, Brownson RC, Mullen EJ, Newhouse RP, Walker BB, Whitlock EP: **Toward a transdisciplinary model of evidence-based practice.** *Milbank Q* 2009, **87**:368–390.
3. Giordano J, Garcia MK, Boatwright D, Klein K: **Complementary and alternative medicine in mainstream public health: a role for research in fostering integration.** *J Altern Complement Med* 2003, **9**:441–445.
4. Coulter ID, Hurwitz EL, Adams AH, Genovese BJ, Hays R, Shekelle PG: **Patients using chiropractors in North America: who are they, and why are they in chiropractic care?** *Spine (Phila Pa 1976)* 2002, **27**:291–296.
5. Davis MA, Sirovich BE, Weeks WB: **Utilization and expenditures on chiropractic in the United States from 1997 to 2006.** *Health Serv Res* 2010, **45**:748–761.
6. Cooper RA, McKee HJ: **Chiropractic in the United States: trends and issues.** *Milbank Q* 2003, **81**:107–138.
7. Meeker WC, Haldeman S: **Chiropractic: a profession at the crossroads of mainstream and alternative medicine.** *Ann Intern Med* 2002, **136**:216–227.
8. Murphy D, Justice B, Paskowski I, Perle S, Schneider M: **The establishment of a primary spine care practitioner and its benefits to health care reform in the United States.** *Chiropr Man Therap* 2011, **19**:17.
9. Murphy DR, Schneider MJ, Seaman DR, Perle SM, Nelson CF: **How can chiropractic become a respected mainstream profession? The example of podiatry.** *Chiropr Osteopat* 2008, **16**:10.
10. Myburgh C, Hartvigsen J, Grunnet-Nilsson N: **Secondary legitimacy: a key mainstream health care inclusion strategy for the danish chiropractic profession?** *J Manipulative Physiol Ther* 2008, **31**:392–395.
11. Redwood D, Hawk C, Cambron J, Vinjamury SP, Bedard J: **Do chiropractors identify with complementary and alternative medicine? Results of a survey.** *J Altern Complement Med* 2008, **14**:361–368.
12. Busse JW, Jacobs C, Ngo T, Rodine R, Torrance D, Jim J, Kulkarni AV, Petrisor B, Drew B, Bhandari M: **Attitudes toward chiropractic: a survey of North American orthopedic surgeons.** *Spine (Phila Pa 1976)* 2009, **34**:2818–2825.
13. Meeker WC: **Public demand and the integration of complementary and alternative medicine in the US health care system.** *J Manipulative Physiol Ther* 2000, **23**:123–126.
14. Villanueva-Russell Y: **Caught in the crosshairs: Identity and cultural authority within chiropractic.** *Soc Sci Med* 2011, **72**:1826–1837.
15. Reggars J: **Chiropractic at the crossroads or are we just going around in circles?** *Chiropr Man Therap* 2011, **19**:11.
16. Hunnisett A, Cunliffe C: **Chiropractic treatment as a primary care intervention for better musculoskeletal health in the aging population in the United Kingdom: an opinion and positioning paper.** *Front Physiol* 2012, **3**:87.
17. LeFebvre R, Peterson D, Haas M: **Evidence-based practice and chiropractic care.** *JEBCAM* 2013, **18**(1):75–79.
18. Kreitzer MJ, Sierpina VS: **NCCAM awards grants to CAM institutions to enhance research education.** *EXPLORE* 2008, **4**(1):74–76.
19. Haas M, Leo M, Peterson D, LeFebvre R, Vavrek D: **Evaluation of the effects of an evidence-based practice curriculum on knowledge, attitudes, and self-assessed skills and behaviors in chiropractic students.** *J Manipulative Physiol Ther* 2012, **35**(9):701–709.
20. Harvey PJ, Goodell KJ: **Development and evolution of an information literacy course for a doctor of chiropractic program.** *Commun Info Lit* 2008, **2**(1):52–61.
21. Shreeve MW: **Evidence-based chiropractic education: are we equipping graduates for clinical practice with improved patient outcomes?** *J Chiropr Educ* 2012, **26**(2):184.
22. Banzai R, Derby DC, Long CR, Hondras MA: **International web survey of chiropractic students about evidence-based practice: a pilot study.** *Chiropr Man Therap* 2011, **19**(1):6.
23. Hall G: **Attitudes of chiropractors to evidence-based practice and how this compares to other healthcare professionals: a qualitative study.** *Clin Chiropr* 2011, **14**(3):106–111.
24. Suter E, Vanderheyden LC, Trojan LS, Verhoef MJ, Armitage GD: **How important is research-based practice to chiropractors and massage therapists?** *J Manipulative Physiol Ther* 2007, **30**(2):109–115.
25. Hadley J, Hassan I, Khan K: **Knowledge and beliefs concerning evidence-based practice amongst complementary and alternative medicine health care practitioners and allied health care professionals: a questionnaire survey.** *BMC Complement Altern Med* 2008, **8**(1):45.
26. Maylahn C, Fleming D, Birkhead G: **Health departments in a brave new world.** *Prev Chronic Dis* 2013. 10:130003:
27. Hawk C, Meeker W, Hansen D: **The national workshop to develop the chiropractic research agenda.** *J Manipulative Physiol Ther* 1997, **20**(3):147.
28. Lawrence DJ, Meeker WC, Commentary: **The national workshop to develop the chiropractic research agenda: 10 years on, a new set of white papers.** *J Manipulative Physiol Ther* 2006, **29**(9):690–694.
29. Mootz RD, Hansen DT, Breen A, Killinger LZ, Nelson C: **Health services research related to chiropractic: review and recommendations for research prioritization by the chiropractic profession.** *J Manipulative Physiol Ther* 2006, **29**(9):707–725.
30. Haas M, Bronfort G, Evans RL: **Chiropractic clinical research: progress and recommendations.** *J Manipulative Physiol Ther* 2006, **29**(9):695–706.
31. Bogdan RCBS: *Qualitative Research for Education: An Introduction to Theories and Methods.* 4th edition. New York: Pearson Education Group, Inc.; 2003.
32. Leach MJ, Gillham D: **Are complementary medicine practitioners implementing evidence based practice?** *Complement Ther Med* 2011, **19**(3):128–136.
33. Cadmus E, Van Wynen EA, Chamberlain B, Steingall P, Kilgallen ME, Holly C, Gallagher-Ford L: **Nurses' skill level and access to evidence-based practice.** *J Nurs Adm* 2008, **38**(11):494–503.
34. Green ML, Ruff TR: **Why do residents fail to answer their clinical questions? A qualitative study of barriers to practicing evidence-based medicine.** *Acad Med* 2005, **80**(2):176–182.
35. Bronfort G, Haas M, Evans R, Leininger B, Triano J: **Effectiveness of manual therapies: the UK evidence report.** *Chiropr Osteopat* 2010, **18**:3.
36. Pickar JG: **Neurophysiological effects of spinal manipulation.** *Spine J* 2002, **2**(5):357–371.
37. Cassidy JD, Boyle E, Cote P, He Y, Hogg-Johnson S, Silver FL, Bondy SJ: **Risk of vertebrobasilar stroke and chiropractic care: results of a population-based case-control and case-crossover study.** *J Manipulative Physiol Ther* 2009, **32**(2 Suppl):S201–S208.
38. Walker BF, French SD, Grant W, Green S: **Combined chiropractic interventions for low-back pain.** *Cochrane Database Syst Rev* 2010, **4**, CD005427.
39. Ianuzzi A, Khalsa PS: **Comparison of human lumbar facet joint capsule strains during simulated high-velocity, low-amplitude spinal manipulation versus physiological motions.** *Spine J* 2005, **5**(3):277–290.
40. Chou R, Qaseem A, Snow V, Casey D, Cross JT Jr, Shekelle P, Owens DK: **Diagnosis and treatment of low back pain: a joint clinical practice guideline from the American College of Physicians and the American Pain Society.** *Ann Intern Med* 2007, **147**:478–491.
41. Childs JD, Fritz JM, Flynn TW, Irrgang JJ, Johnson KK, Majkowski GR, Delitto A: **A clinical prediction rule to identify patients with low back pain most likely to benefit from spinal manipulation: a validation study.** *Ann Int Med* 2004, **141**:920–928.
42. Chou R, Huffman LH: **Nonpharmacologic therapies for acute and chronic low back pain: a review of the evidence for an american pain society/ american college of physicians clinical practice guideline.** *Ann Intern Med* 2007, **147**(7):492–504.
43. UK BEAM Trial Team: **United Kingdom back pain exercise and manipulation (UK BEAM) randomised trial: effectiveness of physical treatments for back pain in primary care.** *BMJ* 2004, **329**(7479):1377.
44. Senstad O, Leboeuf-Yde C, Borchgrevink C: **Frequency and characteristics of side effects of spinal manipulative therapy.** *Spine* 1997, **22**:435–441.
45. Hurwitz EL, Carragee EJ, van der Velde G, Carroll LJ, Nordin M, Guzman J, Peloso PM, Holm LW, Cote P, Hogg-Johnson S: **Treatment of neck pain: noninvasive interventions: results of the bone and joint decade 2000–2010 task force on neck pain and its associated disorders.** *Spine* 2008, **33**(4 Suppl):S123–S152.

46. Nelson CF, Bronfort G, Evans R, Boline P, Goldsmith C, Anderson AV: **The efficacy of spinal manipulation, amitriptyline and the combination of both therapies for the prophylaxis of migraine headache.** *J Manipulative Physiol Ther* 1998, **21**(8):511–519.
47. Olafsdottir E, Forshei S, Fluge G, Markestad T: **Randomised controlled trial of infantile colic treated with chiropractic spinal manipulation.** *Arch Dis Child* 2001, **84**(2):138–141.
48. Skyba DA, Radhakrishnan R, Rohlwing JJ, Wright A, Sluka KA: **Joint manipulation reduces hyperalgesia by activation of monoamine receptors but not opioid or GABA receptors in the spinal cord.** *Pain* 2003, **106**(1–2):159–168.
49. Haldeman S, Carroll L, Cassidy JD, Schubert J, Nygren A: **The bone and joint decade 2000–2010 task force on neck pain and its associated disorders: executive summary.** *Spine (Phila Pa 1976)* 2008, **33**(4 Suppl):S5–S7.
50. Dagenais S, Tricco AC, Haldeman S: **Synthesis of recommendations for the assessment and management of low back pain from recent clinical practice guidelines.** *Spine J* 2010, **10**(6):514–529.
51. Legorreta AP, Metz RD, Nelson CF, Ray S, Chernicoff HO, Dinubile NA: **Comparative analysis of individuals with and without chiropractic coverage: patient characteristics, utilization, and costs.** *Arch Intern Med* 2004, **164**(18):1985–1992.
52. Cramer GD, Gregerson DM, Knudsen JT, Hubbard BB, Ustas LM, Cantu JA: **The effects of side-posture positioning and spinal adjusting on the lumbar Z joints: a randomized controlled trial with sixty-four subjects.** *Spine* 2002, **27**(22):2459–2466.
53. Haas M, Groupp E, Kraemer DF: **Dose–response for chiropractic care of chronic low back pain.** *Spine J* 2004, **4**(5):574–583.
54. Carroll LJ, *et al*: **Research priorities and methodological implications: the bone and joint decade 2000–2010 task force on neck pain and its associated disorders.** *Spine (Phila Pa.1976)* 2008, **33**(4 Suppl):S214–S220.
55. Bogduk N, McGuirk B: *Management of Acute and Chronic Neck Pain: An Evidence-Based Approach.* Philadelphia, PA: Elsevier; 2006.
56. Pickar JG, Kang YM: **Paraspinal muscle spindle responses to the duration of a spinal manipulation under force control.** *J Manipulative Physiol Ther* 2006, **29**(1):22–31.
57. Haas M, Spegman A, Peterson D, Aickin M, Vavrek D: **Dose response and efficacy of spinal manipulation for chronic cervicogenic headache: a pilot randomized controlled trial.** *Spine J* 2010, **10**(2):117–128.
58. Reggars J, Pollard HP: **Analysis of zygapophyseal joint cracking during chiropractic manipulation.** *J Manipulative Physiol Ther* 1995, **18**(2):65–71.
59. Murphy DR: **A theoretical model for the development of a diagnosis-based clinical decision rule for the management of patients with spinal pain.** *BMC Musculoskelet Disord* 2007, **8**:75.
60. Bishop PB, Quon JA, Fisher CG, Dvorak MF: **The chiropractic hospital-based interventions research outcomes (CHIRO) study: a randomized controlled trial on the effectiveness of clinical practice guidelines in the medical and chiropractic management of patients with acute mechanical low back pain.** *Spine J* 2010, **10**(12):1055–1064.
61. Little JS, Ianuzzi A, Chiu JB, Baitner A, Khalsa PS: **Human lumbar facet joint capsule strains: II. Alteration of strains subsequent to anterior interbody fixation.** *Spine J* 2004, **4**(2):153–162.
62. Pickar JG, Sung PS, Kang YM, Ge W: **Response of lumbar paraspinal muscles spindles is greater to spinal manipulative loading compared with slower loading under length control.** *Spine J* 2007, **7**(5):583–595.
63. Herzog W: **The biomechanics of spinal manipulation.** *J Bodyw Mov Ther* 2010, **14**(3):280–286.
64. Ianuzzi A, Khalsa PS: **High loading rate during spinal manipulation produces unique facet joint capsule strain patterns compared with axial rotations.** *J Manipulative Physiol Ther* 2005, **28**(9):673–687.
65. Hartman S: **Why do ineffective treatments seem helpful? A brief review.** *Chiropr Osteo* 2009, **17**(1):10.
66. Henderson CN, Cramer GD, Zhang Q, Devocht JW, Fournier JT: **Introducing the external link model for studying spine fixation and misalignment: part 1–need, rationale, and applications.** *J Manipulative Physiol Ther* 2007, **30**(3):239–245.
67. McGinn T, Jervis R, Wisnivesky J, Keitz S, Wyer P: **Tips for teachers of evidence-based medicine: clinical prediction rules (CPRs) and estimating pretest probability.** *J Gen Intern Med* 2008, **23**(8):1261–1268.
68. Cramer GD, Henderson CNR, Little JW, Daley C, Grieve TJ: **Zygapophyseal joint adhesions after induced hypomobility.** *J Manipulative Physiol Ther* 2010, **33**:508–518.
69. Chevan J, Riddle DL: **Factors associated with care seeking from physicians, physical therapists, or chiropractors by persons with spinal pain: a population-based study.** *J Orthop Sports Phys Ther* 2011, **41**(7):467.
70. Bogduk N: **Truth in musculoskeletal medicine: truth in diagnosis - validity.** *Austr J Musculoskeletal Med* 1999, **4**:32–39.
71. Haneline M: **A primer on evidence-based practice for chiropractors.** *Chiropr J Aust* 2011, **41**(3):78.
72. Murphy D, Hurwitz E, Nelson C: **A diagnosis-based clinical decision rule for spinal pain part 2: review of the literature.** *Chiropr Osteopat* 2008, **16**(1):7.
73. Haldeman S, Carroll L, Cassidy JD, Schubert J, Nygren A: **The bone and joint decade 2000–2010 task force on neck pain and its associated disorders.** *Eur Spine J* 2008, **17**(1):5–7.
74. Carroll L, Hurwitz E, Cote P, Hogg-Johnson S, Carragee E, Nordin M, Holm L, Velde G, Cassidy JD, Guzman J, Peloso P, Haldeman S: **Research priorities and methodological implications.** *Eur Spine J* 2008, **17**(1):214–220.
75. Willinsky J, Quint-Rapoport M: *How Complementary and Alternative Medicine Practitioners use PubMed.* Internet Res: J Medical; 2007:9(2).
76. Dillman DA, Smyth JD, Christian LM: *Internet, Mail, and Mixed-Mode Surveys: The Tailored Design Method.* Hoboken: NJ: Wiley & Sons; 2009.
77. Russell ML, Verhoef MJ, Injeyan HS, McMorland DG: **Response rates for surveys of chiropractors.** *J Manipulative Physiol Ther* 2004, **27**:43–48.
78. Schacter DL, Harbluk JL, McLachlan DR: **Retrieval without recollection: an experimental analysis of source amnesia.** *J Verbal Learning Verbal Behav* 1984, **23**(5):593–611.

Who uses Australian chiropractic services?

Simon D French[1,2*], Konstancja Densley[1], Melanie J Charity[1] and Jane Gunn[1]

Abstract

Background: The use of chiropractic services is widespread, however, little is known about the characteristics of people who seek chiropractic care in Australia. This study compared the characteristics of users and non-users of chiropractic services from a cohort of patients sourced from general medical practice in Victoria, Australia.

Methods: This is a secondary analysis of baseline screening data from a prospective adult cohort study beginning in 2005. Thirty randomly selected Australian general medical practices mailed out surveys to 17,780 of their patients. Differences were examined between chiropractic users and others, and between chiropractic users who reported a back problem to those who did not.

Results: Of 7,519 respondents, 15% indicated they had visited a chiropractor in the last 12 months. Chiropractic users were more likely to have their GP located in a rural location and to be born in Australia; they were less likely to be in the older age group (55–76), to be unemployed or to have a pension/benefit as their main source of income. Chiropractic users were more likely to: have a back problem; use complementary or alternative medication; visit another type of complementary health practitioner or a physiotherapist. They were less likely to take medication for certain health problems (e.g. for high blood pressure, high cholesterol or asthma). No important differences were seen between chiropractic users and non-users for other health problems. People who visited a chiropractor and reported a back problem were more likely to: be a current smoker; have a number of other chronic conditions, including arthritis, hypertension, chronic sinusitis, asthma, dermatitis, depression and anxiety; report taking medications, including antidepressants, analgesics (painkillers and arthritis medication) and complementary or alternative medications.

Conclusions: This large cross-sectional study of general medical practice attendees suggests that chiropractors are the most commonly consulted complementary health profession. Chiropractors should ensure they are aware of their patients' health conditions other than musculoskeletal problems and should ensure they are appropriately managed.

Background

The use of complementary and alternative medicine is widespread across most high income countries [1]. Chiropractic services account for a substantial proportion of this use. There are approximately 4,500 registered chiropractors in Australia, the ninth largest registered health profession (out of 12) [2]. During 2005, 16% of Australians consulted a chiropractor at least once at a cost of $AU905 million [3]. Further, in 2011, Australian private insurers paid approximately AUD$225 million for more than 9 million chiropractic services, almost as much as was paid for physiotherapy services (AUD$258 million) [4].

Most previous studies of chiropractic users have been conducted in the United States and European countries [5-9]. These studies included patients from chiropractic practices rather than from the general population.

Despite a high level of use of chiropractic in Australia, little is known about the characteristics of people who use chiropractic care. Two previous Australian population-based studies about people who consult chiropractors found that chiropractic users, compared to non-users, have a higher income, were more likely to be born in Australia, and were more likely to have also visited a general medical practitioner [3,10]. A study of chiropractic patients in Victoria, Australia, demonstrated that although chiropractors see patients with a range of

* Correspondence: s.french@unimelb.edu.au
[1]General Practice and Primary Health Care Academic Centre, The University of Melbourne, 200 Berkeley Street, Carlton, VIC 3072, Australia
[2]Centre for Health, Exercise and Sports Medicine, School of Health Sciences, The University of Melbourne, Level 7, 161 Barry St, Carlton, VIC 3053, Australia

conditions, most commonly these conditions are musculoskeletal-related [11].

This paper offers a view on how current users of general medical practice use chiropractic services. For general practitioners, it is important to know which of their patients use chiropractic services; more than half of people who use complementary and alternative services and treatments do not reveal this to their general practitioner [12]. For chiropractors, this analysis can reveal important characteristics of the patients who seek their care. The aim of this study was to compare the characteristics of users and non-users of chiropractic services from a cohort of patients sourced from general medical practice. For those people who saw a chiropractor, we also compared the characteristics of those who reported a back problem to those who did not.

Methods

We undertook a secondary analysis of screening data from *diamond*. The *diamond* study began in 2005 and was large prospective study exploring depression, stress and worries in people presenting to primary care. Full details of the study are reported elsewhere [13,14], and the methods are briefly outlined below. Ethics approval for the *diamond* study was granted by the University of Melbourne's Human Research Ethics Committee.

Participant sample

Thirty randomly selected general practices located in Victoria, Australia, mailed out surveys to randomly selected patients. Patients were eligible if they were: aged 18–75 years; able to read English; not terminally ill; and did not reside in a nursing home.

Table 1 Participant demographic characteristics (N = 7,519)

	Visit to chiropractor in last 12 months[1]					
	No (N = 6385)		Yes (N = 1134)			
Participant characteristics	Number	%	Number	%	OR (95% CI)[2]	P
General practitioner location[3]:						
- Urban (RRMA 1 and 2)	4363	*68*	711	*63*	REF	0.03
- Rural (RRMA 3 to 5)	2022	*32*	423	*37*	1.29 (1.03 – 1.62)	
Age group:						
18-34	974	*15*	185	*16*	REF	<0.001
35-54	2631	*42*	562	*50*	1.11 (0.92 – 1.35)	
55-76	2712	*43*	378	*34*	0.73 (0.62 – 0.87)	
Gender: Female	4231	*67*	757	*67*	1.02 (0.87 – 1.20)	0.81
Marital status:						
- Never married/single	1139	*18*	202	*18*	REF	0.24
- Widowed/divorced/separated	1149	*18*	179	*16*	0.88 (0.74 – 1.06)	
- Married	4027	*64*	741	*66*	1.03 (0.87 – 1.23)	
Born in Australia	5104	*80*	972	*86*	1.44 (1.21 – 1.72)	<0.001
English is first language	6012	*95*	1087	*96*	1.24 (0.88 – 1.75)	0.22
Lives alone	877	*14*	130	*12*	0.82 (0.69 – 0.97)	0.02
Highest level of education:						
- Completed year 12 or less	3605	*57*	618	*55*	REF	0.07
- Certificate/diploma	1292	*20*	260	*23*	1.19 (1.02 – 1.38)	
- Bachelor degree or higher	1448	*23*	254	*22*	1.04 (0.89 – 1.21)	
Employment:						
- Employed/student	3970	*62*	815	*72*	REF	<0.001
- Not employed	2018	*32*	286	*25*	0.69 (0.59 – 0.82)	
- Unable to work[4]	372	*6*	32	*3*	0.42 (0.31 – 0.57)	
Pension/benefit is main source of income	1724	*27*	200	*18*	0.58 (0.47 – 0.71)	<0.001

1. Denominators may vary due to missing data.
2. Odds ratios (*OR*), 95% confidence intervals (*CI*) and P values using logistic regression using generalised estimating equations with robust standard errors.
3. *RRMA* Rural Remote and Metropolitan Areas classification [16,17].
4. Includes home duties, unpaid work and maternity leave.

Measures

The survey included questions on general demographic information, general health, medication use and health service use in the previous 12 months. Participants were asked whether they had seen any traditional health professionals (hospital doctor, specialist doctor, physiotherapist, psychologist, counsellor, psychiatrist, nurse, social worker, alcohol or drug worker or family therapist) or a complementary therapist (chiropractor, naturopath, homeopath, acupuncturist or other natural therapist) in the previous 12 months.

Statistical analysis

Data were analysed using Stata version 12 [15] and summarised using frequencies and percentages. Participants were divided into two groups according to whether they had consulted a chiropractor or not in the past 12 months. Logistic regression using generalised estimating equations with robust standard errors was used to examine the demographic characteristics, health issues, and medications taken of people who had consulted a chiropractor and to investigate the association between visiting a chiropractor and other health service use. A

Table 2 Participant health characteristics (N = 7,519)

	Visit to chiropractor in last 12 months[1]					
	No (N = 6385)		Yes (N = 1134)			
Participant health characteristics	Number	%	Number	%	OR (95% CI)[2]	P
Health rate (SF 12) [18]:						
- Fair/poor	1056	*17*	165	*15*	REF	0.16
- Good/excellent	5253	*83*	956	*85*	1.16 (0.94 –1.43)	
Current smoker	1153	*18*	202	*18*	0.97 (0.82 – 1.15)	0.73
Hazardous drinking [19]	1033	*16*	197	*17*	1.06 (0.92 – 1.23)	0.42
Long term health problem limits daily activities	2021	*33*	345	*31*	0.94 (0.84 – 1.06)	0.29
Back problem in last 12 months[3]	1542	*24*	543	*48*	2.90 (2.53 – 3.31)	<0.001
Arthritis in last 12 months	1142	*18*	183	*16*	0.88 (0.74 – 1.06)	0.19
Cardiovascular disorder in last 12 months[4]	1543	*24*	241	*21*	0.84 (0.72 – 0.98)	0.03
Respiratory disorder in last 12 months[5]	948	*15*	190	*17*	1.15 (0.97 – 1.38)	0.12
Dermatitis in last 12 months	414	*7*	99	*9*	1.38 (1.12 – 1.71)	0.003
Diabetes in last 12 months	333	*5*	54	*5*	0.92 (0.68 – 1.24)	0.58
Cancer in last 12 months	162	*3*	26	*2*	0.91 (0.61 – 1.35)	0.63
Depression in last 12 months	1138	*18*	206	*18*	1.03 (0.86 – 1.23)	0.78
Depression and antidepressant use in last 12 months	591	*9*	94	*8*	0.89 (0.75 – 1.05)	0.15
Told by Dr you have depression	1821	*31*	337	*32*	1.07 (0.92 – 1.24)	0.38
Anxiety in last 12 months	1040	*16*	201	*18*	1.11 (0.96 – 1.29)	0.16
Told by doctor you have anxiety	1382	*25*	254	*26*	1.05 (0.90 – 1.23)	0.53
Afraid of partner	1003	*16*	184	*16*	1.02 (0.84 – 1.24)	0.81
Medication use in last 12 months:						
- Analgesics[6]	1677	*27*	279	*25*	0.92 (0.80 – 1.07)	0.28
- Medications for physical problems[7]	2412	*38*	381	*34*	0.83 (0.72 – 0.95)	0.009
- Depression medications	876	*14*	150	*13*	0.97 (0.79 – 1.19)	0.77
- Sedatives	466	*7*	77	*7*	0.95 (0.79 – 1.15)	0.61
- Other medications[8]	1476	*33*	256	*32*	0.96 (0.80 – 1.16)	0.70
- Complementary & alternative medication[9]	1488	*24*	395	*35*	1.79 (1.54 – 2.07)	<0.001

1. Denominators may vary due to missing data.
2. Odds ratios (*OR*), 95% confidence intervals (*CI*) and P values using logistic regression using generalised estimating equations with robust standard errors.
3. Includes back problem, chronic back pain or sciatica.
4. Includes stroke, hypertension, heart disease, lipid disorder.
5. Includes sinusitis, asthma and emphysema.
6. Includes painkillers and arthritis medication.
7. Includes blood pressure, cholesterol lowering & asthma medication.
8. Includes contraceptives and indigestion medication.
9. Includes vitamins, minerals and herbs.

Table 3 Health service use in last 12 months of users of chiropractic compared to non-users

	Non-chiropractic user (N = 6385)[1]		Chiropractic user (N = 1134)[1]		Unadjusted		Adjusted[2]	
	Number	%	Number	%	OR (95% CI)[3]	P	OR (95% CI)[3]	P
12 or more visits to GP[4]	597	9	85	8	0.78 (0.61 - 0.99)	0.04	0.82 (0.65 - 1.04)	0.11
One or more visits to traditional[5]	4510	71	808	71	1.00 (0.90 - 1.10)	0.98	1.03 (0.92 - 1.14)	0.64
One or more visits to complementary[6]	974	15	351	31	2.53 (2.24 - 2.86)	<0.001	2.51 (2.22 - 2.84)	<0.001
One or more visits to physiotherapist	1276	20	246	23	1.19 (1.02 - 1.37)	0.03	1.20 (1.03 - 1.39)	0.02

1. Denominators may vary due to missing data.
2. Adjusted for age, gender, general practice location and health rate.
3. Odds ratios (*OR*), 95% confidence (*CI*) intervals and *P* values using logistic regression using generalised estimating equations with robust standard errors.
4. *GP* general practitioner.
5. Traditional includes: hospital doctor; specialist doctor; physiotherapist; psychologist; counsellor; psychiatrist; nurse; social worker; alcohol and drug worker; family therapist.
6. Complementary includes: naturopath; homeopath; acupuncturist; other natural therapist.

further two groups were formed consisting of those who had a back problem, chronic back pain or sciatica and saw a chiropractor, compared to those who saw a chiropractor and didn't have a back problem.

Analyses allowed for the clustering effect due to recruiting participants from the same general practices. Results are reported as odds ratios (ORs) with 95% confidence intervals (CI) and p values (P). Analyses investigating the association between visiting a chiropractor and other health service use were controlled for the effects of age, sex, general practice location and health rating.

Results

Of the 17,780 patients initially sent a screening survey, 7,667 (43%) returned a completed survey. The mean age of patients who were sent the screening survey was 46.2 years (SD, 15.3) and 61% were women. Patients who returned the survey were on average older (50.9 years; SD, 14.2) and more likely to be female (67%).

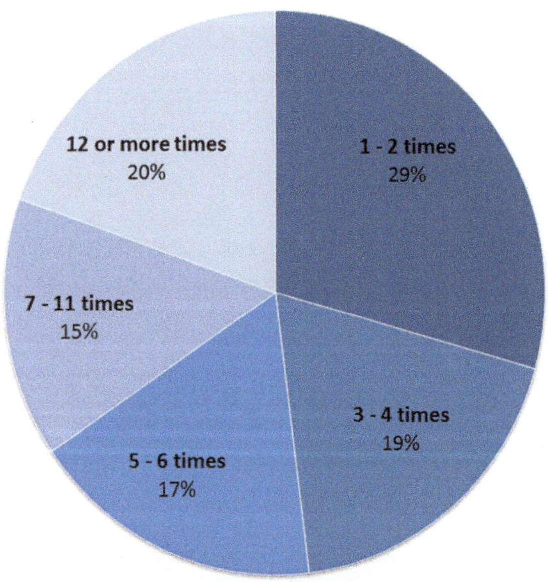

Figure 1 Number of visits to a chiropractor (N = 1,134).

A total 7,519 participants answered the question on whether they had consulted a chiropractor in the past 12 months and of those, 7,477 people responded to the question related to back problem, chronic back pain or sciatica. Fifteen per cent of respondents (N = 1,134) indicated they had visited a chiropractor in the last 12 months. Chiropractors were the fifth most common health professional visited after specialist doctor (47%), nurse (29%), hospital doctor (21%) and physiotherapist (21%) and the most commonly visited complementary health professional.

Important differences in demographic characteristics between people who reported they had consulted a chiropractor in the last 12 months, compared to people who didn't, included that they were more likely to have their GP located in a rural location (Odds Ratio (OR) 1.29, 95% Confidence Intervals (CI) 1.03, 1.62) and to be born in Australia rather than another country (OR 1.44, 95% CI 1.21, 1.72). They were less likely to be in the age group of 55–76 (OR 0.73, 95% CI 0.62, 0.87), to have a pension or benefit as their main source of income (OR 0.58, 95% CI 0.47, 0.71) or to be unemployed (OR 0.69, 95% CI 0.59, 0.82) (Table 1).

Participant health characteristics are shown in Table 2. People who saw a chiropractor in the last 12 months were more likely to have a back problem, chronic back pain or sciatica (OR 2.90, 95% CI 2.53, 3.31). No important differences were seen between chiropractic users and non-users for other health variables, including health rating, arthritis, smoking or drinking rates, history of depression or anxiety, cardiovascular disorder, respiratory disorder and cancer. Chiropractic users, compared to non-users, were slightly less likely to use medications for certain health problems such as for blood pressure, cholesterol lowering and asthma (34% versus 38%; OR 0.83, 95% CI 0.72, 0.95) and were more likely to use complementary and alternative medication (35% versus 24%; OR 1.79, 95% CI 1.54, 2.07).

People who reported seeing a chiropractor were more likely to report also visiting another type of complementary health practitioner (Adjusted OR 2.51, 95% CI 2.22, 2.84). They were also more likely to visit a physiotherapist (Adjusted OR 1.20, 95% CI 1.03, 1.39). They were not more or less likely to visit their GP more than 12 times in the last 12 months, nor more or less likely to have seen another "traditional" health practitioner (Table 3).

For those people who consulted a chiropractor, Figure 1 shows the number of visits over the last 12 months. About a third of people saw a chiropractor once or twice over the last 12 months, and one fifth saw a chiropractor 12 or more times. Figure 2 shows the number of visits to a chiropractor for people with and without back pain. The more often a person saw a chiropractor, the more likely it was that they had back pain; for example, 38% of people who saw a chiropractor 1 to 2 times in the last 12 months reported having back pain, whereas of those who saw a chiropractor 12 or more times in the last 12 months, 58% reported having back pain.

Table 4 shows participant health characteristics for people who visited a chiropractor and compares those who reported a back problem in the last 12 months to those who did not. People who had a back problem were more likely to report they had a long term health problem that limits their daily activities. They were also more likely to report a number of other chronic health conditions including arthritis, hypertension, chronic sinusitis, asthma, dermatitis, depression and anxiety, and were more likely to be a current smoker. They were not more or less likely to report a history of a stroke, heart disease, lipid disorder, emphysema, diabetes or cancer, nor more or less likely to report being afraid of their partner. Chiropractic users with a back problem were more likely to report taking medications, including analgesics, and complementary of alternative medications, and less likely to report taking medications for physical problems such as for blood pressure, cholesterol lowering and asthma. People with a back problem who reported seeing a chiropractor in the last 12 months were more likely to report having depression and to be taking antidepressant medication than those without a back problem.

Discussion

This large cross-sectional study of patients of general practitioners suggests that 15% of people saw a chiropractor in the last 12 months and that chiropractors are the most commonly consulted complementary health profession. People who visit chiropractors are on the whole less disadvantaged (they are employed and they have completed secondary school education), and are more likely to be experiencing back problems. People who saw a chiropractor were also more likely to use complementary and alternative medication and to have visited another type of complementary or alternative health practitioner. People with back problems who visit

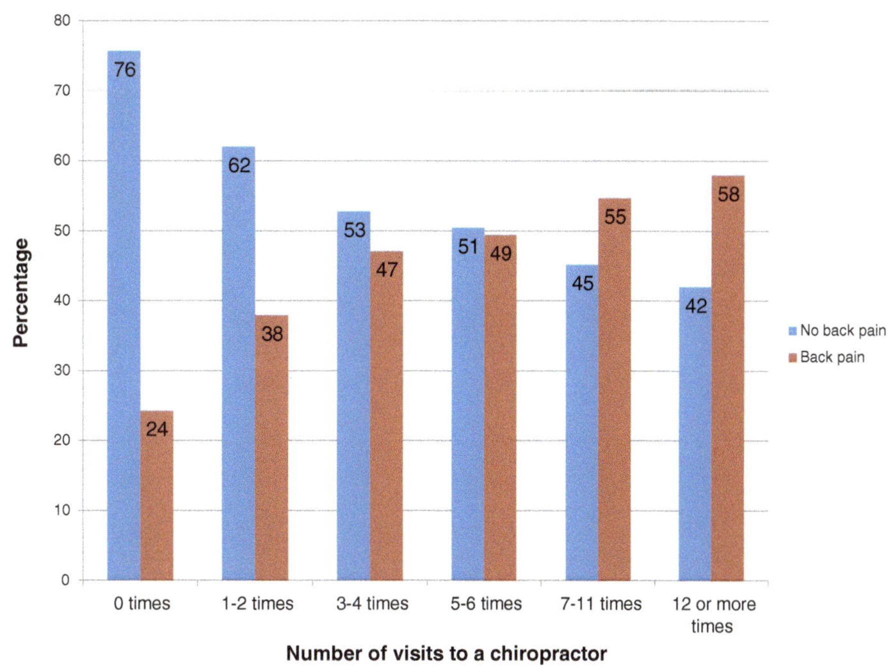

Figure 2 Number of visits to a chiropractor for people with and without back pain (back problem, chronic back pain or sciatica) (N = 7,477).

Table 4 Participant health characteristics for those who visited a chiropractor comparing those who reported a back problem (back problem, chronic back pain or sciatica) in last 12 months to those who did not (N = 1,129)

	Visited chiropractor and had self reported back problem in the last 12 months[1]					
	No (N = 586)		Yes (N = 543)			
Participant health characteristics	**Number**	**%**	**Number**	**%**	**OR (95% CI)[2]**	**P**
Health rate (SF 12) [18]:						
- Fair/poor	82	*14*	83	*15*	REF	0.56
- Good/excellent	498	*86*	453	*85*	0.90 (0.63 - 1.29)	
Current smoker	87	*15*	114	*21*	1.53 (1.15 - 2.03)	0.003
Hazardous drinking [19]	99	*17*	98	*18*	1.09 (0.79 - 1.51)	0.61
Long term health problem limits daily activities	145	*25*	200	*38*	1.78 (1.33 - 2.37)	<0.001
Arthritis in last 12 months	60	*10*	123	*23*	2.57 (1.91 - 3.46)	<0.001
Cardiovascular disorder in last 12 months						
Stroke	2	*0*	4	*1*	2.14 (0.46 - 10.02)	0.34
Hypertension	71	*12*	89	*16*	1.43 (1.05 - 1.96)	0.02
Heart disease	8	*1*	19	*3*	2.59 (1.03 - 6.53)	0.04
Lipid disorder	57	*10*	63	*12*	1.21 (0.87 - 1.67)	0.26
Respiratory disorder in last 12 months						
Chronic sinusitis	26	*4*	53	*10*	2.33 (1.35 - 4.05)	0.003
Asthma	44	*8*	69	*13*	1.78 (1.21 - 2.61)	0.003
Emphysema	9	*2*	11	*2*	1.28 (0.47 - 3.52)	0.63
Dermatitis in last 12 months	38	*6*	61	*11*	1.81 (1.12 - 2.92)	0.02
Diabetes in last 12 months	28	*5*	26	*5*	1.00 (0.57 - 1.73)	0.99
Cancer in last 12 months	14	*2*	12	*2*	0.91 (0.49 - 1.68)	0.76
Depression in last 12 months	81	*14*	125	*23*	1.85 (1.30 - 2.64)	0.001
Depression and antidepressant use in last 12 months	32	*6*	62	*12*	2.23 (1.27 - 3.90)	0.005
Told by Dr you have depression	158	*30*	179	*36*	1.30 (0.99 - 1.71)	0.06
Anxiety in last 12 months	81	*14*	120	*22*	1.76 (1.22 - 2.55)	0.002
Told by doctor you have anxiety	127	*25*	126	*26*	1.08 (0.84 - 1.40)	0.52
Afraid of partner	97	*17*	87	*16*	0.95 (0.71 - 1.28)	0.73
Medication use in last 12 months:						
- Analgesics[3]	121	*21*	157	*29*	1.56 (1.17- 2.08)	0.003
- Medications for physical problems[4]	210	*36*	170	*32*	0.81 (0.64 - 1.03)	0.008
- Depression medications	71	*12*	79	*15*	1.24 (0.85 - 1.82)	0.23
- Sedatives	34	*6*	43	*8*	1.39 (0.81 - 2.38)	0.24
- Other medications[5]	119	*29*	135	*35*	1.36 (1.03 - 1.78)	0.03
- Complementary & alternative medication[6]	187	*32*	206	*38*	1.30 (1.02 - 1.64)	0.03

1. Denominators may vary due to missing data.
2. Odds ratios (*OR*), 95% confidence intervals (*CI*) and P values using logistic regression using generalised estimating equations with robust standard errors.
3. Includes painkillers & arthritis medication.
4. Includes blood pressure, cholesterol lowering & asthma medication.
5. Includes contraceptives and indigestion medication.
6. Includes vitamins, minerals and herbs.

a chiropractor are more likely to be depressed and to have some other chronic health problems.

These findings have important implications for chiropractors. If a consumer seeks their care for a back problem then that consumer is more likely to have a number of other chronic health conditions, including being a smoker, have arthritis, have hypertension, chronic sinusitis or asthma, dermatitis and depression or anxiety. Chiropractors should be aware of this and ensure that these people are assessed and appropriately managed for these other health conditions. In particular, people with an increasing number of chronic health problems are more likely to have depressive symptoms [20], so chiropractors should be particularly cognisant of this significant health problem.

The strength of this study is the large, representative sample of people living in the community. Even though the sample was drawn from general medical practice, four out of five Australians (82%) aged 15 years and over see their GP at least once per year [21].

The limitations of this study include that all data were collected by self-report. This may have led to recall bias in the respondent correctly identifying that the practitioner they consulted was a chiropractor, and also in remembering accurately the number of times they attended over the last 12 months. Also, because this study included analysis of secondary data, the study is limited by scope of questions, in that, the purpose of the questionnaire was not specifically designed to measure differences between people who did and didn't see a chiropractor over the previous 12 months.

In a large study in the United States using National Health Survey data, 9% of respondents consulted a chiropractor in the last 12 months. Those that did were 2.4 times more likely to have low back pain [22]. Our results were similar to this with people visiting a chiropractor 2.9 times more likely to have low back pain. Other studies conducted in the United States have shown that people who visit chiropractors are more likely to be middle aged and to have high school as their highest level of education. Chiropractic patients were also more likely to have significantly worse health status than the general population sample [5]. We did not see these differences in our population.

Conclusion

This large Australian cross-sectional study of general practice attendees suggests that chiropractors are the most commonly consulted complementary health profession. People who report seeing a chiropractor are more likely to be employed, have a back problem, have visited another type of complementary health practitioner and have a GP in a rural location. People who see a chiropractor and have a back problem are likely to have other chronic health conditions. Chiropractors should ensure they are aware of their patients' health conditions other than musculoskeletal problems and should ensure these are appropriately managed.

Competing interests

SF is an Associate Editor with Chiropractic & Manual Therapies and had no involvement in the editorial process for this paper. Otherwise, the authors declare that they have no competing interests.

Authors' contributions

SF and JG conceived and designed the study. KD and MC undertook the analysis. SF wrote the first draft of the manuscript. All authors contributed to revisions of the manuscript and read and approved the final version.

Acknowledgements

The named authors submit this publication on behalf of the *diamond* study investigators which include: Prof Jane Gunn, Prof Helen Herrman, Prof Mike Kyrios, A/Prof Kelsey Hegarty, Prof Christopher Dowrick, Dr Gail Gilchrist, A/Prof Grant Blashki, Prof Dimity Pond, Dr Patty Chondros, A/Prof Renata Kokanovic and Dr Victoria Palmer. The *diamond* study was initiated with pilot funding from the beyondblue Victorian Centre of Excellence and the main cohort has received project grant funding from the National Health and Medical Research Council (grant IDs 299869, 454463, 566511 and 1002908). The one year Computer Assisted Telephone Interview was funded by a Stream 3 grant from the Australian Primary Health Care Research Institute (APHCRI). No funding body had a role in study design; the collection, analysis, and interpretation of data; the writing of the manuscript; or the decision to submit this manuscript for publication. We acknowledge the 30 dedicated GPs, their patients and practice staff for making this research possible. We thank the cohort participants for their ongoing involvement in the study. We also thank the *diamond* project team and associate investigators involved in the study: A/Prof Lena Sanci, A/Prof Catherine Mihalopoulos, Ms Maria Potiriadis, Ms Konstancja Densley, Dr Sandra Davidson, Ms Aves Middleton, and the casual research staff.

References

1. Harris PE, Cooper KL, Relton C, Thomas KJ: **Prevalence of complementary and alternative medicine (CAM) use by the general population: a systematic review and update.** *Int J Clin Pract* 2012, **66:**924–939.
2. Australian Health Practitioner Regulation Agency (AHPRA): *Chiropractic Registrant Data: December 2012. Chiropractic Board of Australia.* Australia: AHPRA; 2013.
3. Xue Ĉ, Zhang AL, Lin V, Da Costa C, Story DF: **Complementary and alternative medicine use in Australia: a national population-based survey.** *J Altern Complement Med* 2007, **13:**643–650.
4. Private Health Insurance Administration Council (PHIAC): *The Operations of Private Health Insurers Annual Report 2010–11.* Canberra: PHIAC; 2011.
5. Coulter ID, Hurwitz EL, Adams AH, Genovese BJ, Hays R, Shekelle PG: **Patients using chiropractors in North America: who are they, and why are they in chiropractic care?** *Spine* 2002, **27:**291–296. discussion 297–298.
6. Hartvigsen J, Sorensen LP, Graesborg K, Grunnet-Nilsson N: **Chiropractic patients in Denmark: a short description of basic characteristics.** *J Manipulative Physiol Ther* 2002, **25:**162–167.
7. Rubinstein S, Pfeifle CE, Van Tulder MW, Assendelft WJ: **Chiropractic patients in the Netherlands: a descriptive study.** *J Manipulative Physiol Ther* 2000, **23:**557–563.
8. Leboeuf-Yde C, Hennius B, Rudberg E, Leufvenmark P, Thunman M: **Chiropractic in Sweden: a short description of patients and treatment.** *J Manipulative Physiol Ther* 1997, **20:**507–510.
9. Ailliet L, Rubinstein SM, De Vet HC: **Characteristics of chiropractors and their patients in Belgium.** *J Manipulative Physiol Ther* 2010, **33:**618–625.
10. Sibbritt D, Adams J, Young AF: **A profile of middle-aged women who consult a chiropractor or osteopath: findings from a survey of 11,143 Australian women.** *J Manipulative Physiol Ther* 2006, **29:**349–353.
11. French SD, Charity M, Forsdike K, Gunn J, Polus B, Walker B, Chondros P, Britt H: **Chiropractic Observation and Analysis STudy (COAST): providing an understanding of current chiropractic practice.** *Med J Aust* 2013. in press.
12. MacLennan AH, Myers SP, Taylor AW: **The continuing use of complementary and alternative medicine in South Australia: costs and beliefs in 2004.** *Med J Aust* 2006, **184:**27–31.
13. Gunn JM, Gilchrist GP, Chondros P, Ramp M, Hegarty KL, Blashki GA, Pond DC, Kyrios M, Herrman HE: **Who is identified when screening for depression is undertaken in general practice? Baseline findings from the Diagnosis, Management and Outcomes of Depression in Primary Care (diamond) longitudinal study.** *Med J Aust* 2008, **188:**S119–S125.
14. Potiriadis M, Chondros P, Gilchrist G, Hegarty K, Blashki G, Gunn JM: **How do Australian patients rate their general practitioner? A descriptive study using the General Practice Assessment Questionnaire.** *Med J Aust* 2008, **189:**215–219.
15. *Stata Statistical Software: Release 12 [program].* College Station, TX: StataCorp LP; 2011.

16. Department of Primary Industries and Energy and Department of Human Services and Health: *Rural remote and metropolitan areas classification 1991 census edition.* Canberra: AGPS; 1994.
17. Australian Institute of Health and Welfare: Rural, regional and remote health: *A guide to remoteness classifications (AIHW cat no: PHE 53).* Canberra: AIHW; 2004.
18. Ware J Jr, Kosinski M, Keller SD: **A 12-Item Short-Form Health Survey: construction of scales and preliminary tests of reliability and validity.** *Med Care* 1996, **34**:220–233.
19. Hodgson R, Alwyn T, John B, Thom B, Smith A: **The FAST Alcohol Screening Test.** *Alcohol Alcohol* 2002, **37**:61–66.
20. Gunn JM, Ayton DR, Densley K, Pallant JF, Chondros P, Herrman HE, Dowrick CF: **The association between chronic illness, multimorbidity and depressive symptoms in an Australian primary care cohort.** *Soc Psychiatry Psychiatr Epidemiol* 2012, **47**:175–184.
21. Australian Bureau of Statistics: **Health Services: patient Experiences in Australia 2009.** *Commonwealth Aust* 2010.
22. Ndetan HT, Bae S, Evans MW Jr, Rupert RL, Singh KP: **Characterization of health status and modifiable risk behavior among united states adults using chiropractic care as compared with general medical care.** *J Manipulative Physiol Ther* 2009, **32**:414–422.

Breast size, thoracic kyphosis & thoracic spine pain - association & relevance of bra fitting in post-menopausal women: a correlational study

Linda Spencer* and Kathy Briffa

Abstract

Background: Menopause would seem to exist as a period of accelerated changes for women and their upper torso mechanics. Whether these anthropometric changes reflect changes in pain states remains unclear. Plausible mechanisms of pain exist for the independent and combined effect of increasing breast size and thoracic kyphosis. Bra fit has the potential to change when the anthropometric measures (chest circumference and bust circumference) used to determine bra size change, such as postmenopausally.

Identifying an association between breast size, thoracic kyphosis and thoracic spine pain in postmenopausal women and identifying the relevance of bra fit to this association may be of importance to the future management and education of post-menopausal women presenting clinically with thoracic spine pain.

Methods: A cross-sectional study design. Fifty-one postmenopausal bra-wearing women were recruited. Measures included breast size (Triumph International), thoracic kyphosis (flexible curve), bra fitted (Y/N) and pain (Short Form McGill Pain Questionnaire) and tenderness on palpation (posteroanterior pressure testing). These measures were collected in one session at a physiotherapy clinic.

Results: The majority of the women in this study were overweight or obese and wearing an incorrect sized bra. Pain was significantly related to breast size, body weight and BMI at mid thoracic levels (T7-8). In contrast self-reported thoracic pain was not correlated with age or index of kyphosis (thoracic kyphosis). Women with thoracic pain were no more likely to have their bra professionally fitted whereas women with a higher BMI and larger breasts were more likely to have their bra professionally fitted.

Conclusion: The findings of this study show that larger breasts and increased BMI are associated with thoracic pain in postmenopausal women. This is unrelated to thoracic kyphosis. Increasing breast size and how a bra is worn may have biomechanical implications for the loaded thoracic spine and surrounding musculature. Post-menopause women present with a spectrum of anthropometrical changes that have the potential to contribute to altered biomechanics and affect pain states in the thoracic spine.

Keywords: Breast size, Thoracic spine pain, Post-menopausal women

Background

Menopause represents a period of accelerated changes for women which is pivotal in the development of osteoporosis [1], obesity [2] and some pain states [3].

Ageing and menopause are closely allied but different variables. Symptoms created by both often lack definition and distinction. Changes in spinal posture and breast size are of interest in this study.

* Correspondence: Lindaspeedyspencer@gmail.com
School of Physiotherapy, Faculty of Health Sciences, Curtin University, Bentley Campus, Perth, Western Australia

Progressive change in adult spinal sagittal posture is a well-documented characteristic feature of the ageing process [4-6]. In the thoracic spine these changes have been attributed to gradual changes in the structure and mechanics of connective tissues including loss of elasticity, a reduction in back extensor strength and concurrent collapse of vertebral bodies resulting from low bone mineral density. Accentuated kyphosis is a noticeable postural change, which has a higher incidence in women post menopause [4,6,7].

Changes in breast size have been shown to vary throughout life. Descriptive evidence suggests that breast size changes are prevalent after menopause. These changes in breast size have been described and measured in several different ways including breast mass; a breast size score; cup size and bra size. Breast mass and breast size score are indicators of absolute breast size, that is, they are independent of the size of the woman. Cup size also indicates breast size, but it is relative to the size of the woman as indicated by her under-breast chest circumference. Cup size has the advantage of being an indicator that is meaningful to most people and therefore is widely used where communication with a lay audience is important. All of these indicators are used in the literature, with the selection often influenced by the research question. For example, cup size is often used for studies of breast augmentation or reduction mammoplasty, whereas breast mass may be more appropriate for biomechanical studies. Increases in breast size post-menopause have been reported together with increases in body weight (and BMI) [8]. Mechanisms - involving a reduction in lypolitic response have been proposed for these changes [9,10]. Whilst it might be assumed that an increase in breast size might be proportionate to an increase in BMI, this has been challenged with evidence that women who lose weight after menopause still show an increase in breast size [8].

Menopause is a period of accelerated changes for women in their upper torso mechanics. Whether these anthropometrical changes reflect changes in pain states remains unclear. Plausible mechanisms for pain exist for the independent and combined effect of increasing breast size and thoracic kyphosis. Breast hypertrophy (macromastia) and associated symptomatology for example, have been well-evidenced [11]. Back pain, neck pain and discomfort during physical activity exist as predominant symptoms causing women to seek help in the form of reduction mammoplasty surgery [11]. Significant reduction of shoulder grooving, back and neck pain have been reported with a mean reduction of 2.6 cup sizes in symptomatic women post reduction mammoplasty [12]. These findings suggest that larger breast sizes do indeed equate with a greater health burden, which is amenable to change. These studies also highlight that a greater proportion of older women (menopausal age and above) undergo such surgery [11,13]. While a number of psychosocial factors might contribute to decisions by older women to have reduction surgery this might also be interpreted as a greater desire for symptomatic relief from large breasts amongst this population.

Static spinal postures have been shown to differ according to breast size [14], suggesting a biomechanical basis for some macromastic symptoms. It has been proposed that anteriorly located breast mass acts to shift the centre of gravity away from the spine thus presenting as a clinical prologue to the development of an increased cervical lordosis and thoracic kyphosis. Emotional factors might also be considered with the impact of upper torso changes as women protract the shoulders to disguise cup size. The addition of a poorly fitting bra with tight shoulder straps and excessive elevation of breast tissue acts to increase the downward drag of breast weight and alter mechanics further [15]. Pain produced by such mechanisms would intuitively be dependent on the size and weight of the breast and surrounding cutaneous tissue, which potentially implicates overall body weight & BMI in the symptom pathway.

A large proportion of large breasted women wear incorrectly sized bras [16]. To date bra fit appears unrelated to pain in normal healthy individuals despite the theory that a poorly fitting bra would compromise bra function (breast support and minimisation of breast bounce) and contribute to unfavourable spinal mechanics [16]. Pain related to bra fit may manifest as shoulder grooving, back or neck pain and neuropathic symptoms in the upper limbs.

Eliciting whether bra fit contributes to pain in an 'at risk' population may be more fruitful. Bra fit has the potential to change when the anthropometrical measures (chest circumference and bust circumference) used to determine bra size change, such as post-menopausally. One in five women have reported that after menopause they had to buy a larger bra because of changes in breast size [8]. Evidence has identified that women show a concomitant increase in thoracic kyphosis and BMI post-menopausally which may also alter chest circumference measures. Therefore, both breast size and chest circumference are likely to change post-menopausally. This may result in the redundancy of a previously well-fitting bra and an appearance of macromastic symptomatology which operates through the mechanism of an ill-fitting bra. It however, remains unknown whether a woman changes cup size, band size or both when selecting a new bra post-menopusally.

In this study we examined thoracic spine pain and tenderness in relation to breast size, thoracic kyphosis and bra fit in post-menopausal women in order to begin exploring the question of whether breast size, thoracic kyphosis and bra fit have consistent independent or combined associations with thoracic spine pain in this population. Clarification of these associations may aid the care of postmenopausal women presenting with thoracic pain.

Methods

This study was approved by the Human Research Ethics Committee at Curtin University. All participants provided written informed consent for their participation in the study.

Participants

Fifty-one post-menopausal women (50-84 years) with and without thoracic pain, who wore a bra on a daily basis, volunteered to participate in this study. Post-menopause was defined as having had their last menstrual period more than one year ago [17]. Thoracic pain was defined as pain felt anywhere in the posterior aspect of the thoracic cage (region bordered by the first thoracic vertebrae and rib superiorly, and the twelfth thoracic vertebrae and rib inferiorly).

Recruitment posters for this study, displayed in community halls and physiotherapy clinics in the Mandurah local area, invited post-menopausal women, who wore a bra on a daily basis to volunteer for this study. Volunteers were excluded if they: (a) were not post-menopausal, (b) had undergone any form of thoracic spine surgery, (c) had a known pathology involving the breast, lung or thoracic spine, (d) had had any form of cancer, (d) were using or had had prolonged use of steroid medication, or (e) were unable to read or understand English.

Data collection and measures

Data collection for this study comprised two parts:

(1) Participants completed a screening questionnaire to ensure inclusion criteria were met and to collect descriptive data, bra size and fitting details. This self-report measure identified the current bra size worn by the women and whether they routinely had their bra fitted by a trained professional (yes/no response).
(2) Eligible participants attended a Physiotherapy clinic on one occasion for the collection of anthropometrical (breast size & thoracic kyphosis) and thoracic pain measurements.

Breast size

Correct bra size was established for each woman according to Triumph guidelines using under-bust and over-bust circumferences [18]. Under-bust circumference (band size) indicated the bra size (10 to 20, analogous to sizes for other clothing) and the difference between under- and over-bust circumferences indicated cup-size (A to G). A tabulated conversion chart provided by Triumph Australia was used to convert the measured bra size to a continuous breast size score (3 to 15). These scores are indicative of cup volume, and consequently breast volume, independent of the band size of the woman and based on calculations of the cup/breast volume as the volume of half a sphere [19]. This method is analogous to those used in the sizing of breast prostheses whereby a size of 4 (for example) is approximately equivalent to a breast volume of 400 cm^3. Tabulated conversions simplify application of the system [18] (see Additional file 1 for calculation table adapted from Triumph). It appears this method was used in a previous study examining relationships between breast size, bra fit and thoracic pain [16]. The application of a continuous numerical scale in less sophisticated ways to indicate cup size is also apparent in literature examining breast size [20]. The bra size measured according to the Triumph guidelines was compared with the self-reported bra size to indicate whether or not the participants in this study were wearing a bra of the correct size.

Thoracic kyphosis

A Flexible Curve (Faber-Castell, Germany) was used to measure the size of the sagittal plane curve (i.e. kyphosis) in the thoracic spine. Denoted by an index of Kyphosis (IK), with higher scores indicating greater degrees of thoracic kyphosis. The intra- and inter-rater reliability of flexible curve measures of thoracic kyphosis are acceptable with reported coefficients of 0.88 and higher [21,22].

Thoracic spine pain

Short form McGill Pain Questionnaire (SF-MPQ) [23]: A total pain score (0-38) was derived from the three subscales (Sensory, Affective & Visual Analogue Scale) of the short form McGill Pain Questionnaire. Satisfactory test–retest reliability and responsiveness values of the NSF-MPQ have been reported [24].

Tenderness on palpation

PA Pressure Testing: Provocation and the behaviour of localised tenderness in the thoracic spine was assessed using a central posteroanterior (PA) applied pressure (grade III) through the spinous processes of the thoracic (T4-10) spine [25]. Each vertebrae producing tenderness with a large- amplitude, through-range oscillatory mobilisation after ten seconds or less were recorded.

Data analysis

Data were analysed using SPSS version 17. Univariate and multivariate relationships between breast size, thoracic kyphosis (IK) and thoracic spine pain (SF-MPQ) were examined using Pearson's correlation co-efficients (r) and stepwise multiple regression analysis respectively.

Tenderness at each thoracic spinal segment tested was plotted using frequency histograms. T-tests were used to compare breast size variables between women with and without tenderness at each thoracic vertebra.

Chi squared analyses were used to examine associations between the categorical variables of bra fitted and thoracic tenderness on palpation at each level. The relationship between breast size and the likelihood of having bras fitted was examined with logistic regression analysis.

Level of significance was set as $p < 0.05$. There were no adjustments for multiple comparisons as these were likely to increase the chances of type II error [26].

Results

Fifty-one women (50-84 years) volunteered for this study.

Seven women were excluded. Six because they did not meet the selection criteria and one because she did not return the screening questionnaire. Consequently data from 44 women were included in the analyses.

The majority of the sample were overweight (32%) (BMI 25-30) or obese (23%) (BMI >30) (Table 1). No women were underweight. Bra sizes ranged from 10A to 22E (median 16B). The average under-bust circumference (band size) was 87 cm and over-bust circumference 102, equivalent to a bra size of 16C (Figure 1). Thoracic Kyphosis indices ranged from 5.9 to 19.1 with a mean thoracic kyphosis of 11.7. Thoracic pain scores ranged from 0 to 38 with a mean score of 8.3 on the SF-MPQ.

Just over half of the women sampled (52%) reported having their bra fitted. The expense associated with bra fitting and the perception that women were able to self-select bras reasonably well were the main reasons given by participants in this study for not having their bra fitted.

Comparisons between measured bra size and bra size worn regardless of whether or not the bras worn had been professionally fitted suggested that the majority (93%) of participants were wearing incorrectly sized bras, with 57% wearing bras that were too small and 36% wearing bras that were too big. The brand of bra worn and the timing of when participants last had their bra fitted were not known.

Tenderness on palpation was more prevalent at higher thoracic levels with 73% reporting pain at T4, decreasing to 18% reporting pain at T10 (Figure 2). There was no difference in the index of kyphosis or BMI between those with or without tenderness on palpation at any of the thoracic levels ($p > 0.05$). Breast size was significantly associated with pain at T7 ($p = 0.007$) and T8 ($p = 0.02$).

There was a positive correlation between body weight and breast size (Table 2). This was mirrored by a strong positive correlation between BMI and breast size. Body weight, BMI and breast size were correlated with thoracic pain indicating that larger women with larger breasts reported more thoracic pain. In contrast, thoracic pain was not correlated with age or thoracic kyphosis (IK) (Table 2).

Table 1 Descriptive data

	Mean (SD)
Age	69 (9.1)
Height	162 (5.0)
Weight	71 (11.0)
BMI	26.5 (4.7)
Breast size score	7.8 (2.8)
Pain(SF-MPQ)	8.3 (8.7)
Thoracic kyphosis(IK)	11.7 (2.9)

Note: *IK* Index of Kyphosis.
SK-MPQ Short form Mc Gill pain questionnaire.
Mean (standard deviation) shown.

In stepwise multiple regression analysis including breast size, IK, and BMI as independent variables, only breast size was significantly associated with thoracic pain ($p = 0.002$).

Women with thoracic spine pain were no more or less likely to have their bra fitted ($p = 0.31$) than women without pain. In contrast, women with larger breasts were more likely to have their bra fitted. For every 1-point increase in breast size score, a woman was 1.3 times more likely to get her bra fitted (CI = 1.04-1.74).

Discussion

The purpose of this study was to explore the relationship between breast size, thoracic kyphosis, bra fit and thoracic pain in post-menopausal women. Menopause and ageing are similar but distinct variables. Menopause exists as period of rapid transition for women in terms of lean tissue mass [27], bone mineral density [28], fat tissue distribution [27], and a range of subsequent anthropometrical dimensions. Identifying if and how these changes might impact on pain experienced by post-menopausal women will help direct future clinical practice.

The sample of women who participated in this study were relatively healthy, community dwelling individuals who were not self-selected on the basis of seeking treatment for pain.

The majority of women were overweight (BMI > 25-30) or obese (BMI > 30), which is coherent with national statistics showing this to be the largest and most rapidly expanding category in women, particularly post-menopausally [29]. Body weight and BMI were significantly associated with breast size, indicating somewhat intuitively that larger women have larger breasts. Women with a greater BMI and larger breasts were more likely to have their bra fitted but the majority of women in this study were not wearing the correct bra size.

Wearing incorrectly sized bras has also been reported in young women with thoracic pain [16]. The procedure for fitting a bra is reasonably universal but due to the constraints on how it can be measured, some random error cannot be excluded in the process. Assumed differences between bra brands together with other substantiated variables such as measurement methodology and chest expansion during measuring [30] are factors affecting the inter-rater reliability in bra measurements.

Breast hypertrophy has been associated with menopause with many women reporting an increase in breast size post-menopause [8]. Women of post-menopausal age are more likely to seek reduction mammoplasty surgery

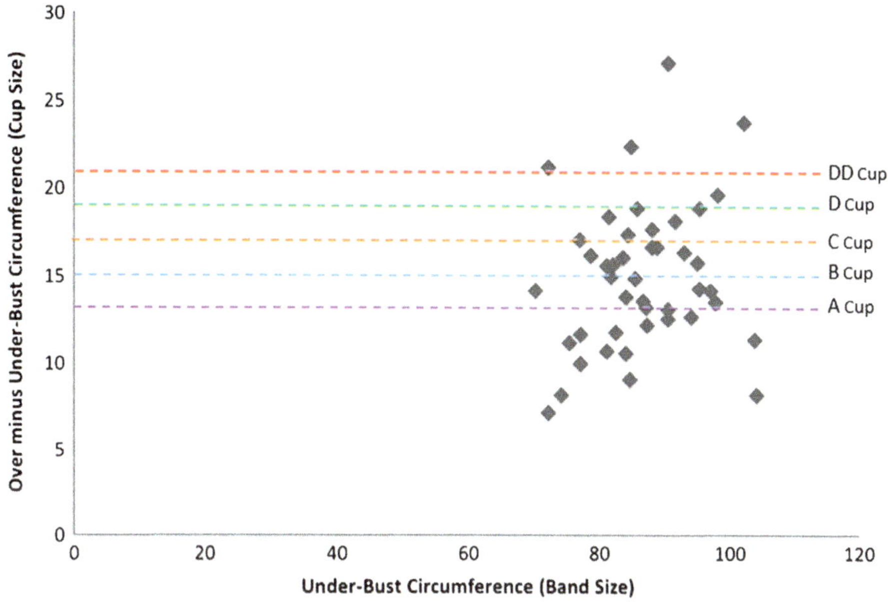

Figure 1 Distribution of bra sizes.

[11,13], suggesting that the postmenopausal increase in breast size is pertinent to symptoms leading women to seek such surgery. There was large variation in the bra size of participants in this study, varying as it did from 10A to 22E with an average size of 16C. Whilst there is no consensus on the definition of macromastia, women with bra cup sizes exceeding DD appear most frequently in reduction mammoplasty studies [11]. If bra cup size is taken as an indicator of breast size, it might be assumed that the DD cup size is a threshold at, or above which, common symptoms associated with macromastia develop. This might be usefully regarded by clinicians treating this category of women but further clarification is needed as to whether breast size, mass, shape and position are influential in part or combination to this relationship.

Large breast size has been purported to exist as a significant health burden in some postmenopausal women, operating mainly through the mechanism of pain [13]. The two procedures used for the assessment of pain in this study provided both localised and global subjective indications of thoracic tenderness and pain respectively. A significant moderate relationship was found between

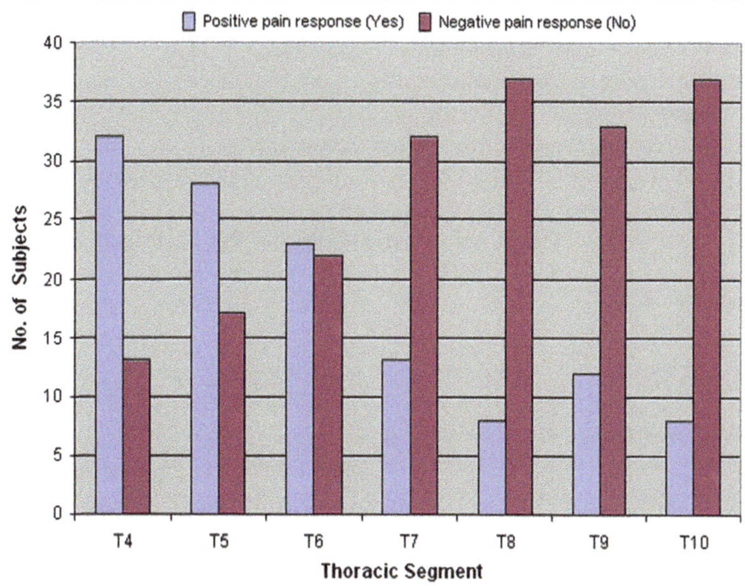

Figure 2 Thoracic spine segmental pain frequency.

Table 2 Relationships (Pearson's) between age, anthropometric variables and self reported thoracic pain

	Weight	BMI	IK	Breastr size	Pain
Age	−0.26 (p = 0.09)	−0.22 (p = 0.16)	−1.0 (p = 0.34)	−0.11 (p = 0.48)	−0.14 (p = 0.35)
Weight		0.88 (p < 0.001)	0.066 (p = 0.68)	0.67 (p < 0.001)	0.47 (p = 0.001)
BMI			0.03 (p = 0.87)	0.57 (p < 0.001)	0.41 (p = 0.005)
IK				0.20 (p = 0.20)	0.08 (p = 0.60)
Breast size					0.46 (p = 0.002)

Note: *IK* Index of Kyphosis.
P = values are from Pearson's correlation co-efficients calculated between variables.

breast size and global thoracic pain. Localised tenderness on palpation at the thoracic levels T7 and T8 was significantly associated with breast size. Although a series of t-tests was used to examine these relationships and no corrections for multiple comparisons were implemented, the p-value for T7 was very small ($p < 0.007$) and the finding of significant associations at two adjacent levels add plausibility to the finding.

Whilst a causal relationship between breast size and thoracic pain (particularly at T7 and T8) cannot be concluded from these cross-sectional data, it is encouraging to find that existing literature has highlighted potential mechanisms that are consistent with the findings of this study. The pulley-like action of brassiere straps and associated downward drag of breast weight has been implicated in the cause of pain in the scapular elevator muscles [15]. It might be speculated that scapular retractor muscles (regional to T7/8) are also a potential source of pain as the shoulder girdle protracts with a larger anterior load (larger breasts). These findings and those produced in the present study provide anatomical, clinical and statistical confirmation and consensus of the plausibility of such a mechanism and highlight the mid thoracic region as one which is implicated with increased stress afforded by larger breasts. Further investigation into the shape and volume of breast tissue in post-menopausal women would help clarify the specific biomechanical impact of breast size relative to overall upper body size/fat distribution which could be used to further elucidate possible pain mechanisms.

Collectively the results of this study support the general consensus of reduction mammoplasty research indicating that breast size is indeed instrumental in producing symptoms of upper back pain in post-menopausal women. With the majority of women undergoing breast reduction surgery being overweight or obese [13] and knowing that pain prevalence has been linked to obesity [31] with the relative odds of chronic pain increasing with every unit of BMI [32], it is helpful that the present study has identified an association between breast size and pain which appears independent of body weight and BMI. If breast size had not been shown to be the most important independent predictor of thoracic pain in this study then it might be speculated that the improvements in symptoms seen in reduction mammoplasty studies are less contingent on actual breast size but more so on breast weight, particularly since some studies report the removal of up to 2330 g per breast [12]. This could arguably translate into a somewhat significant immediate reduction in body weight (and BMI) post-surgery and thus explain the symptom improvement based on the aforementioned relationships.

The results of this study indicate that upper thoracic pain exists in women of postmenopausal age with 82% of participants indicating some pain in the upper back (SF-MPQ score >0). Progressive change in adult spinal sagittal posture is a characteristic feature of the ageing process which is accentuated in women, around the menopause through osteoporosis [6]. Conversely, It is now well-established that the sagittal curvatures of the spine are geometric parameters that are known to have a significant influence on mechanical properties during compression loading [33,34]. Sagittal posture imbalance has been shown to elevate loads and intervertebral disc stresses, thus posing as a plausible mechanism for pain in persons with an increased thoracic kyphosis [6]. Whilst the results of this study cannot confirm the association between increasing kyphosis and global or localised thoracic pain in post-menopausal women, it does highlight the existence of thoracic pain in this population. Breast size is associated with this pain at thoracic levels T7 and T8, which are levels that have been previously identified in postmenopausal women as being frequently deformed (due to wedging or fracture) [4,6] and close to the apex of kyphosis (T6) [5]. Given the abundance of existing literature that has identified relationships between increasing age [6], BMI [7] and pain [35] with accentuated thoracic kyphosis, further examination of these variables in post-menopausal women is suggested.

In summary, the findings of this study show a correlation between breast size and upper back pain in postmenopausal women. This is unrelated to thoracic kyphosis and appears independent of co-existing associations between increasing BMI and thoracic pain. Whilst women with larger breasts are more likely to have their bra fitted, this appears unrelated to thoracic pain.

This study has identified a handful of correlates associated with thoracic pain in post-menopausal women. It is acknowledged that additional possible correlates exist and in this study it was not possible to account for all of these. Bone mineral density, physical activity levels, emotion and in some instances, occupational stresses, are factors that were not measured and may have confounded our results. Random error associated with breast size and thoracic kyphosis measurement should be considered as limitations of this study. In addition, the results of this study were reliant on the accuracy of responses to self-reported measures of pain, bra wear and fitting. Collectively the under or over-reporting of details pertaining to these measures cannot be discounted and should also be considered limitations of this study.

Further research is required to examine women post-menopausally. It exists as a transitional time for women in terms of breast size and BMI, which could also reflect a transitional time in terms of pain. An intuitive and proven relationship exists between breast size and body weight and this is related to thoracic pain. Elucidating possible mechanisms to explain these relationships would be a logical progression to understanding why they exist and how clinical practice might be improved in the treatment of post-menopausal women presenting with thoracic pain.

Conclusions

Multiple factors could determine the prevalence of thoracic pain in postmenopausal women. Based on the results of this study, breast size, body weight, BMI appear important. Thoracic kyphosis and whether the bra is of correct size show little meaningful correlation with thoracic pain in this population. Additional potentially causal factors are plentiful and inter-related. Whilst many of these factors are a feature of normal ageing, most are amenable to change and potentially responsive to conservative measures and therefore are worthy of future investigation.

Additional file

Additional file 1: The calculation table shown below was used in the conversion of bra size to a breast size score (1-15) [18]. This elicited an estimate of breast volume and provided a continuous variable for statistical analysis.

Competing interests

The authors declare that they have no competing interests.

Authors' contributions

This study was completed by LS in partial fulfilment of a Masters degree. KB acted as supervisor to this study. LS conceived the idea for the study. LS and KB designed the study and sought ethical approval. LS collected the data. LS and KB analysed the data. All authors contributed to the writing of this manuscript. All authors read and approved the final manuscript.

Acknowledgments

Dr Helen Slater for assisting with the selection of thoracic spine pain outcome measures.

References

1. Johannes DeVilliers T: **Bone health and osteoporosis in postmenopausal women.** *Best Pract Res Clin Obstet Gynaecol* 2009, **23**:73–85.
2. Dubnov G, Brzezinski A, Berry EM: **Weight control and the management of obesity after menopause: the role of physical activity.** *Maturitas* 2003, **44**:89–101.
3. Rousseau ME, Gottlieb SF: **Pain at midlife.** *J Midwifery Womens Health* 2004, **49**:529–538.
4. Puche RC, Morosano M, Masoni A, Jimeno NP, Bertoluzzo SM, Podadera JC, Podadera MA, Bocanera R, Tozzini R: **The natural history of kyphosis in postmenopausal women.** *Bone* 1995, **17**:239–246.
5. Boyle JJW, Milne N, Singer KP: **Influence of age on cervicothoracic spinal curvature: an ex vivo radiographic survey.** *Clin Biomech* 2002, **17**:361–367.
6. Goh S, Price RI, Leedman PJ, Singer KP: **The relative influence of vertebral body and intervertebral disc shape on thoracic kyphosis.** *Clin Biomech* 1999, **14**:439–448.
7. Hinman MR: **Comparison of thoracic kyphosis and postural stiffness in younger and older women.** *Spine J* 2004, **4**:413–417.
8. Den Tonkelaar I, Peeters PHM, Van Noord PAH: **Increase in breast size after menopause: prevalence and determinants.** *Maturitas* 2004, **48**:51–57.
9. Sowers MR, Wildman RP, Mancuso P, Eyvazzadeh AD, Karvonen-Gutierrez CA, Rillamas-Sun E, Jannausch ML: **Change in adipocytokines and ghrelin with menopause.** *Maturitas* 2008, **59**:149–157.
10. Gompel A, Levy D, Chaouat M, Forgez P, Rostene W: **Apoptosis and aging: breast cells and apoptosis.** *Maturitas* 2001, **38**:39–44.
11. Rogliani M, Gentile P, Labardi L, Donfrancesco A, Cervelli V: **Improvement of physical and psychological symptoms after breast reduction.** *J Plast Reconstr Aesthet Surg* 2009, **62**:1647–1649.
12. Brown AP, Hill C, Khan K: **Outcome of reduction mammaplasty - a patients' perspective.** *Br J Plast Surg* 2000, **53**:584–587.
13. Saariniemi KMM, Keranen UH, Salminen-Peltola PK, Kuokkanen HOM: **Reduction mammaplasty is effective treatment according to two quality of life instruments. A prospective randomised clinical trial.** *J Plast Reconstr Aesthet Surg* 2008, **61**:1472–1478.
14. Findikcioglu K, Findikcioglu F, Ozmen S, Guclu T: **The impact of breast size on the vertebral column: a radiologic study.** *Aesthetic Plast Surg* 2007, **31**:23–27.
15. Edward R: **Pectoral girdle myalgia in women: a 5-year study in a clinical setting.** *Clin J Pain* 2000, **16**:298–303.
16. Wood K, Cameron M, Fitzgerald K: **Breast size, bra fit and thoracic spine pain in young women: a correlational study.** *Chiropr Osteopat* 2008, **16**:1340–1347.
17. *Glossary of Terms.* http://www.menopause.org.au/.
18. Triumph International: *Brastylist: Book of Bras.* Australia: Triumph International Australia; 2005.
19. Brassieres: *An Engineering Miracle.* http://www.firstpr.com.au/show-and-tell/corsetry-1/nanas/engineer.html.
20. Wade TZ G, Martin N: **Body mass index and breast size in women: same or different genes?** *Twin Res Hum Genet* 2010, **13**:450–454.
21. Lundon K, Li A, Bibershtein S: **Interrater and intrrater reliability in the measurement of kyphosis in postmenopausal women with osteoporosis.** *Spine* 1998, **23**:1978–1985.
22. Caine M, McConnell A, Taylor D: **Asessment of spinal curvature: an evaluation of the flexicurve and associated means of analysis.** *Int J Rehabil Res* 1996, **19**:271–278.
23. Melzack R: **The short-form McGill pain questionnaire.** *Pain* 1987, **30**:191–197.
24. Strand LI, Ljunggren AE, Bogen B, Ask T, Johnsen TB: **The short-form McGill pain questionnaire as an outcome measure: test-retest reliability and responsiveness to change.** *Eur J Pain* 2008, **12**:917–925.
25. Maitland G, Hengeveld E, Banks K: *Maitland's Vertebral Manipulation.* 7th edition. Oxford: Butterworth Heinemann; 2005.
26. Perneger TV: **What's wrong with Bonferroni adjustments.** *Br Med J* 1998, **18**:1236–1238.
27. Svendsen OL, Hassager C, Christiansen C: **Age- and menopause-associated variations in body composition and fat distribution in healthy women as measured by dual-energy x-ray absorptiometry.** *Metabolism* 1995, **44**:369–373.

28. Mazzuoli G, Diacinti D, D'Erasmo E, Alfò M: **Cyclical changes of vertebral body heights and bone loss in healthy women after menopause.** *Bone* 2006, **38:**905–910.
29. *4719.0 - Overweight and Obesity in Adults, Australia.* http://www.abs.gov.au/ausstats/abs@.nsf/mf/4719.0/.
30. McGhee D, Steele J: **How do respiratory state and measurement method affect bra size calculations?** *Br J Sports Med* 2006, **40:**970–974.
31. Ray L, Lipton RB, Zimmerman ME, Katz MJ, Derby CA: *Mechanisms of association between obesity and chronic pain in the elderly.* USA: In Press; 2011.
32. Hitt HC, McMillen RC, Thornton-Neaves T, Koch K, Cosby AG: **Comorbidity of obesity and pain in a general population: results from the southern pain prevalence study.** *J Pain* 2007, **8:**430–436.
33. Edmondston SJ, Aggerholm M, Elfving S, Flores N, Ng C, Smith R, Netto K: **Influence of posture on the range of axial rotation and coupled lateral flexion of the thoracic spine.** *J Manipulative Physiol Ther* 2007, **30:**193–199.
34. Polga D, Beaubien B, Kallemeier P, Schellhas K, Lew W, Buttermann G, Wood K: **In vivo measurement of intradiscal pressure in healthy thoracic intervertebral discs.** *Spine J* 2003, **3:**83–84.
35. Ryan PJ, Blake G, Herd R, Fogelman I: **A clinical profile of back pain and disability in patients with spinal osteoporosis.** *Bone* 1994, **15:**27–30.

25

How to proceed when evidence-based practice is required but very little evidence available?

Charlotte Leboeuf-Yde[1,2*], Olivier Lanlo[3] and Bruce F Walker[4]

Abstract

Background: All clinicians of today know that scientific evidence is the base on which clinical practice should rest. However, this is not always easy, in particular in those disciplines, where the evidence is scarce. Although the last decades have brought an impressive production of research that is of interest to chiropractors, there are still many areas such as diagnosis, prognosis, choice of treatment, and management that have not been subjected to extensive scrutiny.

Discussion: In this paper we argue that a simple system consisting of three questions will help clinicians deal with some of the complexities of clinical practice, in particular what to do when clear clinical evidence is lacking. Question 1 asks: are there objectively tested facts to support the concept? Question 2: are the concepts that form the basis for this clinical act or decision based on scientifically acceptable concepts? And question three; is the concept based on long-term and widely accepted experience? This method that we call the *"Traffic Light System"* can be applied to most clinical processes.

Summary: We explain how the Traffic Light System can be used as a simple framework to help chiropractors make clinical decisions in a simple and lucid manner. We do this by explaining the roles of biological plausibility and clinical experience and how they should be weighted in relation to scientific evidence in the clinical decision making process, and in particular how to proceed, when evidence is missing.

Keywords: Chiropractic, Evidence based practice, Biological plausibility

Background

The clinical encounter has many aspects – evidence-based practice expected

For health care practitioners, the first clinical encounter has several important goals, two of these are: 1) to get an idea of what is wrong with the patient and 2) to detect any cases that should be directed elsewhere. Chiropractors, and other professionals who often provide manual therapies, will also work out a "technical" diagnosis in relation to where and what to treat. Thereafter follows the treatment itself, any follow-up procedure, and the long-term strategy. This is a relatively complex process, as many different pieces of information must be considered, brought into a coherent picture and acted upon. In addition, clinicians are expected to keep updated on that part of dynamic knowledge – research – that concerns their area of practice and to apply this knowledge on each patient.

All clinicians of today know that scientific evidence is the base on which clinical practice should rest. However, this is not always easy, in particular in those disciplines, where the evidence is scarce. There is also the issue of the definition of "evidence". Textbooks have been devoted to this. Throughout this text we shall assume that "evidence" equals the "best evidence" available at the time, when evaluating the value of a clinical procedure.

Although the last decades have brought an impressive production of research that is of interest to chiropractors, there are still many areas such as diagnosis, prognosis, choice of treatment, and management that have not been subjected to extensive scrutiny. Therefore, some aspects of health care are accepted on their logic and face value and through their repeated and successful use over time.

* Correspondence: clyde@health.sdu.dk
[1]The Spine Research Centre, Hospital Lillebaelt, and Institute for Regional Health Research, University of Southern Denmark, Middelfart, Denmark
[2]Complexité, Innovation et Activités Motrices et Sportives, Bâtiment 335, UFR STAPS, Université Paris Sud-11, Orsay Cedex 91405, France
Full list of author information is available at the end of the article

If no evidence: plausibility and experience

This lack of specific evidence, however, is not always worrying, as it is considered acceptable to extrapolate from generally acknowledged scientific concepts, and it follows that procedures and concepts will, generally, not be questioned when this happens.

If the underlying rationale is plausible, in addition to the procedure or concept being accepted by many clinicians, then it is likely that it will be considered relatively "acceptable". However, the level of acceptance is lower for only logic and experience than it is for scientific evidence. This means that decisions and actions based solely on logic and experience usually cannot stand on their own. An example is that the plausible and frequently used test for an acutely injured lumbar disc, antalgia on flexion of the lumbar spine, can be used to help diagnose this disc problem [1], but that other corroborating information is needed before the diagnosis is accepted.

Lack of generally acceptable logical concept

However, if the concept, act or procedure is not biologically plausible, as judged by the scientific community in general, then experience is not enough to justify its use. This is not surprising, because if a procedure or decision is based on a biologically implausible rationale, it is unlikely that it will be clinically valid.

An example of a non-acceptable procedure is the use of a pendulum in order to define the gender of the unborn baby. This method lacks an acceptable contemporary scientific rationale, so even if some people think that this method is useful, it cannot be introduced in an obstetrics department, unless several well carried out studies have shown, unequivocally, that the vast majority of unborn babies can be correctly classified by gender using a pendulum. Thus a very heavy onus of proof would rest upon any person who would claim that this method can be used for this purpose.

On the other hand, if, against all odds, a test or treatment that lacks (contemporary) plausibility is shown to be clinically valid in several well designed and appropriately performed studies, then it will be considered "acceptable". The reason for this is, that the contemporary knowledge may not be sufficient to explain why this is so. An historical example of how, sadly, "the evidence" won over common sense and repeated observations is how dirty hands were dismissed as a cause of puerperal fever in childbirth, because its pathogens had not been discovered [2].

Sometimes the question on whether a concept is logical or not will be answered differently by different groups of practitioners. It is, however, outside the scope of this article to define further "logical" and "biologically plausible" in relation to various chiropractic concepts; this discussion belongs elsewhere. However, the plausibility here refers to that which would be acknowledged as such by the contemporary general scientific community.

Easy clinical decisions vs. difficult decisions

Obviously, there are many aspects in clinical practice that lurk in the areas of no specific evidence yet considered to be perfectly acceptable because they are based on sound and generally accepted biological/physiological/anatomical/pathological concepts combined with longstanding and widespread experience.

For example within spinal care it would be considered acceptable to advise a patient with a very painful and antalgic lumbar spine against digging up his garden whilst in such a state. The rationale for this advice is that such activity would be likely to aggravate the affected spinal structures. This advice has never been tested in a randomized controlled clinical trial; instead it is based on our present understanding of the pathology of the disc and backed up by our experience of outcome in relation to whether this type of patients avoid aggravating activities or not.

However, there are other times when clinicians may become confused. For example, when the above patient asks how many treatments he will need and how frequently these should be administered, the rationale for this is not so clear. Should there be frequent treatments over a short period of time (rationale: the more the better) or does it suffice with few treatments (rationale: a few treatments will help the process on its way and healing takes the time it takes)? Further, the experiences of various clinicians may be difficult to evaluate, as each of them probably predominantly acknowledges their own specific rationale and therefore has limited experiences to draw on. Each is likely to assume that their specific approach and experiences represents the gold standard. We contend that the same uncertainty will arise over and over, as other unstudied cases present themselves in the practice.

What to do in these cases?

It can be challenging and confusing to make clinical decisions in situations where clear evidence is lacking. Many people find it uncomfortable and difficult to deal with uncertainty and feel safer if they can follow an algorithm of thought, some sort of recipe on how to proceed. This probably explains the plethora of more or less complicated experience-based recipe-type techniques that are available in the chiropractic profession.

On the other hand, attempts have been made since the early 1990s to assist chiropractors to perform in an evidence-based and streamlined manner. Most manual and/or observational tests in many health care fields would probably be classified under this category. Examples are visual inspections of radiographs, orthopedic and neurological tests, and auscultation of the abdomen and heart.

Other examples would be those chiropractic tests that have been poorly studied or studied with conflicting results yet based on a seemingly logical patho-anatomical concept.

Over the past 25 years, particular since the Mercy Guidelines [3] substantial efforts have resulted in several clinical algorithms pertinent to chiropractic practice in specific domains [4-7], but we have been unable to find a simplistic, general algorithm, applicable to chiropractic practice in general.

In this paper we argue that a simple system consisting of three questions will help clinicians deal with some of the complexities of clinical practice, in particular what to do when clear clinical evidence is lacking. This method, the *"Traffic Light System"*, can be applied to most clinical processes. We shall explain how the Traffic Light System can be used as a framework to help chiropractors make clinical decisions in a simple and lucid manner. We do this by explaining the roles of biological plausibility and clinical experience and how they should be weighted in relation to scientific evidence in the clinical decision making process.

According to the Traffic Light System, decision making is based on some simple concepts. First, scientific evidence carries more weight than biological plausibility and experience and, in particular, when there is lack of biological plausibility, there is a much stronger need for evidence. On the other hand, if there is biological plausibility, strong evidence may not always be needed, provided that the concept is also backed up by considerable clinical experience. This concept is illustrated in Figure 1.

We shall present two clinical situations in which the Traffic Light approach can be used: 1) when examining a patient, and 2) when choosing an appropriate method of treatment. However, we propose that the same approach can be used throughout the entire clinical decision-making process.

Discussion

The three questions in the traffic light system

The Traffic Light System is a method of approach that can be used to deal with the triad of: *evidence, plausibility and clinical experience.* We suggest that three questions be asked, whenever facing a clinical task, and that the continued activities should be based on a set method to interpret the answers to these questions. In order to provide a simple and easy-to-remember algorithm, we have incorporated the three traffic light colors into the system, green (go), yellow (go with care), and red (stop). The three questions are presented below together with their traffic light interpretations in three steps:

Step 1: Are there objectively tested facts to support the concept? In other words, is there sufficient sound research (evidence) supporting this? If the answer is "yes", the light is *green,* and you can go on with your procedure or decision. If the answer is "no", go to the second question.

Step 2: Are the concepts that form the basis for this clinical act or decision based on scientifically acceptable concepts? In other words, is it logical and lucid, biologically plausible? If the answer is "yes", go to question three. If the answer is "no", the light is *red* and you should stop here.

Step 3: Is the concept based on long-term and widely accepted experience? In other words, is 'everybody' doing it? If also this answer is "yes", the light is *yellow* and you can proceed with care. If the answer is "no", then stop for the *red* light.

The use of these three questions will now be demonstrated for two specific clinical aspects, 1) in the examination of the patient, and 2) in the choice of method of treatment. Depending on the answers to these questions, the case will be categorized with one of the three Traffic Light System colors (red, green or yellow).

Two examples on how to apply the Traffic Light System

Example 1: Examining the patient

All questions, observations, and clinical examination procedures that are performed in order to obtain an answer to a clinical question can be classified as "tests". Without discussing details, in general, tests should be used only if they are in some way useful, i.e. if they can help obtain a diagnosis, direct the type of treatment or hint to the prognosis. Tests that provide no such messages are a waste of time, and are to be considered meaningless rituals that may even confuse the issue. The only exception to this would be tests that are used to describe status over the course of treatment to see how the case progresses but play no role in the diagnosis, treatment or initial indications of prognosis. For example, information on particular positions (e.g. bending forward) or activities (e.g. turn in bed) which are painful.

We propose that these are *red light* tests:

1) The test has been submitted to scientific study and found not to "work" (step 1). This is regardless of whether it can be considered to be a plausible test (step 2) or if it is frequently used (step 3); we suggest that this is not a test to be used. In other words, if the test has been shown to be useless, it is not relevant to proceed to steps 2 and 3.
2) The test is illogical (step 2) and it has not been submitted to scientific study to prove its value (step 1). Because it is an illogical test, it would be necessary to have positive evidence to make this test

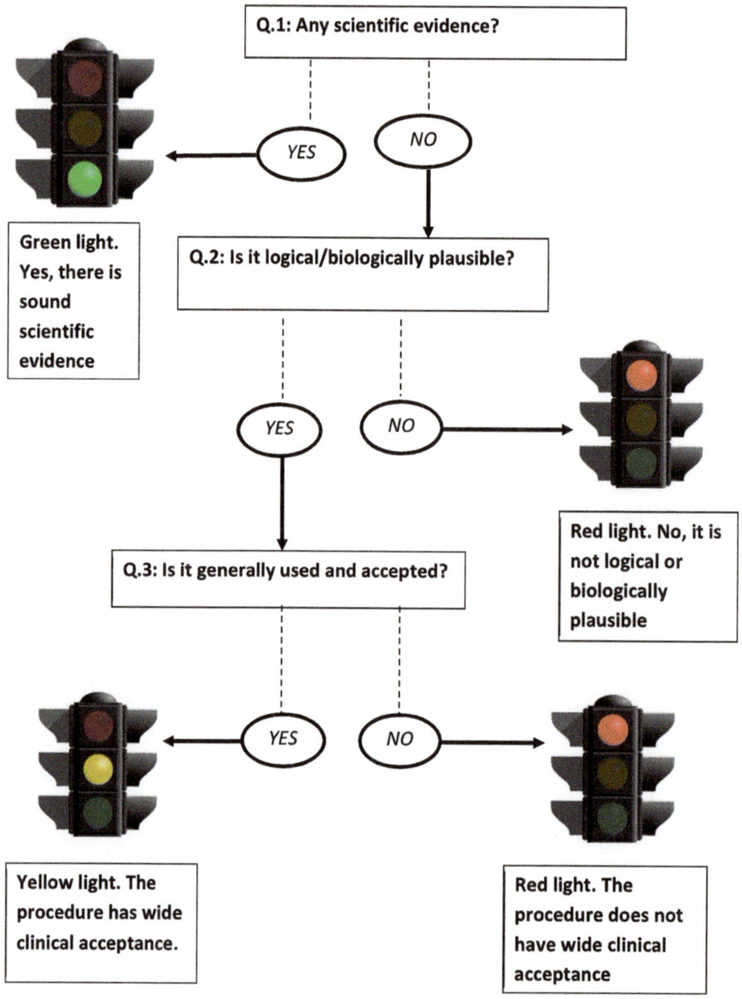

Figure 1 The Traffic Light System, a three-step algorithm for clinical reasoning in chiropractic practice.

acceptable. Therefore, it is not relevant to continue to step 3.
Some tests that make up the examination procedure of various chiropractic technique "systems" belong to this category.

Using the same approach, we propose that the following cases are considered to be *yellow light* tests:

1) The test has not been submitted to scientific scrutiny (step 1) but it is a logical test (step 2) that is generally found to be useful (step 3).
2) The test, which is logical (step 2), has been studied scientifically with differing results or with only moderate success (e.g.low to moderate sensitivity and/or specificity, or low to moderate reliability) (step 1). Most manual and/or observational tests in many health care fields would probably be classified under this category of insufficient evidence. Examples are visual inspections of radiographs, orthopedic and neurological tests, and auscultation of the abdomen and heart. Another example would be the reliability and validity of the identification of a vertebral segment requiring manipulation by using, for example, various types of palpation; generally incompletely studied and/or with conflicting research results but for many seemingly logical.

According to our method of approach, *green light* tests are the following:

1) All tests that have been studied scientifically and found to work (step1), regardless of whether they are plausible or not (step 2).
2) Several moderately useful tests that, when combined, are found to 'work' (step 1).
Manual and observation tests in the green category are uncommon.

To conclude, illogical tests must be shown to be valid before they can be used, whereas logical and commonly used but 'untested' tests are relatively acceptable provided that major decisions are not based entirely on one such single test.

Example 2: Selecting the treatment

Once patients who are unsuitable for treatment have been excluded (because they have either a contra-indication or a non-indication to treatment), and patients who are thought suitable for treatment have been accepted (usually with a tentative diagnosis), the next question to be dealt with is: How should this patient be treated?

Again, we suggest that the Traffic Light System can be used in relation to the choice of treatment method. We shall assume that the chiropractor wishes to select a particular manual technique, either one that includes an analytic method (e.g. sacro-occipital technique [8]) or one that consists of a therapeutic method that stands on its own without the necessity of a special pre-determined analytic approach.

Using the same theoretical approach as previously, *red light* techniques are those that are 1) illogical and untested or 2) logical but tested and found not to "work". *Yellow light* techniques are logical and used extensively with seemingly good results but "unproven" or with research findings indicating only moderately good results or with fluctuating study results between studies. *Green light* techniques are logical (or illogical), tested and found to "work".

"Ordinary" generic manipulation has been used in randomized clinical trials in which the value of spinal manipulation was studied. The results of these studies generally indicate that there is some clinical effect albeit small and not much different to other modalities including sham [9]. So it could be concluded that spinal manipulation is ineffective. However, these trials usually direct the manipulation at a symptom i.e. non-specific back pain and not a diagnosis. Accordingly, it is possible that future research may establish a role for back manipulation for a subset of patients with pain amenable to this type of treatment. So what do we do in the meantime while we await further research? We believe that "ordinary" manipulation for back pain satisfies step 2 and 3 and can be proceeded with as a "Yellow light therapy". However, it should be noted that there is presently scarcity of data on which type of technique (if any) is best for specific cases.

In the case where a treatment technique is encapsulated within a "system" such as the Sacro-Occipital Technique, it would be relevant to separate the analytical (diagnostic) part from the therapeutic part. The reason for this is that it would be possible for the analytical part (e.g. the body sway test, as performed in this technique) to be a "red light" test whilst the therapeutic aspect of the technique (for example pelvic blocking) could be yellow or even potentially green.

Summary

With these explanations we hope to have shown how the Traffic Light System can be used to guide chiropractors through a simple thought process, in which they should habitually consider three questions: Is there specific sound research evidence in favor of this clinical procedure? If not, is it at least logical/biologically plausible? And if so, has it gained wide clinical acceptance? Positive or negative answers to these questions will then be interpreted as one of the three lights, red, yellow or green. Green light means "go ahead", yellow means "proceed with care", whereas red means "stop".

After having applied this method for a while, it will become clear that most clinical procedures in chiropractic practice (diagnostic tests and choice of specific techniques) probably belong under the yellow light.

This abundance of yellow lights makes it obvious that, although the "science of chiropractic practice" is very important, what the clinician often has to deal with is the "art of chiropractic", in the general absence of evidence. This demands an ability to deal with uncertainty. How well this can be handled would depend on patient values and circumstances, but the practitioner's own clinical experience and his/her own ethical stamina are also very important. These additional issues, therefore, deserve careful consideration.

Competing interests

The authors declare that they have no competing interests.

Authors' contributions

CLY presented the concept and all authors discussed this, CLY drafted the manuscript, OL performed a literature review, and all authors reviewed, revised and accepted the final version. The concept has been previously partially presented at professional conferences. All authors read and approved the final manuscript.

Authors' information

Professor Charlotte Leboeuf-Yde, DC, MPH, PhD. The Spine Research Centre, Hospital Lillebaelt, and Institute for Regional Health Research, University of Southern Denmark, Middelfart, Denmark, and Visiting Professor, Complexité, Innovation et Activités Motrices et Sportives, Bâtiment 335, UFR STAPS, Université Paris Sud-11, Orsay Cedex 91405, France

Olivier Lanlo, DC, LLM, Executive President Institut Franco-Européen de Chiropraxie, Paris and Toulouse, France

Associate Professor Bruce Walker, School of Health Professions, Discipline of Chiropractic, Murdoch University, Perth, Western Australia, Australia

Funding

Charlotte Leboeuf-Yde's position in Denmark was until the 31.12.2012 partially funded by'Fonden til fremme for kiropraktisk forskning og postgraduat uddannelse'.

Author details

[1]The Spine Research Centre, Hospital Lillebaelt, and Institute for Regional Health Research, University of Southern Denmark, Middelfart, Denmark. [2]Complexité, Innovation et Activités Motrices et Sportives, Bâtiment 335, UFR STAPS, Université Paris Sud-11, Orsay Cedex 91405, France. [3]Institut Franco-Européen de Chiropraxie, Paris, France. [4]School of Health Professions, Murdoch University, Perth, Western Australia, Australia.

References

1. Miller KJ: **Physical assessment of lower extremity radiculopathy and sciatica.** *J Chiropr Med* 2007, **6**(2):75–82.
2. Hebra, Ferdinand: **"Höchst wichtige Erfahrungen über die Aetiologie der an Gebäranstalten epidemischen Puerperalfieber".** *Zeitschrift der k k Gesellschaft der Ärzte zu Wien* 1847, **4**(1):242–244.
3. Guidelines for Chiropractic Quality Assurance and Practice Parameters: *The mercy conference.* New York: Aspen Publishers, Inc; 1993.
4. Anderson-Peacock E, Blouin JS, Bryans R, Danis N, Furlan A, Marcoux H, Potter B, Ruegg R, Stein JG, White E, Guidelines Development Committee: **GDCJ chiropractic clinical practice guideline: evidence-based treatment of adult neck pain not due to whiplash. Canadian chiropractic association, Canadian federation of chiropractic regulatory boards, clinical practice guidelines development initiative.** *J Can Chiropr Assoc* 2005, **49**(3):158–209.
5. Hulberg JR, Printon R, Osterbauer P, Davis PT, Lamaack R: **Chiropractic treatment of hand and wrist pain in older people: a systematic protocol development. Part 1: informant interviews.** *J Chiropr Med* 2005, **4**(3):144–151.
6. Bryans R, Descarreaux M, Duranleau M, Marcoux H, Potter B, Ruegg R, Shaw L, Watkin R, White E: **Evidence-based guidelines for the chiropractic treatment of adults with headache.** *J Manipul Physiol Ther* 2011, **34**(5):274–289.
7. Kaminski M, Boal R, Gillette RG, Peterson DH, Villnave TJ: **A model for the evaluation of chiropractic methods.** *J Manipul Physiol Ther* 1987, **10**(2):61–64.
8. *Sacro-occipital technique.* http://www.soto.net.au/.
9. Rubinstein SM, Terwee CB, Assendelft WJJ, de Boer MR, van Tulder MW: **Spinal manipulative therapy for acute low-back pain.** *Cochrane Datab Syst Rev* 2012, **Art. No**(Issue 9):CD008880.

A randomized, placebo-controlled double-blinded comparative clinical study of five over-the-counter non-pharmacological topical analgesics for myofascial pain: single session findings

Daniel Avrahami[1,3*], Amanda Hammond[1,4], Ceara Higgins[1,5] and Howard Vernon[2]

Abstract

Objectives: To investigate the effects of topical agents for the treatment of Myofascial Pain Syndrome (MPS) and Myofascial Trigger Point (MTRP).

Methods: Subjects with an identifiable trigger point in the trapezius muscle, age 18-80 were recruited for a single-session randomized, placebo-blinded clinical study. Baseline measurements of trapezius muscle pressure pain threshold (PPT: by pressure algometer) along with right and left cervical lateral flexion (rangiometer) were obtained by a blinded examiner. An assessor blinded to the outcomes assessments applied one of 6 topical formulations which had been placed in identical plastic containers. Five of these topicals were proposed active formulations; the control group was given a non-active formulation (PLA). Five minutes after the application of the formula the outcome measures were re-tested. Data were analyzed with a 5-way ANOVA and Holms-adjusted t-tests with an alpha level of 0.05.

Results: 120 subjects were entered into the study (63 females; ages 16-82); 20 subjects randomly allocated into each group. The pre- and post-treatment results for pressure threshold did show significant intra-group increases for the Ben-Gay Ultra Strength Muscle Pain Ointment (BG), the Professional Therapy MuscleCare Roll-on (PTMC roll-on) and Motion Medicine Cream (MM) with an increased threshold of 0.5 kg/cm^2 (+/-0.15), 0.72 kg/cm^2 (+/-0.17) and 0.47 Kg/cm^2 (+/-0.19) respectively. With respect to the inter-group comparisons, PTMC roll-on showed significant increases in pressure threshold compared with Placebo (PLA) ($p = 0.002$) and Icy Hot Extra Strength Cream (IH) ($p = 0.006$). In addition, BG demonstrated significant increases in pressure threshold compared with PLA ($p = 0.0003$).

Conclusions: With regards to pressure threshold, PTMC roll-on, BG and MM showed significant increases in pain threshold tolerance after a short-term application on a trigger points located in the trapezius muscle. PTMC roll-on and BG were both shown to be superior vs placebo while PTMC was also shown to be superior to IH in patients with trigger points located in the trapezius muscle on a single application.

CMCC Research Ethics Board Approval # 1012X01, 2011

Introduction

Myofascial Pain Syndrome (MPS) is exceedingly common in Western society [1-3]. Vernon and Schneider note that MPS is thought to be the leading diagnosis among pain management specialists [4,5] and the leading diagnosis in pain patients reporting to general practitioners [4,6]. MPS can be viewed as a regional pain syndrome such as, neck, low back and upper quadrant pain syndromes. MPS can also be found focally in discrete painful sites known as Myofascial Trigger Point (MTrP). Locations of MTrP's have been characterized on clinical grounds throughout the musculoskeletal system, starting with the seminal work of Travell and Simons [6,7]. MTrP's have been described as active (clinically active with pain referral upon palpation) or

* Correspondence: dr.danavrahami@gmail.com
[1]Toronto, ON, Canada
Full list of author information is available at the end of the article

latent (not clinically active, but tender on manual palpation) [7-9]. The presence of associated features such as "local twitch sign" and palpable taut bands is thought to confirm the presence of an active MTrP, while latent TP's may not present with the classic features.

Numerous treatments are currently available for MPS and MTrP's. Several systematic reviews have recently been published on a variety of treatments [4,10-14], including pharmacologic agents, physical agents, complementary and alternative therapies. One commonly used therapy is the application of topical agents to relieve pain [15-17]. These agents can be classified as pharmacologic or non-pharmacologic. The former category includes non-steroidal anti-inflammatory agents (such as ketaprofen), opioid agents, classical analgesic agents (such as lidocaine), novel analgesic agents such as capsaicin and rubefascient agents (containing salicylates or nicotinamides) [15-17]. Non-pharmacologic agents generally fall into the complementary and alternative medicine (CAM) category for MPS and MTrP treatments. They may contain putative analgesic agents or counterirritant agents and they may exert cold, hot or neutral effects.

Several studies have investigated the effect of such topicals in the treatment of osteoarthritis, particularly of the knee [18,19]. However, there appears to be a lack of studies investigating the effects of topical agents for the treatment of MPS or MTrP. A randomized, placebo-blinded clinical trial of non-pharmacological topical analgesics was conducted comparing leading national and professional brands in the treatment of a myofascial trigger point.

Materials and methods

Subjects

Subjects were selected from consecutive clinical presentations of patients for treatment in a multidisciplinary health clinic. Subjects aged 18-80, male or female, with or without neck pain were included. Subjects were excluded for the following reasons: acute pain presentation preventing comfortable participation and absence of a palpable tender spot in the right upper trapezius region. Subjects were informed of the nature of the experiment and consented to participate. This protocol was approved by the Research Ethics Board of the Canadian Memorial Chiropractic College.

Randomization

A random number sequence was generated by an independent party and kept in the care of the clinic administrator until required for subject allocation. The randomization schedule was concealed from all other study staff prior to selection and prior to group allocation.

Outcome measures

Pre- and post-intervention measures consisted of 1) tenderness at an MTrP in the upper trapezius and, 2) right and left cervical spine lateral flexion. Tenderness was measured using a manual pressure algometer and was reported in kg/cm^2 [20]. Once identified by palpation and marked on the skin, the MTrP was subjected to vertical pressure with the pressure algometer at the rate of 1 kg/cm^2 per second. The subject was instructed to indicate verbally when the first instance of tenderness was felt. A single trial was used. Right and left cervical spine lateral flexions were measured using a cervical rangiometer [21] and were reported in degrees. A single trial was used. Both measures have proven reliable and valid in the assessment of MTrP's [9,21-27]. Following the intervention, subjects were asked to rate their level of satisfaction on a verbal satisfaction scale (P = poor, F = fair, G = good, E = excellent).

Interventions

Six topical products were tested: three were ointments, two were roll-on gels and one a non-medicinal placebo cream (PLA) which served as the control. The comparative topicals were Professional Therapy MuscleCare Roll-on[a] (PTMC roll-on), Motion Medicine cream[b] (MM cream), Bengay Ultra Strength Muscle Pain ointment[c] (BG), Icy Hot Extra Strength Cream[d] (IH), and Biofreeze roll-on gel[e] (BF). All of these products were placed in identical 0.5 ounce white plastic screw top containers or 3 ounce generic white roll-on bottles. Only a coded letter was applied as a label. The master code for these products was kept with the clinic administrator and was unknown to all study participants and assessors.

Procedures

Subjects were seated erect in a comfortable ergonomic chair in a private room. Subjects wore a nose clip for the entire duration of the study so they could not smell any of the scents from the topical analgesics. Subjects were not allowed to view the application of the topical analgesics and they were not permitted to look at their shoulder during the entire process. Assessor #1 entered the room and palpated the subject's right shoulder in order to determine the presence and location of an MTrP in the upper trapezius muscle adjacent to the 7th cervical vertebrae and the 1st thoracic vertebrae. This was marked with a black dot. Assessor #1 exited the room and assessor #2 entered and performed the baseline testing of the outcome measures (Figure 1). The rangiometer was placed on the subject's head. From a neutral position, right and left active end-range lateral flexion measurements were recorded. The pressure algometer was applied over the marked trapezius trigger

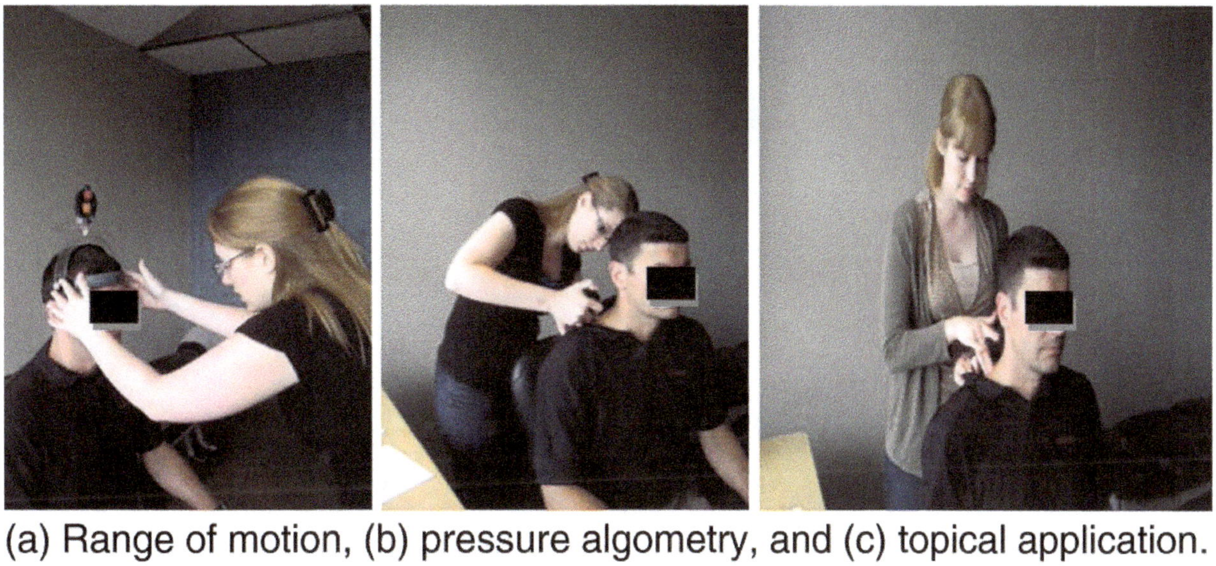

Figure 1 (a) Range of motion, (b) pressure algometry, and (c) topical application.

point for the baseline pressure reading. The subject was instructed to indicate when the pressure point was painful.

Following the initial outcome measurements, assessor #1 re-entered the room and applied one of the six samples according to the randomization schedule which was revealed only at that time in the area of the marked pressure point (Figure 1). The subject was instructed to stay seated in the chair with little head movement for five to seven minutes, following which, assessor #2 reassessed and recorded the pain and range of motion outcome measures. The study was conducted over a 7-day period.

Analyses

Data were first analyzed descriptively–baseline, post-intervention and change scores. Change scores for each of the three measurements (Pressure pain threshold, Right and Left lateral flexion) were analyzed using a 5-way ANOVA. Statistically significant ANOVA's ($p > 0.05$) were then subjected to multiple t-tests with Holm's adjustment of the p-value. As such, the alpha levels were set at 0.007.

Results

120 subjects were entered into the study, 20 in each group (63 females; ages 18-80). Fifty-six percent (56%) of patients presented with clinical shoulder or neck pain. Group demographics and clinical baseline values can be found in Table 1. There were no significant differences regarding group demographics and clinical baseline values.

The pre- and post-treatment results for pressure threshold are displayed in Table 2. ANOVA for inter-group differences was significant ($F = 5.2$, $p = 0.002$). Significant intra-group increases for BG, PTMC roll-on and MM cream were obtained with an increased threshold of 0.5 kg/cm^2 (+/-0.15), 0.72 kg/cm^2 (+/-0.17) and 0.47 Kg/cm^2 (+/-0.19) respectively.

With respect to the inter-group comparisons, PTMC roll-on showed significant increases in pressure threshold compared with PLA ($p = 0.002$) and IH ($p = 0.006$). In addition, BG demonstrated significant increases in pressure threshold compared with PLA ($p = 0.0003$).

The pre- and post-treatment results for right and left lateral flexion did not show significant increases in range of motion for any of the topical analgesics (Table 3).

Patient satisfaction ratings were high in each group and there were no significant differences between groups. There were no adverse reactions or complaints of pain aggravation reported in this study.

Discussion

This study investigated the immediate effect of six different topical analgesic creams on pressure pain threshold at a single trapezius MTrP and on bilateral cervical lateral flexions. We found that the topical analgesics BG, PTMC roll-on and MM cream demonstrated significant and clinically important increases in pressure threshold when comparing short-term MTrP tenderness. In addition, PTMC roll-on was better than placebo and Icy Hot Extra Strength Cream in reducing short-term MTrP tenderness. BG was better than placebo at reducing short-term MTrP tenderness.

Table 1 Group demographics and clinical baseline values

Variable	Group A	Group B	Group C	Group D	Group E	Group F	Statistic
AGE	48.5 (17.7)	48.5 (14.7)	47.9 (15.1)	47.1 (14.7)	45.0 (12.5)	51.1 (15)	NS F = 0.3 p = 0.89
GENDER	M = 8 F = 12	M = 8 F = 12	M = 11 F = 9	M = 11 F = 9	M = 11 F = 9	M = 7 F = 13	NS CSq = 4.0, p = 0.97
NECK and SHOULDER PAIN	Y = 11 N 9	Y = 12 N = 8	Y = 11 N = 9	Y = 10 N = 10	Y = 12 N = 8	Y = 11 N = 9	NS CSq = 2.2, p = 0.99
Pressure Pain Threshold (kg/in^2)	4.5 (2.2)	4.6 (1.5)	4.9 (2.4)	4.2 (1.3)	4.1 (0.9)	4.5 (2.4)	NS F = 0.41 p = 0.83

None of the groups demonstrated a statistically significantly increase in right or left lateral flexion.

The effectiveness of the topical analgesics that showed clinically significant improvements in cervical spine pressure threshold may be due to several factors. Eucalyptus oil, that was found in the PTMC solution, has been shown to transport active ingredients deep into the subcutaneous tissues [28,29]. Camphor and menthol, found in both BG and PTMC, have been proven to provide immediate pain relief [19,30,31]. Glucosamine sulfate, chondroitin sulfate, dimethyl sulfoxide and Boswellia serrata extract, found in the PTMC roll-on formulation, have been shown to improve circulation and reduce inflammation, thus reducing pain in the short-term [19,32,33]. In addition, magnesium chloride, which is unique to the PTMC roll-on, has been shown to be effectively absorbed through the dermis into muscle [34,35].

Topical analgesics are typically easy to self-apply. While this is a feature of many non-pharmacologic topicals, evidence of the effectiveness of the topical analgesics tested in this study is significantly lacking in the research literature. The results from the study demonstrate promising results for patients with myofascial pain. Since the topical analgesics are easy to use, they may improve the patients' self-care through increased compliance and help alleviate the painful symptoms they experience from MTrPs.

Many clinicians use these topical analgesics during multiple sessions or in combination with other proven therapies. Many clinicians theorize that the combination therapy or multiple session uses will result in long-term benefits. The intervention in this study was applied in one single session with only short-term outcomes measured. A similar study has been published on the outcomes from a single manual therapy session for patients with neck pain [36]. A clinical prediction rule has been formulated for single-session response to manual therapy for neck pain. Our findings show similar benefits compared with the manual therapy neck pain study and provides support for further research. Future studies with multiple sessions over several treatment days or in combination with other therapies are needed to validate the effects of the topical analgesics commonly used in clinical settings.

Limitations

This study used participants with and without cervical spine and trapezius pain. This may have attenuated the outcomes measured in this study. Future research should separately evaluate pain and non-painful groups to eliminate any confounding factors.

Table 2 Pressure pain thresholds.

Group	Pre-Tx (kg/cm^2)	Post-Tx (kg/cm^2)	Change (kg/cm^2)	Intra-group Significance	Inter-group Significance*
A	4.5 (+/-0.48)	5.0 (+/-0.56)	0.5 (+/-0.15)	p = 0.002	A > C (p = 0.0003)
B	4.6 (+/-0.33)	4.5 (+/-0.35)	-0.45 (.12)	p = 0.37 NS	
C	4.9 (+/-0.53)	4.6 (+/-0.54)	-0.3 (+/-0.19)	p = 0.067 NS	
D	4.2 (+/-0.28)	4.96 (+/-0.39)	0.72 (+/-0.17)	p = 0.0002	D > C (p = 0.002) D > E (p = 0.006)
E	4.1 (+/-0.20)	4.4 (+/-0.32)	0.35 (+/-0.23)	p = 0.07 NS	
F	4.4 (+/-0.55)	4.9 (+/-0.59)	0.47 (+/-0.19)	p = 0.01	

A = Bengay Ultra Strength Muscle Pain ointment, B = Biofreeze roll-on gel, C = Placebo, D = Professional Therapy Muscle Care roll-on, E = Icy Hot Extra Strength Cream, F = Motion Medicine

*Bonferroni corrected p value = 0.007

Table 3 Right Lateral Flexion.

Group	Pre-Tx (Degrees)	Post-Tx (Degrees)	Change (Degrees)	Significance
A	39.4 (+/-3.3)	44.9 (+/-2.6)	5.45 (+/-1.7)	NS
B	45.9 (+/-2.3)	46.7 (+/-2.9)	.8 (+/-1.5)	NS
C	40.6 (+/-2.8)	40.1 (+/-2.4)	-0.45 (+/-1.1)	NS
D	44.4 (+/-2.9)	48.3 (+/-3.0)	3.95 (+/-1.6)	NS
E	46.9 (+/-2.7)	48.4 (+/-2.7)	1.4 (+/-1.5)	NS
F	44.5 (+/-1.7)	44.7 (+/-1.6)	0.2 (+/-1.1)	NS

A = Bengay Ultra Strength Muscle Pain ointment, B = Biofreeze roll-on gel, C = Placebo, D = Professional Therapy Muscle Care roll-on, E = Icy Hot Extra Strength Cream, F = Motion Medicine

Subjects were not excluded if they had prior experience, nor, was prior experience measured as an explanatory variable. However, our efforts to blind subjects to the nature of the topicals used should have reduced the effect of any prior treatment experience.

Only one trial of pressure algometery and cervical ranges of motion was obtained pre-post intervention for each patient. As there is likely to be some variability with examiner testing, multiple recordings should be obtained in future studies.

It is unknown if any of the significant results obtained immediately post-intervention would be sustained over a longer period of time. Future studies should measure longer term outcome measures, such as a few hours after treatment.

Conclusions

This study demonstrated that some topical analgesic products do reduce myofascial pain or tenderness. The results of this study demonstrated that there were clinically important and significant differences between the topical analgesics tested. The BG, MM and the PTMC roll-on ointment demonstrated significant increases in pressure threshold levels. PTMC roll-on and BG were significantly superior to the placebo in the short-term reduction of myofascial tenderness. Furthermore, the PTMC roll-on demonstrated that it was significantly superior to the IH in the short-term reduction of myofascial tenderness.

There were no significant differences in range of motion testing for any of the topical analgesics. Future studies are needed to evaluate the effect of topical analgesics on the duration of effects of topical pain relief.

Endnotes

[a]Professional Therapy Muscle Care® Extra Strength Pain Relief Roll-on, Muscle Care Products (div. of Active & Innovative Inc.) Toronto, ON M4T 2V7

[b]MM Cream, Motion Medicine Inc., Calgary, AB T2Y 2Z7

[c]Bengay Ultra Strength Muscle Pain non-greasy, non-staining cream, Johnson & Johnson Inc. Markham, ON L3R 5L2, Canada.

[e]Icy Hot Extra Strength Pain Relieving Cream, Chattem Canada, Mississauga, ON L5N 2K7, Canada

[f]Biofreeze Pain Relieving Roll-on Gel with Ilex, Royal Cross, Concord, ON L4K 2L9, Canada

Acknowledgements
We thank Roslyn Manchee for her help as project administrator.

Author details
[1]Toronto, ON, Canada. [2]Canadian Memorial Chiropractic College, 6100 Leslie Street, Toronto, ON M2H 3J1, Canada. [3]204 Parkmount, Toronto, ON M4J 4V6, Canada. [4]Lakeview Chiropractic Health and Wellness, 2B 3602 Taylor St. E, Saskatoon, SK S7H 5H9, Canada. [5]777 Woodbine Ave, Toronto, ON M4E 2J5, Canada.

Authors' contributions
DA have made substantial contributions to the acquisition of data, analysis and interpretation of data, have been involved in drafting the manuscript or revising it critically for important intellectual content and have given final approval of the version to be published. AH and CH have made substantial contributions to conception and design, acquisition of data, analysis and interpretation of data, have been involved in drafting the manuscript or revising it critically for important intellectual content and have given final approval of the version to be published. HV made substantial contributions to the design of this study as well as to the analyses and interpretations of the findings. He was substantially involved in drafting the manuscript or revising it critically for important intellectual content and has given final approval of the version to be published. All authors read and approved the final manuscript.

Competing interests
The authors declare that they have no competing interests.

References

1. Skootsky SA, Jaeger B, Oye RK: **Prevalence of myofascial pain in general internal medicine practice.** *West J Med* 1989, **151**:157-160.
2. Gerwin RD: **Classification, epidemiology, and natural history of myofascial pain syndrome.** *Curr Pain Headache Rep* 2001, **5**:412-420.
3. Gerwin RD: **A review of myofascial pain and fibromyalgia-factors that promote their persistence.** *Acupunct Med* 2005, **23**:121-134.
4. Vernon H, Schneider M: **Chiropractic management of myofascial trigger points and myofascial pain syndrome: a systematic review of the literature.** *J Manipulative Physiol Ther* 2009, **32**:14-24.
5. Norman HR: **Muscle pain syndromes.** *Am J Phys Med Rehabil* 2007, **86**: S47-S58.
6. Harden RN, Bruehl SP, Gass S, Niemiec C, Barbick B: **Signs and symptoms of the myofascial pain syndrome: a national survey of pain management providers.** *Clin J Pain* 2000, **16**:64-72.
7. Travell J, Rinzler SH: **The myofascial genesis of pain.** *Postgrad Med* 1952, **11**:425-434.
8. Travell J, Simons D: *Myofascial Pain and Dysfunction: The Trigger Point Manual* Baltimore MD: Williams and Wilkens; 1983.
9. Cummings M, Baldry P: **Regional myofascial pain: diagnosis and management.** *Best Pract Res Clin Rheumatol* 2007, **21**:367-387.
10. Fernandez de las Penas C, Sohrbeck Campo M, Fernandez Carnero J, Miangolarra Page JC: **Manual therapies in myofascial trigger point treatment: a systematic review.** *J Bodyw Mov Ther* 2005, **9**:27-34.

11. Cummings TM, White AR: **Needling therapies in the management of myofascial trigger point pain: a systematic review.** *Arch Phys Med Rehabil* 2001, **82**:986-992.
12. Harris RE, Clauw DJ: **The use of complementary medical therapies in the management of myofascial pain disorders.** *Curr Pain Headache Rep* 2002, **6**:370-374.
13. Rickards LD: **The effectiveness of non-invasive treatments for active myofascial trigger point pain: a systematic review of the literature.** *Inter J Osteop Med* 2006, **9**:120-136.
14. Bronfort G, Haas M, Evans R, Leininger B, Triano J: **Effectiveness of manual therapies: the UK evidence report.** *Chiropr Osteopat* 2010, **18**:3.
15. Mason L, Moore RA, Edwards JE, Derry S, McQuay HJ: **Topical NSAIDs for acute pain: a meta-analysis.** *BMC Fam Pract* 2004, **5**:10.
16. Argoff CE: **A review of the use of topical analgesics for myofascial pain.** *Curr Pain Headache Rep* 2002, **6**:375-378.
17. Matthews P, Derry S, Moore RA, McQuay HJ: **Topical rubefacients for acute and chronic pain in adults.** *Cochrane Database Syst Rev* 2009, **8(3)**: CD007403.
18. Sontakka S, Thawani V, Pimpalkhute S, Kabra P, Babhulkar S, Hingorani L: **Open, randomized, controlled clinical trial of Boswellia serrata Extract as compared to Valdecoxib in osteoarthritis of knee.** *Indian J Pharmacol* 2006, **39**:27-29.
19. Cohen M, Wolfe R, Mai T, Lewis D: **A randomized, double blind, placebo controlled trial of a topical cream containing glucosamine sulfate, chondroitin sulfate, and camphor for osteoarthritis of the knee.** *J Rheumatol* 2003, **30**:523-528.
20. Fischer AA: **Pressure algometry over normal muscles. Standard values, validity and reproducibility of pressure threshold.** *Pain* 1987, **30**:115-126.
21. Piva SR, Erhard RE, Childs JD, Browder DA: **Inter-tester reliability of passive intervertebral and active movements of the cervical spine.** *Man Ther* 2006, **11**:321-330.
22. Al Shenqiti AM, Oldham JA: **Test-retest reliability of myofascial trigger point detection in patients with rotator cuff tendonitis.** *Clin Rehabil* 2005, **19**:482-487.
23. Bendtsen L, Jensen R, Jensen NK, Olesen J: **Pressure-controlled palpation: a new technique which increases the reliability of manual palpation.** *Cephalalgia* 1995, **15**:205-210.
24. Boline PD, Haas M, Meyer JJ, Kassak K, Nelson C, Keating JC Jr: **Interexaminer reliability of eight evaluative dimensions of lumbar segmental abnormality: Part II.** *J Manip Physiol Ther* 1993, **16**:363-374.
25. Gerwin RD, Shannon S, Hong CZ, Hubbard D, Gevirtz R: **Interrater reliability in myofascial trigger point examination.** *Pain* 1997, **69**:65-73.
26. Gerwin R, Shannon S: **Interexaminer reliability and myofascial trigger points.** *Arch Phys Med Rehabil* 2000, **81**:1257-1258.
27. Levoska S, Keinanen-Kiukaanniemi S, Bloigu R: **Repeatability of measurement of tenderness in the neck-shoulder region by a dolorimeter and manual palpation.** *Clin J Pain* 1993, **9**:229-235.
28. Yamane MA, Williams AC, Barry BW: **Terpene penetration enhancers in propylene glycol/water co-solvent systems: effectiveness and mechanism of action.** *J Pharm Pharmacol* 1995, **47**:978-989.
29. Narishetty ST, Panchagnula R: **Effect of L-menthol and 1,8-cineole on phase behavior and molecular organization of SC lipids and skin permeation of zidovudine.** *J Control Release* 2005, **102**:59-70.
30. Patel T, Ishiuji Y, Yosipovitch G: **Menthol: a refreshing look at this ancient compound.** *J Am Acad Dermatol* 2007, **57**:873-878.
31. Cliff MA, Green BG: **Sensory irritation and coolness produced by menthol: evidence for selective desensitization of irritation.** *Physiol Behav* 1994, **56**:1021-1029.
32. Beilke MA, Collins-Lech C, Sohnle PG: **Effects of dimethyl sulfoxide on the oxidative function of human neutrophils.** *J Lab Clin Med* 1987, **110**:91-96.
33. Kimmatkar N, Thawani V, Hingorani L, Khiyani R: **Efficacy and tolerability of Boswellia serrata extract in treatment of osteoarthritis of knee-a randomized double blind placebo controlled trial.** *Phytomedicine* 2003, **10**:3-7.
34. Nagai I, Gebrewold A, Altura BT, Altura BM: **Magnesium salts exert direct vasodilator effects on rat cremaster muscle microcirculation.** *Arch Int Pharmacodyn Ther* 1988, **294**:194-214.
35. Nishio A, Gebrewold A, Altura BT, Altura BM: **Comparative vasodilator effects of magnesium salts on rat mesenteric arterioles and venules.** *Arch Int Pharmacodyn Ther* 1989, **298**:139-163.
36. Vernon H, Humphreys BK: **Chronic mechanical neck pain in adults treated by manual therapy: a systematic review of change scores in randomized controlled trials of a single session.** *J Man Manip Ther* 2008, **16**:E42-E52.

Radial neck fracture presenting to a Chiropractic clinic: a case report and literature review

Clinton J Daniels[1*], Jordan A Gliedt[2] and Dennis E Enix[3]

Abstract

Objective: The purpose of this case report is to describe a patient that presented with a Mason type II radial neck fracture approximately three weeks following a traumatic injury.

Clinical features: A 59-year old female presented to a chiropractic practice with complaints of left lateral elbow pain distal to the lateral epicondyle of the humerus and pain provocation with pronation, supination and weight bearing. The complaint originated three weeks prior following a fall on her left elbow while hiking.

Intervention and outcome: Plain film radiographs of the left elbow and forearm revealed a transverse fracture of the radial neck with 2mm displacement–classified as a Mason Type II fracture. The patient was referred for medical follow-up with an orthopedist.

Conclusion: This report discusses triage of an elbow fracture presenting to a chiropractic clinic. This case study demonstrates the thorough clinical examination, imaging and decision making that assisted in appropriate patient diagnosis and management.

Keywords: Elbow fracture, Radial head fracture, Chiropractic

Background

Traumatic injuries to the forearm are a common occurrence in the emergency room setting. They occasionally present in the private practice setting, especially as a chronic presentation. It is easy for the clinician to ignore the obvious diagnosis of fracture due to the length of time the patient has endured this condition. Fractures of the radial head are relatively common. They represent approximately 5.4 percent of all fractures, between 1.5 and 4.5 percent of fractures in adults, and approximately one third of all fractures of the elbow [1-5]. The vast majority of these fractures occur in individuals between the ages of 30-60 years, with a mean age between 45 and 45.9 years and are more common in women than men [6]. It has been reported that in children the incidence of radial head and neck fractures is up to 1.3% [6]. Mechanism of injury is usually a fall on an outstretched arm, and in rare cases, direct trauma [1-3,6-9]. These fractures are typically seen in isolation, but may be accompanied by other fractures, dislocations or soft tissue injuries. Because of their proximity, the medial collateral ligament, lateral collateral ligament and interosseous ligaments are most prone to injury with radial head fractures. The radial head of the elbow acts as a secondary stabilizer of the joint creating 30% of the elbow's resistance to valgus forces as such it is prone to compressive forces and hyperextension injuries.

Symptoms typically include pain and tenderness along the lateral aspect of elbow and a limited range of motion (ROM) in the elbow, forearm or wrist. A thorough physical exam should include an inspection of ROM and longitudinal and rotational joint stability, evaluating the joint for resistance to elbow flexion and extension and forearm pronation and supination; stressing varus and valgus positions of the joint. Particular attention should be paid to the presence of pain and tenderness in the interosseous membrane.

Patients presenting with a mechanism of injury consistent with known fractures should be examined radiographically. Radial head fracture presentations are described by the Mason classification guideline. Mason, originally described three types: non-displaced fractures (Type I); displaced partial head fractures (Type II); and

* Correspondence: clintdanielsdc@gmail.com
[1]Private Practice, St. Louis, MO, USA
Full list of author information is available at the end of the article

comminuted, displaced fractures involving the entire head (Type III) [10]. In an attempt to quantify the extent of radial head involvement, Broberg and Morrey proposed that a partial radial head fracture (Type II) must be of adequate size and movement to be considered displaced, suggesting fracture of at least 30 percent of the auricular surface and 2 mm of displacement [11,12]. Further modification was proposed by Johnston who sought to include fractures of the radial head with associated elbow dislocation (Type IV) [13]. This modified Mason classification system (Figure 1) is widely considered the principal radial head fracture subgrouping system, and is often referenced at time of diagnosis and treatment.

Case presentation

Clinical history

A 59 year-old female presented to a private chiropractic clinic complaining of a three week history of generalized left elbow pain with no symptomatic referral to the upper extremity. The injury began immediately following a fall onto the left elbow while hiking. She could not recall the exact mechanism of her fall. The pain was described as deep and was exacerbated by weight bearing exercise and twisting motions such as opening a door. She had attempted to self-manage her symptoms with home use of a transcutaneous electrical nerve stimulation (TENS) unit, which increased her symptoms, and over the counter non-steroidal anti-inflammatory (NSAID's) medications which had no apparent effect. She denied any history of swelling, numbness/tingling, locking sensation, or previous elbow injuries.

Physical examination

Relevant examination findings revealed an alert and oriented, non-distressed, patient with no signs of upper extremity bracing or splinting. Active range of motion (ROM) of the left elbow was full in all directions and pain was present at end-range supination and pronation of the forearm. Palpation revealed significant tenderness slightly distal to the left radial head and along the lateral forearm, and hypertonicity of the forearm extensor muscle group was noted. To assess for lateral epicondylitis

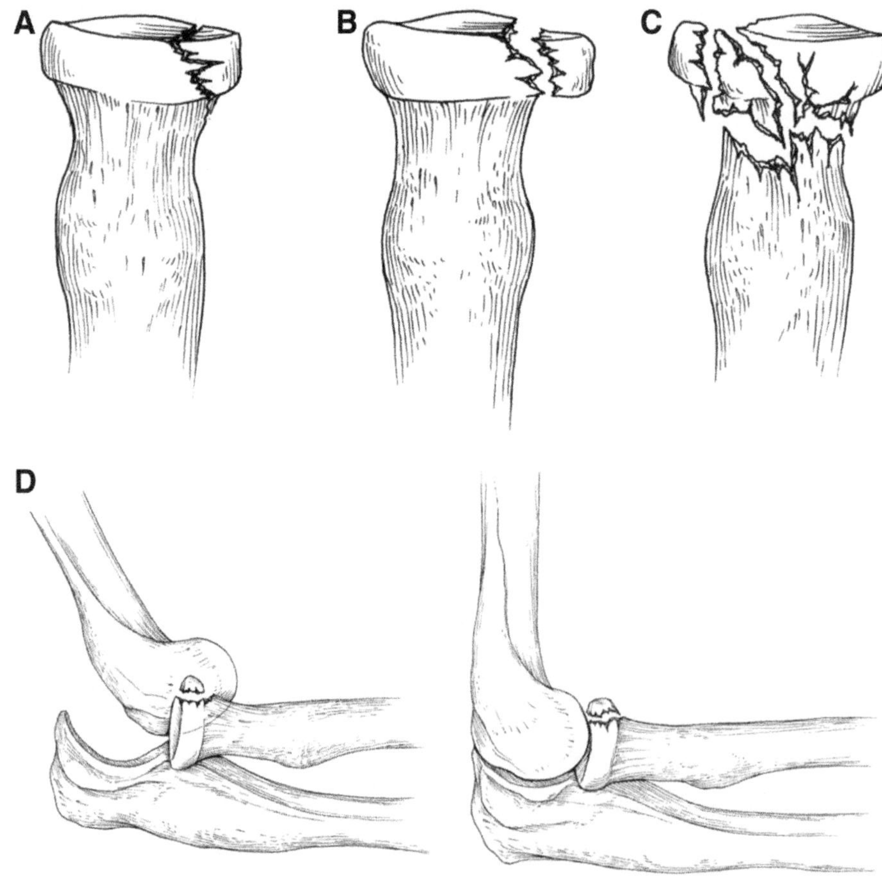

Figure 1 Mason classification of radial head/neck fractures. **A**, Type I, nondisplaced. **B**, Type II, displaced partial articular fracture of ≥2mm displacement or ≥30% of the articular surface. **C**, Type III, comminuted fracture. **D**, A type IV injury, described by Johnson [14] in 1962, indicates an associated ipsilateral ulnohumeral dislocation. Image from Terrible Triad Injury of the Elbow: Current Concepts, JAAOS March 2009 vol. 17 no. 3 137-151 [15].

Mill's and Cozen's tests were performed, both provoking discomfort in the proximal forearm. The discomfort could not be reproduced at the lateral epicondyle. Valgus and varus stress testing of the elbow provoked significant discomfort distal to the lateral epicondyle, but again were not consistent with expected positive testing.

Bilateral upper extremity neurological examination was within normal limits, revealing 2+ triceps, biceps, and wrist reflexes, intact sensation to light touch of C5 to T1 dermatomes, and 5/5 motor testing of C5 to T1 myotomes. Upper limb tension test was negative for upper extremity radicular pain provocation.

Imaging

Due to the traumatic nature of the injury and the examination that was inconsistent for myofascial condition, she was referred to a local imaging center. Radiographs of the elbow and forearm revealed a transverse fracture through the neck of the proximal radius. There was an approximately 2mm medial displacement of the radius distal to the fracture, no evidence of dislocation, and there was suspected joint effusion (Figures 2 and 3).

Case management

Three days post initial consultation, the patient's X-ray results were received from the imaging center and the patient was referred to a general medical specialist for care. A clinical report and the radiologists report were forwarded to the referred physician. Verbal follow-up with the patient two-weeks later revealed that she had been referred to an orthopedic specialist by her primary care physician. The orthopedist elected not to cast the fracture due to small degree of displacement, lack of significant swelling, and range of motion within normal limits. She was restricted from performing any weight bearing exercise and was instructed to return in one month for follow-up X-ray to assess the healing of the fracture site. At four-weeks following the initial evaluation, a repeated radiographic examination demonstrated healing of the fracture site. At three month telephone follow-up the patient reported full use of her elbow with no pain in any ranges of motion.

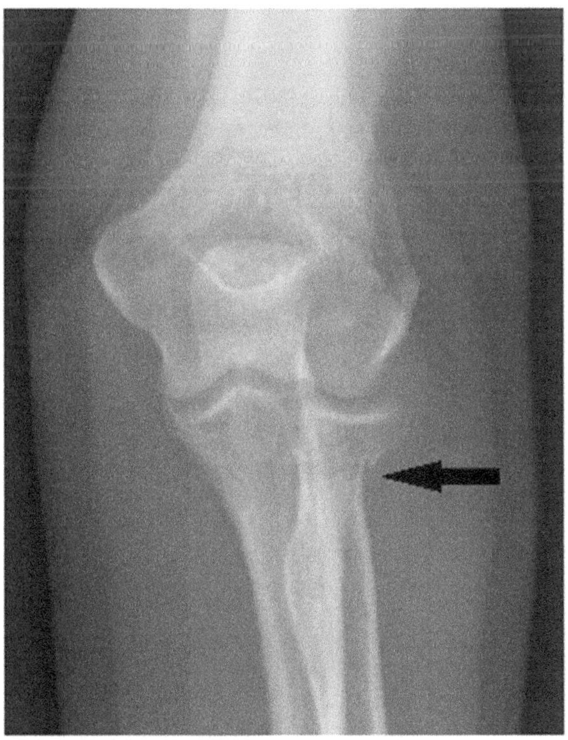

Figure 2 Antero-posterior X-ray elbow view. Note the approximately 2mm displacement of the radial head. Mason Type II Fracture.

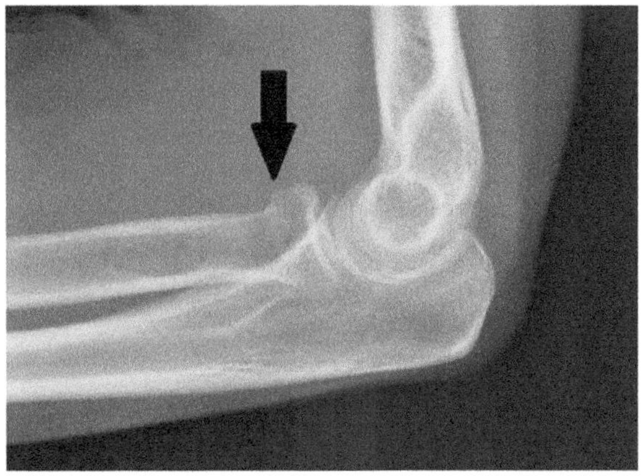

Figure 3 Lateral X-ray elbow view.

Discussion

The Mason classification system is used to classify radial head and neck fractures and is useful when assessing further treatment options [16]. The classification system consists of three types: Type I, non-displaced (or small marginal) radial head or neck fracture; Type II, marginal fractures with displacement including impaction, depression and angulation; and Type III, comminuted fractures involving the entire radial head [10,16,17]. Type I fractures are initially treated with 3 to 5 days of immobilization. After pain has subsided, gentle active range of motion at the elbow should begin. The immobilizing splint should be replaced by a sling as range of motion exercises begin. Follow-up radiographs are obtained to ensure that no further displacement has occurred. The patient may return to full, unrestricted activity in 3 to 4 weeks in most cases. The criterion used for return to activity is the level of comfort reported by the patient.

When Type II fractures have only a single displacement with greater than 3mm, or when the articular surface of the fracture fragment diverges more than 30 degrees, open reduction internal fixation surgery with small screws is recommended [18]. In most Mason Type II and III fractures in which displacement and/or comminution are noted on radiographs the elbow joint should be aspirated and injected with local anesthetic. This allows for careful passive range of motion examination to determine the presence or absence of mechanical blockage due to displaced fragments through the articular surface. If no mechanical blockage is identified, and if the fracture is not displaced or angulated extensively, conservative treatment is appropriate [19].

The anterior and posterior fat pads are intracapsular structures that may provide valuable information on intracapsular injuries [19]. Hemarthrosis from intra-articular fractures commonly cause the anterior fat pad to bulge further anteriorly, and the posterior fat pad will be displaced posteriorly and proximally, rendering it visible on the standard lateral x-ray projection [19]. In addition, potential injury to the supporting ligamentous structures in the elbow include sprain strain, ligament ruptures and tendon entrapments must always be considered (Table 1). The distal radioulnar joint should be examined for obvious bruising and tenderness, with special attention to the area around the medial collateral ligament and Interosseous ligament. The lateral collateral ligament stabilizes the joint against posterolateral rotational instability and is prone to injury. It is difficult to properly assess level of damage to the interosseous membrane and the resultant radioulnar instability by exam only. Diagnostic ultrasonography is a valuable tool for assessing soft tissue injuries and should be considered if ligament damage is suspected. Injuries to the median, ulnar and radial nerves as well as serious vascular claudication is possible and have been reported in Type III fractures. Therefore a thorough neurological exam of the region should be included in the patient work up.

Conservative treatment of Type II and Type III fractures of the radial head consists of immobilization for 7 to 10 days in a posterior splint. Splinting the elbow in flexion versus extension does not affect outcome [20]. The elbow should be splinted at the angle of greatest comfort. [21] Radiographs should be repeated at appropriate intervals to ensure that further displacement or loose body formation has not occurred. Graduated mobilization may be achieved using a functional fracture brace with controlled hinges and active range of motion exercises. Several reports show excellent results using conservative treatment measures for even the most extensive comminuted radial head fractures [22,23]. The keys to success are exclusion of cases in which mechanical blockage is present and the implementation of early, controlled active range of motion [20]. After the orthopedic goals of stabilization have been achieved, the rehabilitative objectives of restoring normal ranges of motion and restoring muscle strength to the supporting musculature should be met.

Table 1 Sites of injuries with radial head fractures

Osseous injuries	Soft tissue injuries
Distal radioulnar joint fractures	Interosseous membrane disruption
Coronoid fractures	Lateral collateral ligament injuries
Carpal fractures	Medial collateral ligament injuries
Distal radioulnar joint and radial head fracture (Essex-Lopresti)	Elbow dislocation
Radial head fx, coronoid fx, elbow dislocation (terrible triad)	Vascular injuries

The complex motion of the proximal radioulnar joint includes both pronation and supination. These movements occur in conjunction with simultaneous movement of the distal radioulnar joint [24]. Proximally, supination and pronation occur with spinning of the radial head within the fibro-osseous ring formed by the annular ligament and radial notch of the ulna [24]. During supination, the proximal surface of the articular disc remains in contact with the ulna head and at end range the palmar capsular ligament is stretched to its maximal length creating stiffness and stabilization of the joint. [24]. Whereas full pronation elongates the dorsal capsular ligament at the distal radioulnar joint and slackens the palmar capsular ligament [24]. Rehabilitation is an important part in re-establishing normal kinematics of the joint.

Conclusion

Radial head fractures are relatively common and therefore it is important for the chiropractic physician to have knowledge of their diagnosis and treatment strategies. The clinical presentation, classification, and treatment options of radial head fractures vary depending on the amount of radial head displacement and soft tissue injury. This case study demonstrates thorough clinical examination, imaging and triage to assist in appropriate patient diagnosis and management. In this case the minimally displaced Type II Mason fracture did not require surgical intervention to return to full functionality.

Consent

Written informed consent was obtained from the patient for publication of this case report and accompanying images. A copy of written consent is available for review by the Editor-in-Chief of this journal.

Competing interests
The authors declare that they have no competing interests.

Authors' contributions
CD cared for the patient, performed the literature review, and prepared the manuscript. JG performed the literature review and assisted in preparation of the manuscript. DE assisted in manuscript preparation, developing figures and revision. All authors' read and approved the final manuscript.

Author details
[1]Private Practice, St. Louis, MO, USA. [2]Private Practice, Chandler, AZ, USA. [3]Logan University, Chesterfield, MO, USA.

References

1. Morrey BF: **Radial Head Fracture.** In *The Elbow and Its Disorders.* 3rd edition. Philadelphia, Pa: Saunders; 2000.
2. Black WS, Becker JA: **Common forearm fractures in adults.** *Am Fam Physician* 2009, **80**(10):1096–1102.
3. Ditsios KT, Stavridis SI, Christodoulou AG: **The effect of haematoma aspiration on intra-articular pressure and pain relief following Mason I radial head fractures.** *Injury.* 2011, **42**:362–365.
4. Herbertsson P, Josefsson PO, Hasserius R, Karlsson C, Besjakov J, Karlsson M: **Uncomplicated Mason type-II and III fractures of the radial head and neck in adults. A long-term follow-up study.** *J Bone Joint Surg Am* 2004, **86-A**:569–574.
5. Herbertsson P, Josefsson PO, Hasserius R, Besjakov J, Nyqvist F, Karlsson MK: **Fractures of the radial head and neck treated with radial head excision.** *J Bone Joint Surg Am* 2004, **86-A**:1925–1930.
6. Kovar FM, Jaindl M, Thalhammer G, Rupert S, Platzer P, Endler G, Vielgut I, Kutscha-Lissberg F: **Incidence and analysis of radial head and neck fractures.** *World J Orthop* 2013, **4**(2):80–84.
7. van Riet RP, Morrey BF: **Documentation of associated injuries occurring with radial head fracture.** *Clin Orthop Relat Res* 2008, **466**:130–134.
8. Kaas L, van Riet RP, Vroemen JP, Eygendaal D: **The epidemiology of radial head fractures.** *J Shoulder Elbow Surg* 2010, **19**:520–523.
9. Karlsson MK, Herbertsson P, Nordqvist A, Besjakov J, Josefsson PO, Hasserius R: **Comminuted fractures of the radial head.** *Acta Orthop* 2010, **81**:224–227.
10. Mason ML: **Some observations on fractures of the head of the radius with a review of one hundred cases.** *Br J Surg* 1954, **42**(172):123–132.
11. Ruchelsman DE, Christoforou D, Jupiter JB: **Fractures of the radial head and neck.** *J Bone Joint Surg Am* 2013, **95**(5):469–478.
12. Broberg MA, Morrey BF: **Results of treatment of fracture-dislocations of the elbow.** *Clin Orthop Relat Res* 1987, **216**:109–119.
13. Thomas TT: **Fractures of the head and neck of the radius.** *Ann Surg* 1907, **46**:280–291.
14. Johnston GW: **A follow-up of one hundred cases of fractures of the head of the radius with a review of the literature.** *Ulster Med J* 1962, **31**:51–56.
15. Matthew PK, Athwal GS, King GJ: **Terrible triad injury of the elbow: current concepts.** *J Am Acad Orthop Surg* 2009, **17**(3):137–151.
16. Iannuzzi NP, Leopold SS: **In brief: the mason classification of radial head fractures.** *Clin Orthop Relat Res* 2012, **470**:1799–1802.
17. Mason JA, Shutkin NM: **Immediate active motion treatment for fractures of the head and neck of the radius.** *Surg Gynecol Obstet* 1943, **76**:731–737.
18. Shmueli O, Herold HZ: **Compression screwing of displaced fractures of the head of the radius.** *J Bone Joint Surg Br* 1981, **63**:535–538.
19. Doerr GH, Carmichael JP, Buchberger DJ, Pajaczkowski J, Spina AA: **The Elbow, Wrist, and Hand.** In *Conservative Management of Sports Injuries.* 2nd edition. Edited by Hyde T. Boston: Jones and Bartlett Publishers; 2007:543–611.
20. Thompson DJ: **Comparison of flexion versus extension splinting in the treatment of Mason type I radial head and neck fractures.** *JOrthop Trauma* 1988, **2**:117–119.
21. Watson JT: **Fractures of the forearm and elbow.** *Clin Sports Med* 1990, **9**:59–83.
22. Miller KG, Drennan DB, Mavlahn DJ: **Treatment of displaced segmental radial head fractures.** *J Bone Joint Surg Am* 1984, **63**:712–717.
23. Weseley MS, Barenfield PA, Eisenstein HL: **Closed treatment of isolated radial head fractures.** *J Trauma* 1983, **23**:36–39.
24. Neumann D: **Elbow and Forearm Complex.** In *Kinesiology of the Musculoskeletal System: Foundations for Physical Rehabilitation.* Edited by Neumann D. St. Louis, MO: Mosby; 2012:133–171.

Outcomes of pregnant patients with low back pain undergoing chiropractic treatment: a prospective cohort study with short term, medium term and 1 year follow-up

Cynthia K Peterson*, Daniel Mühlemann and Barry Kim Humphreys

Abstract

Background: Low back pain in pregnancy is common and research evidence on the response to chiropractic treatment is limited. The purposes of this study are 1) to report outcomes in pregnant patients receiving chiropractic treatment; 2) to compare outcomes from subgroups; 3) to assess predictors of outcome.

Methods: Pregnant patients with low back or pelvic pain, no contraindications to manipulative therapy and no manual therapy in the prior 3 months were recruited.
Baseline numerical rating scale (NRS) and Oswestry questionnaire data were collected. Duration of complaint, number of previous LBP episodes, LBP during a previous pregnancy, and category of pain location were recorded. The patient's global impression of change (PGIC) (primary outcome), NRS, and Oswestry data (secondary outcomes) were collected at 1 week, 1 and 3 months after the first treatment. At 6 months and 1 year the PGIC and NRS scores were collected. PGIC responses of 'better' or 'much better' were categorized as 'improved'.
The proportion of patients 'improved' at each time point was calculated. Chi-squared test compared subgroups with 'improvement'. Baseline and follow-up NRS and Oswestry scores were compared using the paired t-test. The unpaired t-test compared NRS and Oswestry scores in patients with and without a history of LBP and with and without LBP during a previous pregnancy. Anova compared baseline and follow-up NRS and Oswestry scores by pain location category and category of number of previous LBP episodes. Logistic regression analysis also was also performed.

Results: 52% of 115 recruited patients 'improved' at 1 week, 70% at 1 month, 85% at 3 months, 90% at 6 months and 88% at 1 year. There were significant reductions in NRS and Oswestry scores ($p < 0.0005$). Category of previous LBP episodes number at one year ($p = 0.02$) was related to ‚improvement' when analyzed alone, but was not strongly predictive in logistic regression. Patients with more prior LBP episodes had higher 1 year NRS scores ($p = 0.013$).

Conclusions: Most pregnant patients undergoing chiropractic treatment reported clinically relevant improvement at all time points. No single variable was strongly predictive of, improvement' in the logistic regression model.

Keywords: Pregnancy, Low back pain, Pelvic pain, Outcomes, Chiropractic, Treatment

* Correspondence: cynthia.peterson@balgrist.ch
Department of Chiropractic Medicine, Orthopaedic University Hospital Balgrist, University of Zürich, Forchstrasse 340, Zürich, Switzerland

Background

Low back and pelvic pain in pregnant women is such a common phenomenon that it is often considered a normal part of the pregnancy [1-3]. However, the high prevalence of this problem (50-80% of women) and the impact that this may have on their quality of life, as well as the fact that back pain during pregnancy is commonly linked to low back pain persisting after pregnancy, mandates that it be taken seriously by health care practitioners [1-6]. Many of these patients rate their back pain as moderate to severe with a small percentage claiming to be significantly disabled by the pain [6-8].

Pregnancy-related low back pain is most often divided into 3 categories based on location. These are: lumbar spine pain (LP), posterior pelvic pain (PPP), or a combination of these two [1,2,9], with posterior pelvic pain reported to be the most common presentation [1,10] and the location most specific for pregnant patients [9]. However, other authors have used 4 categories for pelvic only pain, including anterior pain at the pubic symphysis (symphysiolysis) but excluding lumbar spine pain [11].

Although the etiology of low back pain associated with pregnancy is not definitively known, the predominate theories include biomechanical changes due to the enlarging uterus resulting in an increasing lumbar lordosis and the influence of the hormone relaxin on stabilizing ligaments leading to hypermobility of joints [12-14].

The treatment of pregnancy-related low back pain has often been a 'watch and wait' approach, as medication use in pregnancy is strongly discouraged in many cases [15] and it is assumed that the pain will disappear after delivery. Two recent systematic reviews of the literature looked specifically at the evidence for chiropractic treatment of pregnancy-related low back pain and both reviews concluded that there is research evidence demonstrating that chiropractic care is associated with improved outcomes, but that the evidence is limited due to the low to moderate quality of the studies [4,6]. A prospective cohort outcomes study on pregnant patients with low back pain receiving chiropractic treatment from a single practitioner published since the systematic reviews evaluated data from 78 patients [16]. Seventy three percent of that cohort reported 'good' or 'excellent' outcomes from chiropractic treatment performed by a single chiropractor and his physical therapist. However, the outcomes varied depending upon the specific location of the pain.

Finally a prospective randomized trial was published in 2013 which compared routine obstetrical care for pregnant patients suffering from low back pain with chiropractic treatment consisting of manual therapy, stabilization exercises and patient education [17]. The chiropractic treatment group reported statistically and clinically significant improvement compared to patients in the routine obstetrical care group. However, outcome data was only collected between 5 and 9 weeks after the baseline data and prior to delivery of the baby.

Additional research is therefore needed from a larger number of chiropractors to assess outcomes as would be obtained in routine chiropractic practice and to follow the patients for a longer time period. Furthermore, it is desirable to see if factors associated with improvement or failure to improve identified in previous studies will also be found in this current study [16]. Thus, the purposes of this study are 1) to report outcomes at various time points up to 1 year in pregnant patients undergoing chiropractic treatment for low back and pelvic pain; 2) to compare outcomes from various subgroups of patients; and 3 to investigate the various demographic factors as predictors out outcome.

Methods

This is a prospective, cohort, outcomes study. Patients with baseline and 1 year data are included in the study. Cantonal ethics approval was obtained prior to the start of the study and all patients signed informed consent.

Pregnant patients over the age of 18 with low back pain, pelvic pain, or both of any duration who have not undergone chiropractic or manual therapy in the prior 3 months were recruited from chiropractic practices in Switzerland. All chiropractors in the German and French speaking regions of the country were invited to submit patients but 2 multi-clinician practices in particular that receive a high number of referrals from gyaecologists were targeted specifically. These two practices were asked to recruit all consenting pregnant patients. Patients with specific pathologies of the lumbar spine that are contraindications to chiropractic manipulative treatment, such as tumors, infections, inflammatory spondylarthropathies, acute fractures, Paget's disease and severe osteoporosis, were excluded.

Chiropractic treatment was not standardized to any specific treatment methods or frequencies and was left to the discretion of the treating clinician. However, it is known from the Swiss job analysis study that the Diversified method of high velocity, low amplitude spinal manipulative therapy (SMT) is the most common SMT method used in this country [18].

Baseline data and outcome measures

The numerical rating scale (NRS) for pain, where 0 = no pain and 10 = the worst pain imaginable, and the Oswestry questionnaire, which has been validated in German and French [19,20] were administered to the patient immediately prior to the first treatment by the office staff of the practice. Additional information provided by the treating chiropractor at the initial consultation included: patient age, gestational week, number of previous pregnancies, work status, whether or not the patient smokes, duration of current complaint, number of previous LBP episodes, LBP during a previous pregnancy (yes/no), location category of pain (lumbar pain only (LP), pelvic pain only (PP), both areas) and exercise level (regular, occasional, none). The number of previous episodes of LBP was further categorized into one of three groups: None, 1 – 4 episodes, ≥ 5 episodes.

One week after the first consultation/treatment, data from the NRS, patient's global impression of change (PGIC) scale, and the Oswestry questionnaire were collected from the patient via a short telephone interview. Similarly, these same data were collected at 1 month and 3 months after the start of chiropractic treatment via telephone interviews. At 6 months and 1 year after the first chiropractic treatment, the NRS and PGIC scores were collected, but not the Oswestry data. These telephone interviews were conducted by trained research assistants at the university, unknown to the patients or clinicians. The PGIC scale was a 7 point verbal scale, including the options 'much worse', 'worse', 'slightly worse', 'no change', 'slightly better', 'better', and 'much better'. Patients responding 'better' or 'much better' were categorized as 'improved' and all other patients as 'not improved'. This was considered the primary outcome measure. Additionally, one question was included on the 1 year follow-up data collection concerning the patient satisfaction with their treatment. The options included: 'very happy', 'happy', 'neutral', 'unhappy' and 'very unhappy'.

The time frame within which each data collection telephone interview was allowed was narrow. If a patient could not be reached within the window of time allowed, that data collection time point was missed but the patient remained in the study. However, if 3 consecutive data collection telephone interviews were missed, the patient was deleted from the study.

Statistical methods

Descriptive statistics were calculated. The proportion (%) of patients improved at each data collection time point was calculated. Subgroup analysis was carried out using 'improved' or 'not improved' as categorical variables. The chi-squared test was used to compare the presence/absence of LBP during a previous pregnancy, category of the number of previous episodes of LBP, and the category of the location of LBP with 'improvement'. The scores on the baseline and follow-up NRS for pain and Oswestry questionnaire were compared using the paired t-test. The unpaired t-test was used to compare NRS and Oswestry scores in patients with and without a prior history of LBP and for patients with and without LBP during a previous pregnancy. Anova was used to assess for differences in baseline and follow-up NRS and Oswestry scores by location category of the LBP and category of the number of previous episodes of LBP. NRS and Oswestry change scores were also calculated for each follow-up time period compared to the baseline scores.

Logistic regression analysis was also performed to determine statistically significant predictors of improvement using the 10 baseline variables (age, number of previous pregnancies, chronicity category, history of LBP, LBP during a previous pregnancy, gestational week, location category for LBP, work status, exercise level category, smoking status) at 1 month, 3 months, 6 months and 1 year after start of treatment. The full model containing all predictors was also assessed for statistical significance and ability to distinguish between patients who improved or did not improve as well as the proportion of correctly classified cases.

Results

Baseline and 1 year data were available on 115 patients. In order to obtain 1 year outcomes data on these 115 patients, 143 were enrolled with baseline data. Seven of these 143 patients requested to drop out of the study prior to the 1 year data collection time point and 28 other patients were not able to be contacted for 3 consecutive telephone data collection time periods. Thus they were deleted from the study. The patients came from a total of 15 different chiropractors. One hundred of the 115 patients came from the 2 practices specifically targeted. One of these sites has 4 chiropractors and the other 3 and all referred pregnant patients to the study.

The mean patient age was 32.96 (SD = 4.64) years and the mean gestational week was 26.21 (SD = 6.98). Table 1 shows the results of the various baseline demographic factors. A slight majority of patients (53.1%) were in their 3rd trimester of pregnancy (Table 1) and thus would have delivered their babies by the 3 month follow-up time point. There was a fairly even distribution in the percentage of patients complaining of lumbar pain only, pelvic pain only or a combination of the two areas. Of the 53 patients who had at least one previous pregnancy, 31 (58%) reported having experienced back pain during the previous pregnancies.

Over half of the patients reported clinically relevant 'improvement' at 1 week, with the vast majority 'improved' at all subsequent data collection time points (Table 2). Statistically significant reductions in NRS and Oswestry scores ($p < 0.0005$) at all follow-up time points compared to the baseline scores was also noted (Table 2). Comparing the category of the number of previous episodes of LBP with 'improvement' found a significant relationship at 1 week ($p = 0.035$) and especially at 1 year ($p = 0.02$). Patients who 'improve' have fewer episodes of prior LBP. Patients with more previous episodes (≥ 5, n = 29) of LBP also had significantly higher 1 year NRS scores

Table 1 Percentage of patients with the various baseline demographic factors

Baseline variable				
Previous Pregnancy number	None = 51.3% (N = 59)	1 = 35.4% (N = 41)	2 = 12.4% (N = 14)	3 = 0.9% (N = 1)
Chronicity LBP	0-4 Weeks = 58.3% (N = 67)	4-12 Weeks = 30.4% (N = 35)	More than 12 Weeks = 11.3% (N = 13)	
History of LBP	No = 46% (N = 53)	Yes = 54% (N = 62)		
Number of Prior LBP episodes	None = 36.5% (N = 42)	1 - 3 = 27.0% (N = 31)	4 or more = 36.5% (N = 42)	
LBP during previous pregnancy	No previous pregnancy = 53.0% (N = 61)	Yes = 27.0% N = 31)	No = 20.0% (N = 23)	
Location of LBP	LBP only = 32.2% (N = 37)	Pelvic pain only = 31.3% (N = 36)	Combination = 35.7% (N = 41)	
Work Status	Working = 71.3% (N = 82)	Off due to LBP = 10.4% (N = 12)	Not working = 18.3% (N = 21)	
Smoker	No = 96.5% (N = 111)	Yes = 3.5% (N = 4)		
Exercise	Regular = 58.5% (N = 68)	Occasional = 18.4% (N = 21)	None = 22.8% (N = 26)	
Gestational Week Category	1st Trimester = 5.3% N = 6)	2nd Trimester = 41.6% (N = 48)	3rd Trimester = 53.1% (N = 61)	

LBP low back pain, *N* number or patients.

with a mean of 2.16 (SD = 2.36) compared to a score of 0.60 (SD = 1.07) for patients with no prior LBP history (n = 30) (p = 0.013). Patients who reported having LBP in a previous pregnancy had significantly lower baseline NRS scores (5.22, SD = 2.10) compared to those who did not have LBP in a previous pregnancy (6.35, SD = 1.84) (p = 0.01). However, there was no significant difference in the NRS scores between these two groups at any follow-up time point. There was no significant link between the category of location of LBP (i.e. low back pain only, pelvic pain only, or both) and 'improvement' at any of the follow-up time points.

At 1 year, 85.2% of patients (n = 98) were 'very happy' or 'happy' with their chiropractic treatment and 6% (n = 7) were 'unhappy'.

Logistic regression analysis using the 10 independent variables (Table 1) compared to the primary outcome of, improvement' showed that the full model was statistically significant, X^2 (5, N = 115) = 40.71, p < 0.009 at 1 month, indicating that the model could distinguish between patients 'improved' and 'not improved'. Between 55.7% and 79.0% of the variability is explained by this set of variables at 1 month after start of treatment. However, no single independent variable made a unique statistically

Table 2 Baseline and outcome data for all patients at the various time points

	Baseline data (115 PTS)	1 week (100 PTS)	1 month (106 PTS)	3 months (104 PTS)	6 months (110 PTS)	1 year (115 PTS)
PGIC		*52% = Much better or better*	*70% = Much better or better*	*85% = Much better or better*	*90% = Much better or better*	*88% = Much better or better*
		6% = worse	*8% = worse*	*3% = worse*	*4% = worse*	*1% = slightly worse*
NRS (Mean (SD))	6.07 (1.91)	4.22* (2.13)	3.06* (2.63)	1.58* (2.15)	1.10* (2.0)	1.19* (1.86)
NRS Change (Mean (SD))		1.85 (2.32)	3.06 (3.27)	4.54 (2.85)	5.07 (2.78)	4.92 (2.59)
OSWESTRY (Mean (SD))	14.33 (8.01)	11.48* (7.27)	8.36* (7.18)	4.97* (6.84)		
Oswestry Change (Mean (SD))		2.85 (5.79)	6.36 (8.35)	9.70 (10.29)		

NRS numerical rating scale for pain, *PGIC* patient's global impression of change, *SD* Standard deviation, *PTS* patients.
* = p < 0.0001 compared to baseline score.

significant contribution to the model. Additionally, at 3 months, 6 months and 1 year the model was not statistically significant as the vast majority of patients were 'improved'.

Discussion

The results of this current study which showed that a high proportion of pregnant patients with LBP undergoing chiropractic treatment reported clinically relevant 'improvement' support those published in a recent cohort study as well as the recent randomized clinical trial (RCT) looking at chiropractic treatment for pregnant patients with low back or pelvic pain [16,17]. The most recent systematic reviews of the literature for interventions for preventing and treating pelvic and back pain in pregnancy [5] and more specifically chiropractic treatment for these patients [4,6] unanimously concluded that the available research evidence at that time was low to moderate quality at best. However, these reviews were published prior to the cohort study by Murphy et al. published in 2009 [16] and the excellent RCT by George et al. published in 2013 [17].

In the RCT by George et al. one treatment arm of the trial on pregnant women suffering from LB, PP or both included treatment by a chiropractor. The results clearly showed a statistically and clinically significant greater level of improvement for the patients who received the additional chiropractic treatment [17]. However, outcomes in that RCT were only measured at one time point between 5 and 9 weeks after the start of treatment and while the patients were still pregnant whereas this current study measured outcomes at 5 different and consistent time points during the pregnancy and after delivery. Comparing the baseline scores between this current cohort study with the baseline scores for the patients in the RCT who were treated with chiropractic shows that they were nearly identical, including the standard deviations (5.8 +/- 2.2 in the RCT, 6.07 +/- 1.91 in this current study). Additionally, the mean gestational weeks were also nearly identical in the two studies. Comparing the 1 month NRS pain scores in this current study with the NRS scores in the RCT measured between 5 and 9 weeks after the start of treatment for those patients in the treatment arm that received chiropractic treatment also shows that they are nearly identical. The NRS change score in the RCT was 2.9 and in this cohort study it was 3.06 [17]. When looking at the mean NRS score at 3 months after the first treatment in this current study it is less than 1/3 of the original baseline score. However, approximately half of the patients would have delivered their babies by this 3 month data collection time point and this likely had a positive impact on this outcome. Therefore, although this cohort study is not a randomized clinical trial and thus the outcomes cannot be attributed to the chiropractic treatment, the strong similarity between these results and those from the recently published RCT supports their validity.

Comparing the outcomes from this study on Swiss patients with those from a very similarly designed outcomes study on patients in the United States (US) [16], shows that they are also quite similar. At 1 month after the start of treatment 70% of the patients in this current study reported clinically relevant improvement of 'much better' or 'better' compared to 73% of patients in the Murphy et al. [16] study. However, the precise time of their outcome data collection is not specified. It was done at the end of active treatment, and this time frame varied between patients. By 3 months after the start of treatment 85% of the patients in this current study reported being clinically significantly improved. It is important to point out that the option 'slightly better' on the PGIC scale was not considered clinically relevant improvement in this current study and these patients were classified as unchanged. Unfortunately it is not possible to compare disability scores or other quality of life factors between these two studies because the Murphy et al. paper used the Bournemouth questionnaire [16] whereas our current study used the Oswestry pain and disability questionnaire. The Bournemouth questionnaire would have been a better choice as an outcome measure for these types of patients as it measures more relevant domains, including psychosocial factors, compared to the Oswestry questionnaire. However, at the time that this current study was conducted the Bournemouth questionnaire was not yet translated and validated into German so could not be used whereas the Oswestry questionnaire had been translated and validated into both German and French.

Another relevant, although perhaps not surprising finding from this current cohort study includes the fact that patients who reported a higher number of previous LBP episodes (≥ 5) were less likely to report clinically relevant improvement, particularly at 1 year after the first treatment. However, this factor was not predictive in the logistic regression model. This is consistent with other studies that show that back pain is commonly recurrent [21-23]. However, the location category of the LBP (LB, PP, both) in this current study was not linked with the likelihood of improvement at any data collection time point nor in the logistic regression model. This is different from what Murphy et al. [16] found. They reported that patients with pain in both areas were significantly less likely to report clinically significant improvement in disability, at least in the short-term, compared to the other two groups. Furthermore, the majority of patients in the Murphy et al. [16] study had posterior pelvic pain (58.3%) whereas the location of the LBP in this current Swiss study was quite evenly distributed between the three locations, with approximately 1/3 of the patients reporting pelvic pain. Another difference between the Murphy et al. [16] study and this current one is that Swiss patients with a history of LBP during a previous pregnancy did not have worse outcomes compared to patients without LBP in a prior pregnancy whereas US patients without LBP in a previous pregnancy were more likely to report improvement compared to US patients with LBP in a previous pregnancy. Reasons for the differences in these outcomes between US and Swiss patients can only be speculated upon. Obesity is much more common in the US than in Switzerland and this may result in a higher proportion of women experiencing both LBP and pelvic pain during pregnancy as this could further increase the lumbar lordosis and place additional stresses on the pelvic joints [24].

The literature states that 94% of women who have LBP in a previous pregnancy have recurrent pain with subsequent pregnancies [23]. However, in this current cohort study only 58% of the patients who had experienced a previous pregnancy reported that they had suffered from back pain at that time. The reason for this discrepancy in proportions is unclear. It is also somewhat surprising that patients with more episodes of previous LBP have worse outcomes at the 1 week and 1 year time points but not at the 1, 3 and 6 month time points. Obviously at the 1 year data collection point all patients would have delivered their babies several months before and would likely then fall into the category of 'usual' low back pain patients where recurrence is not unusual.

No serious adverse events were reported in this study and over 85% of the patients were happy or very happy with their chiropractic treatment. Adverse events from spinal manipulation to pregnant women or those in the early post-partum period are very rare with only 7 cases found in the literature [25]. All seemed to be related to treating the cervical spine rather than the low back however, and the practitioners involved included chiropractors, a physiotherapist, and a general medical practitioner. A recent qualitative study evaluating the treatment experience of pregnant women under chiropractic care reported that chiropractors' approach to these patients is patient-centered rather than symptom centered [26]. This may explain why such a high percentage of the patients in this current study were happy with their treatment.

Some of the limitations to this study have been alluded to above. Because this is a cohort study without a control group or other treatment group for comparison, the outcomes reported cannot be assumed to arise from the treatment. Additionally, the patients in this study were treated primarily at two practice sites but by different chiropractors and the details of the types of treatments and treatment dosage are not known. No attempt was made to compare outcomes by practitioner or style of treatment. This would be interesting for future studies. As previously stated, the use of the Oswestry questionnaire was not the best choice for this patient population, but was the best available that was translated and validated in both German and French. Additionally, the assessment of symphysis pubis pain in these pregnant patients was not specifically assessed as it was desired to use those same categories of low back pain in pregnancy that previous papers used in order to make direct comparisons.

Conclusions

A large proportion of pregnant patients with LBP or pelvic pain undergoing chiropractic treatment report clinically relevant improvement in their symptoms at all time points up to 1 year. There is a relationship between the number of prior episodes of LBP and 'improvement' with patients reporting more episodes being less likely to improve. However, this was not a strong predictor of, improvement' when placed into a logistic regression model.

Abbreviations

LBP: Low back pain; LP: Lumbar spine pain; n: Number; NRS: Numeric rating scale for pain; PGIC: Patient's global impression of change; PPP: Posterior pelvic pain; PTS: Patients; SD: Standard deviation; SMT: Spinal manipulative therapy.

Competing interests

The authors declare that they have no competing interests.

Authors' contributions

CP: Ethics approval submission, Literature search, data entry, analysis and interpretation of data, drafting and revising the manuscript, final approval of the manuscript. DM: Patient recruitment, baseline data collection, patient treatment, final approval of the manuscript. BKH: Concept and design of the study, manuscript preparation and final approval of the manuscript.

References

1. Perkins J, Hammer RL, Loubert PV: **Identification and management of pregnancy-related low back pain.** *J Nurse Midwifery* 1998, **43**:331–340.
2. Skaggs CD, Prather H, Gross G, George JW, Thompson PA, Nelson DM: **Back pain and pelvic pain in an underserved United States pregnant population: a preliminary descriptive survey.** *J Manipulative Physiol Ther* 2007, **30**:130–134.
3. Mohseni-Bandpei MA, Fakhri M, Ahmad-Shirvani M, Bagheri-Nessami M, Khalilian AR, Shayesteh-Azar M, Mohseni-Bandpei H: **Low back pain in 1,100 Iranian pregnant women: prevalence and risk factors.** *Spine J* 2009, **9**:795–801.
4. Khorsan R, Hawk C, Lisi AJ, Kizhakkeveettil A: **Manipulative therapy for pregnancy and related conditions: a systematic review.** *Obstet Gynecol Surv* 2009, **64**:416–427.
5. Pennick V, Young G: **Interventions for preventing and treating pelvic and back pain in pregnancy (Review).** *Cochrane Database Syst Rev* 2007, **18**:CD001139.
6. Stuber KJ, Smith DL: **Chiropractic treatment of pregnancy-related low back pain: a systematic review of the evidence.** *J Manipulative Physiol Ther* 2008, **31**:447–454.
7. Sabino J, Grauer JN: **Pregnancy and low back pain.** *Curr Rev Musculoskelet Med* 2008, **1**:137–141.

8. Stapleton DB, MacLennan AH, Kristiansson P: **The prevalence of recalled low back pain during and after pregnancy: a South Australian population survey.** *Aust N Z J Obstet Gynaecol* 2002, **42**:482–485.
9. Gutke A, Östgaard C, Öberg B: **Association between muscle function and low back pain in relation to pregnancy.** *J Rehabil Med* 2008, **40**:304–311.
10. Röst CC, Jacqueline J, Kaiser A, Verhagen AP, Koes BW: **Pelvic pain during pregnancy.** *Spine* 2004, **29**:2567–2572.
11. Albert HB, Godskesen M, Korsholm L, Westergaard JG: **Risk factors in developing pregnancy-related pelvic girdle pain.** *Acta Obstet Gynecol Scand* 2006, **85**:539–544.
12. Keriakos R, Bhatta SR, Morris F, Mason S, Buckley S: **Pelvic girdle pain during pregnancy and puerperium.** *Obstet Gynecol* 2011, **31**:572–580.
13. Mogren IM, Pohjanen AI: **Low back pain and pelvic pain during pregnancy.** *Spine* 2005, **30**:983–991.
14. Wijnhoven HA, de Vet HC, Smit HA, Picavet HS: **Hormonal and reproductive factors are associated with chronic low back pain and chronic upper extremity pain in women–the MORGEN study.** *Spine* 2006, **31**:1496–1502.
15. Sihvonen T, Huttunen M, Makkonen M, Airaksinen O: **Functional changes in back muscle activity correlate with pain intensity and prediction of low back pain during pregnancy.** *Arch Phys Med Rehabil* 1998, **79**:1210–1212.
16. Murphy DR, Hurwitz EL, McGovern EE: **Outcome of pregnancy-related lumbopelvic pain treated according to a diagnosis-based decision rule: a prospective observational cohort study.** *J Manipulative Physiol Ther* 2009, **32**:616–624.
17. George JW, Skaggs CD, Thompson PA, Nelson DM, Gavard JA, Gross GA: **A randomized controlled trial comparing a multimodal intervention and standard obstetrics care for low back and pelvic pain in pregnancy.** *Am J Obstet Gynecol* 2013, **295**:e1–e7.
18. Humphreys BK, Peterson CK, Muehlemann D, Haueter P: **Are Swiss chiropractors different than other chiropractors? Results of the job analysis survey 2009.** *J Manipulative Physiol Ther* 2010, **33**:519–535.
19. Mannion AF, Junge A, Fairbank JCT, Dvorak J, Grob D: **Development of a German version of the Oswestry disability index: part 1: cross-cultural adaptation, reliability, and validity.** *Eur Spine J* 2006, **15**:55–65.
20. Vogler D, Paillex R, Norberg M, de Goumoëns P, Cabri J: **Cross-cultural validation of the Oswestry disability index in French.** *Ann Readapt Med Phys* 2008, **51**:379–385.
21. Axén I, Bodine L: **The Nordic maintenance care program: the clinical use of identified indications for preventive care.** *Chiropr Man Therap* 2013, **21**:10.
22. Mannion AF, Wieser S, Elfering A: **Association between beliefs and care-seeking behavior for low back pain.** *Spine* 2013, **38**:1016–1025.
23. Brynhildsen J, Hansson A, Persson A, Hammar M: **Follow-up of patients with low back pain during pregnancy.** *Obstet Gynecol* 1998, **91**:182–186.
24. Vesco KK, Karanja N, King JC, Gillman MW, Perrin N, McEvoy C, Eckhardt C, Smith KS, Stevens VJ: **Healthy moms, a randomized trial to promote and evaluate weight maintenance among obese pregnant women: study design and rationale.** *Contemp Clin Trials* 2012, **33**:777–785.
25. Stuber KJ, Wynd S, Weis CA: **Adverse events from spinal manipulation in the pregnant and postpartum periods: a critical review of the literature.** *Chiropr Man Therap* 2012, **20**:8.
26. Sadr S, Pourkiani-Allah-Abad P, Stuber KJ: **The treatment experience of patients with low back pain during pregnancy and their chiropractors: a qualitative study.** *Chiropr Man Therap* 2012, **20**:32.

The provision of chiropractic, physiotherapy and osteopathic services within the Australian private health-care system: a report of recent trends

Roger M Engel*, Benjamin T Brown, Michael S Swain and Reidar P Lystad

Abstract

Background: Chiropractors, physiotherapists, and osteopaths receive training in the diagnosis and management of musculoskeletal conditions. As a result there is considerable overlap in the types of conditions that are encountered clinically by these practitioners. In Australia, the majority of benefits paid for these services come from the private sector. The purpose of this article is to quantify and describe the development in service utilization and the cost of benefits paid to users of these healthcare services by private health insurers. An exploration of the factors that may have influenced the observed trends is also presented.

Methods: A review of data from the Australian Bureau of Statistics, Australian Health Practitioner Regulation Agency, and the Australian Government Private Health Insurance Administration Council was conducted. An analysis of chiropractic, physiotherapy and osteopathic service utilisation and cost of service utilisation trend was performed along with the level of benefits and services over time.

Results: In 2012, the number of physiotherapists working in the private sector was 2.9 times larger than that of chiropractic, and 7.8 times that of the osteopathic profession. The total number of services provided by chiropractors, physiotherapists, and osteopaths increased steadily over the past 15 years. For the majority of this period, chiropractors provided more services than the other two professions. The average number of services provided by chiropractors was approximately two and a half times that of physiotherapists and four and a half times that of osteopaths.

Conclusions: This study highlights a clear disparity in the average number of services provided by chiropractors, physiotherapists, and osteopaths in the private sector in Australia over the last 15 years. Further research is required to explain these observed differences and to determine whether a similar trend exists in patients who do not have private health insurance cover.

Keywords: Chiropractic, Physiotherapy, Osteopathy, Allied health, Healthcare utilisation

Introduction

In Australia health care costs are covered by the private and public sectors. In 2009–2010 the private health insurance sector provided $13.5 billion towards the total cost of the Australian health care system. This represented about 12% of total health funding [1]. These funds came from two sources: insurance premium payments by members ($9.2 billion) and premium rebates from the Australian Government ($4.3 billion). Of the $9.2 billion paid by members, 5.3% went to payment for non-hospital, non-medical treatment such as chiropractic, physiotherapy and osteopathic services.

Australian chiropractors, physiotherapists and osteopaths are all trained to diagnose and treat musculoskeletal (MSK) conditions [2-4]. It is therefore reasonable to assume a degree of overlap in the types of conditions treated by each of these professions. A recent cross-sectional study of chiropractors from Victoria, Australia reported that MSK conditions were the most common reason for patients seeking chiropractic care. Chiropractors who participated in the study stated that MSK

* Correspondence: roger.engel@mq.edu.au
Department of Chiropractic, Macquarie University, Balaclava Rd, North Ryde 2109, Australia

conditions were the main reason for the practitioner-patient encounter in 60 per 100 encounters (95% CI, 54–67 per 100 encounters) [5]. The Australian Physiotherapy Association's 'Scope of Practice' states that physiotherapy involves the prevention, diagnosis, and management of movement disorders that involve the MSK system [6]. In addition, physiotherapists also provide other services including, but not limited to, post-fracture, post-surgery and pre- and post-natal care. It is a similar scenario for osteopaths with nine of the twelve conditions listed under 'Treatment' by the Australian Osteopathic Association being MSK in nature [3].

Musculoskeletal conditions such as back and neck pain cause significant disability and loss of productivity and represent a considerable portion of healthcare expenditure in Australia. The Global Burden of Disease study 2010 ranks low back pain and neck pain first and third respectively in Australasia as the cause of years lived with disability [7]. The prevalence of these conditions increases up to the age of 60 [8] and the demand for health care services associated with managing them is likely to increase significantly over the next three decades. It is therefore important to quantify and describe current trends in service utilisation in order to assist future planning of healthcare service provision and expenditure.

In Australia, the provision of chiropractic, physiotherapy and osteopathic services is driven by a number of factors that can be classified as internal or external. Internal factors encompass graduate capabilities, code of conduct and self-regulated professional behaviour and practice, while external factors include government legislation, private health insurance policies, individual/community preference, population demographics, economic circumstances such as the level of household disposable income and the health status of the population [9]. These factors operate in a state of dynamic equilibrium, whereby change in one factor produces an alteration in one or more of the others. Understanding the dynamics of these changes is not always straightforward. The aims of this article are to A) quantify and describe developments in service utilisation and total cost of service benefits for chiropractic, physiotherapy and osteopathic services in the Australian private health sector, and B) to discuss factors that may account for any observable trends in the development.

Methods

Data sources

Data were obtained retrospectively from the Australian Bureau of Statistics (ABS) [10], Australian Health Practitioner Regulation Agency (AHPRA) [11-13], and the Australian Government Private Health Insurance Administration Council (PHIAC) [14,15] with a review period of 15 years (1998–2012) chosen for convenience. The PHIAC is the regulatory body for the private health insurance industry in Australia. It protects the consumer by ensuring a safe, efficient, compliant, and competitive health insurance industry. The PHIAC collects key information and monitors activity from all health insurers in Australia on a quarterly basis.

In this study data was gathered from PHIAC pertaining to total cost of services, ancillary benefits, and number of services provided to all Australians with private health insurance by chiropractors, physiotherapists and osteopaths. The total 'cost of service' represents the sum total of the fees charged at the time of consultation (fee for service) to individuals with private health insurance. An 'ancillary benefit' relates to the portion of the total fee for service that is reimbursed by the health insurer. A 'service' represents one visit to a healthcare provider. The number of general treatment policies held during the review period was also retrieved from the PHIAC databases. A 'general treatment policy' represents insurance for treatment that is intended to manage or prevent a disease, injury or condition, and is separate to hospital treatment cover.

Total numbers of registered, practising practitioners in 1998 and 2012 were collated using data from the ABS and AHPRA. Data regarding the total number of hours worked by registered physiotherapists, in both the public and the private sector, were obtained from the ABS and from three Australian state government agencies (New South Wales 2009, Queensland 2005, and Victoria 2006) [16-19]. The ABS data described the percentage of hours worked by physiotherapists in the private sector in 1998.

Quarterly data relating to the majority of these key variables was available for the review period for the chiropractic, physiotherapy and osteopathic professions. In this study, quarterly services, cost of services, and ancillary benefits data were summated to give yearly statistics for that period. No other transformations were required.

Data analyses

Each discipline's service utilisation and cost of service utilisation trend was plotted showing the level of services and benefits over time. The percentage change from one year to the next for both total service cost and number of services was calculated for chiropractic, physiotherapy and osteopathy. The percentage change in practitioner numbers between 1998 and 2012 was also calculated. As chiropractors and osteopaths work exclusively in the private sector, an estimate of the number physiotherapists working in the private sector was required. The estimate for the total number of physiotherapists working in the private sector in 2012 was based on data from the three state government agencies. The proportion of 53.5% was calculated by taking the average number of hours worked by physiotherapists in the private sector across these three states and applying it to the total number of registered, practising physiotherapists in 2012. The average yearly number of services delivered was calculated for each profession by dividing the total number of services by the total number of registered, practising practitioners in the private sector for each profession. The percentage change from the previous yearly figures was calculated for all the key variables.

Results

Number of practitioners

Table 1 shows the number of chiropractors, physiotherapists and osteopaths in Australia in 1998 and 2012 working in private practice and the proportional change over time [11-13,19-21]. As the number of physiotherapists working in the private sector in 2012 was not directly available we used the estimate referred to previously for the analysis. There were just under three times (2.9) as many physiotherapists as chiropractors in 2012 and 2.6 times as many chiropractors as osteopaths. The osteopathic profession experienced a four-fold increase in practitioner numbers during the review period which was considerably larger than the increases in the number of chiropractors and physiotherapists. It is however important to note that despite this large increase in the practitioner numbers during the review period, the overall number of osteopaths is much smaller when compared to the number of chiropractors and physiotherapists working in the private sector.

Level of services

Figure 1 reports the total number of chiropractic, physiotherapy and osteopathic services provided to individuals with private health insurance between 1998 and 2012 [22]. Profession service figures have been provided in Additional file 1 [15]. Figure 2 illustrates the total private health insurance expenditure for chiropractic, physiotherapy and osteopathic services between 1998 and 2012. A detailed breakdown of this data is provided in Additional file 2 [22]. There was an overall trend towards increasing expenditure for all three providers during the review period. While the total number and dollar value of osteopathic services was less compared to chiropractic and physiotherapy services the percentage change in osteopathic services exceeded chiropractic and physiotherapy for the majority of the review period. The expenditure on osteopathic services must be interpreted with the knowledge that the overall level of services for the osteopathic profession represents a small percentage of the total expenditure for services rendered by the three services providers.

Table 1 Total number of registered, practising practitioners in the private sector by profession in 1998 and 2012

Provider	1998	2012	Proportion change
Chiropractors	2,053	4,221	2.1
Physiotherapists	5,187	12,230*	2.4
Osteopaths	395	1,608	4.1

*Estimated figure: 53.5% of total registered, practising physiotherapists (24,304).
Source: 1998 figures ABS [19,21], 2012 figures AHPRA [11-13].

Average number of services per practitioner

In 1998 the average number of services per practitioner provided to individuals with private health insurance per practitioner was 1,901 for chiropractors, 691 for physiotherapists and 141 for osteopaths. Using the estimated figure for the number of physiotherapists working in the private sector, the average number of services per registered, practising practitioner in 2012 was 2,252 for chiropractors, 796 for physiotherapists and 483 for osteopaths [11-13]. The average number of services provided by chiropractors was more than two and a half times that of physiotherapists and four and a half times that of osteopaths working in the private sector in 1998 and 2012.

Discussion

The purpose of this study was to quantify and describe developments in service utilisation and total cost of service benefits for chiropractic, physiotherapy and osteopathic services in the private healthcare sector in Australia between 1998 and 2012. There has been a substantial increase in the number of chiropractors, physiotherapists and osteopaths in the last 15 years, with physiotherapy being the largest of the three providers in terms of practitioner numbers in the private sector. This growth in practitioner numbers has been accompanied by a steady increase in the utilisation of these services, a scenario that has been most pronounced for osteopathic services. Chiropractors have delivered more services to individuals with private health insurance compared to physiotherapists and osteopaths for the majority of the review period. Chiropractors deliver, on average, a higher number of services each year in the private sector compared to physiotherapists and osteopaths. With respect to expenditure, there has been a trend towards an increasing cost of chiropractic, physiotherapy and osteopathic services, as well as an increase in the benefits paid for these services by private health insurers. Both the total cost and the benefits paid for osteopathic services have accelerated dramatically over the review period when viewed alongside the data for the other two service providers.

The secondary aim of this study was to discuss the factors that may account for the development in the figures relating to total cost of services, benefits paid by private health insurers, and utilisation rates for chiropractic, physiotherapy and osteopathic services. While it is not possible, based on the data, to provide definitive explanations

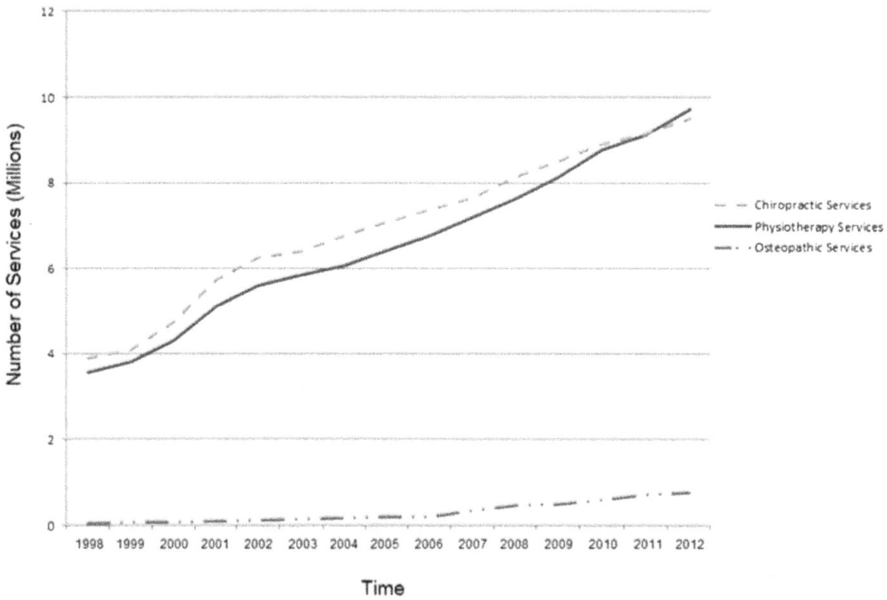

Figure 1 Total number of services provided to individuals with private health insurance by profession: 1998 – 2012. Source: PHIAC [15].

for the observed trends a discussion of the factors that may have contributed to changes in these areas is presented below.

With respect to service utilisation, the increases observed during the review period cannot be fully explained by the increase in practitioner numbers. Between 2005 and 2010, the total number of workers across all health occupations in Australia increased by 26%. During the same period, the number of chiropractors and osteopaths increased by 17% while the number of physiotherapists increased by 42% [23].

The number of chiropractic services provided to patients with private health insurance was higher than for physiotherapy for the majority of the review period (1998–2011). If the two professions were compared on size alone it would make sense that the profession with the largest private sector presence (physiotherapy) would have also provided the most number of services. However, this was not the case for the majority of the review period. Data from 2012 highlights a change to this trend with the total number of services provided by physiotherapists exceeding those provided by chiropractors. It

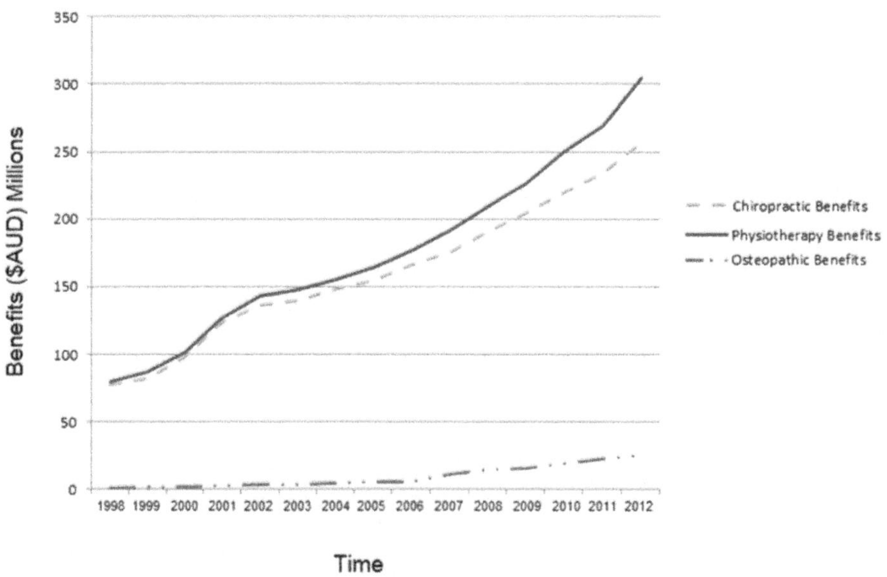

Figure 2 Private health insurance rebates by profession: 1998–2012. Source: PHIAC [15].

is yet to be seen whether this increase will continue into the future.

Factors that could explain the disparity in the number of services provided by chiropractors and physiotherapists during the review period include internal factors such as code of conduct and self-regulated professional behaviour and practice, and/or external factors such as government legislation, changes in private health insurance policy or economic factors.

Code of conduct and self-regulated professional behaviour and practice includes elements such as fees charged for services, and the location of practices. With respect to the fees charged for chiropractic services, the average fee declined in real terms between 2007 and 2012 [9]. The opposite situation occurred regarding fees for physiotherapy services with average fee in real terms increasing between 2007 and 2012 [24]. However, the benefit paid by private health insurers declined by approximately 1% in the same period for both chiropractic and physiotherapy services [9,24]. The size of the difference in both fee for service, and benefits paid by insurers over this period is therefore unlikely to account for the disparity between the average number of chiropractic and physiotherapy services.

While there is a general consensus regarding the types of conditions that fall within the scope of practice for each profession, the precise case-mix for each profession is not well-described in the literature. It could be argued that physiotherapists, through their involvement in areas such as post-surgical rehabilitation, may see patients who justifiably require more frequent and intensive care. This could have created a scenario where there is considerable heterogeneity in case-mix between the three professions. This scenario could also potentially alter the length of time required to treat each patient, with patients seeing a physiotherapist experiencing greater disability requiring more care and attention equating to longer 'service' duration.

The data presented in this study describe a higher average number of services provided per chiropractic practitioner compared to physiotherapists and osteopaths. This finding does not necessarily mean that chiropractors delivered more services per patient. Instead, it may be that chiropractors see more new patients or a greater proportion of their existing client base more often. Recent industry estimates suggest that Australian chiropractors see approximately 300,000 patients per week [9]. Using this estimate, each chiropractor (4402 in June 2013) would be seeing on average 68.1 patients per week. Based on a 48 week working year these estimates are higher than the estimates detailed in this study. More accurate point prevalence data on service utilization for each of these professions is required before any meaningful predictions can be made about the level of chiropractic, physiotherapy and osteopathic services in the future.

Results from a 2005 Australian survey of 1,067 adults over the age of 18 found that 16.1% reported using chiropractic services during the previous 12 months [25]. The most common reasons given for seeking chiropractic and osteopathic treatment were back and/or neck pain, non-specific musculoskeletal problems and enhancement of general health and well-being [25]. While the response rate for each of these categories did differ between the two professions the size of the differences are not enough to explain the disparity in the average number of services for each profession.

A recent survey of 1,427 Australian women showed high utilisation of chiropractors in non-urban compared to urban settings [26]. It may be the case that there is a different pattern in the utilisation of chiropractic, physiotherapy and osteopathic services in rural areas. It is important to note that there has not been any research into the utilisation of these services by males in non-urban regions. However, we do not believe that a preference for chiropractic in non-urban settings would be sufficient to explain the magnitude of the disparity in average servicing as the number of chiropractors practising in rural and remote regions of Australia (30%) is substantially less than the number of chiropractors practising in urban regions (70%) [27].

With respect to the previously identified external factors that could explain the utilisation disparity between the three disciplines, the Australian Federal Government does not regulate the level of chiropractic, physiotherapy or osteopathic services provided in the private sector. As for private health insurance coverage, the increased uptake in general treatment cover over the review period does not match the increase in service provision by the three professions. There have not been any changes in private health insurance policies during the review period that favoured one discipline over the other or any economic factors that may have influenced the Australian economy in a way that would have impacted on the three disciplines differently.

An absence of practice guidelines for the chiropractic profession could account for a high average number of services provided per practitioner. This absence may have unwittingly led to the acceptance of a wide variation in the level of servicing among chiropractors in Australia. However, the problem is not unique to the chiropractic profession, and would therefore exist to some extent in both the physiotherapy and osteopathic professions. This is an area in which further research is required. While our analysis cannot identify whether the average number of services per chiropractor can be uniformly applied across the profession, it is possible that a section of the profession practices in a manner so different to the rest that the average for the entire profession becomes distorted. Anecdotally, there are large differences between chiropractors in the average number of services provided per patient. It must be acknowledged that the same scenario could also exist within the physiotherapy and osteopathic professions. However, if this were the case for chiropractic, it would be of interest to the private health insurance sector as they provide the majority of benefits for chiropractic services. In the current economic climate, it is hard to imagine insurers continuing to support such high levels of utilisation without evidence to support the premise that a higher level of servicing delivers increased benefit to their members. This point is especially pertinent to insurance companies as there has been a steady increase in the number of Australians with general treatment insurance over the review period [15]. It must be noted however that while an individual may have had general treatment cover, this does not mean that they have coverage for chiropractic, physiotherapy, or osteopathic treatment within that general treatment cover.

The differences observed between the three service providers with respect to service utilisation, and average number of services provided per practitioner cannot be adequately explained by the data presented here. It is possible that factors that were not measured in this research such as working hours, full-time equivalent working status, capacity of a profession to treat patients, patient demographics, and treatment type/content may be salient. Further research that includes these metrics is required to more accurately account for the observed trends.

Limitations

There are several limitations to this study. Firstly, the estimate for the number of physiotherapists working in the private sector was based on figures from only three states at different time periods. It is unknown how these estimates relate to full-time practitioners as there are no current reports that detail the full-time equivalent status of practitioners working in these three professions. Secondly, PHIAC collects data on the cost of benefits for services and the number of services received by individuals with private health insurance. However, if a patient had exceeded their yearly benefit limit for a particular service, any additional services provided by a treating practitioner after that point would not have been recorded. Furthermore, not all Australians have private health insurance. In fact, only 54.6% of Australians had general treatment policies in December 2012 [28]. Of the patients with private health insurance, not all had a level of cover that included ancillary services such chiropractic, physiotherapy or osteopathy. Currently, chiropractic, physiotherapy, and osteopathy services are bundled together in the majority of ancillary health cover packages. Patients are therefore not given the option to select health insurance coverage for an individual profession, despite any preference they may have. The reasons for seeking chiropractic treatment are quite diverse and readers are directed to a recent review paper by Hurwitz [29] for a more detailed discussion on the topic. It must be acknowledged that the data presented in this paper does not fully reflect the various reasons for why patients choose a particular modality and that this may be a salient factor in the observed trends in service utilization. Further research, including an analysis of the social and cultural reasons that drive care seeking behaviour, is required to accurately profile/explain the trends in utilisation across the three professions.

The data presented in this study do not include data from the Chronic Disease Management arm of the Enhanced Primary Care Program. Under this program, patients with a chronic medical condition, e.g. chronic musculoskeletal condition, who would benefit from multidisciplinary care, are eligible to receive five allied health services in conjunction with standard GP care. These services are rendered under a GP management plan and are covered publicly under the Medical Benefits Schedule in Australia [30]. Services provided under this program are not included in the data from PHIAC. It is possible that a proportion of patients that would ordinarily be recorded in the private system have not been identified in this study due to their involvement in this program. This may have influenced the figures relating to total cost of services, level of services and the number of average services provided per practitioner. It is however important to note that chiropractors, physiotherapists and osteopaths are involved in this program.

The estimate for the point prevalence of chiropractic service utilisation obtained in this study is lower than the utilisation figures obtained from a recent industry report [9]. This finding highlights a need for accurate data regarding point prevalence of chiropractic service utilisation. There is also a paucity of data pertaining to point prevalence of service utilisation for physiotherapy and osteopathy services. Targeted research into service utilisation rates amongst those with and without private health insurance is required to accurately explain the observed trends in service utilisation for these three professions.

Conclusion

This article describes the development in the utilisation of chiropractic, physiotherapy and osteopathic services in Australia over the past 15 years. While there is a paucity of data to inform the drivers of this change the authors have provided some hypotheses for the identified disparity in service provision and identified areas where further research is warranted. While this study highlights a clear disparity in service utilisation in the Australian private sector, further research is required to determine if a similar trend exists in patients who do not have private health insurance cover. De-identified individual patient data and de-identified individual clinician data regarding variability in frequency of services per patient are required to better explain the observed trends.

Additional files

Additional file 1: Number of services provided by profession: 1998 - 2012.

Additional file 2: Total cost ($AUD) of services provided by profession: 1998 - 2012.

Abbreviations

ABS: Australian Bureau of Statistics; AHPRA: Australian Health Practitioner Regulation Agency; PHIAC: Private Health Insurance Administration Council; MSK: Musculoskeletal.

Competing interests

The authors declare that they have no competing interests.

Authors' contributions

All authors contributed equally to the design, analysis, writing, and review of the final manuscript.

Acknowledgements

Thank you to Petra Graham for her help and advice with the statistical analyses.

References

1. Australian Institute of Health and Well-being: **Health expenditure Australia 2009–10.** [http://www.aihw.gov.au/publication-detail/?id=10737420435]
2. Australian Physiotherapy Association: **What is Physiotherapy?** [http://www.physiotherapy.asn.au/APAWCM/Physio_and_You/physio/APAWCM/Physio_and_You/physio.aspx?hkey=25ad06f0-e004-47e5-b894-e0ede69e0fff]
3. Australian Osteopathic Association: **Treatment.** [http://www.osteopathy.org.au/pages/osteopathy-and-you.html]
4. Chiropractor's Association of Australia: **Fact sheet - about chiropractic.** [http://chiropractors.asn.au/index.php?option=com_k2&view=item&layout=item&id=107&Itemid=233]
5. French S, Charity MJ, Forsdike K, Gunn JM, Polus BI, Walker BF, Chondros P, Britt HC: **Chiropractic Observation and Analysis Study (COAST): providing an understanding of current chiropractic practice.** *Med J Aust* 2013, **10**(199):687–691.
6. Australian Physiotherapy Association: **Scope of Practice.** [http://www.physiotherapy.asn.au/APAWCM/Advocacy/Position_Statements/APAWCM/Advocacy/Position_Statements.aspx?hkey=5eb019e2-29f9-40a0-bd4d-f98605d23da5]
7. Vos T, Flaxman AD, Naghavi M, Lozano R, Michaud C, Ezzati M, Shibuya K, Salomon JA, Abdalla S, Aboyans V, Abraham J, Ackerman I, Aggarwal R, Ahn SY, Alvarado M, Anderson HR, Anderson LM: **Years lived with disability (YLDs) for 1160 sequelae of 289 diseases and injuries 1990–2010: a systematic analysis for the Global Burden of Disease Study 2010.** *Lancet* 2012, **380**(9859):2163–2196.
8. Fejer R, Leboeuf-Yde C: **Does back and neck pain become more common as you get older? A systematic literature review.** *Chiropr Man Therap* 2012, **20**(24):1–6.
9. Fitzpatrick N: **IBIS World Industry Report Q8534: chiropractic and osteopathic services in Australia.** [http://www.ibisworld.com.au/industry/default.aspx?indid=620]
10. Australian Bureau of Statistics: **Homepage.** [http://www.abs.gov.au/websitedbs/D3310114.nsf/home/home?opendocument#frombanner=GT]
11. Australian Health Practitioner Regulatory Agency - Chiropractic Board of Australia Data tables: June 2012 Chiropractic. [http://www.chiropracticboard.gov.au/About-the-Board/Statistics.aspx]
12. Australian Health Practitioner Regulatory Agency - Physiotherapy Board of Australia Data tables: June 2012. [http://www.physiotherapyboard.gov.au/About/Statistics.aspx]
13. Australian Health Practitioner Regulatory Agency - Osteopathy Board of Australia Data tables: June 2012. [http://www.osteopathyboard.gov.au/About/Statistics.aspx]
14. Private Health Insurance Administration Council: **Industry Statistics.** [http://phiac.gov.au/industry/industry-statistics/statistical-trends/]
15. Private Health Insurance Administration Council: **Statistical trends in membership and benefits data tables.** [http://phiac.gov.au/consumers/consumer-statistics/]
16. New South Wales Health: **Physiotherapy Labour Force Profile NSW - 2009.** [www0.health.nsw.gov.au/pubs/2011/pdf/physio_2009.pdf]
17. Department of Human Services: **Physiotherapy labour force - Victoria 2006: a report by Service and Workforce Planning.** [docs.health.vic.gov.au/docs/doc/.../$FILE/physio-report-2007-final.pdf]
18. Health Statistics Centre: **Workforce characteristics: physiotherapists re- registered in Queensland, 2005.** [www.health.qld.gov.au/hic/labour_force/physio_05.pdf]
19. Australian Bureau of Statistics: **Physiotherapy services - 8552.0.** [http://www.abs.gov.au/ausstats/abs@.nsf/mf/8552.0/]
20. Australian Bureau of Statistics: **Complementary therapies.** [http://www.abs.gov.au/AUSSTATS/abs@.nsf/Lookup/4102.0Chapter5202008]
21. Australian Bureau of Statistics: **Chiropractic and osteopathic services - 8550.0.** [http://www.abs.gov.au/ausstats/abs@.nsf/mf/8550.0/]
22. Private Health Insurance Administration Council: **All states benefits.** [http://phiac.gov.au/industry/industry-statistics/statistical-trends/]
23. Australian Institute of Health and Welfare: **Australia's health 2012.** [www.aihw.gov.au/publication-detail/?id=10737422172]
24. Fitzpatrick N: **IBIS World Industry Report Q8535: Physiotherapy services in Australia.** [http://www.ibisworld.com.au/industry/default.aspx?indid=619]
25. Xue CC, Zhang AL, Lin V, Da Costa C, Story DF: **Complementary and alternative medicine use in Australia: a national population-based survey.** *J Altern Complement Med* 2007, **13**(6):643–650.
26. Adams J, Sibritt D, Broom A, Loxton D, Wardle J, Pirotta M, Lui C-W: **Complementary and alternative medicine consultations in urban and nonurban areas: a National Survey of 1427 Australian women.** *J Manipulative Physiol Ther* 2013, **36**:12–19.
27. Eaton S, Bonello R, Strkalj G, Brown BT, Green H, Graham PL: **Demographic characteristics and perceptions of supply and demand of chiropractic services in Australia: results from stage 1 of the Work Force Study Survey.** *Chiroprac J Aust* 2012, **42**(3):82–90.
28. Private Health Insurance Administration Council: **Quarterly statistics December 2012.** [http://phiac.gov.au/industry/industry-statistics/statistical-trends/]
29. Hurwitz EL: **Epidemiology: spinal manipulation utilization.** *J Electromyogr Kinesiol* 2012, **22**(5):648–654.
30. The Department of Health: **Chronic Disease Management (CDM) medicare items.** [http://www.health.gov.au/internet/main/publishing.nsf/Content/mbsprimarycare-chronicdiseasemanagement]

The relation of experience in osteopathic palpation and object identification

Rosanna C Sabini[1*], Chadwick S Leo[2] and Alton E Moore II[3]

Abstract

Background: To determine whether osteopathic medical students, fellows, residents, and practicing physicians differ in their ability to identify inanimate objects and if these skills relate to palpatory experience.

Methods: Fifteen commonly known objects were fixed to a board and blinded with a cotton cloth. In Part I of testing, participants were asked to identify 9 objects, with choices provided. In Part II participants were asked to identify 6 objects using one word only. Part III consisted of identifying the shape of an object in Part II.

Results: Eighty-nine osteopathic medical students, fellows, residents, and practicing physicians participated in the study. Overall, correct identification of objects was higher in Part I with choices than in Part II without choices available. No statistically significant difference was found among osteopathic medical students, fellows, residents, and practicing physicians in the correct identification of the objects.

Conclusions: Accuracy in tactile identification of objects among varying levels of palpatory experience was not found. Correlation with clinical palpation cannot be made as it requires a subset of palpatory skills not tested in this study. Accuracy and measurement of palpation should be studied further to demonstrate if palpatory experience improves palpatory accuracy.

Keywords: Palpation, Experience, Osteopathy, Manual Medicine

Background

Like other forms of manual medicine osteopathic philosophy requires palpation as a method for diagnosing and treating disease. To obtain these abilities, osteopathic medical schools teach first and second year students the palpatory skills needed to assess and administer osteopathic manipulation in a laboratory setting. Students then spend two years in the clinical setting to refine their skills in taking a complete history, performing a physical examination and improving their palpation.

With continued use of manual medicine, students should improve their palpatory skills and learn to filter insignificant observations [1]. Testing palpation accuracy is challenging because different clinicians vary in their treatment paradigm and professional experience, even though there is standardized medical school training. Moir et al [2] notes that each clinician develops his or her own criteria by which to determine standards of any given test procedure, and there can be a difference in interpretation of the findings [2] and difficulty with these findings being objectively measured [3]. Therefore, it is not surprising that studies showing that palpatory accuracy is related to experience have been conflicting in their findings [2,4-6].

Most articles have failed to show the reliability of palpation in evidence-based clinical practice [7]. Assessing tenderness with palpation can have higher reliability [5,6,8] because patients may contribute to the abnormal findings, whereas identifying anatomical landmarks and other diagnostic tests have been inconsistent [2,4,6,9-13]. Some studies state that the reliability of the palpatory examination has been shown to improve if consensus training is performed prior to testing [5,6,8]. However, a review by Seffinger et al [5] discussed that this was not always demonstrated. Degenhardt et al [7] explained that because patients' bodies are not static, reliability of palpation can be difficult. The author continued to state that "the neuromusculoskeletal system changes according to

* Correspondence: drsabini@gmail.com
[1]Department of Physical Medicine & Rehabilitation, North Shore LIJ - Southside Hospital, 301 East Main Street, Bay Shore, NY 11706, USA
Full list of author information is available at the end of the article

the impulses or stresses that an individual experiences and this inherent neurophysiologic variability occurs in both the examiner and subject" [7]. Even if motionless, human tissues respond to touch and change in texture where findings initially diagnosed may no longer be present after multiple examinations via palpation.

Despite the paucity of evidence, professionals continue to use palpation for diagnosis and treatment. Given the difficulties with testing the accuracy of palpatory skills in patients, simplifying the testing conditions to identify objects could help objectively measure haptic skills. Haptic perception is thought to be the perceptual system mediated by active cutaneous and kinesthetic manual exploration [14]. Visual imagery and verbal processing are also proposed theories for identifying the palpatory stimulus [15]. This study sought to investigate the accuracy of object identification using a blinded board as the testing medium of common objects. Haptics, visual imagery and verbal processing of the objects being palpated, processes which are possibly used to palpate clinically, would be assessed. The goal of the study was to show whether osteopathic medical students, fellows, residents, and practicing physicians differ in the accuracy of object identification due to palpatory experience. The statistical null hypothesis was that there would be no difference. No known similar studies have been identified in the literature.

Methods

Two identical boards were constructed containing fifteen secured items and covered with a one-eighth of an inch cotton cloth (Figure 1). The objects used are common in day to day activities and were chosen for their similar, yet distinct features. All but one investigator and all participants were blinded to the objects. The unblinded investigator chose the objects tested and constructed the board. The study was exempt by the Institutional Review Board.

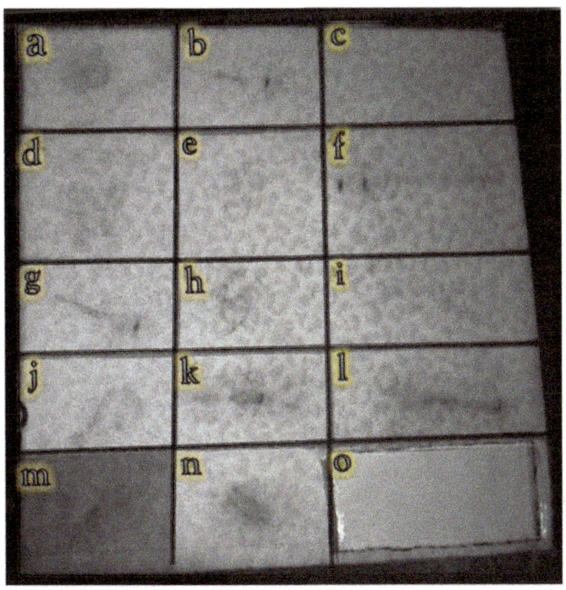

Figure 1 Palpation board covered.

Testing was administered during a national osteopathic conference in the exhibit hall. All osteopathic medical students, fellows, residents, and practicing physician attendees were invited to participate. Prior to testing, each participant was given both written and verbal instructions:

- In order to participate, you must agree to the honor code.
- Do not discuss the test with others, regardless if they have or have not taken the test.
- Fill out only one answer sheet.
- Use light but meaningful touch, as too much pressure may damage delicate items.
- All data submitted will be held confidential.

Each participant was required to sign their name on the answer sheet (Figure 2), agreeing to the honor code for inclusion in the study. No practice time was given and test taking was limited to 10 minutes to complete.

Part I of testing consisted of identifying 9 objects 'a-i' and choosing the answers from 15 choices provided. Part II consisted of identifying 6 objects 'j-o' and providing one word answers for the object. No acceptable alternate answers were determined prior to the study. Finally, Part III required participants to draw object 'o'. There was no partial credit given for answers to this item, with the exception of spatial orientation. The uncovered board and item list are shown in Figure 3. Inspection of both boards after completion of the test revealed no alteration from its original form.

After completion, data from answer sheets was converted into an MS Excel Spread sheet. Statistical analysis was conducted using a nonparametric Wilcoxon–Mann–Whitney test, a two-sample rank-sum test. Two-tailed statistical significance was set to a $P < 0.05$.

Results and discussion

A total of eighty-nine osteopathic medical students ($n = 45$), fellows ($n = 16$), residents ($n = 6$), and practicing physicians ($n = 22$) participated in the study. The accuracy of identifying the blinded objects was 82% (SD 17.4%) in Part I, 33% (SD 35%) in Part II, and 0% in Part III for all participants. Overall accuracy for each object is shown in Figure 4.

Accuracy of object identification based on osteopathic level of experience is shown in Figure 5. No statistically significant difference was found in the accuracy of object identification among osteopathic medical students, fellows, residents and practicing physicians.

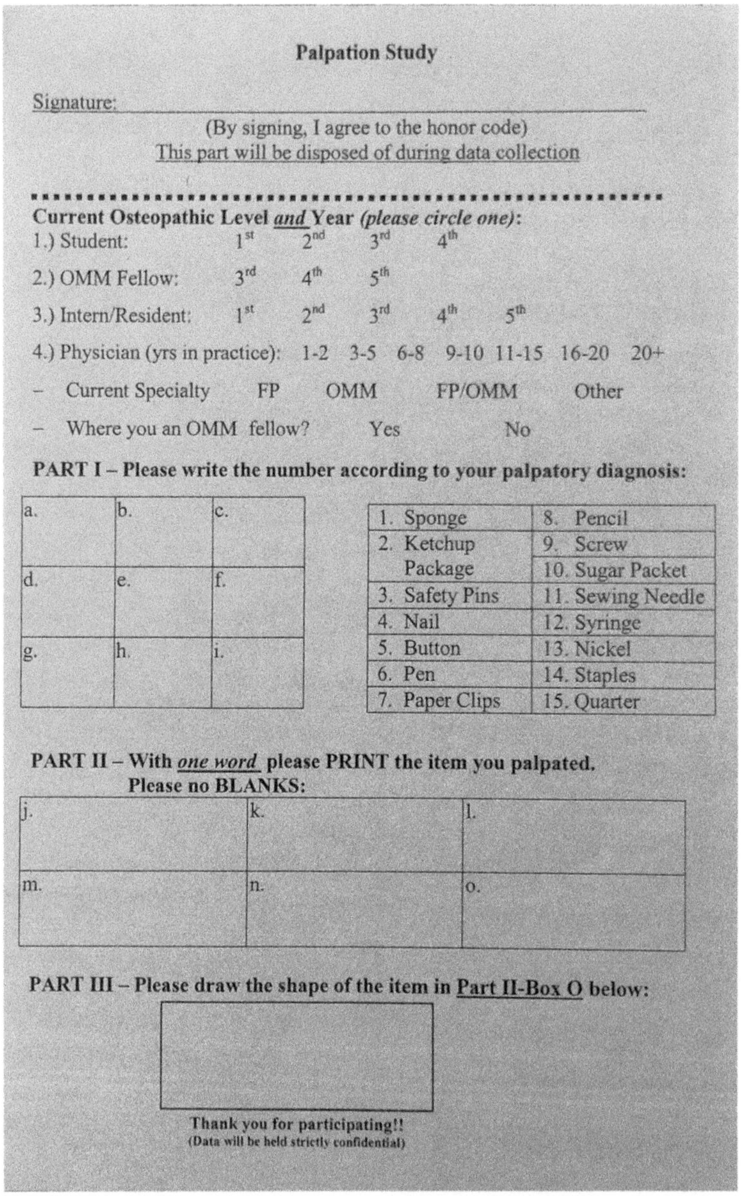

Palpation Study

Signature: ______________________________

(By signing, I agree to the honor code)

This part will be disposed of during data collection

Current Osteopathic Level *and* Year *(please circle one)*:

1.) Student: 1st 2nd 3rd 4th

2.) OMM Fellow: 3rd 4th 5th

3.) Intern/Resident: 1st 2nd 3rd 4th 5th

4.) Physician (yrs in practice): 1-2 3-5 6-8 9-10 11-15 16-20 20+

- Current Specialty FP OMM FP/OMM Other
- Where you an OMM fellow? Yes No

PART I – Please write the number according to your palpatory diagnosis:

a.	b.	c.
d.	e.	f.
g.	h.	i.

1. Sponge	8. Pencil
2. Ketchup Package	9. Screw
	10. Sugar Packet
3. Safety Pins	11. Sewing Needle
4. Nail	12. Syringe
5. Button	13. Nickel
6. Pen	14. Staples
7. Paper Clips	15. Quarter

PART II – With *one word* please PRINT the item you palpated.
Please no BLANKS:

j.	k.	l.
m.	n.	o.

PART III – Please draw the shape of the item in Part II-Box O below:

Thank you for participating!!
(Data will be held strictly confidential)

Figure 2 Questionnaire sheet.

In this study, accuracy of object identification among all participants was higher in Part I than Part II. This was expected because Part I provided choices, whereas Part II required participants to identify the objects without cues. For Part II, because alternate answers were not determined prior to the study, only absolute answers were accepted. Alternate answers chosen post-testing would have biased result interpretation.

Correct identification was unexpectedly low for some objects. In Part I, 54% of participants accurately identified object 'a' as a button and 40% incorrectly identified it as a nickel. Yet when evaluating answers for object 'e,' 92% of participants correctly identified the item as a quarter. A possible explanation may be that participants may not have reviewed all fifteen choices available prior to beginning Part I. Thus, participants were not mindful of the subtle difference in the objects. For example, the button was the first item and participants may not have identified the holes and incorrectly answered nickel, thereby eliminating nickel as a future choice. If this is in fact the case, the order of objects and resultant elimination of choices becomes an issue.

Insufficient time dedicated to meaningful touch or lack of reexamination may have also been the cause for low accuracy in object identification. For example in Part III, although 35% correctly identified the item as "hair," 0%

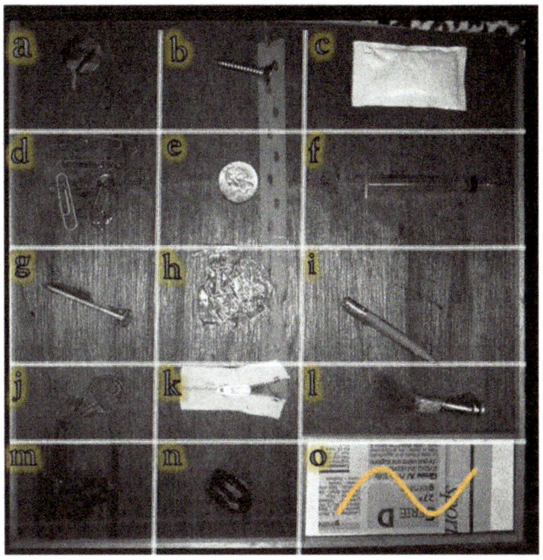

a) Button
b) Screw
c) Ketchup Packet
d) Paper Clips
e) Quarter
f) Syringe
g) Nail
h) Staples
i) Pencil
j) Key
k) Zipper
l) Brush
m) Raisins
n) Pecan
o) One hair strand in a distinct pattern placed under 3 sheets of newspaper

Figure 3 Palpation board uncovered (Part "o" shows graphic shape of item) with item list.

of the participants were able to determine how the hair was arranged. In addition in Part I, about two-thirds of the participants correctly identified object 'd' as paper clips, while the remaining incorrectly identified the object as safety pins. Although similar, there are characteristics that help distinguish between these two objects. Irrespective of there being a 10 minute time limit, no participant required additional time for testing. It is possible that the amount of time dedicated to each object varied. This leads to the question of how much time should an examiner palpate? With increased palpatory experience, it is assumed that less time is needed.

While a novel study design, affixing objects against a board created a two-dimensional surface, and the cloth blinding the objects may have further impeded tactile abilities. Three-dimensional testing could have improved accuracy if participants freely handled an object in a blinded container. In this experiment, haptic perception was limited by the cloth and is considered to be indirect palpation because the cutaneous feedback has been limited [14]. In addition, accuracy of object identification may have been poor because despite the objects being "common," participants may not have had intentional experience in handling these objects. Ability to perform this task could possibly rely more on the ability to visually imagine or mentally represent the object and/or the ability to verbally describe the object being palpated [15]. Familiar objects are more likely to be accurately recognized, but even unfamiliar objects are possibly recognized at levels significantly above chance [16]. Therefore, each palpatory experience of an object should improve accuracy with palpations of that object.

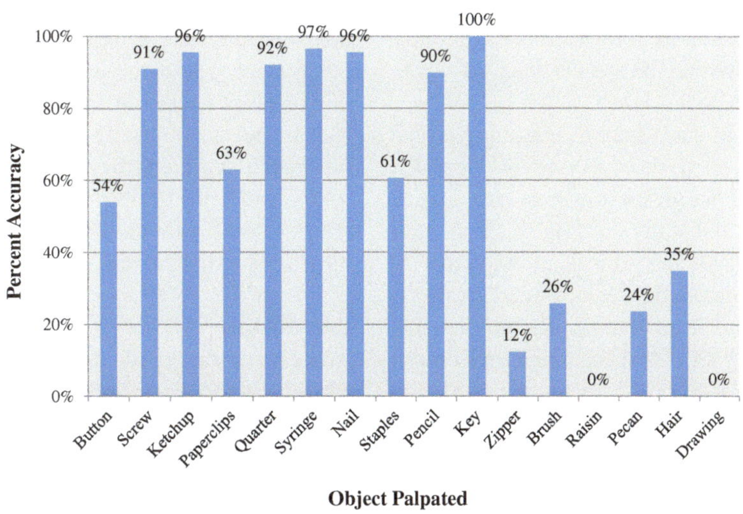

Figure 4 Overall accuracy of each object palpated.

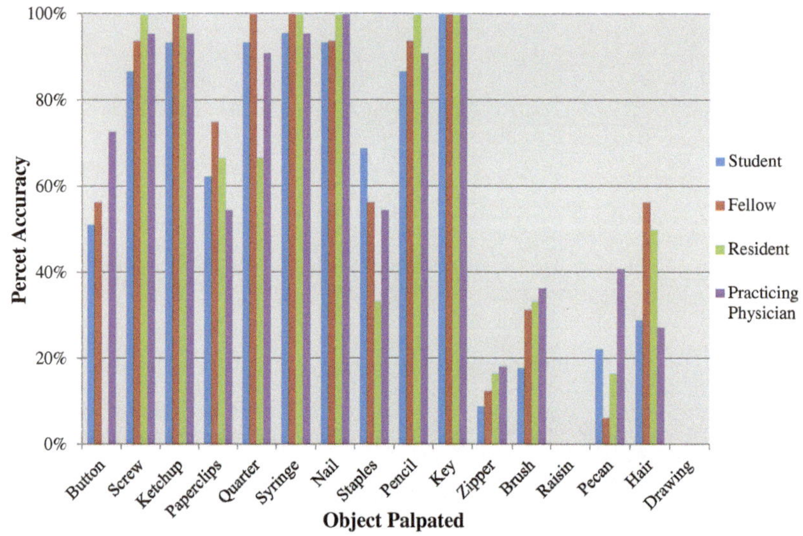

Part I.

	Button	Screw	Ketchup	Paperclips	Quarter	Syringe	Nail	Staples	Pencil
Student	51%	87%	93%	62%	93%	96%	93%	69%	87%
Fellow	56%	94%	100%	75%	100%	100%	94%	56%	94%
Resident	0%	100%	100%	67%	67%	100%	100%	33%	100%
Practicing Physician	73%	95%	95%	55%	91%	95%	100%	55%	91%

Part II & III.

	Key	Zipper	Brush	Raisin	Pecan	Hair	Drawing
Student	100%	9%	18%	0%	22%	29%	0%
Fellow	100%	13%	31%	0%	6%	56%	0%
Resident	100%	17%	33%	0%	17%	50%	0%
Practicing Physician	100%	18%	36%	0%	41%	27%	0%

Figure 5 Accuracy of palpation between osteopathic medical students, fellows and practicing physician.

Accuracy of object identification may have improved if a training session was performed prior to testing. Conclusions as to whether the results stemmed from pre-testing training would then need to be addressed. Equal amount of training may result in no difference in accuracy of object identification among different levels of osteopathic experience. However, having clinical palpatory experience may generate a measurable difference because the learning curve may be steeper than for someone with less palpatory experience.

Although this study was successful in obtaining a high number of participants in a short period of time, the population was heavily weighted towards osteopathic medical students. Given the study's setting this may have been unavoidable, because the American Academy of Osteopathy Annual Convocation is attended more by students than interns and residents. On the other hand, testing at such an event was ideal for attracting practitioners who are actively using osteopathic manipulation and are a better population for measuring a difference in tactile skills.

The finding that no statistically significant difference was found between accuracy of object identification and levels of experience is still surprising. However, measuring clinical palpatory accuracy is more difficult to assess. Osteopathic philosophy and teachings focus on palpation of living and moving tissue, a component of palpation which this study did not undertake. In addition, multiple variables are involved in the evolution of one's clinical palpatory experience and clinicians depend upon a milieu of clinical skill sets learned from experience that is beyond palpation alone. This study was a simple design, and the complexity of palpatory skills evident among varying levels of experience was not measured and contributed to the lack of perceivable difference. However, future studies on measuring palpatory accuracy as it relates to palpatory experience should be performed. Better designed studies could provide light on how training can lead to improved palpatory accuracy.

Conclusion

Accuracy in tactile identification of objects did not differ among osteopathic medical students, fellows, residents, and practicing physicians. Measuring palpatory skills such as palpation of patients requires a subset of palpatory skills that were not tested in this study. Therefore, accuracy and measurement of palpation needs to be studied further to demonstrate changes with palpatory experience.

Competing interests

No financial support was received for this manuscript.
All of the authors have no financial disclosure or conflict of interest to report.

Author's contributions

All authors conceived the study, participated in its design and coordination and helped to draft the manuscript. All authors read and approved the final manuscript.

Author details

[1]Department of Physical Medicine & Rehabilitation, North Shore LIJ - Southside Hospital, 301 East Main Street, Bay Shore, NY 11706, USA. [2]Tioga OB/Gyn Center, 15 Meade Street Suite L1, Wellsboro, PA 16901, USA. [3]C/O MH Northeast Hospital, 18951 N Memor, Humble, TX 77338, USA.

References

1. Mann M, Glasheen-Wray M, Nyberg R: **Therapist agreement for palpation and observation of iliac crest heights.** *Phys Ther* 1984, **64**(3):334–338.
2. Mior SA, McGregor M, Schut B: **The role of experience in clinical accuracy.** *J Manipulative Physiol Ther* 1990, **13**(2):68–71.
3. Meijne W, van Neerbos K, Aufdemkampe G, van der Wurff P: **Intraexaminer and interexaminer reliability of the Gillet test.** *J Manipulative Physiol Ther* 1999, **22**(1):4–9.
4. O'Haire C, Gibbons P: **Inter-examiner and intra-examiner agreement for assessing sacroiliac anatomical landmarks using palpation and observation: pilot study.** *Man Ther* 2000, **5**(1):13–20.
5. Seffinger MA, Najm WI, Mishra SI, *et al*: **Reliability of spinal palpation for diagnosis of back and neck pain: a systematic review of the literature.** *Spine (Phila Pa 1976)* 2004, **29**(19):E413–425.
6. Hestbaek L, Leboeuf-Yde C: **Are chiropractic tests for the lumbo-pelvic spine reliable and valid? A systematic critical literature review.** *J Manipulative Physiol Ther* 2000, **23**(4):258–275.
7. Degenhardt BF, Snider KT, Snider EJ, Johnson JC: **Interobserver reliability of osteopathic palpatory diagnostic tests of the lumbar spine: improvements from consensus training.** *J Am Osteopath Assoc* 2005, **105**(10):465–473.
8. Herzog W, Read LJ, Conway PJ, Shaw LD, McEwen MC: **Reliability of motion palpation procedures to detect sacroiliac joint fixations.** *J Manipulative Physiol Ther* 1989, **12**(2):86–92.
9. Holmgren U, Waling K: **Inter-examiner reliability of four static palpation tests used for assessing pelvic dysfunction.** *Man Ther* 2008, **13**(1):50–56.
10. Hawk C, Phongphua C, Bleecker J, Swank L, Lopez D, Rubley T: **Preliminary study of the reliability of assessment procedures for indications for chiropractic adjustments of the lumbar spine.** *J Manipulative Physiol Ther* 1999, **22**(6):382–389.
11. Mootz RD, Keating JC Jr, Kontz HP, Milus TB, Jacobs GE: **Intra- and interobserver reliability of passive motion palpation of the lumbar spine.** *J Manipulative Physiol Ther* 1989, **12**(6):440–445.
12. Leboeuf C: **The reliability of specific sacro-occipital technique diagnostic tests.** *J Manipulative Physiol Ther* 1991, **14**(9):512–517.
13. Haneline M, Cooperstein R, Young M, Birkeland K: **An annotated bibliography of spinal motion palpation reliability studies.** *J Can Chiropr Assoc* 2009, **53**(1):40–58.
14. Lederman SJ, Klatzky RL: **Haptic perception: a tutorial.** *Atten Percept Psychophys* 2009, **71**(7):1439–1459.
15. Lacey S, Campbell C: **Mental representation in visual/haptic crossmodal memory: evidence from interference effects.** *Q J Exp Psychol* 2006, **59**(2):361–376.
16. Bushnell EW, Baxt C: **Children's haptic and cross-modal recognition with familiar and unfamiliar objects.** *J Exp Psychol Hum Percept Perform* 1999, **25**(6):1867–1881.

Permissions

 Every chapter published in this book has been scrutinized by our experts. Their significance has been extensively debated. The topics covered herein carry significant findings which will fuel the growth of the discipline. They may even be implemented as practical applications or may be referred to as a beginning point for another development.

The contributors of this book come from diverse backgrounds, making this book a truly international effort. This book will bring forth new frontiers with its revolutionizing research information and detailed analysis of the nascent developments around the world.

We would like to thank all the contributing authors for lending their expertise to make the book truly unique. They have played a crucial role in the development of this book. Without their invaluable contributions this book wouldn't have been possible. They have made vital efforts to compile up to date information on the varied aspects of this subject to make this book a valuable addition to the collection of many professionals and students.

This book was conceptualized with the vision of imparting up-to-date information and advanced data in this field. To ensure the same, a matchless editorial board was set up. Every individual on the board went through rigorous rounds of assessment to prove their worth. After which they invested a large part of their time researching and compiling the most relevant data for our readers.

The editorial board has been involved in producing this book since its inception. They have spent rigorous hours researching and exploring the diverse topics which have resulted in the successful publishing of this book. They have passed on their knowledge of decades through this book. To expedite this challenging task, the publisher supported the team at every step. A small team of assistant editors was also appointed to further simplify the editing procedure and attain best results for the readers.

Apart from the editorial board, the designing team has also invested a significant amount of their time in understanding the subject and creating the most relevant covers. They scrutinized every image to scout for the most suitable representation of the subject and create an appropriate cover for the book.

The publishing team has been an ardent support to the editorial, designing and production team. Their endless efforts to recruit the best for this project, has resulted in the accomplishment of this book. They are a veteran in the field of academics and their pool of knowledge is as vast as their experience in printing. Their expertise and guidance has proved useful at every step. Their uncompromising quality standards have made this book an exceptional effort. Their encouragement from time to time has been an inspiration for everyone.

The publisher and the editorial board hope that this book will prove to be a valuable piece of knowledge for researchers, students, practitioners and scholars across the globe.

List of Contributors

Janine S Riksman
School of Chiropractic and Sports Science, Murdoch University, South Street, Murdoch WA, 6151, Australia

Owen D Williamson
Department of Epidemiology and Preventive Medicine Monash University, The Alfred Centre, 99 Commercial Road, Melbourne VIC, 3004, Australia

Bruce F Walker
School of Chiropractic and Sports Science, Murdoch University, South Street, Murdoch WA, 6151, Australia

John W Reggars
Suite1/593 Whitehorse Road, Mitcham, Victoria, 3132 Australia
School of Chiropractic and Sports Science, Faculty of Health Sciences, Murdoch University. Murdoch, Western Australia, 6150

Ryunosuke Banzai
Palmer Center for Chiropractic Research, Palmer College of Chiropractic, 741 Brady Street, Davenport, IA 52803-5209, USA

Dustin C Derby
Institutional Planning & Research, Palmer College of Chiropractic, 723 Brady Street, Davenport, IA 52803-5209, USA

Cynthia R Long
Palmer Center for Chiropractic Research, Palmer College of Chiropractic, 741 Brady Street, Davenport, IA 52803-5209, USA

Maria A Hondras
Palmer Center for Chiropractic Research, Palmer College of Chiropractic, 741 Brady Street, Davenport, IA 52803-5209, USA

Naomi D McKay
Anglo-European College of Chiropractic, 13-15 Parkwood Road, Bournemouth, UK

Jennifer Langworthy
Anglo-European College of Chiropractic, 13-15 Parkwood Road, Bournemouth, UK

Nadège Lemeunier
Institut Franco-Européen de Chiropratique, Toulouse, France

Alice Kongsted
Nordic Institute of Chiropractic and Clinical Biomechanics, Odense, Denmark

Iben Axén
Unit of Intervention and Implementation Research, Institute of Environmental Medicine, The Karolinska Institutet, Stockholm, Sweden

Shawn Williams
Department of Health Professions, CUNY York College, 94 - 20 Guy R. Brewer Blvd, Jamaica, NY 11451, USA

Stanley Innes
35 Maroondah Highway, Lilydale 3140, Australia

Stacey A Page
Office of Medical Bioethics, RM 93, HMRB, Faculty of Medicine, University of Calgary, 3330 Hospital Drive NW, Calgary AB. T2N-4N1, Canada

Jaroslaw P Grod
Private practice, Toronto, ON

D Gordon McMorland
National Spine Care, #300 - 301 14th Street NW, Calgary, Alberta T2N 2A1, Canada

Cynthia Peterson
University of Zürich and Orthopaedic University Hospital Balgrist, Forchstrasse 340, 8008 Zürich, Switzerland

Jennifer Bolton
Anglo-European College of Chiropractic, 13-15 Parkwood Road, Bournemouth, England BH5 2DF, UK

B Kim Humphreys
University of Zürich and Orthopaedic University Hospital Balgrist, Forchstrasse 340, 8008 Zürich, Switzerland

Martin Wangler
European Academy of Chiropractic, Bahnhofstrasse 15, CH-3400 Burgdorf, Switzerland

Cynthia Peterson
University of Zürich and Orthopaedic University Hospital Balgrist, Forchstrasse 340, 8008 Zürich, Switzerland
Swiss Academy for Chiropractic, Sulgenauweg 38, 3007 Bern, Switzerland

Beatrice Zaugg
ChiroSuisse, Eidgenössische Prüfung Chiropraktik, Johann-Verresisus Strasse 18, CH-2502 Biel, Switzerland

Haymo Thiel
Anglo-European College of Chiropractic, 13-15 Parkwood Road, Bournemouth BH5 2DF, UK

Rob Finch
The Royal College of Chiropractors, Chiltern Chambers, St Peters Avenue, Reading RG4 7DH, UK

J Keith Simpson
School of Chiropractic & Sports Science Murdoch University, Perth, Australia

Martin Wangler
European Academy of Chiropractic, academic dean and private practice, Bahnhofstrasse 15, 3400 Burgdorf, Switzerland

Ricardo Fujikawa
Real Centro Universitario Maria Cristina-College of Chiropractic, Paseo de los Alamillos 2, 28200 San Lorenzo de El Escorial, Spain

Lise Hestbæk
Nordisk Institut for Kiropraktik og Klinisk Biomekanik Forskerparken 10, 5230 Odense M, Denmark

Tom Michielsen
European Academy of Chiropractic, Department of Research and private practice, St. Paulusstraat 15, 2400 Mol- Belgium

Timothy J Raven
European Council on Chiropractic Education and private practice, Kiropraktorklinikken Strandgården, Havnegt. 1, 4790 Lillesand, Norway

Haymo W Thiel
Anglo-European College of Chiropractic, 13-15 Parkwood Road, Bournemouth BH5 2DF, UK

Beatrice Zaugg
Swiss Academy of Chiropractic and private practice, Johann-Verresius-Str. 18 2502 Biel, Switzerland

Shabnam Sadr
Canadian Memorial Chiropractic College, 6100 Leslie Street, Toronto, Ontario M2H 3J1, Canada

Neda Pourkiani-Allah-Abad
Canadian Memorial Chiropractic College, 6100 Leslie Street, Toronto, Ontario M2H 3J1, Canada

Kent Jason Stuber
Canadian Memorial Chiropractic College, 6100 Leslie Street, Toronto, Ontario M2H 3J1, Canada

Melanie J Charity
General Practice and Primary Health Care Academic Centre, University of Melbourne, 200 Berkeley St, Carlton, VIC 3010, Australia

Simon D French
General Practice and Primary Health Care Academic Centre, University of Melbourne, 200 Berkeley St, Carlton, VIC 3010, Australia
Centre for Health Exercise and Sports Medicine, Melbourne School of Health Sciences, University of Melbourne, 200 Berkeley St, Carlton, VIC 3010, Australia

Kirsty Forsdike
General Practice and Primary Health Care Academic Centre, University of Melbourne, 200 Berkeley St, Carlton, VIC 3010, Australia

Helena Britt
Family Medicine Research Centre, Sydney School of Public Health, Sydney Medical School, The University of Sydney, Level 7, 16-18 Wentworth Street, Parramatta, NSW 2150, Australia

Barbara Polus
Research & Innovation, RMIT University, 110 Victoria Street, Melbourne, VIC 3000, Australia

Jane Gunn
General Practice and Primary Health Care Academic Centre, University of Melbourne, 200 Berkeley St, Carlton, VIC 3010, Australia

Iben Axén
Karolinska Institutet, Unit of Intervention & Implementation Research, Institute of Environmental Medicine, Nobels väg 13, S-171 77 Stockholm, Sweden

Charlotte Leboeuf-Yde
Research Department, Spinecenter of Southern Denmark, Institute of Regional Health Research, University of Southern Denmark, Hospital Lillebælt, Østre Hougvej 55, DK-5500 Middelfart, Denmark

Matthew A Davis
Center for Health Policy Research, The Dartmouth Institute for Health Policy & Clinical Practice, 35 Centerra Parkway, Lebanon, NH 03766, USA

Todd A Mackenzie
Geisel School of Medicine at Dartmouth, Section of Clinical Research, HB 7505, Dartmouth Hitchcock Medical Center, One Medical Center Drive, Lebanon, NH 03766, USA

Ian D Coulter
University of California at Los Angeles, CA, Senior Health Policy Analyst, RAND Corporation, Santa Monica, CA 90401, USA

James M Whedon
The Dartmouth Institute for Health Policy & Clinical Practice, 35 Centerra Parkway, Lebanon, NH 03766, USA

William B Weeks
The Dartmouth Institute for Health Policy & Clinical Practice, 35 Centerra Parkway, Lebanon, NH 03766, USA

Olivier Guenoun
Institute Franco-Européen de Chiropratique, 24 blv Paul Vaillant Couturier, F- 94200 Ivry sur Seine, France

Michel Debarle
Institute Franco-Européen de Chiropratique, 24 blv Paul Vaillant Couturier, F- 94200 Ivry sur Seine, France

Coralie Garnesson
Institute Franco-Européen de Chiropratique, 24 blv Paul Vaillant Couturier, F- 94200 Ivry sur Seine, France

Sylvie Proisl
Institute Franco-Européen de Chiropratique, 24 blv Paul Vaillant Couturier, F- 94200 Ivry sur Seine, France

Delphine Ray
Institute Franco-Européen de Chiropratique, 24 blv Paul Vaillant Couturier, F- 94200 Ivry sur Seine, France

Charlotte Leboeuf-Yde
Institute Franco-Européen de Chiropratique, 24 blv Paul Vaillant Couturier, F- 94200 Ivry sur Seine, France

Daniel Westin
Anglo European College of Chiropractic, 13-15 Parkwood Road, Bournemouth, UK

Tine Tandberg
Elverum Kiropraktikk & Rehabilitering, Storgata 7B 2408, Elverum, Norway

Carol John
Anglo European College of Chiropractic, 13-15 Parkwood Road, Bournemouth, UK

Iben Axén
Karolinska Institutet, Institute for Environmental Medicine, Unit of Intervention and Implementation Research, Nobels v 13, 171 77, Stockholm, Sweden

Bjorn J Hennius
Parkwood Chiropractic Clinic, 93, Cathedral Road, Cardiff CF11 9PG, UK
Welsh Institute of Chiropractic (WIOC), University of South Wales, Treforrest, Wales, UK

Stephen M Foreman
Private practice of chiropractic, West Hills, California, USA

Michael J Stahl
Private practice of chiropractic, West Hills, California, USA

Gary D Schultz
University of Western States, Portland, Oregon, USA

Cheryl Hawk
Logan College of Chiropractic, 1851 Schoettler Rd, 63017 Chesterfield, MO, USA

Marion Willard Evans Jr
University of Western States, 2900 NE 132nd Ave, 97230 Portland, OR, USA

John J Triano
Canadian Memorial Chiropractic College, 6100 Leslie St., Toronto, Ontario, Canada

Brian Budgell
Canadian Memorial Chiropractic College, 6100 Leslie St., Toronto, Ontario, Canada

Angela Bagnulo
Private Practice of Chiropractic, Burlington, Canada

Benjamin Roffey
Private Practice of Chiropractic, Toronto, Canada

Thomas Bergmann
Northwestern Health Sciences University, Bloomington, MN, USA

Robert Cooperstein
Palmer College of Chiropractic, San Jose, CA, USA

Brian Gleberzon
Canadian Memorial Chiropractic College, 6100 Leslie St., Toronto, Ontario, Canada

Christopher Good
University of Bridgeport College of Chiropractic, Bridgeport, CT, USA

Jacquelyn Perron
Private Practice of Chiropractic, Calgary, Canada

Rodger Tepe
Logan College of Chiropractic, Chesterfield, MO, USA

Barbara A Mansholt
Technique Department, Palmer College of Chiropractic, 1000 Brady St, Davenport, IA 52803, USA

John S Stites
Community Clinics, Palmer College of Chiropractic, 2001 52nd Ave, Moline, IL 61265, USA

Dustin C Derby
Institutional Planning & Research, Palmer College of Chiropractic, 723 Brady St, Davenport, IA 52803, USA

Ron J Boesch
Palmer Davenport Clinical Affairs, Palmer College of Chiropractic, 1000 Brady St, Davenport, IA 52803, USA

Stacie A Salsbury
Palmer Center for Chiropractic Research, Palmer College of Chiropractic, 741 Brady St, Davenport, IA 52803, USA

Simon D French
General Practice and Primary Health Care Academic Centre, The University of Melbourne, 200 Berkeley Street, Carlton, VIC 3072, Australia
Centre for Health, Exercise and Sports Medicine, School of Health Sciences, The University of Melbourne, Level 7, 161 Barry St, Carlton, VIC 3053, Australia

Konstancja Densley
General Practice and Primary Health Care Academic Centre, The University of Melbourne, 200 Berkeley Street, Carlton, VIC 3072, Australia

Melanie J Charity
General Practice and Primary Health Care Academic Centre, The University of Melbourne, 200 Berkeley Street, Carlton, VIC 3072, Australia

Jane Gunn
General Practice and Primary Health Care Academic Centre, The University of Melbourne, 200 Berkeley Street, Carlton, VIC 3072, Australia

Linda Spencer
School of Physiotherapy, Faculty of Health Sciences, Curtin University, Bentley Campus, Perth, Western Australia

Kathy Briffa
School of Physiotherapy, Faculty of Health Sciences, Curtin University, Bentley Campus, Perth, Western Australia

Charlotte Leboeuf-Yde
The Spine Research Centre, Hospital Lillebaelt, and Institute for Regional Health Research, University of Southern Denmark, Middelfart, Denmark Complexité, Innovation et Activités Motrices et Sportives, Bâtiment 335, UFR STAPS, Université Paris Sud-11, Orsay Cedex 91405, France

Olivier Lanlo
Institut Franco- Européen de Chiropraxie, Paris, France

Bruce F Walker
School of Health Professions, Murdoch University, Perth, Western Australia, Australia

Daniel Avrahami
Toronto, ON, Canada
204 Parkmount, Toronto, ON M4J 4V6, Canada

Amanda Hammond
Toronto, ON, Canada
Lakeview Chiropractic Health and Wellness, 2B 3602 Taylor St. E, Saskatoon, SK S7H 5H9, Canada

Ceara Higgins
Toronto, ON, Canada
777 Woodbine Ave, Toronto, ON M4E 2J5, Canada

Howard Vernon
Canadian Memorial Chiropractic College, 6100 Leslie Street, Toronto, ON M2H 3J1, Canada

Clinton J Daniels
Private Practice, St. Louis, MO, USA

Jordan A Gliedt
Private Practice, Chandler, AZ, USA

Dennis E Enix
Logan University, Chesterfield, MO, USA

Cynthia K Peterson, Daniel Mühlemann and Barry Kim Humphreys
Department of Chiropractic Medicine, Orthopaedic University Hospital Balgrist, University of Zürich, Forchstrasse 340, Zürich, Switzerland

Roger M Engel, Benjamin T Brown, Michael S Swain and Reidar P Lystad
Department of Chiropractic, Macquarie University, Balaclava Rd, North Ryde 2109, Australia

Rosanna C Sabini
Department of Physical Medicine & Rehabilitation, North Shore LIJ – Southside Hospital, 301 East Main Street, Bay Shore, NY 11706, USA

Chadwick S Leo
Tioga OB/Gyn Center, 15 Meade Street Suite L1, Wellsboro, PA 16901, USA

Alton E Moore II
C/O MH Northeast Hospital, 18951 N Memor, Humble, TX 77338, USA